Lobar Approach to Breast Ultrasound

Dominique Amy
Editor

Lobar Approach to Breast Ultrasound

Springer

Editor
Dominique Amy
Department of Radiology
Breast Center Department of Radiology
Aix-en-Provence
France

ISBN 978-3-030-09666-3 ISBN 978-3-319-61681-0 (eBook)
https://doi.org/10.1007/978-3-319-61681-0

Printed on acid-free paper

This Springer imprint is published by the registered company Springer International Publishing AG part of Springer Nature
The registered company address is: Gewerbestrasse 11, 6330 Cham, Switzerland

To Florence, Aude and Jérôme

Also thanks to Michel Teboul to whom this work owes its existence and to J. Amoros and P. Scaramucci, the three lovers of ductal echography who died too early

With thanks to M.T. Castay and C. Bartoli for their invaluable help

Foreword

In my past residency years, it was quite common for women with a breast finding to enter the operating room both for intraoperative diagnosis and, potentially, immediate treatment. Indeed, it was commonplace for a patient to enter the operating room without knowing if she would emerge with both breasts intact. These indeed were the dark days of breast surgery when removing a breast lump and performing an intraoperative frozen section on a suspect lesion might result, upon awakening, with the loss of a breast.

Imaging technology since that dark period of blind surgical biopsy has undergone refinement in breast imaging, including mammography, MRI, and ultrasound, leading to accurate wire localization of suspicious lesions to guide surgical excision. In a similar fashion, image-guided preoperative biopsy has honed to a fine edge the identification of lesions requiring surgical excision. Breast ultrasound, however, has lagged behind other imaging modalities in recognition of its potential utility in both diagnosis and surgical treatment of breast cancer and, unfortunately, is still considered the handmaiden of mammography by both radiologist and breast surgeon alike. The majority of clinicians view breast ultrasound as an adjunctive imaging examination to both mammography and MRI. Indeed, in many instances, examinations are done by technicians with the review of static images done by a radiologist. All breast imaging techniques have led to increased diagnostic accuracy in identifying recognized signs of suspect malignancy leading to preoperative tissue analysis and as a guide for targeted excision of a geographical site of a biopsy-proven cancer.

A Question

Is image-guided biopsy as practiced today, whether it be via mammography, MRI, or ultrasound, actually a targeted excision of the "entire extent" of a nidus of localized breast cancer? The answer to this question is readily apparent and documented in the oncological literature of both surgical and radiation oncology journals. The re-excision rate for positive margins after partial mastectomy for image-guided targeted lesions is documented in surgical journals as anywhere between 20% and 40%. And, after definitive surgical excision and negative pathological margin assessment followed by a standard course of radiotherapy, both short- and long-term local recurrence rates remain elevated and static.

The Conundrum of Local Recurrence and Re-excision

The dilemma of continued positive postoperative surgical margin rates and static short- and long-term recurrence rates, in many instances, can be decreased with the utilization of an improved technique to identify and target the true extent of a cancerous breast lesion. In the modern operating room, the complete surgical excision of a particular breast cancer is hampered by the inability of a surgeon to identify and resect all cancerous tissue that may be present. This is a fact simply because there are no anatomical landmarks visible to the naked eye in the surgical field that can aid a deliberate and complete surgical excision. The question of what, where, and how much to resect in the performance of a partial mastectomy is the crucial key to the performance of a truly "targeted" surgical operation. The solution to this conundrum is straightforward. Cancer of the breast arises in the ducto-lobular system of the breast. Without visualization of the involved ducto-lobular or ductal segment, any resection will be, although grossly targeted via wire localization or seed implant, a blind excision and one that most certainly has left cancer in the vicinity of some specimens pathologically analyzed as negative.

Ancient Roots: The Anatomical Basis for Surgical Treatment of Breast Cancer

Evidence supporting this assertion has been reported in the literature but obscured by time and, for the most part, not given notice or is unknown to clinical investigators. For the inquisitive, however, unearthing journal papers that are perhaps yellowed with age and covered with dust may offer valuable insight into why some types of breast cancer undergo inadequate resection. A truncated list of investigators who have provided evidence for this assertion includes Wellings, Parks, Gallager, Martin, and Tot. Of particular significance related to the adequate surgical resection of breast cancer are the findings found in a study by Holland et al. entitled "Histologic Multifocality of Tis, T 1-2 Breast Carcinomas." Noteworthy is the finding that not all cancers are confined to a primary site and that a significant proportion of cancers have extension at a distance from the primary cancer. And that distance can extend centimeters beyond the primary. A question: Might today's partial mastectomy [aka lumpectomy], identified as the site of the preoperative biopsy and subsequently used as a marker for excision, not be an accurate guide as to the full ductal or lobular extent of disease? Based on Holland's work alone, one must answer in the affirmative. Nor can one, based on Holland's findings, categorically posit as an inviolable rule that the standard for pathologic specimen analysis for all types of breast cancer is "no tumor on ink." Today, molecular sub-typing of breast cancers into luminal A or B, Her2, and triple-negative categories provides the evidence that not all cancers are bound by the same therapeutic rules, whether they be surgical or those provided in the adjuvant setting. The various molecular subtypes of breast cancer may be the marker that signals that a particular sub-type of cancer does require a negative margin greater than no tumor on ink.

The Problem

How can one accurately and fully excise the limit of involvement of a breast cancer without being able to map its course? The answer, in my opinion, is that without accurate guidance, it cannot be done. And I would point to the statistics on re-excision and local recurrence rates as evidence supporting this statement. Furthermore, the answer to these stubborn statistics, in part, does not lie in more complicated and expensive imaging modalities. Nor does it lie in the accumulation of metadata that sacrifices the individual for the collective in its pronouncements. Breast cancer is defined in a unique anatomical fashion in each patient. And it should be of no surprise that it will be the individual anatomy of a breast cancer patient that can provide the map used in the operating room as a guide to a more rational and complete surgical excision for those patients considered candidates for breast-conserving surgery.

The Solution: Visualization of the Ductal Anatomy of the Breast

In 1995, Dr. Michel Teboul and Michael Halliwell published *Atlas of Ultrasound and Ductal Echography of the Breast*. This seminal work on breast ultrasound is the bedrock upon which the content of this book, *Lobar Approach to Breast Ultrasound*, is based. The technique and interpretation of ultrasound ductal-lobular images were catalogued, described, and conceptually nurtured through lean years of nonacceptance by the single-minded tenacity of Michel Teboul. As a scientific investigator, Dr. Teboul had an uncompromising vision of the true breath of breast ultrasound beyond the further categorization of a breast mass as seen on mammography or felt on physical examination. The visualization of the ductal and lobar anatomy of the breast is now utilized in performing more complete surgical excisions. DE (ductal echography) provides the surgeon with a visual map of the anatomy of the breast revealing not only the extent of disease but also the boundaries required for complete excision. Many will take credit for the development of ductal echography. But those of us fortunate enough to have known Michel and who recognize the enormous amount of energy he expended over so long a period of time in advocating the merits of his technique know who should be recognized for its development. This book celebrates his work with the greatest accolade possible, the practical application of DE to reveal the anatomy of the breast, both normal and pathological, for both diagnosis and treatment. This book is a fitting homage to that man. I consider it a singular privilege to have known and studied with Michel and to have called him my friend.

A final comment: It is perhaps ironic to realize that a man so consumed with sound has paradoxically "shown" us the way forward. Somewhere, somehow, I bet Michel is chuckling at that. I will miss him. Au revoir, mon ami!

Chicago, IL, USA Dario Francescatti

Contents

List of Contributors

Dominique Amy, M.D. Centre du Sein, Aix-en-Provence, France

Jeremy Bercoff, Ph.D. R&D Ultrasound Department, SSI SupersonicImagine, Aix-en-Provence, France

Ellison Bibby, M.Sc. Hitachi Medical Systems UK, Northants, UK

Giovanni Botta, M.D. Department of Pathology, Sant' Anna Hospital, Torino, Italy

Jean-Marie Bourgeois Centre Medical Delta, Nimes, France

Vedrana Buljević, M.D. Spinciceva 2, Split, Croatia

Aristida Colan-Georges, M.D., Ph.D. Imaging Center Prima Medical, County Clinical Emergency Hospital, Craiova, Romania

Giancarlo Dolfin, M.D. Gynecologist, Oncologist, Torino, Italy

Enzo Durante, M.D. Institute of General Surgery, Ferrara, Italy

Dominique Fournier Institut de Radiologie, Sion, Switzerland

Darius Francescatti Department of Surgery, Rush University Medical Center, Chicago, IL, USA

Cornelis A. Hoefnagel, M.D. Nuclear Medicine Consultant, Badhoevedorp, The Netherlands

Jose Parada Clinica por Imagenes Dres. Parada, Montevideo, Uruguay

Norran Hussein Said, M.D., F.R.C.R. Egyptian National Breast Screening Program, Nasser Institute, Cairo, Egypt

Ashraf Selim Radiology Department, Cairo University, Cairo, Egypt

Mona Tan MammoCare, Singapore, Singapore

Tibor Tot, M.D., Ph.D. Pathology & Cytology Dalarna, Falun County Hospital, Falun, Sweden

Ei Ueno Tsukuba International Breast Clinic, Tsukuba, Ibaraki, Japan

1 Introduction

J.M. Bourgeois and D. Amy

This book is a synthesis of knowledge concerning the lobe, which is the mammary anatomic unit.

It indeed gives prime importance to the lobar concept as the basis of breast anatomy, a concept shared by all the co-authors present here.

Tot presents his 'sick lobe theory'.

Fournier studies the mammary nodes by following the full extension of the lobes.

Hoefnagel follows the lymphatic drainage of each lobe.

Parada and Buljevic map out the ductal axes of the lobes in interventional echography for millimetric lesions.

Amy and Dumitru describe lobar anatomy and its variations.

Selim, Said, and Georges present lobar echography and its semiology in detail.

Ueno, a pioneer in lobar echography, describes "no mass, mammo-negative cancers."

Durante, Dolfin, and Tan expound their lobar surgical techniques.

This book propounds the third chapter in the history of mammary echography.

The foundation of the ultrasound diagnosis of mammary lesions was laid in the 1970s (Kobayashi) [12]. The second chapter was provided by the presentation of the lobar anatomy of the breast in the 1990s (Teboul, Stavros). From the year 2000, the lobar concept has been taking up the place it rightly deserves: Tot presented his "sick lobe theory."

This book is not the last word for the whole pathology of the breast. It will not answer all the questions we are faced with on a daily basis in our practice of echography; it is even likely that it will raise questions (which is a form of progressing).

This book is meant to be the complement of many publications; it does not aim at repeating all that has already been published, in mammary echography as well as in ultrasound technique.

It serves as a conclusion to more than three decades of failures, of research, of discoveries, and of exchanges in breast echography, and, by taking up again anatomy as an analytical basis, we wish to redirect the techniques of examination, diagnosis, or treatment so as to achieve a better understanding and a good reproducibility.

In analyzing the earlier work which has been published for decades, in putting together the huge jigsaw of fragmented knowledge left to us by our masters, in adapting the recent technological improvements in the field of echography, we wish to open out a new vision in senology.

J.M. Bourgeois (✉)
CFFE, Centre Medical Delta, Nimes, France
e-mail: jmbourgeois@ultrason.com

D. Amy
Centre du sein, Aix-en-Provence, France
e-mail: domamy@wanadoo.fr

D. Amy (ed.), *Lobar Approach to Breast Ultrasound*, https://doi.org/10.1007/978-3-319-61681-0_1

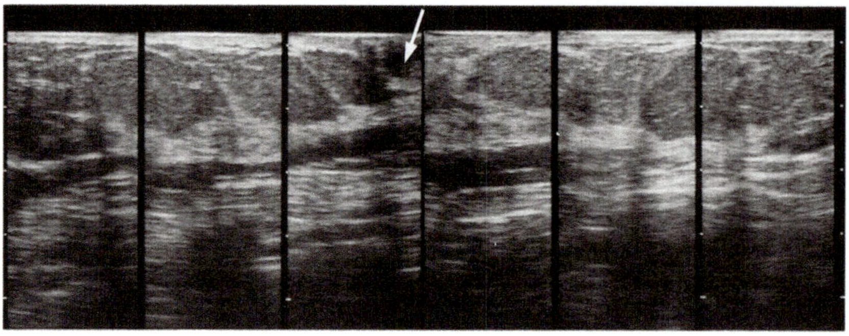

Fig. 1.1 Large reconstructed breast ultrasound section presented by Pr. E.UENO in 1991: radial lobar scanning of two lobes with the nipple in the middle arrow (Courtesy of Pr. E. Ueno, Japan)

Such prestigious names as Cooper [1], Gallager [6], Nakama [9], Going [2], Ueno [10], Tot [7, 8] Stavros [3], Dolfin [4], Francescatti [11] (to quote only these), and more particularly Michel Teboul [5], on a personal level, have been with us all these years. According to Stavros, Michel Teboul "has pioneered the anatomic approach of breast imaging" (sic) (Fig. 1.1).

Tot, lastly, with his huge experience and "sick lobe theory" has come to give a concrete grounding to the work of all these researchers. We hope this book will be worthy of their teachings. We will be castigated for the lack of extensive statistics and analytical surveys. We hope that the success of the concept of the "lobar approach" of the breast will lead many of our colleagues to add their experience to this preliminary presentation of diagnosis and surgery.

This book may make surgeons uncomfortable as they cannot see the lobes and find it hard to delineate their edges, unless they agree to use an echograph in the operating theater.

It may annoy anatomopathologists used to working on 2 cm × 2 cm small sections, which do not allow a good global vision of the lobes and of multifocal pathology, unless they agree to use 10 cm × 10 cm large sections (new technique, new investment).

It may make radiologists uncomfortable if they are not used to the radial technique, if they do not have large probes, and if they do not have anatomic knowledge of the lobes, unless they train in radial scanning and elastography.

It may not interest the oncologist: a new concept and a new approach are not strictly adapted to their protocols. But a good collaboration with the radiologist will be fruitful and will bring in more information with the discovery of a larger number of multifocal and multicentric lesions, an assessment of tumoral aggressiveness and a help in the management of neoadjuvant chemotherapies.

Lastly it may not meet whole-hearted support from the manufacturers of echographs who do not have the adequate equipment or whose automatized breast echographs are imperfectly fitted for the anatomic analysis of the breast and the lobar approach of the diagnosis.

But this book and this concept will meet the full approval of the patients who understand the lobar anatomy of their breasts perfectly and who surmise all the benefits that can be drawn from it. The understanding of anatomy, of the examination technique, and of the possible uncovering of pathology is, for most of these patients, an essential stage in accepting and following their treatment.

We have the experience of decades practicing ducto-radial echography, training colleagues to these techniques, and taking part in very many conferences or symposiums every year. We can assert that we have encountered full approval among the vast majority of colleagues who have made the effort to learn this diagnostic or therapeutic approach: they experienced great enthusiasm in discovering anatomy and other forms of knowledge, and they expressed a real interest in improving their diagnostic technique.

This said, very many questions will not find immediate answers:

Many ask why there has not been a precise anatomic analysis of the breast.

Why do some of our colleagues show so little interest, or even none whatsoever?

Why do ducto-radial echography and the lobar concept remain such well-kept secrets?

Why are the lobules in the upper part of the lobes larger than those in the lower part? Why are those close to the areola more developed than those at the end of the lobes?

Why does pathology develop more specifically in the TDLUs?

Is there a relationship between the morphological type of a lobe (hyper-echogenic or predominantly hypo-echogenic, with an early or late involution) and pathology?

Can elastography and the Doppler vascular study significantly modify the therapeutic decisions?

Is there really a relationship between long-term survival and surgical techniques (lobectomy versus lumpectomy)? Complementary, multicentric studies involving a larger number of cases are necessary.

This list is by no means exhaustive; other answers and other questions will come to us, but we are convinced that the lobar approach and the ducto-radial echographic analysis amount to a real progress in the diagnosis of breast cancers.

Let us now turn briefly to the technical side of things. It is important here to recall in passing some basic principles. In the course of the many tuition sessions, conferences, and exchanges, it has become clear that in the field of echography as well as the one of elastography, the practice of mammary echography in general is characterized by a certain lack of precision, training, and guidelines. In echography, the major basic principle is that the probe must be strictly perpendicular to the skin and perfectly horizontal. One must avoid scanning the breast with the probe in an oblique position (Figs. 1.2 and 1.3).

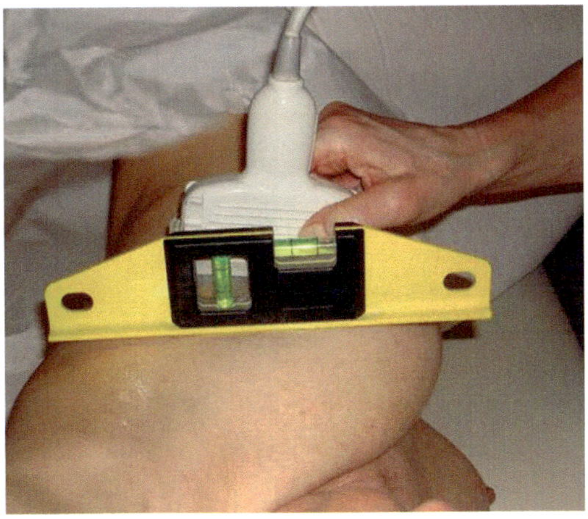

Fig. 1.2 The best ultrasonic technique: horizontal probe strictly perpendicular to the skin, here the external part of the breast and the chest wall

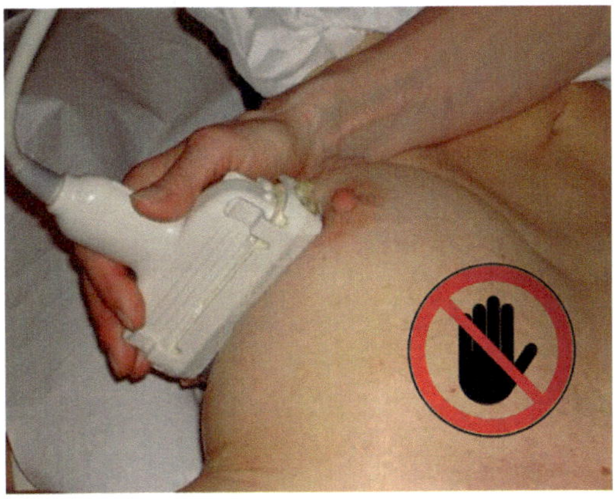

Fig. 1.3 The wrong technique of scanning a breast with the probe in an oblique position. Artifacts (Figs. 1.4, 1.5, 1.6, and 1.7) can be created and elastography will not be efficient (strain and/or SWE)

In mammary echography, it is therefore advisable to move the patient instead of the probe so that the latter can be positioned ideally. Indeed, too oblique a positioning of the probe can result in false pathological images (Figs. 1.4, 1.5, 1.6, and 1.7) when it is only a case of transitory artifacts.

For the breast, one must follow a very strict rule: avoid compressing the breast too much with the probe on the skin. Compressing it too much would lead to a loss of information which could be detrimental as regards superficial elements (fascia and Cooper's elements) and conceal preliminary signs in the case of the development of a breast cancer.

The echographic examination of the breast must be carried out with "the fingers" and not with the hand which would imprison the probe and therefore crush the mammary lobes (Figs. 1.8 and 1.9).

Echographic scanning must be systematic radial scanning (anti-radial scanning only in case of known pathology). Note that the use of a 3D

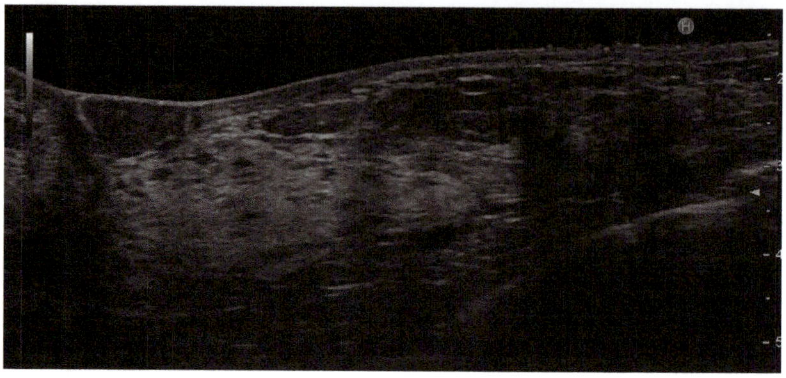

Fig. 1.4 Oblique scanning: at the lobe extremity, two hypoechogenic areas seem very suspicious

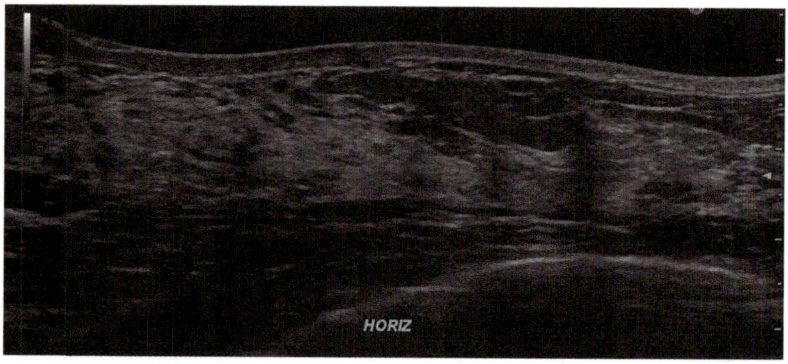

Fig. 1.5 The same lobe with perfectly horizontal probe: disappearance of the artifacts

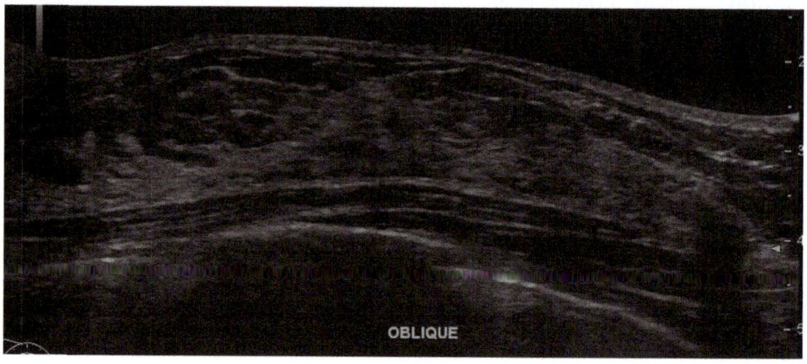

Fig. 1.6 Another oblique lobar scan with an artifact at the distal extremity of the lobe due to the bad probe position

probe is only useful as a means of verification on an already detected anomaly and that a systematic screening of the whole breast in 3D cannot be considered. In the case of a breast tumor, the coronal sections are important especially in a "minimal breast cancer."

The probe must be as long as possible. Since high-frequency probes longer than 10 cm do not exist, Hitachi and SuperSonic Imagine offer ideal (10 cm) probes adapted to breast echography. Shorter 7 cm probes are available and often used by other manufacturers.

Another particular feature to consider in order to obtain the ideal probe in senology is the use of an especially conceived water bag clipped to the probe so that it becomes a component part of the probe but can be removed, cleaned, and changed easily.

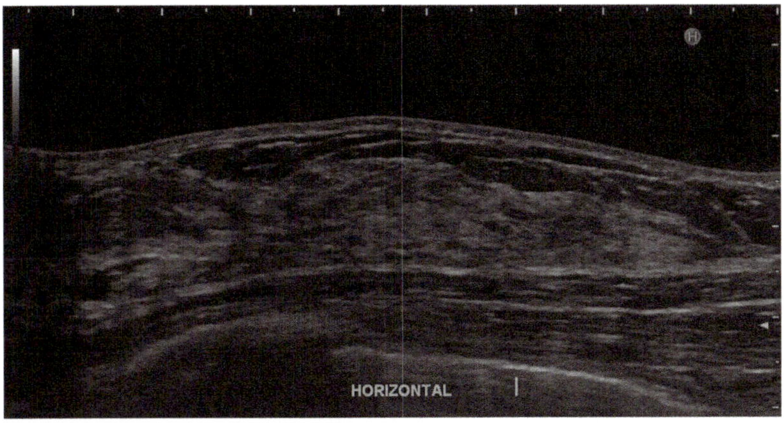

Fig. 1.7 When the probe becomes horizontal, all the dubious areas appear

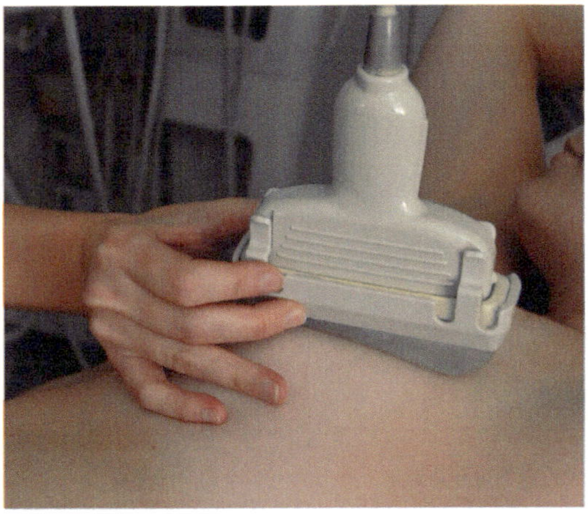

Fig. 1.8 The best position for the probe (with a dedicated water bag) is horizontal and held only with the fingers (no breast compression)

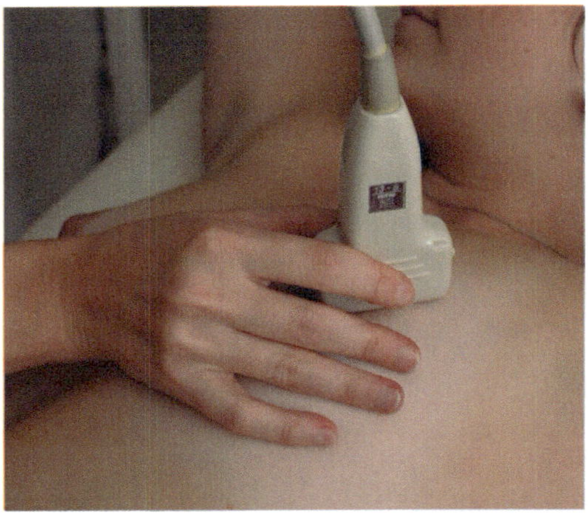

Fig. 1.9 Ideal probe position for both B-mode imaging and elastography (strain and SWE) just in contact with the skin

Although very much debated and derided by manufacturers, the water bag has numerous advantages:

- It allows a better contact between the linear transducer face and the curved body surface (especially with the long L53L linear probe 10 cm).
- It allows a better visualization of very superficial tissue layers where near-field artifact may otherwise obscure the fine detail.
- It can place the near-field area of interest into the best focal zone of the transducer.
- It increases the contrast resolution.
- It allows a better analysis of the nipple, intra-nipple, and retro-nipple structures, even in the cases of scars and retraction of the nipple.
- It clearly limits the retro-areolar or retro-ligamentous artifacts.
- It allows an excellent analysis of the axillary zone.
- It avoids an excessive compression of the breast.
- It prevents the toning down of ultrasound beams noted in the interposition of silicone pads or block, Sonogel, echo kit, etc.

The ideal thing in mammary echography is to avoid the use of the "compound mode" which is recommended for the investigation of a lesion or a tumor but has the drawback of "erasing" the small anatomic structures (ducts and lobules) which are concealed by crossed scanning.

The use of new Doppler techniques is essential in the identification and the assessment of small lesions: at the millimetric stage, classic echographic semiologic signs are not always convincing. The addition of Doppler and elastography becomes essential for an accurate diagnosis. Angio PL.U.S is a new Color Doppler imaging mode, designed to image slow-flow and microvascularization. Like Color Doppler, Angio PL.U.S displays color-coded blood flow maps of the mean Doppler velocity, mean Doppler power, and/or flow direction superimposed on the B-mode grayscale image.

Acquisition: Instead of successively insonifying the medium with focused beams like conventional Color Doppler, Angio PL.U.S relies on Aixplorer UltraFast technology and emits unfocused beams (plane waves) with multiple steering angles followed by coherent compounding of the backscattered signals received from the steered plane waves. The plane wave approach offers significantly higher Doppler acquisition speeds, resulting in longer ensembles and higher frame rates than those achievable in conventional Color Doppler.

Processing: The high-pass wall filters used in conventional Color Doppler to separate tissue motion from blood flow perform poorly at such low-velocity scales, resulting in strong tissue motion (flash) artifacts and loss of low-velocity blood flow information. To overcome this problem, Angio PL.U.S uses an advanced spatial and temporal wall filtering technique which offers significant improvements in the preservation of slow-flow blood signals. The combination of ultrafast plane wave insonification with intelligent wall filtering allows better sensitivity, resolution, and slow-flow extraction than in conventional Doppler. The use of Angio PL.U.S for neoangiogenesis imaging is a very promising application.

TriVu: TriVu combines the SWE and Angio PL.U.S technologies in a single triplex real-time mode. It allows for the first time the simultaneous visualization of morphology, vascularization, and stiffness of tissues. An example of TriVu on a breast lesion is given below (Figs. 1.10, 1.11, and 1.12).

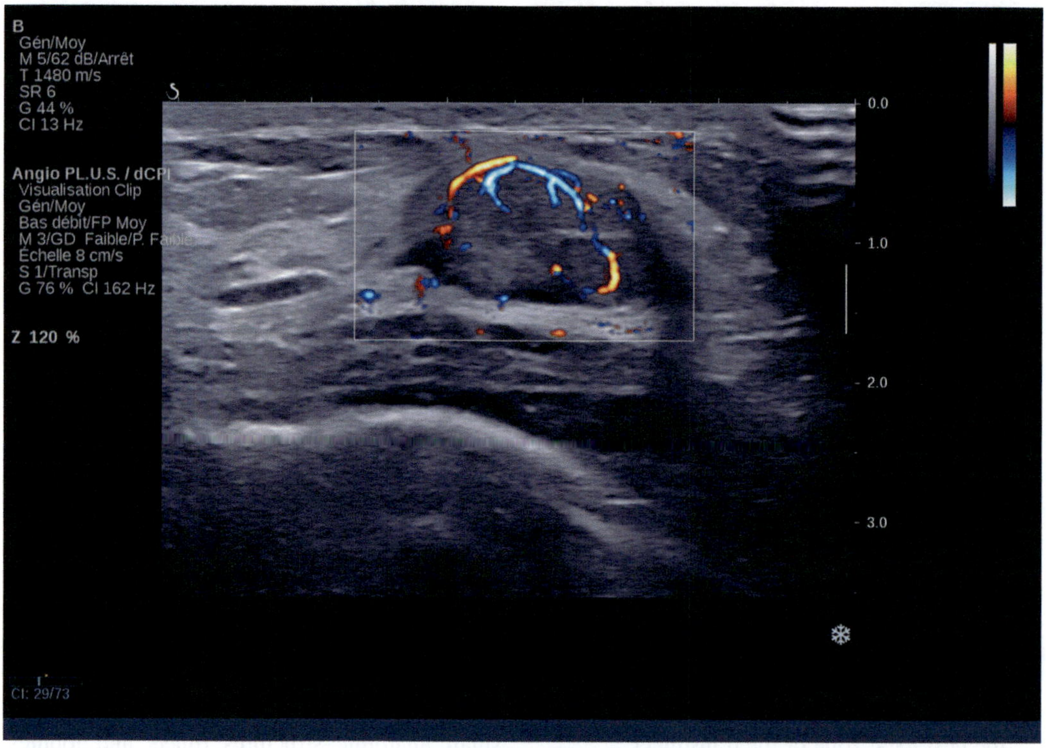

Fig. 1.10 Angio PL.U.S Doppler of a benign lesion with harmoniously curve microvessels in and around the nodule

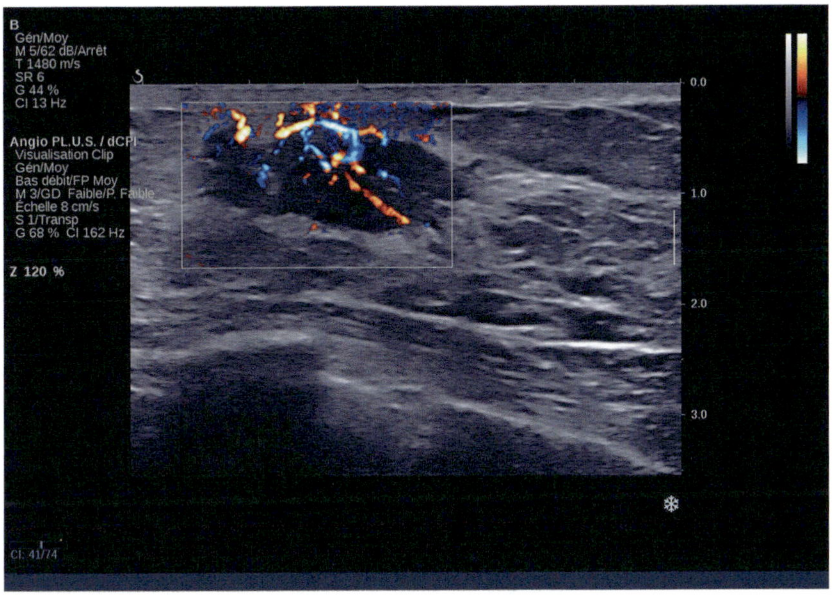

Fig. 1.11 Irregular microvessels (in diameters and orientation) of a lesion obviously malignant (proved minimal breast cancer)

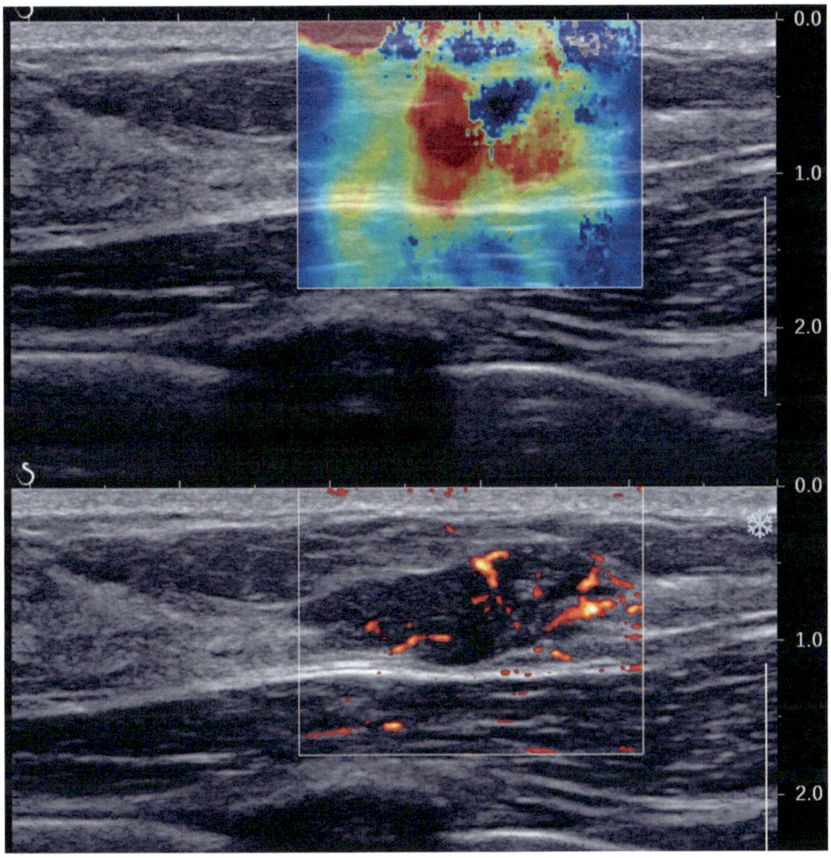

Fig. 1.12 TriVu analysis combining the Angio PL.U.S Doppler (typical irregular microvessels) and the SW elastography stiffness (score 5) indicates the diagnosis of a small malignant lesion

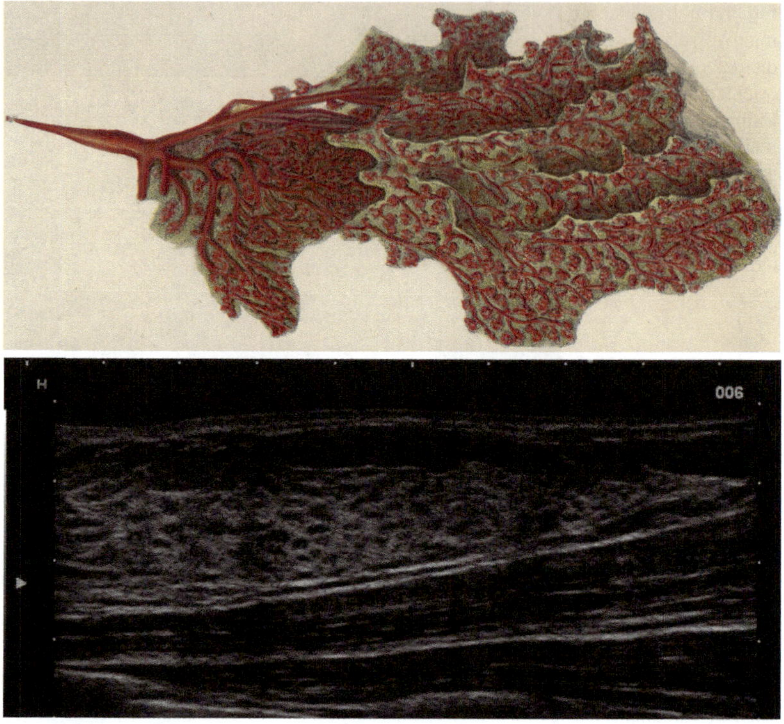

Fig. 1.13 1840/2017: Perfect correlation between the A. COOPER sketch (radial section) and the lobar/radial echographic scanning of a young female with an important epithelial hyperplasia (courtesy of Welcome Institute librairy. London: Cooper A.P. 1840 On the anatomy of the breast)

The possibility to use the new mobile echographic machines for pre- and postoperative scanning (cf Chap. 18) is essential for a good follow-up of the patients. In the near future, the introduction of smartphones connected by WiFi to specific probes will transform the use of preoperative echography or checkups in specialized consultations.

To end on this technical part, the final report of mammary echography cannot but include a lobar analysis, an anatomic description of the morphological type of breast, and an extremely precise mapping out of the lesion(s) (distance of the lesion from the nipple, depth from the skin), achieved in the operating position with the arm at a 90° angle, within the international BI-RADS classification.

References

1. Cooper AP. On the anatomy of the breast. London: Longman, Orme, Green, Brown, and Longmans; 1840.
2. Going JJ, Mohun TJ. Human breast duct anatomy, the 'sick lobe' hypothesis and intraductal approaches to breast cancer. Breast Cancer Res Treat. 2006;97:285–91.
3. Stavros T. Breast ultrasound. Philadelphia, PA: Lippincott; 2006.
4. Dolphin G. The surgical approach to the "sick lobe". In: Francescatti DS, Silverstein MJ, editors. Breast cancer: a new era in management. New York, NY: Springer; 2014. p. 113–32.
5. Teboul M, Halliwell M. Atlas of ultrasound and ductal echography of the breast. Oxford: Blackwell Science; 1995.
6. Gallager S, Martin J. Early phases in the development of breast cancer. Cancer. 1969;24:1170–8.
7. Tot T. The sick lobe concept. In: Francescatti DS, Silverstein MJ, editors. Breast cancer: a new era in management. New York, NY: Springer; 2014a. p. 79–94.
8. Tot T. The sick lobe concept. In: Francescatti DS, Silverstein MJ, editors. Breast cancer: a new era in management. New York, NY: Springer; 2014b. p. 79–94.
9. Nakama S. Comparative studies on ultrasonogram with histological structure of breast cancer: an examination in the invasive process of breast cancer and the fixation to the skin. In: Kasumi F, Ueno E, editors. Topic in breast ultrasound. Tokyo: Shinohara; 1991.
10. Ueno E. Real-time two dimensional Doppler imaging in the breast diseases. Proceedings of the 55th annual scientific meeting of Japan Society of Ultrasonics in Medicine. 1990;73–74.
11. Francescatti DS. Goers, Donalds (Eds) Breast cancer: a new era in management. New York, NY: Springer; 2014.
12. Kobayashi T. Clinical ultrasound of the breast. Berlin: Springer Sciences; 1978.

The Lobar Concept in Imaging the Complex Morphology of Breast Carcinoma

2

Tibor Tot

2.1 Introduction

Breast carcinoma is a heterogeneous and progressive disease, rather than a group of diseases, in which the individual cases deviate from each other in their clinical and radiological manifestations, gross, subgross, and microscopic morphology, in the phenotype and genetic construction of the tumor cells and their sensitivity to the applicable therapy, and also in metastatic capacity of the tumors and prognosis [1]. Basically, three general approaches exist in diagnosing and treating breast carcinomas: (1) focusing on the differences between the individual cases, (2) focusing on common characteristics of the cases, and (3) combining the two aforementioned approaches.

1. The differences between the individual cases are evident at all the levels of diagnostic observations, but the currently most exploited ones are those in protein expression (molecular phenotypes) and in genomic alterations of the tumor cells (intrinsic tumor types). The aim of modern oncological therapy is to damage the tumor cells with drugs that were developed specifically against proteins that are expressed or overexpressed by the tumor cells (targeted therapy). In neoadjuvant settings, the damage may be of such extent that the tumor regresses which allows an easier operation. In adjuvant settings the aim is to damage the tumor cells which remained within the organism after the surgical intervention and to prevent recurrences this way. Unfortunately these attempts are not infrequently compromised by heterogeneity of the tumor cell populations within the same patient and by the ability of tumor cells to develop resistance against the targeting therapy agent(s) [2, 3].
2. All breast carcinomas, irrespective to their histopathologic, phenotypic, and genetic characteristics, are distributed within the breast in unifocal, multifocal, or diffuse fashion; the tumors occupy a certain part of the breast tissue and have a three-dimensional extent; all invasive carcinomas have a size defined as the largest dimension of the largest invasive focus within the breast, and many of them exhibit intra- or intertumoral heterogeneity. These four general characteristics can be revealed with high accuracy with the methods of modern multimodality radiology preoperatively and best with contiguous large-format histology sections which properly document these parameters in the surgical specimens [4, 5]. The aim of the surgical intervention is to remove the diseased part of the breast that

T. Tot, M.D., Ph.D.
Pathology & Cytology Dalarna, Falun County Hospital, Falun, Sweden
e-mail: tibor.tot@ltdalarna.se

D. Amy (ed.), *Lobar Approach to Breast Ultrasound*, https://doi.org/10.1007/978-3-319-61681-0_2

contains all the malignant tumor foci, irrespective to the tumors' molecular or genetic characteristics, and to achieve this with clear surgical margins of a certain width. Unfortunately, these attempts are compromised with the fact that the sensitivity of breast radiology is still under 100% and parts of the cancer may remain preoperatively undetected and left within the breast after a seemingly radical surgical intervention. The aim of postoperative irradiation is to destroy the remaining part of the cancer.

3. The two approaches mentioned above are usually combined in everyday practice, and patients often receive surgical, oncological, and radiation therapy. A multidisciplinary tumor board should discuss every individual case and decide which one of the therapy modalities will be applied. The decision should be based on careful analysis of the parameters provided in the radiology and pathology reports which should include all the elements needed for this decision [6].

Most of the reported studies in the current related scientific literature focus in details on oncological parameters, therapeutic options, and prognosis. Multifocality, disease extent, and tumor heterogeneity are often ignored in these publications. This resulted in the fact that in the mainstream opinion of current breast cancer care, the tumors are regarded for a unifocal non-heterogeneous disease that is sufficiently operated with "no tumor on the ink" and is efficiently treated with targeted therapy [7]. The shortcomings of this approach are frequent reoperations, local recurrences, and development of tumor resistance to the applied therapy. A more balanced approach, taking into the account the general subgross parameters assessed with the same care as the molecular ones, could reduce the mentioned shortcomings of the mainstream approach. High-quality multimodality breast radiology methods are one of the conditions to achieve this balance, the other one is better understanding of the complexity of breast cancer morphology. This chapter aims to support the members of the breast team with describing this complexity and is based on the findings in a large consecutive series of breast cancer cases documented in large-format histology slides and worked up with detailed radiological–pathological correlation in our institution. It will also reintroduce the previously published sick lobe concept [8–12] that indicates the presence of a genetically altered progenitor cell population within a single breast lobe and eventual clustering of the malignant progenies within the area of this lobe. This concept has become the theoretical basis for the lobar approach in breast imaging and surgery [13–16].

2.2 Normal Anatomy and Histology of the Lobes

Breast is an organ with lobar morphology. The breast lobes are complex structures with a central lactiferous duct that opens with a single opening on the nipple, branches in segmental, subsegmental, and terminal ducts that terminate in hundreds and thousands of lobules composed of blindly ending acini. A lobule together with their terminal duct is often designated as terminal ductal–lobular unit (TDLU) as it represents a physiological unit that produces the milk. All these structures are luminated, and their lumen is surrounded by a single inner layer of epithelium, a single outer layer of myoepithelium, and a continuous basement membrane. The surrounding stroma is an active component of the lobe being specialized and more hormone sensitive within the lobules and around the larger ducts [17].

The lobules and the TDLUs are less than a millimeter in size and are hardly visible on radiology images. Distended ducts and lobules are easier to detect. The lobes are several centimeter large structures detectable with galactography but not seen on mammograms, traditional ultrasound, or on magnetic resonance imaging. Ductal echography visualizes the lobes efficiently and demonstrates the variations between the lobes regarding their size and shape [14].

2.3 The Subtle Differences Between Healthy and Sick Lobes

The core idea of the sick lobe concept defines breast cancer being a lobar disease in the meaning that the structures of the tumor develop most often in a single lobe of the breast. The lobes are initiated early during the embryonic development through formation of the main branches from the initial bud. The process is regulated at the level of the progenitor cells their progenies being the source of both normal epithelium and myoepithelium. The hypothetic mechanism of the appearance of a sick lobe is through early genetic alterations of the progenitor cells that become committed this way to potentially develop a malignant progeny. Thus the sick lobe deviates from the healthy lobes of the same breast in the presence of altered (committed) progenitor cells dispersed unevenly within this lobe. The sick lobe has higher sensitivity to oncogenic stimuli presumable due to the presence of the committed progenitor cells [11].

2.4 Early Malignancy Within the Sick Lobe and Patterns of Its Development

Complete malignant transformation of the committed progenitor cells is a result of further accumulation of genetic alterations during decades. Mutations and other genetic alterations appear most commonly during the replication of the cells. For a complete malignant transformation of the committed progenitor cells, a certain number of replication is needed, which indicates that the complete malignant transformation is biologically timed and may happen simultaneously on distant locations within the sick lobe. The process may involve several distant TDLUs (the so-called peripheral growth pattern), a segment of the sick lobe (the so-called segmental pattern), or the entire lobe or large parts of it contiguously (the so-called lobar pattern). These patterns are best recognized in purely in situ carcinomas and in early invasive cancer (defined as those measuring <15 mm in their largest dimension), while in more advanced cases, the tumor often infiltrates beyond the area of the sick lobe. These patterns of development of cancer within the sick lobe have prognostic implications in terms of local recurrences and survival: the peripheral pattern is usually associated with a low-grade slowly progressing disease with low mortality rates but with a substantial potential to locally recur after a long time due to its often multifocal and extensive nature; the lobar pattern of cancer development within the sick lobe indicates an aggressive disease with high mortality and recurrence rates and more rapid course. The segmental disease has a prognosis that is intermediate between these two extremes [11, 12].

2.5 Subgross Parameters in Practice

2.5.1 Definition of the Subgross Parameters

The subgross parameters defined above are essential in guiding the surgical and oncological therapy and should be therefore carefully assessed with radiological methods preoperatively. Careful assessment of the surgical specimen after the operation is necessary to confirm or complete the preoperative radiological findings; assess the results of the surgical intervention; indicate the need, if any, for complete surgery; and provide morphological prognostic and predictive parameters for oncological treatment.

Disease extent is defined as the volume of the breast tissue containing all the malignant structures within the same breast. It is assessed in three dimensions with multimodality radiology methods and in two dimensions histologically. Histology is still a more sensitive method compared to radiology and detects radiologically occult malignant lesions in addition to those that were radiologically evidenced in approximately 15–20% of cases [18]. The radiologically occult lesions are most often non-calcified in situ carcinoma foci or very small invasive foci. Disease extent of 40 mm or larger (regards the larges dimension of the volume of the breast involved by the malignant process) is associated with almost three times higher local recurrence rates after breast conserving surgery and with decreased disease-specific survival compared to the cases with less extensive disease [19, 20]. Diagram 2.1 shows a substantial proportion; 40–50% of the cases are extensive (extent ≥40 mm) in every size category of the tumors.

Tumor size is defined as the largest dimension of the largest invasive tumor focus within the breast. It is relatively easy to measure in cases of circular/oval mass lesions. The size of spiculated masses should be measured without including the spiculations even if they contain invasive tumor structures. Following this rule, the concordance of radiological and pathological tumor size measurements will be high. Regarding categorization of the cases into early and more advanced based on tumor size, this concordance is 85% [21]. Histological tumor size measurement is superior to the radiological one only under the condition that the tumor is embedded into a sufficiently large paraffin block without fragmentation and in the level of its largest dimension at cross section. Histological tumor size measurement is, on the other hand, unreliable in cases with tumor regression after neoadjuvant therapy. Tumor size is a robust prognostic parameter and is also used as indicator of necessity of neoadjuvant therapy.

Tumor foci may show unifocal, multifocal, or diffuse **lesion distribution** within the breast tissue that is defined with the extent of the disease. This regards both the in situ and the invasive components of the tumor; thus both should be assessed individually and also joint into an aggregate growth pattern. **Unifocal tumors** represent a single focus disease (in situ, invasive, or both) comprising 39% of breast carcinoma in our series, as shown in Table 2.1. In these cases the extent of the disease is either equal to tumor size or is slightly larger due to presence of in situ tumor component(s) at the periphery of the lesion. A case of unifocal cancer is illustrated in Figs. 2.1a and 2.2. **Multifocality** is defined as simul-

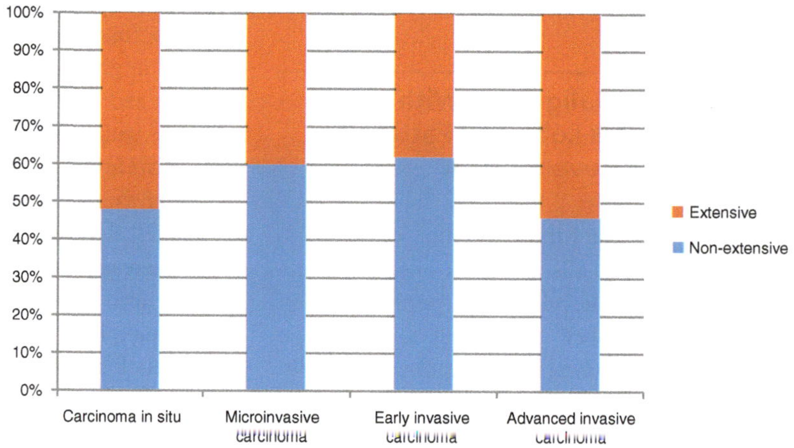

Diagram 2.1 Breast carcinoma cases by tumor stage and disease extent, consecutive series of 1796 cases, Dalarna, Sweden, 2008–2016. Extensive defined as an occupied breast volume ≥40 mm in largest dimension

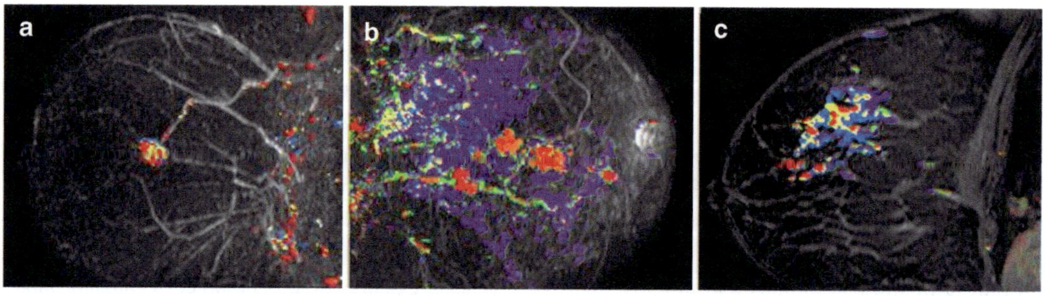

Fig. 2.1 Magnetic resonance imaging demonstrating the three basic growth patterns in breast carcinomas. (**a**) Unifocal cancer, (**b**) multifocal cancer, (**c**) diffuse cancer

taneous presence of multiple well-circumscribed tumor foci (in situ, invasive, or both) within the same breast, irrespective to the distance between the foci, as illustrated in Figs. 2.1b and 2.3e, f. In our consecutive series of large-format histology cases, a third of breast carcinomas comprise multiple invasive tumor foci, while in another third, a unifocal invasive focus is associated with multifocal or diffuse in situ component (Table 2.1). The rates of multifocality, however, differ substantially in published series due to variations in definition of multifocality and the used radiological and pathological methods. Defined as above, multifocality is a robust prognostic parameter associated with doubled frequency of

Table 2.1 Breast carcinoma cases by stage, invasive, and aggregate growth patterns (Dalarna, 2008–2016 September)

		Unifocal	Multifocal	Diffuse	Total
Breast carcinoma in situ		33% (81/242)	27% (64/242)	40% (97/242)	13% (242/1887)
Early invasive breast cancer (<15 mm in size)	Invasive component	70% (485/688)	30% (203/242)	0	36% (688/1887)
	Aggregate pattern[a]	44% (304/688)	31% (212/688)	25% (172/688)	51% (957/1887)
Advanced invasive breast cancer (≥15 mm in size)	Invasive component	50% (481/957)	39% (374/957)	11% (102/957)	
	Aggregate pattern[a]	37% (351/957)	34% (325/975)	29% (281/957)	
All cancers	Invasive component	59% (966/1645)	35% (577/1645)	6% (102/1645)	87% (1645/1887)
	Aggregate pattern[a]	39% (736/1887)	32% (601/1887)	29% (550/1887)	100% (1887/1887)

[a]Aggregate pattern: combined pattern of growth of both in situ and invasive tumor components

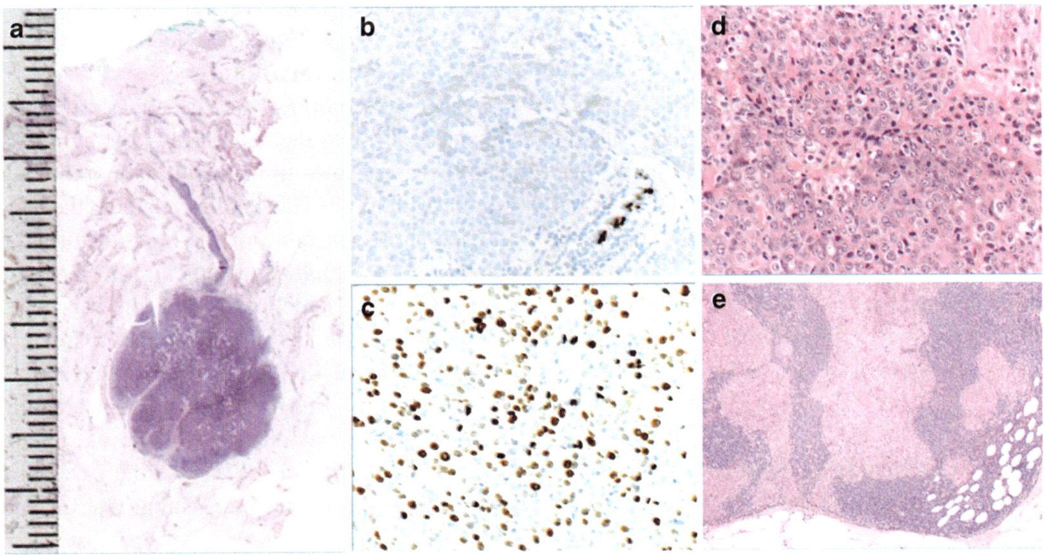

Fig. 2.2 Unifocal invasive breast carcinoma with an in situ component. (**a**) Large-format histopathology image; (**b**) negative estrogen receptor staining in the tumor cells, stained normal glands; (**c**) ki67 staining showing high proliferative activity of the tumor cells; (**d**) microscopic image of the poorly differentiated invasive carcinomas; (**e**) lymph node metastasis

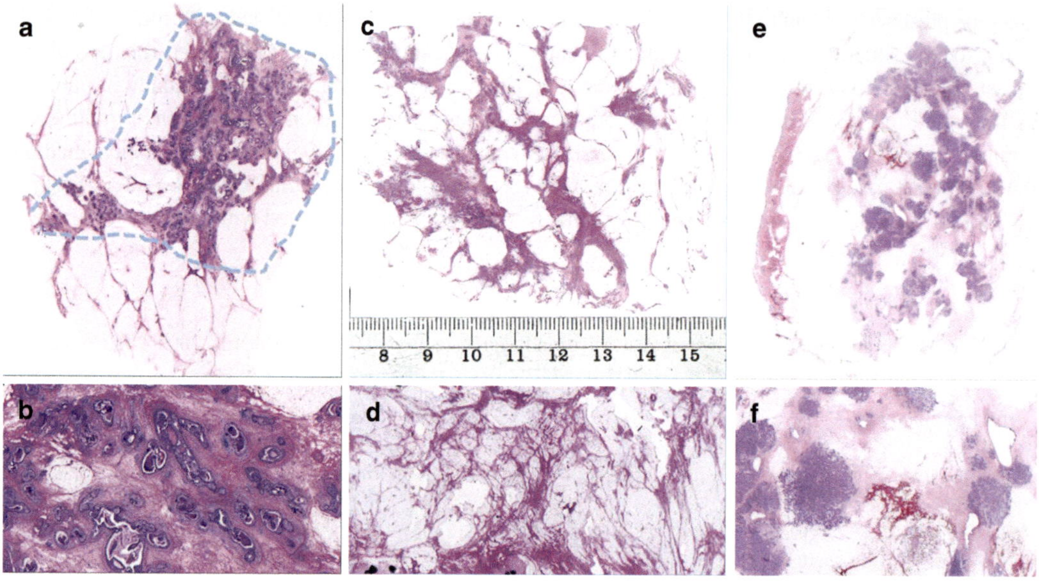

Fig. 2.3 Diffuse and multifocal breast carcinomas. (**a**) Large-format histopathology image of diffuse in situ carcinoma; (**b**) histology detail from image a showing a diffuse network of large ducts that are involved by the in situ cancer; (**c**) large section histology image of a diffuse invasive breast carcinoma; (**d**) histology image showing typical spiders weblike growth pattern in diffuse invasive cancer; (**e, f**) multifocal invasive breast carcinoma

vascular invasion and lymph node positivity and decreased disease-specific survival, compared to unifocal disease [22, 23]. This relates both to multifocality of the invasive component and to multifocal aggregate growth. Meta-analysis of related published series also evidenced the negative prognostic input of multifocality [24]. **Diffuse invasive tumors** are rare comprising about 6% of all cases as shown in Table 2.1. The diffuse growth often results in a poorly defined architectural distortion on the mammograms that is difficult to detect and in a spider's weblike appearance at large-format histopathology (Figs. 2.1e and 2.3c, d). The size of these tumors is difficult to measure; they are better characterized with their extent. Diffuse invasive carcinomas are the most aggressive tumors in the screening era [25].

2.5.2 Subgross Parameters in Early Breast Cancer

Early breast cancer is defined by its excellent prognosis. The category comprises purely in situ carcinomas and invasive carcinomas <15 mm in size (microinvasive carcinomas <1 mm in size are also included). In contrary to the "mainstream opinion" regarding breast carcinoma for "early" if it is operable, our definition is based on the expected favorable long-term outcome in such cases, similar to that of early cancers in other organs [3, 26].

2.5.2.1 In Situ Carcinomas

In situ carcinomas are characterized with retained ability of the malignant progenitor cells and their progenies to maintain the morphology similar to normal. This implies retaining the ductal–lobular architecture of the breast tissue, the biphasic (epithelial–myoepithelial) differentiation of the cells, delineation of the structures from the stroma with a continuous basement membrane, and a limited stromal reaction. Exceptions from this rule exist, although are rare, challenging the pathologists to delineate in situ and invasive cancers. In 75% of the cases, the tumor cells fill in the preexisting TDLUs and ducts leading to their dilatation and distortion. Most in situ carcinomas involve the TDLUs and are either unifocal (if a single TDLU or neighboring TDLUs are involved) or multifocal (if distant TDLUs are involved with uninvolved ones in between). These tumors tend to have a low histological grade and are usually composed of small monomorphic cells that most often express estrogen receptors but not HER2. Diffuse in situ carcinomas, on the other hand, involve mainly the larger ducts and form a network-like structure which is difficult to delineate. They tend to show high histology grade and are composed of large polymorphic cells (Fig. 2.2a, b). Table 2.1 shows the percentage of unifocal, multifocal, and diffuse in situ carcinoma cases in our series, while Diagram 2.2 shows the distribution of these tumors by extent and grade. Clustered calcifications indicate in situ carcinoma within the TDLU(s), while linear branching calcifications are associated with in situ carcinomas involving the ducts. Calcifications are, however, a rather uncertain indicator of presence of in situ cancer as low-grade in situ tumors calcify in approximately 30% while high grade in approximately 50% of the cases [5]. Importantly, in a quarter of the cases, the in situ cancer do not form ducts and TDLUs but develop mass lesions or involves preexisting benign structures (notably papillary lesions) or the skin as in Paget's disease.

Proper preoperative characterization of in situ carcinomas includes the assessment of the extent of the disease, as it is the most important prognostic factor with regard to local recurrences. Histology grade of the in situ component is associated with the risk of developing invasive disease and the risk of fatal outcome (Diagram 2.2), which is much higher in high-grade lesions compared to low-grade ones. All the in situ carcinomas are traditionally divided into "lobular" and "ductal" which may coexist within the sick lobe and also within the same duct or TDLU. This does not indicate the site of origin of the tumor as both lobular and ductal carcinoma in situ may originate in any part of the sick lobe. It indicates genetic differences between the two entities as the lobular ones rarely express E-cadherin.

Although delineated from the stroma, in situ carcinomas are not totally innocent. 3–7% of the patients die of this disease during a 20-year follow-up period, young patients significantly more often, and in half of the cases with poor outcome, no invasive recurrences are seen [27].

2.5.2.2 Early Invasive Breast Carcinoma

The small tumor size of early breast carcinomas does not exclude that they may have complex morphology [28]. In fact, they are almost as often multifocal as their advanced counterparts and as often are associated with multifocal or diffuse in situ components (Table 2.1). The proportion of extensive cases (extent ≥40 mm) is also similar in the early and advanced categories (Diagram 2.1). The invasive tumor component itself forms one or more spiculated or circular/oval mass lesion in the area of the sick lobe.

Early invasive tumor foci have significantly more favorable histological characteristics than the more advanced cancers. They are rarely

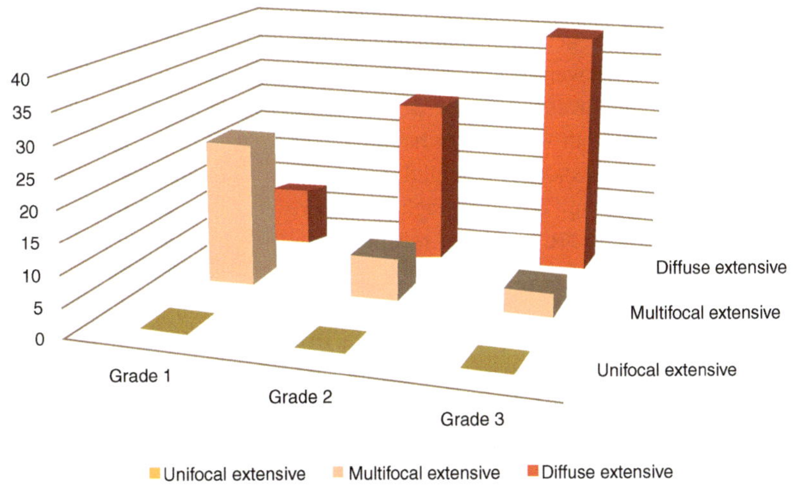

Diagram 2.2 In situ carcinomas by extent, growth pattern, and histology grade (Dalarna, Sweden, 242 consecutive cases, 2008–2016 September). Note the tendency of diffuse cases to be of higher grade and the opposite in multifocal ones. None of the unifocal in situ carcinomas was extensive (extent ≥ 40 mm)

Table 2.2 Histological and molecular characteristics of invasive breast carcinomas by natural history stage

	Early invasive cancer	Advanced invasive cancer	Total	*P* values
Grade III	12% (83/674)	27% (259/950)	21% (342/1624)	$P < 0.0001$
ER-negative	9% (59/664)	15% (147/953)	13% (206/1617)	$P = 0.0003$
PR	21% (168/664)	33% (316/952)	30% (484/1616)	$P < 0.0001$
HER2	**10% (65/667)**	**13% (121/952)**	12% (186/1619)	$P = 0.0653$
High Ki67	22% (146/650)	39% (370/948)	32% (516/1598)	$P < 0.0001$
Luminal A	52% (330/638)	35% (329/952)	41% (659/1590)	$P < 0.0001$
Luminal B	40% (255/638)	50% (480/952)	46% (735/1590)	$P = 0.0001$
HER2-type	**3% (20/638)**	**4% (36/952)**	4% (56/1590)	$P = 0.2942$
Triple negative	5% (33/638)	11% (107/952)	9% (140/1590)	$P < 0.0001$
Basal like	6% (41/663)	14% (129/929)	11% (170/1592)	$P < 0.0001$
Total	42% (688/1645)	58% (957/1645)	100% (1645/1645)	

Significant differences are observed in all parameters except the HER2 status

high-grade, rarely highly proliferative, and rarely triple negative (Table 2.2). Thus, the importance of the subgross morphological parameters is higher than that of the molecular ones in early category. In fact, multifocality of the invasive component and the presence of extensive diffuse in situ component are established prognostic parameters in early breast cancer. HER2-positive tumors, however, represent an exception; they are as frequent among early invasive carcinomas as in the advanced category. This indicates that HER2-positive disease is biologically different from the HER2-negative cancers; it is extensive and aggressive from the beginning of its natural history. Most such cases are typical examples of lobar growth pattern within the sick lobe [29].

The prognosis in early invasive breast carcinoma is, however, generally favorable as mentioned above. The overall survival of the patients having <15 mm invasive cancer is not significantly different from women not having cancer provided that the cancer is detected with mammography screening [26]. Although most early breast carcinomas are estrogen receptor positive, antihormonal therapy seems to have only limited effect on the long-term survival in this category of the patients [30]. The benefit from adjuvant therapy in the rare HER2-positive and triple negative early carcinoma still has to be studied.

2.5.3 Subgross Parameters in Advanced Breast Cancer

The outcome of breast cancer cases is less and less favorable parallel to increase of tumor size with beginning at the 15 mm cutoff point. This indicates that the cases with tumor size ≥15 mm are best categorized separately. As shown in Table 2.2, these tumors are not only larger than their early counterparts but carry unfavorable biological characteristics significantly more often. This may be a result of overgrowth of an aggressive clone or dedifferentiation of the tumor cells during the natural history of the disease, but late detection due to a more rapid growth of the tumor in these cases is also a possible explanation. The histological type of the tumor, its histology grade, and the molecular and genetic characteristics of the tumor cells impact on prognosis substantially more than in early invasive cases. However, the prognostic power of the subgross morphological parameters is retained in this category [21, 31, 32], as demonstrated in Diagram 2.3.

As already mentioned, pathology as a more sensitive method than radiology may detect radiologically occult lesions in a substantial proportion of the cases. Non-calcified in situ foci, small invasive tumor foci, and rarely diffuse invasive cancers may remain radiologically undetected. Detailed pathological work-up of the cases may reveal that a radiologically unifocal

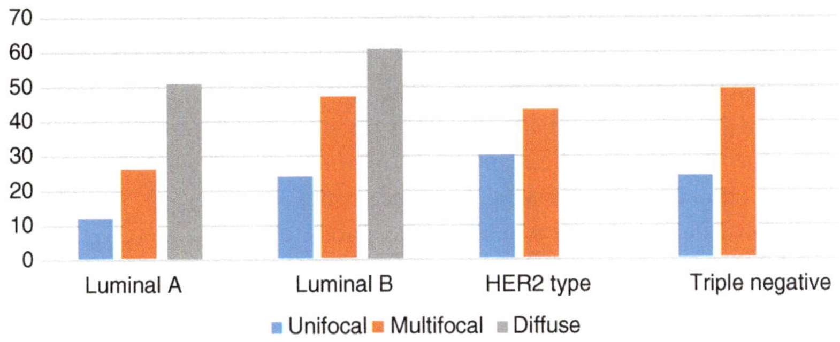

Diagram 2.3 Axillary lymph node macro-metastasis rates (%) by invasive cancer focality and St. Gallen 2013 molecular phenotypes in 1439 consecutive invasive breast cancer cases, Dalarna, Sweden, 2008–2015

lesion with simple morphology is in fact a multifocal or diffuse complex case [18]. Therefore postoperative radiological–pathological correlation is mandatory for definite characterization of the subgross parameters even in advanced cases.

2.5.3.1 Molecular Phenotypes

Detailed genetic characterization of breast carcinomas revealed a few intrinsic categories [33]. For practical reasons, these categories are defined using surrogate clinical–pathological parameters. Although many classification systems have been proposed, the St. Gallen system is the most accepted, despite the fact that it develops over time in terms of definition details. In its version from 2013 [7], this system discriminates luminal A, luminal B, HER2 overexpression, and "basal-like" categories of breast carcinomas. Tumors in the luminal categories are characterized by the expression of estrogen and progesterone receptors, absence of HER2 overexpression, and low proliferative activity. Luminal B-like tumors are subdivided into two categories: luminal B HER2-negative tumors, exhibiting either a high Ki67 proliferation index or low (<20%) levels of progesterone receptors, and luminal B-like HER2-positive tumors. The HER2 overexpression category comprises tumors that are non-luminal (estrogen receptor-negative) and HER2-positive. The "basal-like" intrinsic category is defined as triple negative (ductal); these tumors do not express estrogen or progesterone receptors, neither HER2. The molecular phenotype of breast carcinoma has become the main determinant of oncological therapy in both neoadjuvant and adjuvant settings. However, the obvious relation of the molecular phenotypes to subgross morphological parameters [21] indicates again the need for multiparameter characterization of breast carcinomas even in the advanced cases as it has been stressed in the 2015 version of the St. Gallen recommendations.

2.5.3.2 Intra- and Intertumoral Heterogeneity

The temporal and spatial evolution of the process of malignancy leads to appearance of different tumor cell clones deviating from each other in their genetic and phenotypic characteristics in a considerable number of cases. The different cell clones may be present within the same primary or metastatic tumor focus (intratumoral heterogeneity), in simultaneously or asynchronously developing multiple tumor foci within the same breast (intertumoral heterogeneity in multifocal tumors), or they may manifest as differences between primary tumors and circulating tumor cells and/or metastatic deposits. Intra- and intertumoral heterogeneity is a complex issue, posing obvious impediments to the successful clinical development of targeted therapeutic agents. It is also a real challenge for future developments in diagnostic pathology.

2.6 Concluding Remarks

- Breast carcinoma is a lobar disease; thus the lobar approach in diagnosing breast carcinoma is justified.
- The majority of breast carcinomas are of complex subgross morphology with multiple or

diffuse in situ and/or invasive tumor structures which occupy a breast volume ≥40 mm in largest dimension in almost half of the cases.

- Early breast carcinomas defined as in situ tumors and/or invasive carcinomas <15 mm in size have favorable molecular characteristics and excellent prognosis with a few exceptions.
- Multifocality and diffuse lesion distribution are negative prognostic parameters.
- Adequate radiological methods are needed for proper preoperative characterization of the complex morphology of breast carcinomas.
- The complexity of breast cancer morphology indicates the need for interdisciplinary approach in diagnosing and treating this disease.

References

1. Lakhani SR, Ellis IO, Schnitt SJ, Tan PH, van de Vijver M, editors. WHO classification of tumours of the breast. Lyon: International Agency for Research on Cancer (IARC); 2012.
2. Boros M, Marian C, Moldovan C, Stolnicu S. Morphological heterogeneity of the simultaneous ipsilateral invasive tumor foci in breast carcinoma: a retrospective study of 418 cases of carcinomas. Pathol Res Pract. 2012;208:604–9.
3. Kahán Z, Tot T, editors. Breast cancer, a heterogeneous disease entity. The very early stages. Dordrecht: Springer; 2011.
4. Tabár L, Tot T, Dean PB. Breast cancer: the art and science of early detection with mammography: perception, interpretation, histopathologic correlation. Stuttgart: Thieme; 2005.
5. Tot T, Tabár L, Dean PB. Practical breast pathology. 2nd ed. Stuttgart: Thieme; 2014.
6. Tot T, Viale G, Rutgers E, Bergsten-Nordström E, Costa A. Optimal breast cancer pathology manifesto. Eur J Cancer. 2015;51:2285–8.
7. Goldhirsch A, Winer EP, Coates AS, Gelber RD, Piccart-Gebhart M, Thürlimann B, Senn HJ, Panel members. Personalizing the treatment of women with early breast cancer: highlights of the St Gallen International Expert Consensus on the Primary Therapy of Early Breast Cancer. Ann Oncol. 2013;24:2206–23.
8. Foschini MP, Morandi L, Leonardi E, Ishikawa Y, Masetti R, Eusebi V. Genetic clonal mapping of in situ and invasive ductal carcinoma indicates the field cancerization phenomenon in the breast. Hum Pathol. 2014;44:1310–9.
9. Tot T. DCIS, cytokeratins, and the theory of the sick lobe. Virchows Arch. 2005;447:1–8.
10. Tot T. The theory of the sick breast lobe and the possible consequences. Int J Surg Pathol. 2007a;15:369–3751.
11. Tot T, editor. Breast cancer – a lobar disease. Dodrecht: Springer; 2011a.
12. Tot T. Subgross morphology, the sick lobe hypothesis, and the success of breast conservation. Int J Breast Cancer Article ID. 2011b;2011:634021. https://doi.org/10.4061/2011/634021. 8 pages.
13. Amy D. Lobar ultrasound of the breast. In: Tot T, editor. Breast cancer – a lobar disease. Dodrecht: Springer; 2011. p. 153–62.
14. Amy D, Durante E, Tot T. The lobar approach to breast ultrasound imaging and surgery. J Med Ultrasonics. 2015;42(3):331–9.
15. Tan MP, Sitoh NY, Sitoh YY. Optimising breast conservation treatment for multifocal and multicentric breast cancer: a worthwhile endeavour? World Journal of Surgery. 2016;40(2):315–22.
16. Teboul M, Halliwell M. Atlas of ultrasound and ductal echography of the breast: the introduction of anatomic intelligence into breast imaging. London: Wiley-Blackwell; 1995.
17. Going JJ, Mohun TJ. Human breast duct anatomy, the 'sick lobe' hypothesis and intraductal approaches to breast cancer. Breast Cancer Res Treat. 2006;97:285–91.
18. Tot T, Gere M. Radiologically unifocal invasive breast carcinomas: large-section histopathology correlate and impact on surgical management. J Cancer Sci Ther. 2016;8:050–4.
19. Lindquist D, Hellberg D, Tot T. Disease extent ≥4cm is a prognostic marker of local recurrence in T1-2 breast cancer. Pathol Res Int. 2011;2011:860584.
20. Tot T. The metastatic capacity of multifocal breast carcinomas: extensive tumors versus tumors of limited extent. Hum Pathol. 2009;40:199–205.
21. Tot T. Breast cancer: the relation of some radiological and morphological parameters to molecular phenotypes and prognosis. J OncoPath. 2014;2(4):69–76.
22. Chung AP, Huynh K, Kidner T, Mirzadehgan P, Sim MS, Giuliano AE. Comparison of outcomes of breast conserving therapy in multifocal and unifocal invasive breast cancer. J Am Coll Surg. 2012;215(1):137–46.
23. Pekar G, Gere M, Tarjan M, Hellberg D, Tot T. Molecular phenotype of the foci in multifocal invasive breast carcinomas: intertumoral heterogeneity is related to shorter survival and may influence the choice of therapy. Cancer. 2014;120(1):26–34.
24. Vera-Badillo FE, Napoleone M, Ocana A, Templeton AJ, Seruga B, Al-Mubarak M, Al Hashem H, Tannock IF, Amir E. Effect of multifocality and multicentricity on outcome in early stage breast cancer: a systematic review and meta-analysis. Breast Cancer Res Treat. 2014;146(2):235–44.
25. Tot T. Diffuse invasive breast carcinoma of no special type. Virchows Arch. 2016;468(2):199–206.

26. Otten JDM, Broeders MJM, Den Heeten GJ, Holland R, Fracheboud J, De Koning HJ, Verbeek AL. Life expectancy of screen-detected invasive breast cancer patients compared with women invited to the Nijmegen Screening Program. Cancer. 2010;116:586–91.
27. Narod SA, Iqbal J, Giannakeas V, Sopik V, Sun P. Breast cancer mortality after a diagnosis of Ductal Carcinoma In Situ. JAMA Oncol. 2015;1(7):888–96.
28. Tot T, Pekár G, Hofmeyer S, Sollie T, Gere M, Tarján M. The distribution of lesions in 1-14-mm invasive breast carcinomas and its relation to metastatic potential. Virchows Arch. 2009;455:109–15.
29. Tot T. Early (<10 mm) HER2-positive invasive breast carcinomas are associated with extensive diffuse high-grade DCIS: implications for preoperative mapping, extent of surgical intervention, and disease-free survival. Ann Surg Oncol. 2015;22(8):2532–9.
30. Bustreo S, Osella-Abate S, Cassoni P, Donadio M, Airoldi M, Pedani F, Papotti M, Sapino A, Castellano I. Optimal Ki67 cut-off for luminal breast cancer prognostic evaluation: a large case series study with a long-term follow-up. Breast Cancer Res Treat. 2016;157:363–71.
31. Tot T. The clinical relevance of the distribution of the lesions in 500 consecutive breast cancer cases documented in large-format histological sections. Cancer. 2007b;110:2551–60.
32. Tot T, Gere M, Pekár G, Tarján M, Hofmeyer S, Hellberg D, Lindquist D, Chen TH, Yen AM, Chiu SY, Tabár L. Breast cancer multifocality, disease extent, and survival. Hum Pathol. 2011;42(11):1761–9.
33. Sorlie T, Perou CM, Tibshirani R, Tibshirani R, Aas T, Geisler S, Johnsen H, Hastie T, Eisen MB, van de Rijn M, Jeffrey SS, Thorsen T, Quist H, Matese JC, Brown PO, Botstein D, Lønning PE, Børresen-Dale AL. Gene expression patterns of breast carcinomas distinguish tumor subclasses with clinical implications. Proc Natl Acad Sci USA. 2001;98:10869–74.

3 Lobar Anatomy

Dominique Amy

The purpose of this chapter is to fill in an important gap in breast imaging in general and in recent literature on mammary gland as visualized from the angles of radiology, MRI, and ultrasound.

Mammography is indeed a radiological technique which does not allow an identification of breast anatomy and whose further drawback is that it does not expose mammary epithelium.

MRI uses squared orthogonal slices overlooking the specific analysis of the various lobes. The technique of MRI is based on the modifications of neoangiogenesis following the injection of a contrast-enhancing chemical.

Last to come on the scene of medical imagery, scintigraphy, a nuclear medicine technique, allows the study of the lymph nodes but does not provide any information on anatomic details.

As for conventional echography with its systematic orthogonal ultrasound slices, it fails to make the lobar structures conspicuous. When radial slices occur, they generally concern the study of milk ducts only. It is exceptional to find echographic reports including descriptions of the lobes and of their contents, and the terms lobules, epithelial proliferation, or termino-ducto-lobular units are never used.

D. Amy, M.D.
Centre du sein, Aix-en-Provence, France
e-mail: domamy@wanadoo.fr

Conventional echography analyzes the inner components of the breast: connective and fatty tissue and occasionally epithelium (which unfortunately closely resembles fat in echography). Because of that, a lesion can be overlooked at a millimetric stage if it is not precisely located in a duct or a lobule. Conventional echography is geared to the search for a lesion, a mass, or a gap. The ultrasound semeiology of these lesions, as established by numerous authors, though very useful, sophisticated, and complex, bears no relationship to the anatomy of the breast.

In the 1980s and 1990s, such authors as E. Ueno and M. Teboul next, who were pioneers in their field, initiated us to the systematic radial analysis of the breast, so as to reveal its lobar anatomy [1–5]. Furthermore, the remarkable technological improvements of the last two decades have allowed the study of millimetric mammary structures which were hardly visible previously. The best example lies in the surprising analysis of large echographic slices with 10 cm large anatomo-pathological slices of the breast (Fig. 3.1 [6–9] (see Chaps. 2 and 5). It has become possible to analyze through echography structures which until then had been largely ignored (lobules, Cooper's ligaments, TDLUs, fascia). Lastly the use of water bag attached to large (10 cm) probes has been a decisive factor of improvement in ducto-radial echography.

D. Amy (ed.), *Lobar Approach to Breast Ultrasound*, https://doi.org/10.1007/978-3-319-61681-0_3

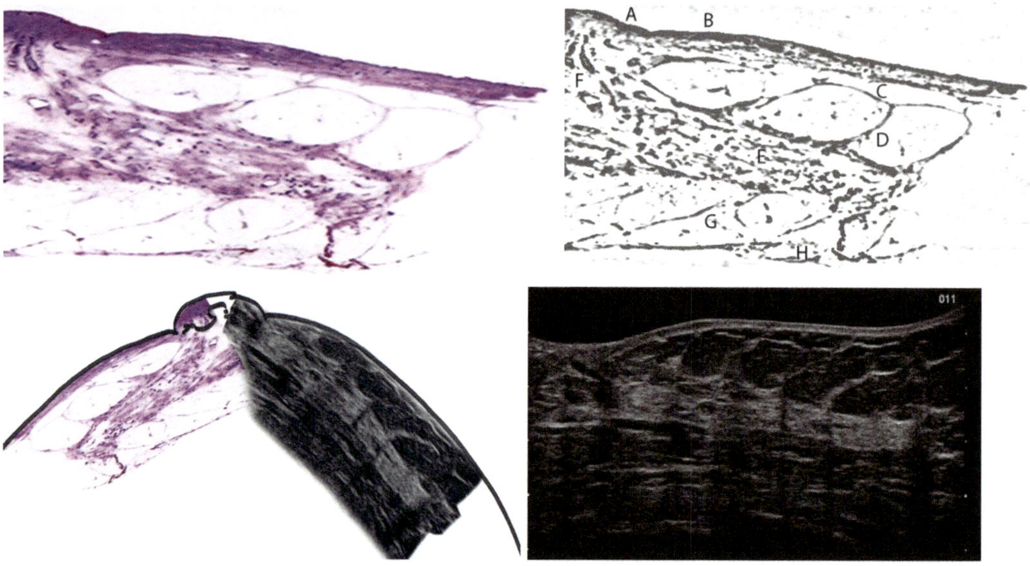

Fig. 3.1 Comparison between the anatomo-pathological section and the ultrasonic scanning. Anatomical elements: (*A*) Nipple. (*B*) Areola. (*C*) Skin. (*D*) Muscle pectoralis. (*E*) Lobe. (*F*) Cooper's ligament. (*G*) Fascia superficialis. (*H*) Retinacula cutis. (*I*) Cooper's ligament inferior. (*J*) Fascia inferior (Courtesy of Pr. T. Tot, Falun)

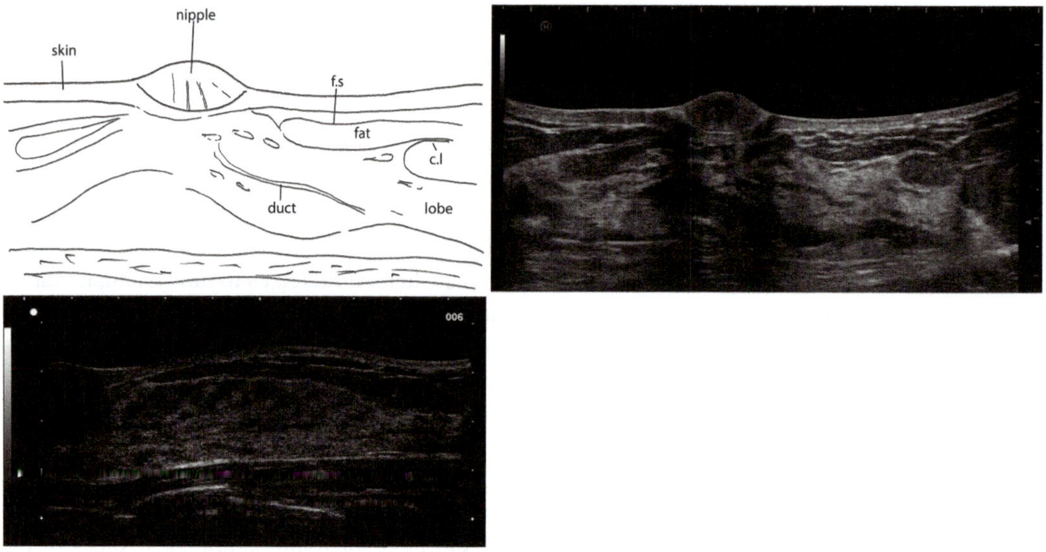

Fig. 3.2 Lobar analysis: nipple in the *upper left* portion of the image, the lobe extremity on the *right* side, skin surface and chest wall at the *bottom*

In order to ensure a better reproducibility of the ultrasound examination of the breast, within our group, it was decided to present all the echographic slices systematically in the same way, whatever the topographic location of the different lobes in the breast may be (Fig. 3.2)

- The nipple is always positioned on the top left side of the echographic screen, the distal end of the lobe resting on the left-hand side, the skin on the upper part of the screen, and the thoracic wall on the lower part. Each of the lobes being an independent anatomic and

functional element with an identical structure, it is logical to analyze them all successively in the same way.
- The technical "check list" (choice of the level of decibels, gain, focal length, contrast, etc.) as well as the analytic one (study of each lobe, of its inner structures and of related indirect peripheral signs) is the same for them all so that the technique is reproducible and totally independent of the operator: the technique is thus no longer operator-dependent but is merely anatomy-dependent.

It is indeed essential to have a perfect knowledge of the precise anatomical lay out so as to be able to understand all the physiological and pathological variations encountered during the various examinations. There are numerous parameters likely to modify the appearance of the ultrasound slices, but a minimum experience makes it possible to integrate them into the phrasing of the examination report.

The understanding of the initial development and formation of the lobes after puberty, of their growth in adulthood, and of their involution after the menopause, as well as of their disappearance in later life, will be presented in Chap. 5.

Within these lobes, mammary echography must focus on the study of the most important anatomic element, that is, the acino-ductal axis, which holds all the epithelium (since epithelium bears mammary pathology) [10–13]. We must remember that mammary pathology can be either ductal, lobular, or mixed, bringing together the two types of pathology.

The ultrasound analysis of the breast starts with the exploration of the ductal axes, the lobules attached to them within the lobes, to move on to the surrounding perilobar connective and fatty tissues, and lastly the cutaneous and subcutaneous cover as well as the deeper muscular planes. It is taken for granted that the exploration of the side-sternal, subclavicular, axillary, and upper and outer side-thoracic zones is an integral part of the examination and should in no way be neglected [14–16].

Before embarking on the actual ultrasound description of the lobes, an important point needs to be underlined.

The usual description of a lobe is that it has a triangular shape structure with a nipple vertex and a large lower base. This appearance, classically described by numerous authors, is not absolutely identical to the one noted "in vivo" during the ultrasound examination. The lobes, for the most part, are spear shaped and elongated like the petals of a daisy, with a thin distal tip ending with one or two ligaments. Only the lobes located between 5 o'clock and 7 o'clock in the lower part of the breast can have a pyramidal or triangular appearance due to the gravity of the breast which causes a relative compression of the lobes.

To confirm what we have just said about the shape of the lobes, we have compared the way in which they appear through MRI and through ultrasound (i.e., "in vivo"). Let us indicate that only the slices concerning the 9 o'clock and 3 o'clock lobes which are the only really radial slices in MRI were compared with the equivalent ultrasound slices produced in the same decubitus position. The comparison of the results reveals a perfect superimposition of the anatomic appearance of the lobes and a confirmation of their elongated spear shape (Fig. 3.3).

There is thus a "theoretical" difference in the anatomic description of the lobes as observed through MRI and/or ducto-radial echography and the surgical or anatomo-pathological descriptions based on anatomic pieces of quadrantectomy or mastectomy [17, 18].

Retraction due to changes in vascularization, temperature, section of the ligaments, and the technical handling and preparation of the anatomo-pathological sections modifies the shape of the lobes which take up a triangular, retracted appearance ("in vitro" appearance). This nevertheless does not alter in any way the nature, structure, and anatomical reality of the lobes.

There are some 12–15 lobes per breast, spread out among the various internal and external quadrants. For a perfect analysis and understanding of lobar echography, they are labelled in

Fig. 3.3 Lobar comparison between MRI and ductal echography: remarkable similarity of the lobar spear shape

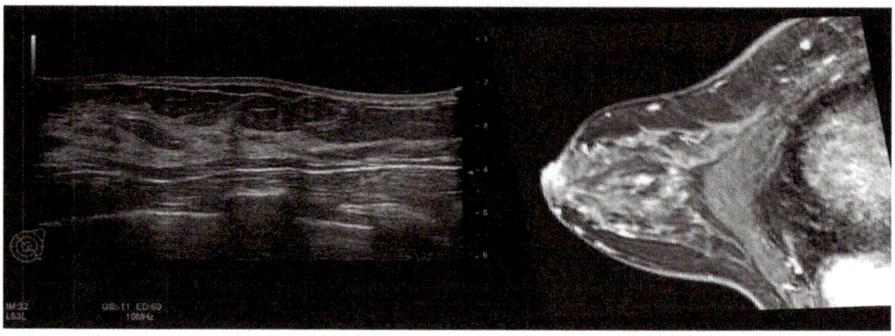

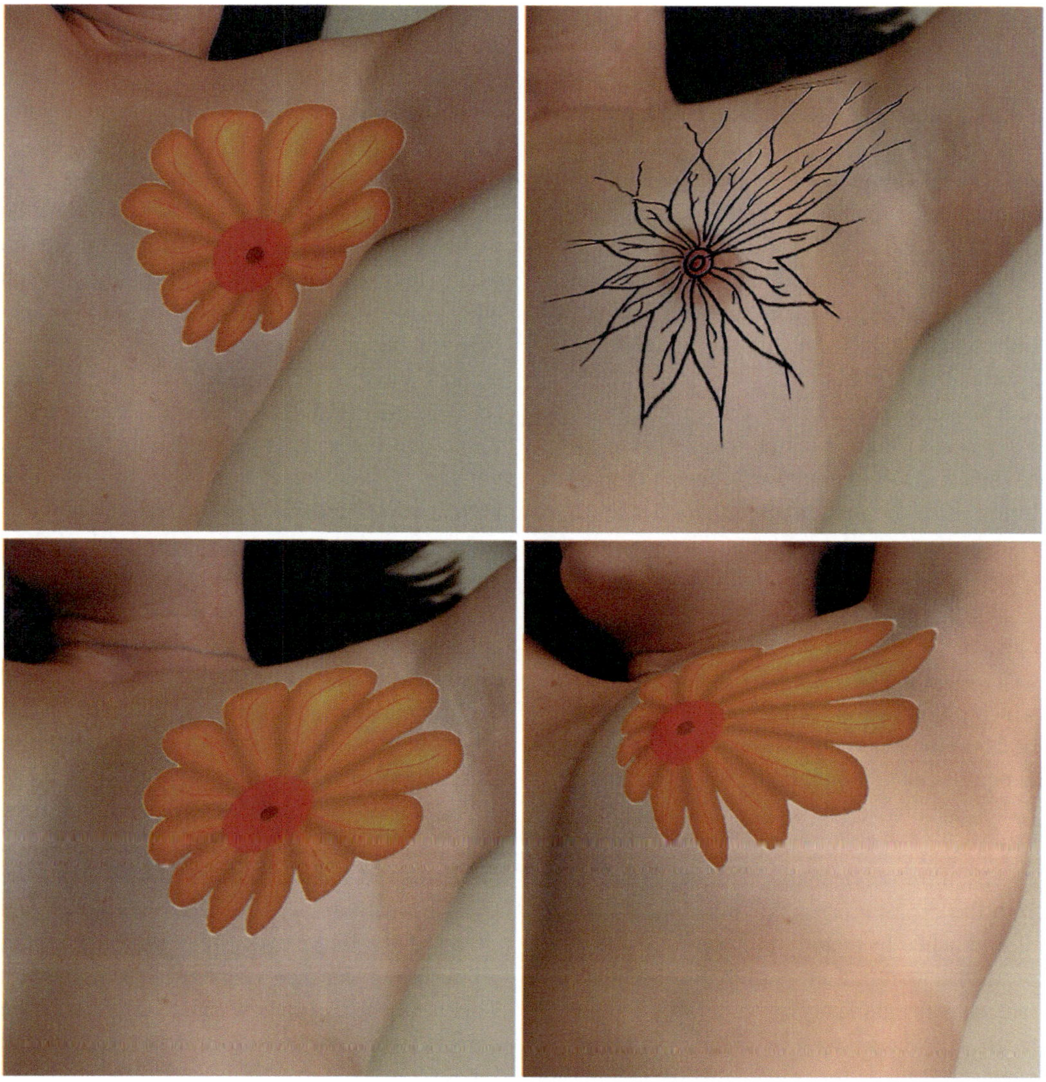

Fig. 3.4 Lobar distribution in the breast with smaller lobes in the inner inferior quadrant and the longer ones in the superior external area toward the axilla

accordance with the classic clock numeration: R12 corresponding to a lobe in the right breast located at 12 o'clock, L6 to a lobe in the left breast at 6 o'clock. This universally accepted method allows perfect reproducibility of ultrasound examinations (Figs. 3.4 and 3.5) [19].

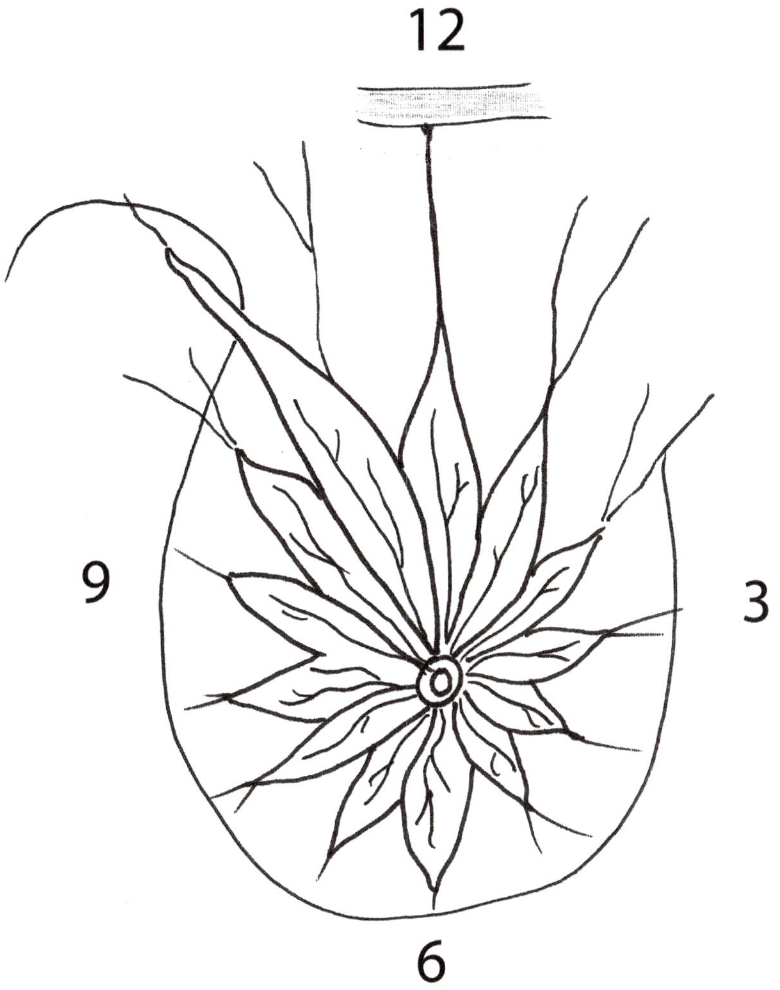

Fig. 3.5 Lobar distribution in the breast with smaller lobes in the inner inferior quadrant and the longer ones in the superior external area toward the axilla

3.1 Ducts

In lobar echography, the ducts are analyzed from the nipple to their distal end. As these ducts are less than a millimeter wide, some are more difficult to analyze, but most of them are nevertheless perfectly visible. The huge technical improvements and the introduction of high frequency large probes, as well as the development of possible more or less pronounced epithelial proliferation or ductal ecstasy, make the identification of the ducts easier. The difference in acoustic impedance with the periductal stroma allows one to follow the main ductal routes. As these are rather twisted, small movements of the probe allow one to straighten them back into the axis of the ultrasound beam and therefore to analyze their contents better.

It may seem a tedious task to analyze three or four ducts in 14 or so lobes, but in reality, only the distended or atypical ducts have to be studied more in detail, and all the others can be considered as normal. Should there be no distension, the examination can be rather swift and straightforward.

The nipple is always carefully analyzed thanks to the waterbags fixed onto the probe. The ducts within the nipple, at the back of it, and at the back of the areola are clearly visible. When they are distended, their ultrasound appearance is hypoechogenic, or anechoic in case of ectasia, and "pseudo-solid" in the case of epithelial proliferation (Figs. 3.6 and 3.7).

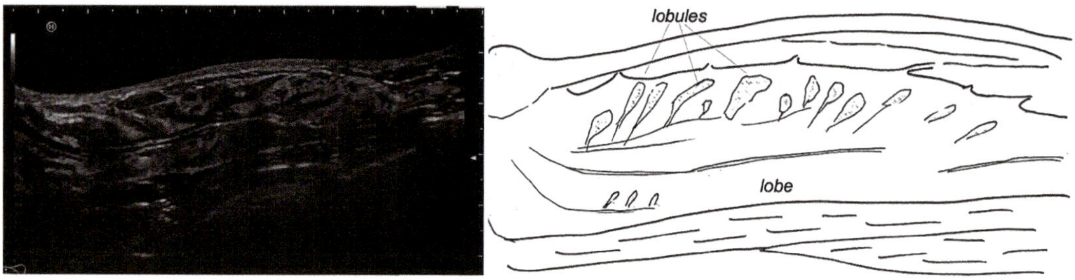

Fig. 3.6 Radial scanning focused on the ductal axis in the medial part of a lobe associated with lobular hyperplasia

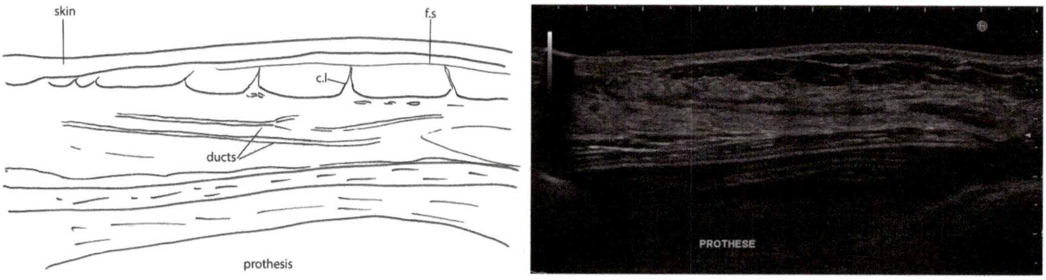

Fig. 3.7 The prothesis is pushing back the main ducts of the lobe; they become linear and perfectly visible

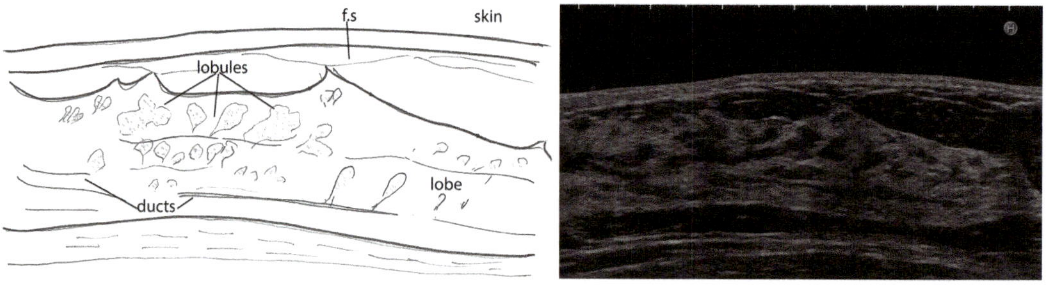

Fig. 3.8 Typical ductal and lobular hyperplasia with hypo-echogenic pattern, solid-like, all along the ductal axis. The lobules are bigger in the *upper part* of the lobe

3.2 Lobules

These are structures difficult to identify without initial training. Located along the ductal axes (above and/or in an oblique position above it), they are often grouped together in a mass of hypo-echogenic echostructures with fine internal echoes. Lobules can be spread out along the ductal axes like trees on a roadside or gathered in small groups like tree copses in the countryside. There are thousands of them in each breast, but only a small proportion of them are visible. There are a few lobules at the back of the ducts located only in the lower part of the lobe, more difficult to study.

The size of lobules depends on their topography: the larger ones are connected with the ducts in the upper part of the lobes and close to the areola; the smaller ones are located along the lower ducts and at their periphery.

The various shapes of lobules have been perfectly described by M. Teboul (trefoil, retort, mushroom, leaf, bag-shaped lobule, group of

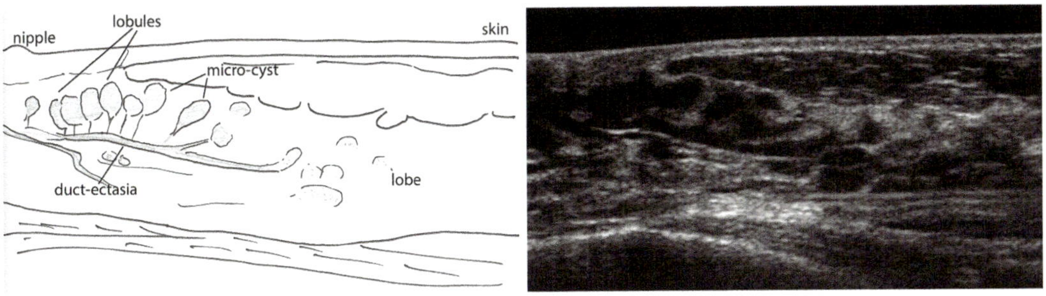

Fig. 3.9 Combination of ductal ectasia, lobular hyperplasia and micro-lobular cysts

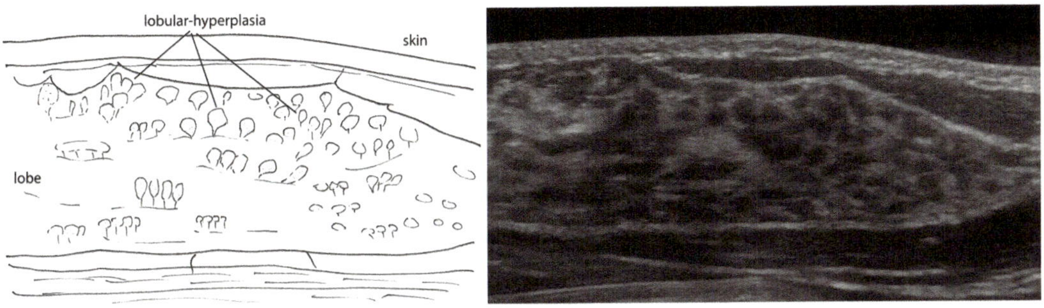

Fig. 3.10 Typical aspect of a young woman with important physiologic hyperplasia distending many lobules. Difficulty to identify the duct among them. The lobe boundaries are well defined in a fatty environment

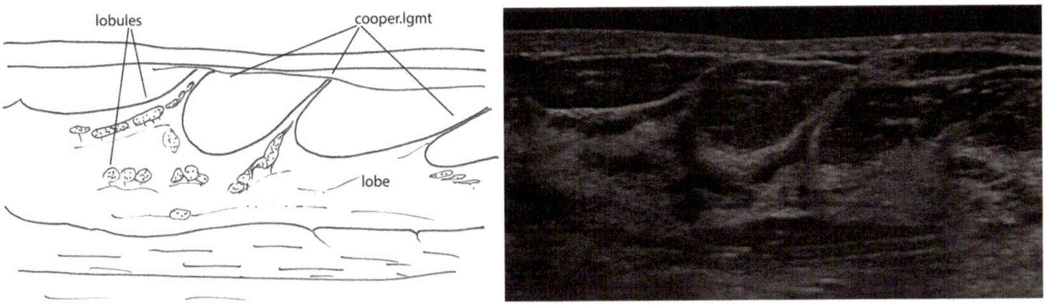

Fig. 3.11 Lobules located in the Cooper's ligament with typical hyperplasia in neck lace segment. The duct lumen is very thin

branching lobules, etc.), but none yet of the variations in the shape of the lobules seems to be directly related to a possible pathology or be a factor of seriousness.

To be able to distinguish a ductal anomaly from a lobular one is often essential in cancerology; it is therefore important to know the various echographic appearances of lobules (Figs. 3.8, 3.9, 3.10, 3.11, 3.12, 3.13, and 3.14).

3.3 Lobes

The lobes are delineated by connective covering membranes called upper and lower fascia. These hyper-echogenic fasciae bristle with spicule corresponding to the base of Cooper's ligaments (upper and lower).

The contents of lobes are predominantly hyper-echogenic and heterogeneous, given the

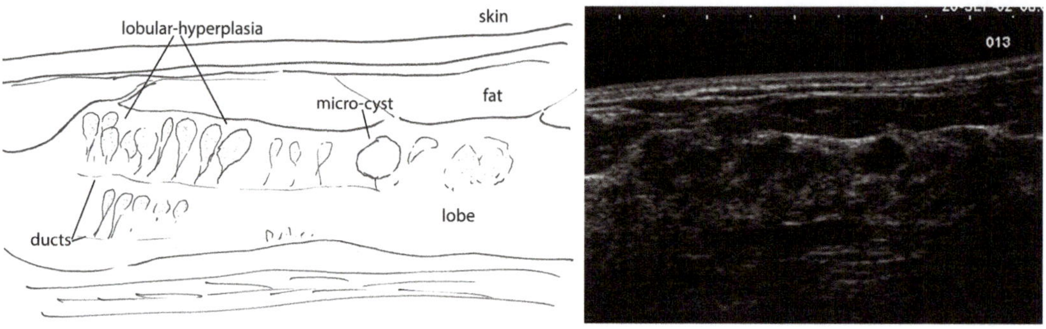

Fig. 3.12 Important lobular hyperplasia in lobules localized along the duct like a hedge of trees on a roadside. One of them, on the right, presents an anechoic pattern corresponding to a small millimetric lobular microcyst, facing the Cooper's ligament axis

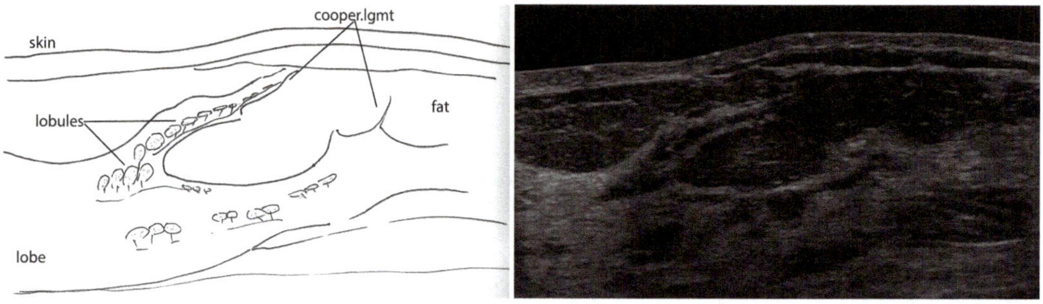

Fig. 3.13 In the segmental part of a lobe, the dilated Cooper's ligament contains several lobules with a chain aspect. The fascia superficialis is well visible under the skin

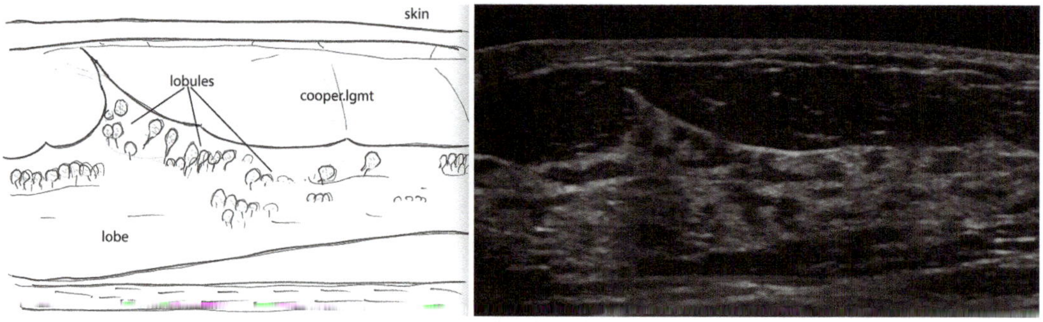

Fig. 3.14 Partial scan of a lobe with small lobules in the cone of the Cooper's ligament: aspect of trees with a hypo-echogenic content. The other lobules in small groups look like tree copses in the country side

presence of a stroma composed of connective tissue, intralobar fat, ducts and lobules, with or without epithelial proliferation, with or without physiological modification or pathological event, and blood and lymph vessels.

The lobes have a radial orientation around the nipple; they are grouped together behind the areola in a mass within which the limits of each individual one cannot be identified. On the other hand, the ductal axes help to guide us in our investigation. In their distal part, the lobes are clearly separated and are prolonged by hyper-echogenic ligamentous structures, clearly visible in their fatty hypo-echogenic environment.

The most tale-telling lobes to be analyzed are those located in the upper outer quadrant of the breast (the first to develop in adolescence), and their study will determine the morphological type

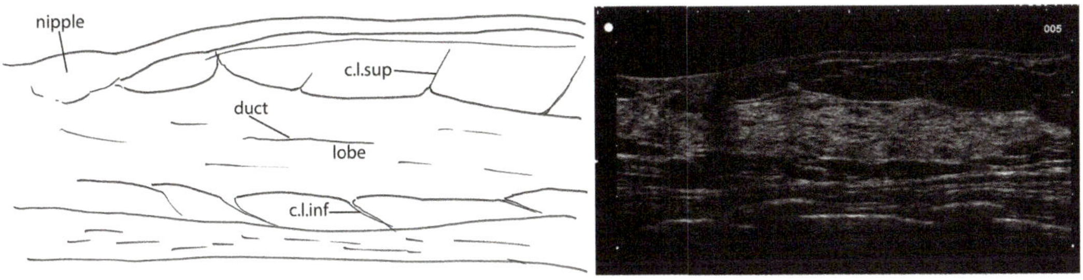

Fig. 3.15 Typical aspect of a hyper-echogenic lobe, with slight heterogeneity combining small lobular groups and thin ducts. The superior and inferior Cooper's ligaments are defined in the fatty tissue around the lobe. Thanks to the waterbag of the probe no ultrasonic artifact in the nipple, behind it and behind the Cooper's ligaments

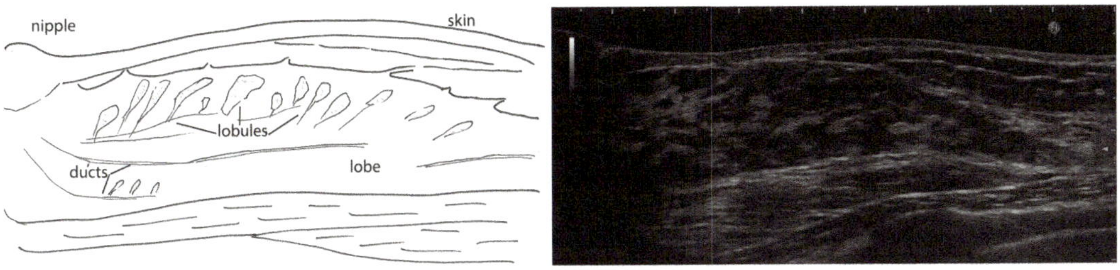

Fig. 3.16 Small lobe with important lobular and ductal hyperplasia. This aspect present in a postmenopausal woman appears in 20/30% of the breast ultrasonic exams (a typical persistence of the lobe after the menopause (Cf. Chap 4))

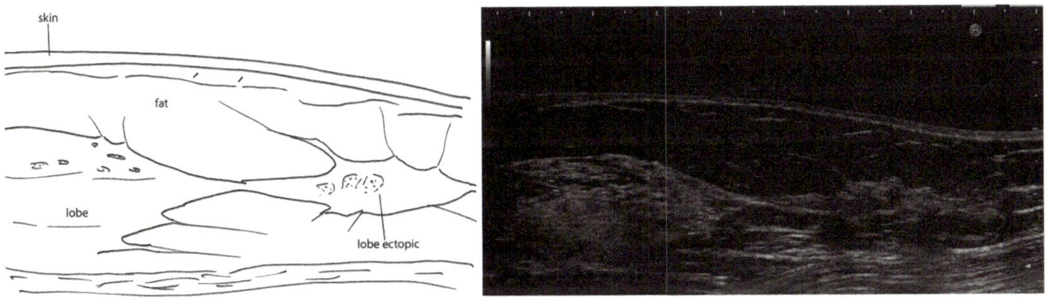

Fig. 3.17 Variation of the lobar anatomy with an atypical lobar development at the extremity of a lobe, in the axilla

of the breast (see Chap. 5), the normality of lobar anatomy, or identify its different variations: very elongated lobe reaching into the armpit, distal swelling of the lobe, atypical location some distance away from a lobar islet or on the contrary lobar atrophia, etc. (Figs. 3.15, 3.16, and 3.17).

3.4 Cooper's Ligaments

The ligaments are clearly visible on longitudinal radial slices as well as antiradial ones (at 90° they have a stellar orientation) [20].

Considered for a long time as mere connective supporting structures (like the rigging of ship sails), Cooper's ligaments really are superficial extensions of the lobes and hold cell matter, lobules, and vessels.

Located in the upper part or upper side of a lobe, their bases appear like connective cones extended upwards by the ligaments themselves. The orientation of the ligaments is either perpendicular or in a diagonal between the lobe and the cutaneous planes. The ligaments end upward against a connective strip called fascia superficialis which is linked to the skin through fine connective subcutaneous thread: the retinacula cutis. They are surrounded with fatty tissue which is more or less important according to the mammary morphological type. This hypo-echogenic fat displays small variations in echogenicity from one woman to another (Fig. 3.19).

In the lower part of the lobe, as in a mirror image, there are lower Cooper's ligaments aiming at the inferior fascia which is often difficult to perceive, as it often is next to the underlying pectoral muscle and flattened out by the lower face of the lobe. In order to visualize the lower ligaments and the inferior fascia accurately, it may be useful to mobilize the patient in a standing position and to clear the under-lobar space (because of the gravity of the breast), but this is only necessary in the case of a suspicion of pathology. These changes in position also allow us better to distend the upper ligaments and "widen" their lobar implantation and their contents for a better analysis.

A particular ligament, located in the upper part of the tip of the 12 o'clock lobe, has been described by Giraldes as the suspensory ligament of the breast. The tip of its upper end is located at the level of the collarbone. Its study guides the examiner toward the nodal territories under and at the back of the collarbone and can reveal the presence of an atypical lobe extending away from the nipple (Figs. 3.18 and 3.19).

In the same way, the ultrasound examination of the area around the nipple must be complemented by a second external scanning of the upper part of the breast in its upper latero-sternal, subclavicular, axillary and latero-thoracic territories (Fig. 3.20).

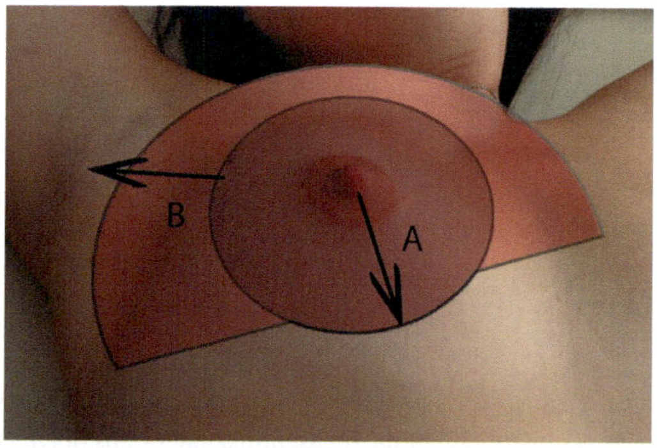

Fig. 3.20 Description of the biradial technique: the first one (**a**) around the nipple and the second (**b**) more external for the *upper part* of the breast

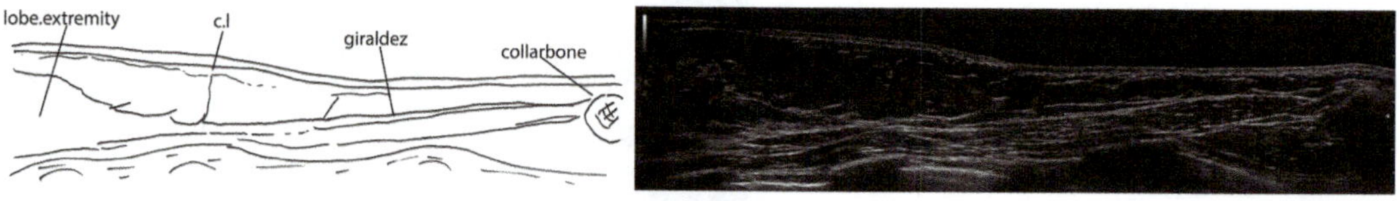

Fig. 3.18 The Giraldes ligament continuing the lobe extremity (lobe at 12 o'clock) joins the collarbone (in this case 19 cm away from the nipple)

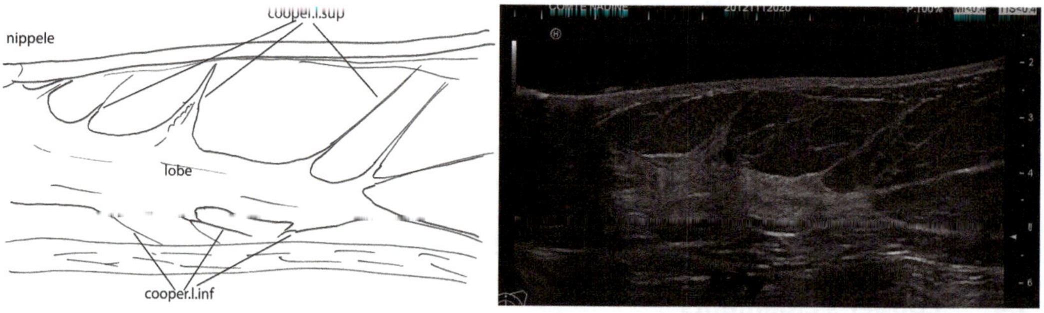

Fig. 3.19 Well-defined Cooper's ligaments (superior and inferior) distended or very thin, connected to the fascia superficialis or the lower fascia (mirror pattern). They have a hyper-echogenic (connective-like) appearance, in a hypo-echogenic fatty environment

Careful observation of Cooper's ligaments is essential in the search for initial signs of millimetric cancer of the breast. At this millimetric stage, there is neither a back ultrasonic shadow nor a lobar alteration attached to it (and no radiological sign either at the mammogram). Pr. T. Tot's remarkable anatomo-pathological slice perfectly reveals the presence of cells within the ligament. These malignant cells go toward the fascia superficialis to the skin. He describes the growth and development of lobular cells already located in the ligaments. They distend the ligament and distort the fascia superficialis. Nakama [21] has indeed described the migration of malignant cells in a Cooper's ligament, toward the skin with histiocytes, fibroblasts, and even lymphocytes at an early stage of cancer development. All this confirms Gallager's conclusion who wrote in "Cancer" as early as 1969 [22] that supportive connective tissue is early affected by the carcinologic agent (Figs. 3.21 and 3.22).

Furthermore, it is to be noted that it is at the junction of the axis of Cooper's ligaments on the one hand and of the ductal axis on the other that a particular zone is located within which the majority of lesions (benign as well as malignant) tend to develop.

Lastly, the analysis of the orientation of Cooper's ligaments is important for it guides us in the search for indirect cutaneous signs away from the initial lesion (perpendicular, centrifugal orientation toward the periphery or centripetal toward the nipple).

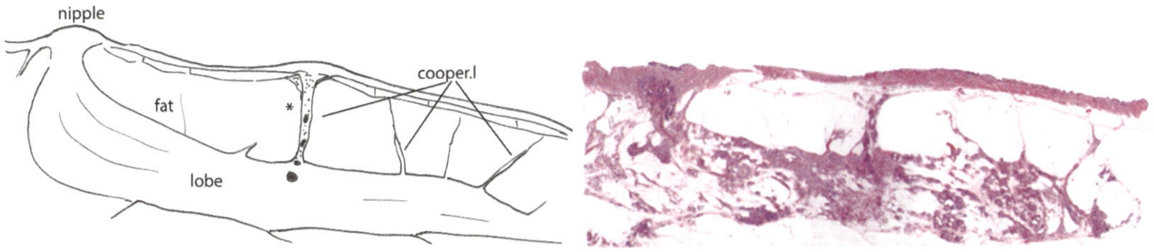

Fig. 3.21 Exceptional radial anatomo-pathological section of a lobe: dilatation of the Cooper's ligament with malignant cells, involvement of the fascia superficialis and the skin. Confirmation of Nakama and Tot's publications and perfect similitude with Fig. 3.22 (Courtesy of Pr. T. TOT, Falun)

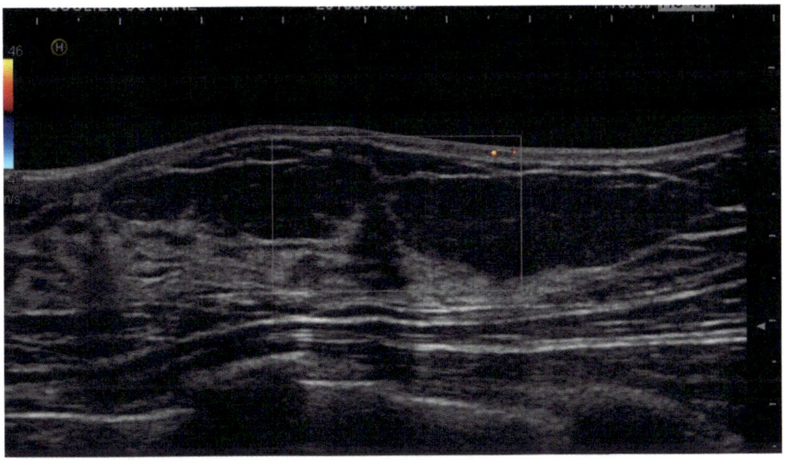

Fig. 3.22 Good ultrasonic correlation with Fig. 3.21: hypo-echogenic millimetric dilatation of a Cooper's ligament, attraction of the fascia superficialis, without classic semiological ultrasonic indirect signs (no projected shadow) at so early a stage. Specific localization of the disease at the junction of the Cooper's ligament axis and the main duct axis

3.5 Blood Vessels and Lymph Ducts

Blood circulation in the breast is threefold:

1. A superficial subcutaneous network
2. A deeper intralobar network and lastly
3. Anastomosis located in the ligaments. The recent fully digitized echographic machines are the only ones which enable us to observe this vascularization accurately thanks to new recent applications (highly detailed real-time microvascular imaging with Angio PLUS) (Figs. 3.23 and 3.24). A marked improvement in the distinction between benignancy and malignancy is made possible thanks to these recent developments.

Lymphatic vessels are not visible in their normal condition. In some exceptional cases of advanced pathology, a lymphatic distension has been observed (without any modification at the Doppler examination).

Lymph nodes are studied in detail (Chaps. 11 and 12).

3.6 Deeper Muscular Planes

The technique of radial echography does not provide any specific information if we compare it to conventional echography and what has already been published on the topic. Let us simply note that the use of a large-size linear probe has facilitated the discovery of costal lesions (costal metastasis) in the follow-up of breast cancers under treatment and of pleural effusion related or not to solid pleural lesions.

A thorough knowledge of the anatomic structures of the lobe and of its physiological as well as pathological modifications is perfectly relevant to the description of these two cases:

1. Our attention is immediately attracted to the distortion of the lobe by a poly-lobulated, solid, homogenous, and hypo-echogenic

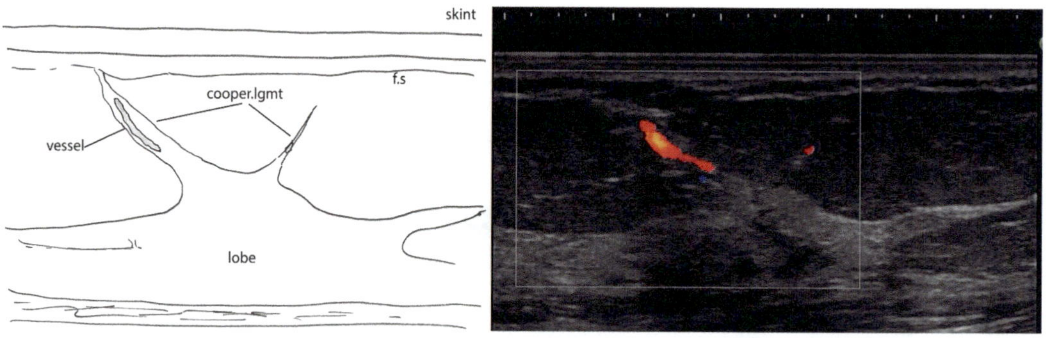

Fig. 3.23 Presence of a vessel in the Cooper's ligament, detected with a classic Doppler (dilated Cooper's ligament linked to the fascia superficialis)

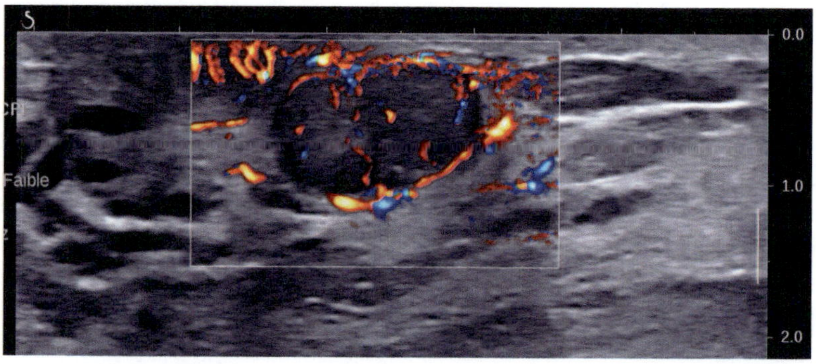

Fig. 3.24 New Doppler technique (Angio PLUS) underlining not visible microvessels with traditional Doppler

structure. It is nevertheless essential to uncover the anatomic relations of this nodule: as a matter of fact, there clearly appears a ductal axis below with little ducts connecting the nodule to the duct. It is therefore a lobular lesion affecting several lobules, hence its bumpy appearance. At the Doppler examination, there is no sign of intra-nodular anarchic vascularization; at elastography, we have a score 2; the anatomo-pathologist confirms the lobular fibro-adenomatous nature of this lesion. Each lobule distorted by the internal growth of small fibroadenomas is going to bend laterally to one side, and their diameter is progressively going to come parallel to the skin; all these lobules side by side will give a poly-lobulated bumpy appearance to this bunch of fibroadenomas (Fig. 3.25).

2. Presence of a solid hypo-echogenic distention of the Cooper's ligament base. Tot and Nakama confirm the early signs of the development of a small cancer migrating in the Cooper's ligament, hence its appearance classically described in echography as taller than large, since it is fixed within the ligament and is migrating vertically toward the cutaneous and subcutaneous planes (Figs. 3.26 and 3.27).

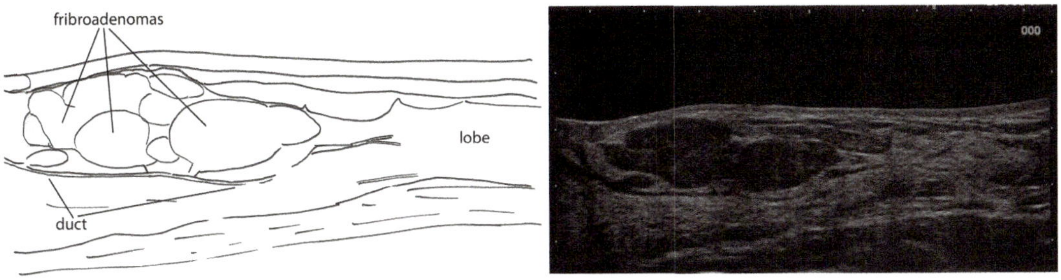

Fig. 3.25 Poly-lobular group of solid structures corresponding to multilobular dilatations, overhanging a main ductal axis with several ductule connections: bunches of proved lobular fibroadenomas with a global horizontal diameter

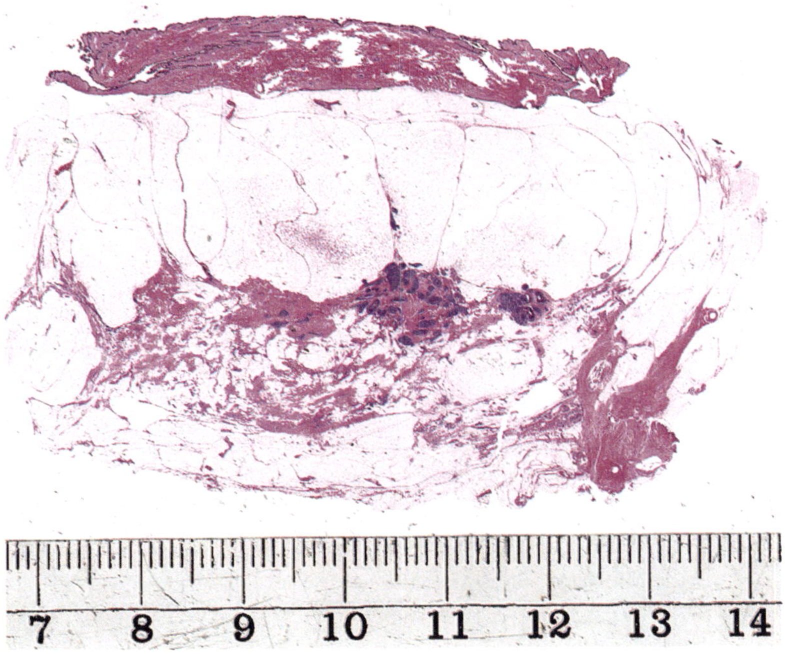

Fig. 3.26 Radial lobar anatomo-pathological section with breast carcinoma foci located at the intersection of ductal axis and Cooper's ligament axis. Multifocal disease (that means several foci in the same lobe) (courtesy of Pr. T.TOT, Falun)

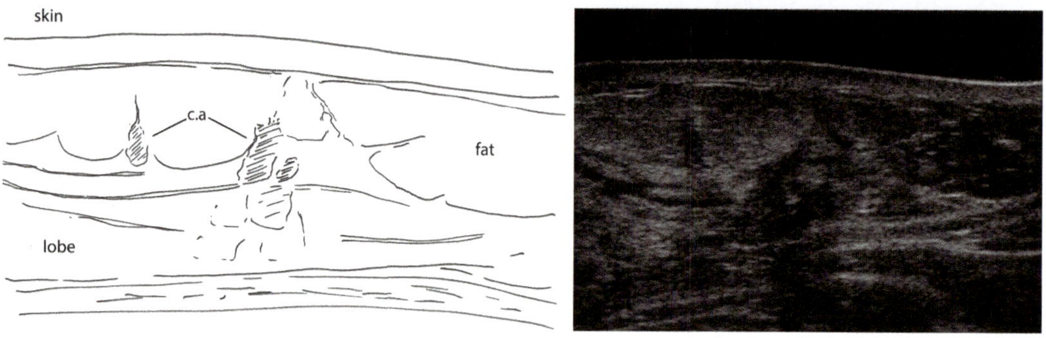

Fig. 3.27 Multifocal breast cancer perfectly correlated with Fig. 3.26: ductal involvement, several hypo-echogenic irregular foci, partially located in the Cooper's ligaments

Presence of several malignant foci along the ductal axis in the same lobe (multifocal disease).

Only a thorough anatomic analysis of the lobe allows the early detection of this millimetric lesion.

References

1. Teboul M, Halliwell M. Atlas of ultrasound and ductal echography of the breast. Oxford: Blackwell Science; 1995.
2. Ueno E. Real time ultrasound; 1991 Printed and Bound in Japan.
3. Teboul M. Practical ductal echography, guide to intelligent and intelligible ultrasonic breast imaging. Madrid: Medgen SA; 2004. p. 240–340.
4. Teboul M. Advantages of ductal echography (DE) over conventional breast investigation: the requirement for an anatomically led breast ultrasonography. Med Ultrason. 2010;12:32–42.
5. Teboul M. A new concept in breast investigation: echohistological acino ductal analysis or analytic echography. Biomed Pharmacother. 1988;42: 289–96.
6. Tot T. DCIS, cytokeratins, and the theory of the sick lobe. Virchows Arch. 2005;447:1–8. 13. Villadsen R. In search of stem cell hierarchy in the human breast and its relevance in breast cancer evolution. APMIS. 2005;113:903–21.
7. Tot T. The role of large-format histopathology in assessing subgross morphological prognostic parameters: a single institution report of 1000 consecutive breast cancer cases. Int J Breast Cancer. 2012;2012:395415.
8. Tot T. The sick lobe concept. In: Francescatti DS, Silverstein MJ, editors. Breast cancer: a new era in management. New York, NY: Springer; 2014. p. 79–94.
9. Tot T. Breast cancer subgross morphological parameters and their relation to molecular phenotypes and prognosis. J OncoPathol. 2014;2:69–76.
10. Amy D. Echographie mammaire: echoanatomie. JL mensuel d'echographie LUS. 2000;10:654–62.
11. Aristida C-G. Atlas of full breast US. Ed. Springer Int. Publishing: Cham; 2016.
12. Stavros AT, Rapp LC, Parker HS. Breast ultrasound. Philadelphia, PA: Lippincott Williams & Wilkins; 2004.
13. Stavros T. Breast ultrasound. Philadelphia, PA: Lippincott; 2006.
14. Amy D. Lobar ultrasound of the breast. In: Tot T, editor. Breast cancer, a lobar disease. New York, NY: Springer; 2011. p. 153–62.
15. Dolfin G, Chebib A, Amy D, Tagliabue P Carcinome mammaire et chirurgie conservatrice. 30e Seminaire FrancoSyrien d'Imagerie Médicale. Tartous, Syrie Durante E; 2006.
16. Going JJ, Mohun TJ. Human breast duct anatomy, the 'sick lobe' hypothesis and intraductal approaches to breast cancer. Breast Cancer Res Treat. 2006;97:285–91.
17. Dolphin G. The surgical approach to the "sick lobe". In: Francescatti DS, Silverstein MJ, editors. Breast cancer: a new era in management. New York, NY: Springer; 2014. p. 113–32.
18. Amoros J, Dolfin G, Teboul M. Atlas de Ecografia de la Mama. Torino: Ananke; 2009.
19. Amy D. Millimetric breast carcinoma ultrasonic detection. In: Leading Edge conference Pr. Goldberg B. USA; 2005.
20. Cooper AP. On the anatomy of the breast. London: Longman, Orme, Green, Bown, and Longmans; 1840.
21. Nakama S. Comparative studies on ultrasonogram with histological structure of breast cancer: an examination in the invasive process of breast cancer and the fixation to the skin. In: Kasumi F, Ueno E, editors. Topic in breast ultrasound. Tokyo: Shinohara; 1991.
22. Gallager S, Martin J. Early phases in the development of breast cancer. Cancer. 1969;24:1170–8.

Physiological Breast Evolution

4

Dominique Amy

A woman's breast experiences constant modifications throughout her life, from its forming at adolescence until its involution in old age. The transformations undergone by the anatomical elements must be analyzed perfectly for a better understanding of the pathological evolutions [1, 2, 3, 4].

(a) In the little girl and during the period of adolescence when the future lobes of the breasts are developing, such an analysis is not easy to carry out. The budding mammary epithelium is compressed in a mass at the back of the nipple, with very little fatty tissue around it. For an easier understanding of the development of the lobes, we have chosen to scan a man's breast in a case of gynecomastia. The growth of breasts for a man is strictly identical to the one observed in a woman. Masculine lobes are a little more voluminous than an adolescent girl's, but above all they have more fatty tissue around, which leads to a better differentiation between the lobar structures.

Below the nipple and at the back of the areola plaque, hypo-echogenic ductal axes appear, wrapped in a hyper-echogenic connective sheath. Their roughly straight 'glove finger like' courses diverge from the nipple. The connective elements, that is the fascias, the outlines of the Cooper's ligaments, the lobar covering membrane, the palleal stroma etc. will become more visible as the breast grows.

The lobes unfurl like the petals of a daisy around the nipple. But there is a certain amount of asymmetry in this development. The first lobes to appear are those located in the upper, outer quadrants of the breasts (from nine o'clock to one o'clock for the right breast), the last lobes to appear are the ones located in the lower, inner quadrants (between three o'clock and seven o'clock, right breast also) (Figs. 4.1, 4.2, 4.3, 4.4, 4.5, 4.6, 4.7, 4.8).

These discrepancies in the sequence of development have a repercussion on the respective sizes of the lobes at adult age as well as during the post-menopausal lobar involution.

The inner structure of the lobes varies in relation to the hormonal environment, hyper-echogenic with fine ductal courses whose diameter thins out very quickly at the periphery in normal development, or, on the contrary, predominantly hypo-echogenic if transitory juvenile hyperplasia is associated to it. The lobules along the ductal axes have a very variable appearance, linked to the amount of proliferation (usual lobar proliferation).

D. Amy, M.D.
Centre du sein, Aix-en-Provence, France
e-mail: domamy@wanadoo.fr

D. Amy (ed.), *Lobar Approach to Breast Ultrasound*, https://doi.org/10.1007/978-3-319-61681-0_4

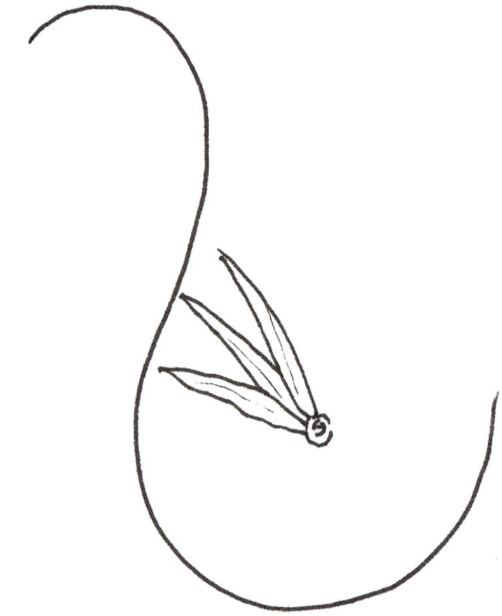

Fig. 4.1 Early development of the first lobes (upper-external quadrant)

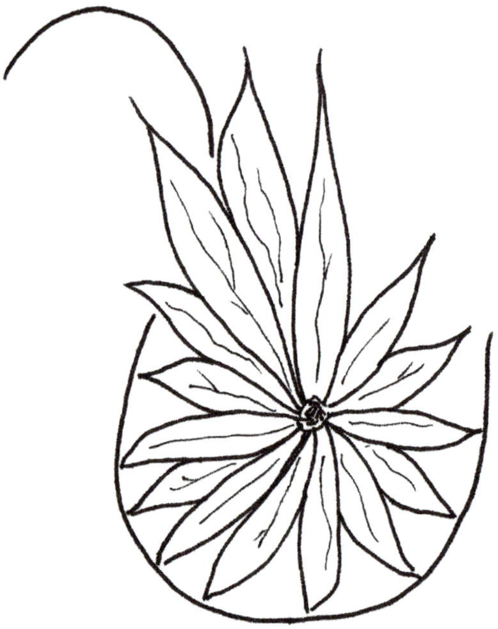

Fig. 4.3 Adult lobes around the nipple

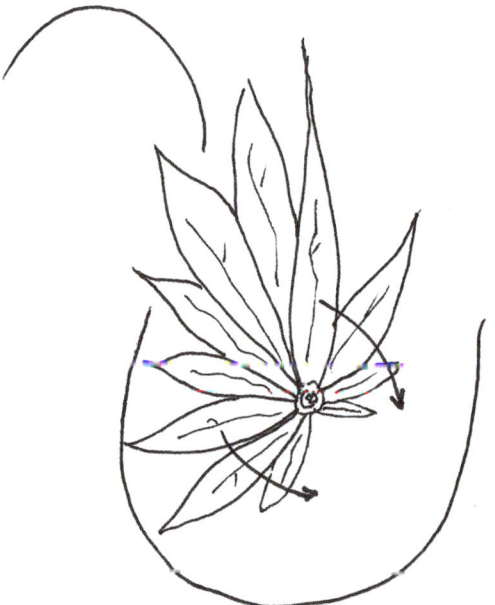

Fig. 4.2 Lobar growth towards the infero-internal quadrant

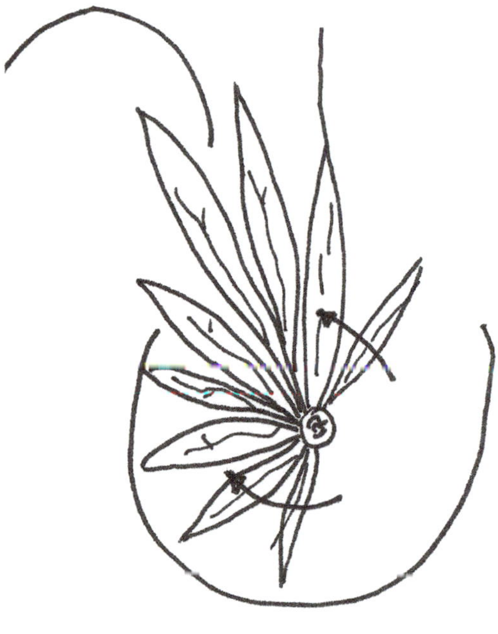

Fig. 4.4 Lobar involution starting in the infero-internal quadrant

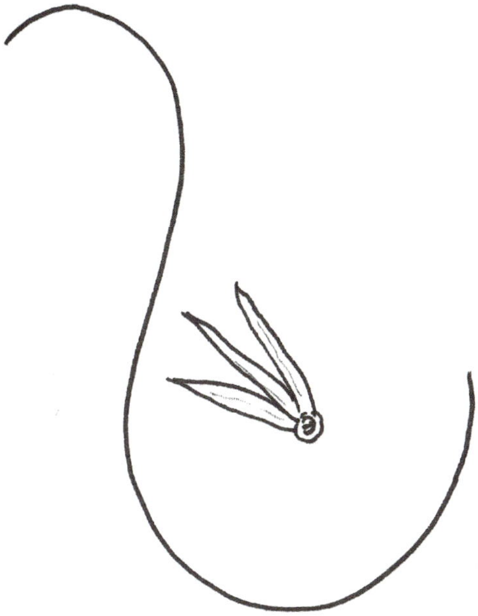

Fig. 4.5 Belated residual lobes in the upper-external quadrant

Cooper's ligaments are hardly or badly visible at adolescence, given the important volume of the lobes and the small amount of fatty tissue around them.

All the vessels (superficial or deep as well as their anastomoses) are very difficult to uncover with traditional Doppler (Figs. 4.9, 4.10, 4.11, 4.12, 4.13, 4.14)

(b) From adolescence until the age of 25 or so, the lobes generally fill in almost the whole of the mammary volume, and the layer of fat around them is fine and not very thick. The lobes have a hyper-echogenic structure with a variable content, roughly hypo-echogenic and becoming more and more differentiated as development progresses: the lobules and ductal axes are more developed in the uppermost part of the lobes and in the lobar zone next to the area around the areola.

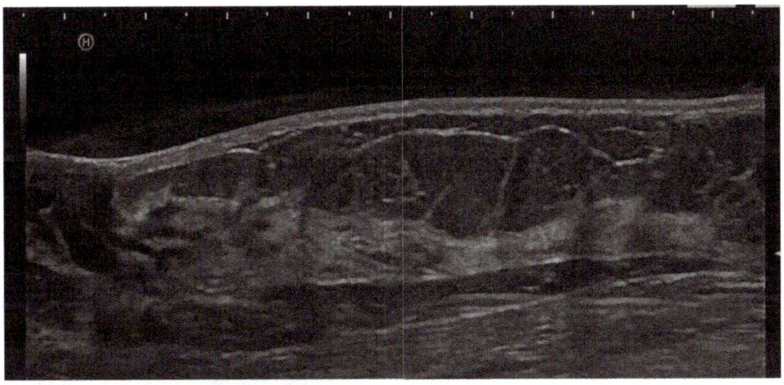

Fig. 4.6 Lobar analysis with Cooper's ligaments and fascia sup et inf

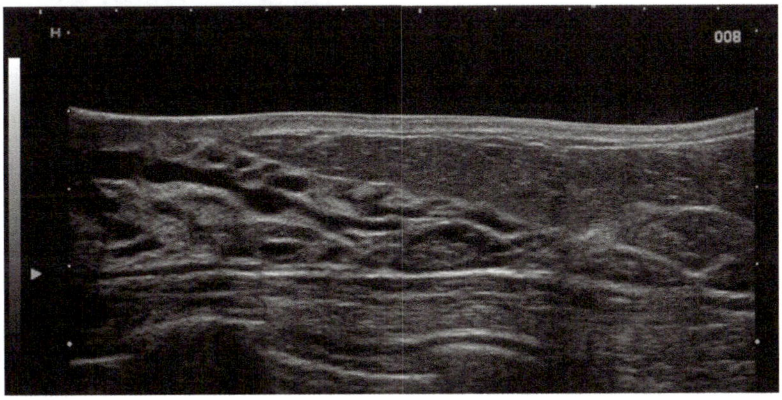

Fig. 4.7 Ductal axis (with ectasia) and lobules (with micro-cysts)

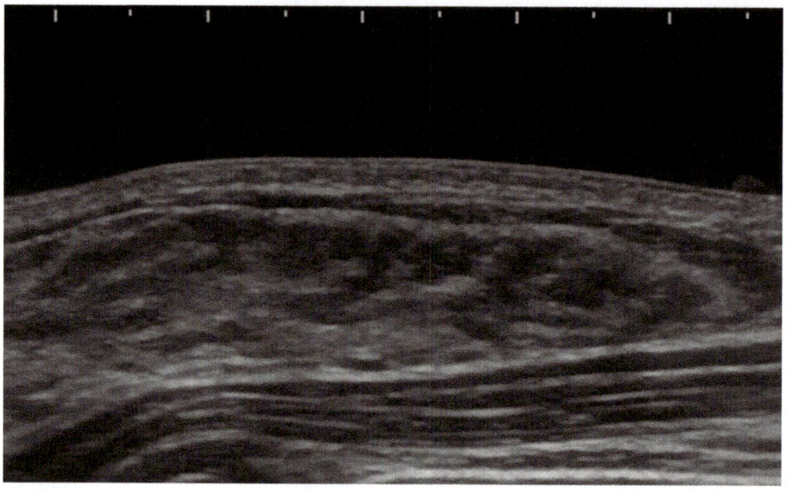

Fig. 4.8 Lobules: lobular hyperplasia along the ductal axis

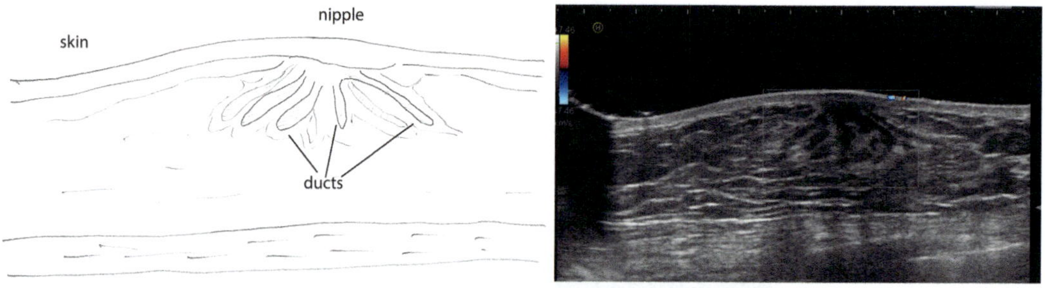

Fig. 4.9 (**a**, **b**) Breast lobe development during adolescence: converging ducts behind the areola

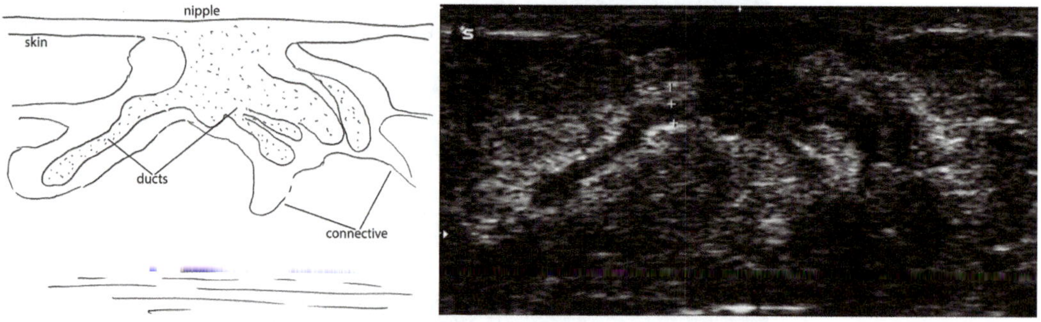

Fig. 4.10 (**a**, **b**) "Glove finger like" development of the lobe with hypo echogenic ductal epithelial proliferation

Cooper's ligaments become much more visible in the course of the development of the breast, but the lower ligaments (mirror image of the two sides of a lobe) are rarely visible in a younger woman, as they are stuck against the pectoral muscle and the lower face of the lobe.

The identification of the exact outlines of the lobes is very difficult to achieve in the central portion at the back of the areola, while it is very clear at the periphery where the end parts of the lobes tend to diverge.

(c) In adulthood, as the lobes very slowly lose some of their thickness and as the fatty tissue in front and at the back of the lobes begins to appear, the outline of each lobe is easier to follow with both types of ultrasound scanning (radial or with anti-radial 90° sections). Cooper's ligaments are

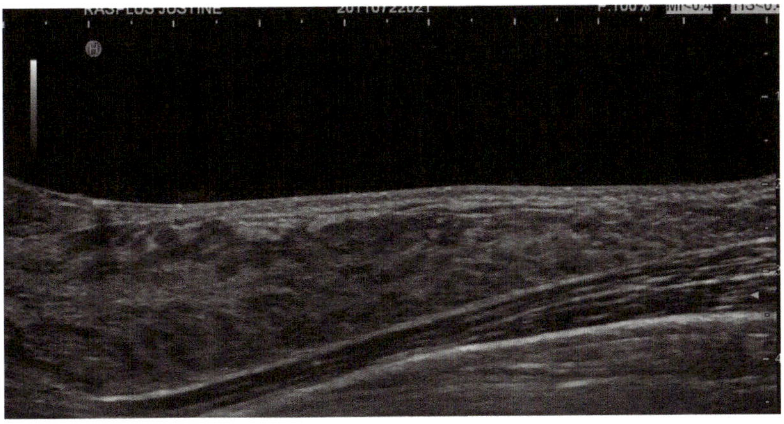

Fig. 4.11 (**a**, **b**) Young female lobe with important physiological lobular epithelial proliferation along the linear ductal axis

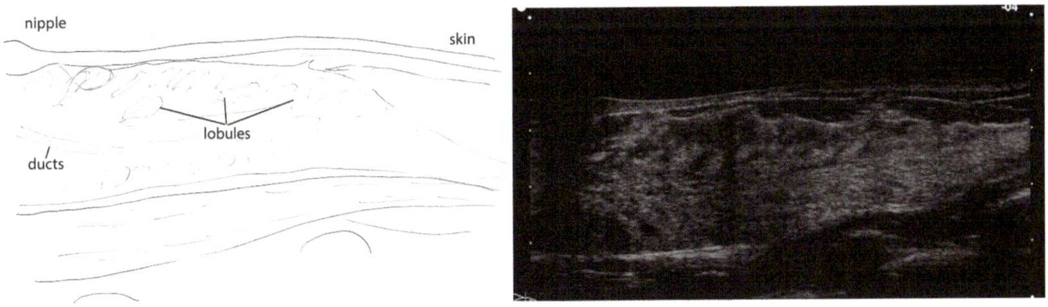

Fig. 4.12 (**a**, **b**) Young adult lobar appearance: hyperechogenic lobe with hypoechogenic lobular epithelial proliferation along the linear ductal axis

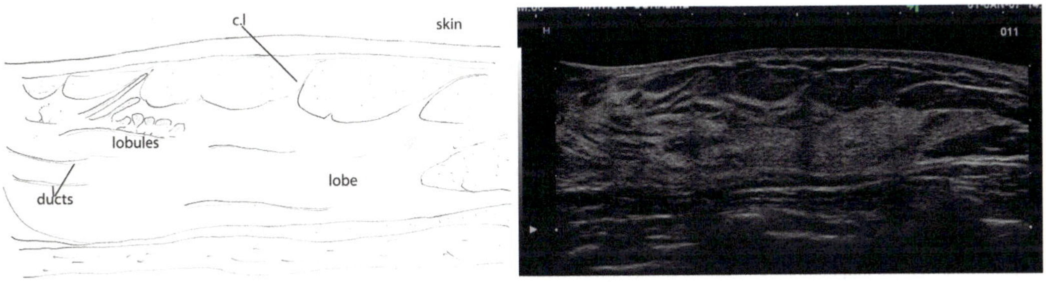

Fig. 4.13 (**a**, **b**) Typical adult lobe with the upper Cooper ligaments connected to the superficial sub-cutaneous fascia

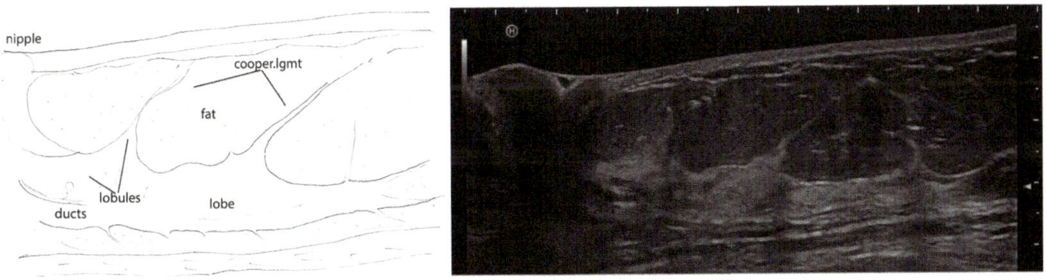

Fig. 4.14 (**a**, **b**) Pre-menopausal lobar involution: decreasing lobar thickness

clearly visible and their internal analysis is more accurate with the presence of lobules either in their implantation zone or within the ligaments themselves, which alters their appearance.

On the upper side of the lobes, the ligaments look like suspension bridges linking each ligament to the concave upper edges of the lobes. The lower side of the lobes is usually more linear and bristles with fine little quills corresponding to the cones of implantation of the lower ligaments aiming at the lower fascia.

The ductal and lobular structures are more or less visible according to the importance or absence of epithelial proliferation. The number of lobules decreases in relation to the patient's age, the first to go being the lobules from the lower and distal zones and the inter ligamentous locations.

The more involuted the lobes are, the easier it is to identify them. On sections carried out at an angle of 90° of the ductal axis, the orientation of Cooper's ligaments is stellar, either perpendicular or diagonal to the surface of the lobe (Figs. 4.15, 4.16, 4.17).

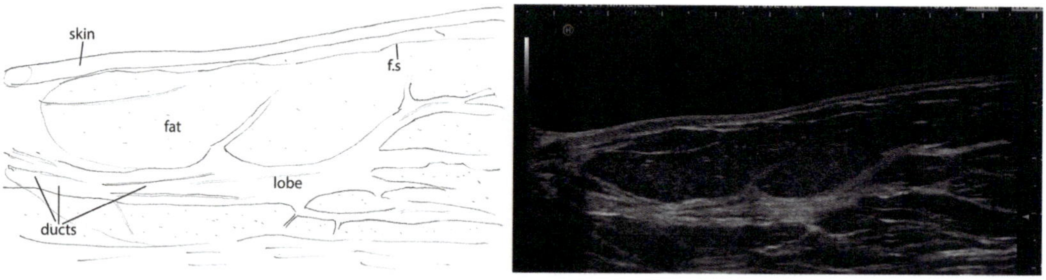

Fig. 4.15 (**a**, **b**) Post-menopausal fatty infiltration between different ductal axes from the periphery toward the nipple

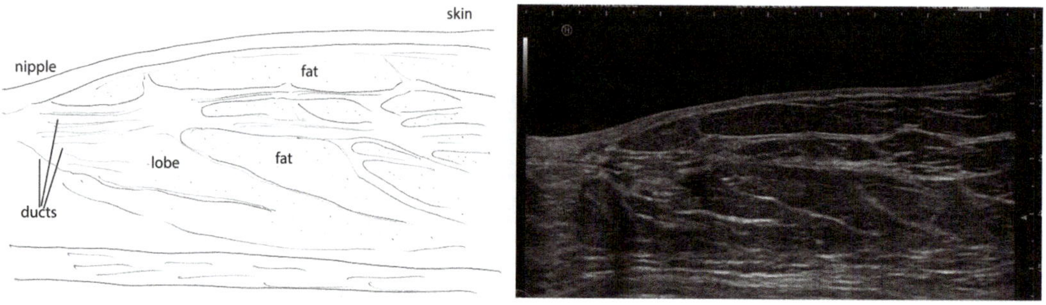

Fig. 4.16 (**a**, **b**) Lobar involution with an important fatty progression splitting the ductal axis (hypoechogenic lines between the hyper-echogenic connective surrounding tissue)

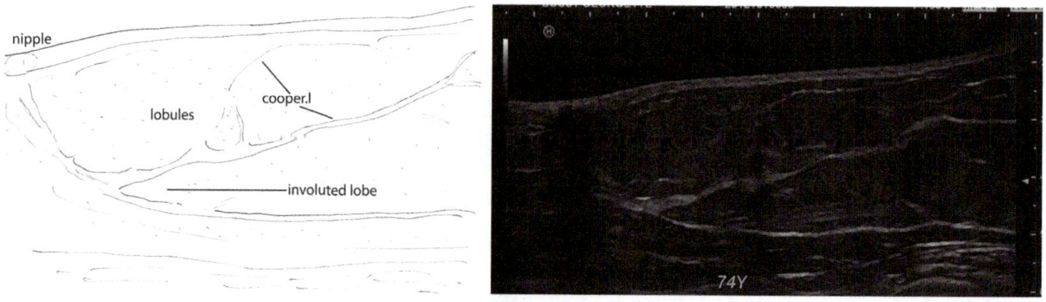

Fig. 4.17 (**a**, **b**) Residual involutive lobar connective structures (74 year old woman)

(d) At menopause and after, lobar involution increases with a decrease in the volume of the lobes and a fatty infiltration filling in the inside of the lobes and pulling apart the ductal axes, starting from the periphery and progressing toward the nipple. This fatty transformation goes with an important reduction in the lobes (even those facing the ligaments), in the number of the ducts and the number of Cooper's ligaments.

The reduction followed by the complete disappearance of the lobes first affects those located in the lower inner quadrant, then the inner quadrants, and only the lobes in the upper outer part of the breast last longer, and, in the end, there only remain a few largely reduced epithelial structures at the back of the nipple. This appearance corresponds to completely emptied breasts in full fatty involution on mammograms.

And so the cycle of the development of the breast going from a little budding nipple onto the asymmetrical production of lobes with their epithelial, connective and ligamentous contents ends on the reversed involution of the whole mammary gland.

The lobar concept of the origin, growth and involution of the breast can only be perceived with that accuracy through echography. This evolutionary pattern can only be understood and analyzed through the technique of ducto-radial ultrasound.

No other technique of breast imaging allows the direct visualization of anatomy, morphological types and lobar evolution.

Nevertheless, to this theoretical pattern (very often encontered in clinical practice), it is necessary to add variations, atypical developments as well as more rarely encountered appearances which it is however important to know (Figs. 4.18, 4.19, 4.20, 4.21, 4.22, 4.23, 4.24).

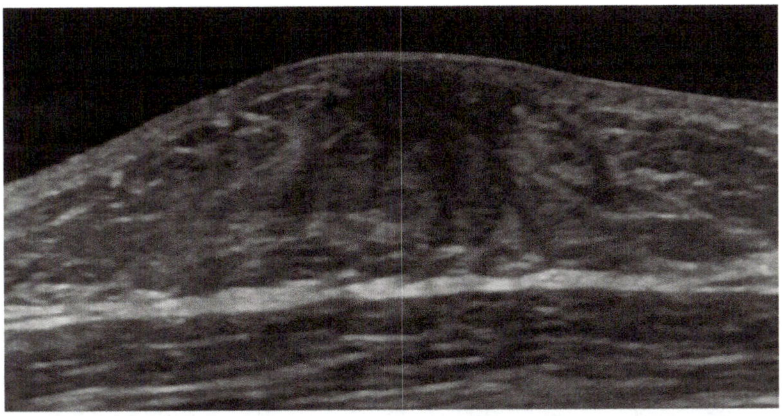

Fig. 4.18 Early ductal development behind the nipple

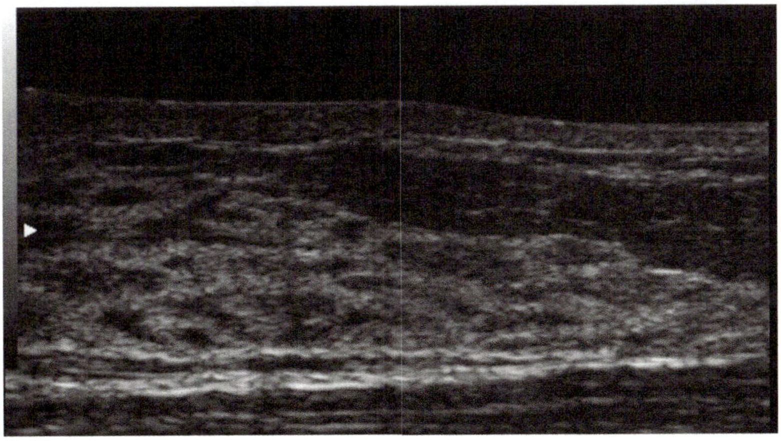

Fig. 4.19 Young woman's lobar aspect

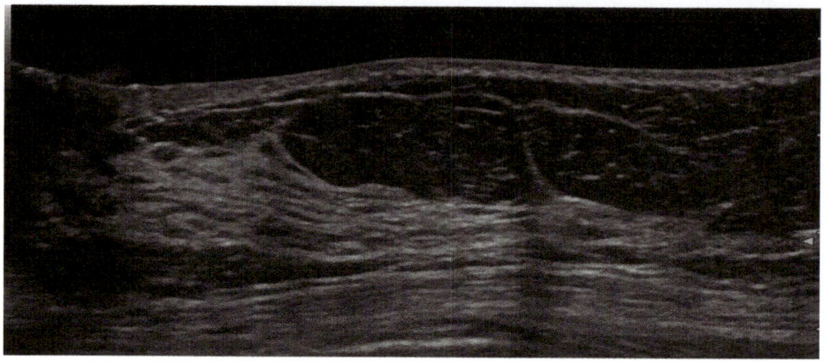

Fig. 4.20 Adult lobar appearance

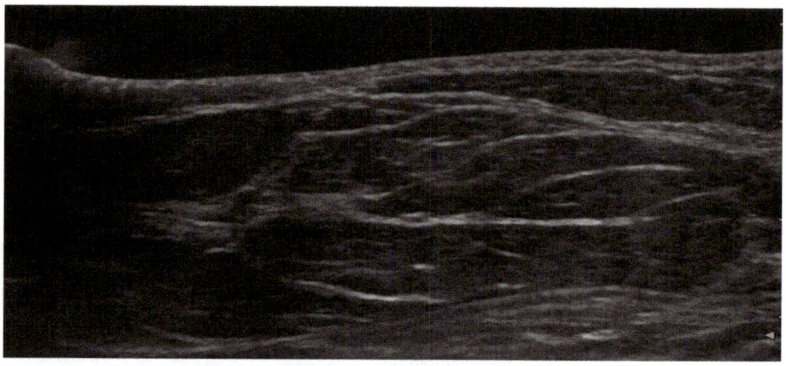

Fig. 4.21 Post menoposal lobar involution

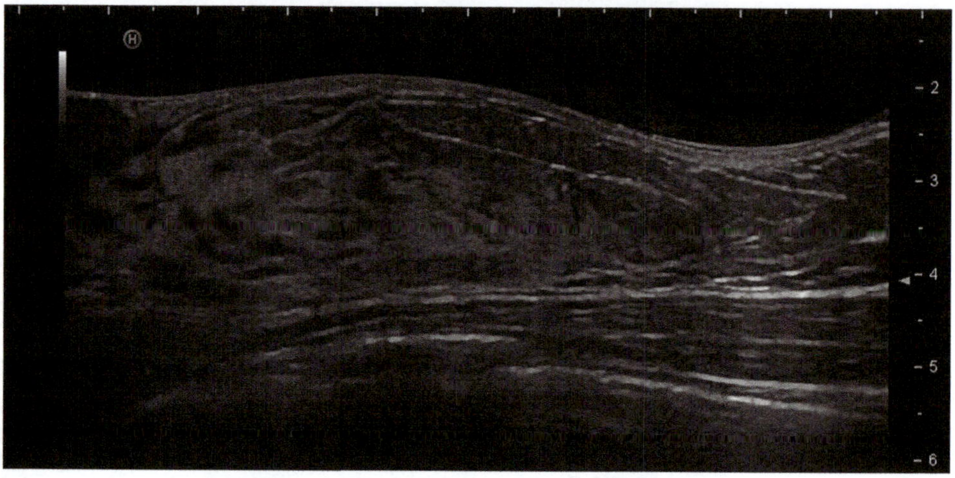

Fig. 4.22 Fibrous lobar morphology

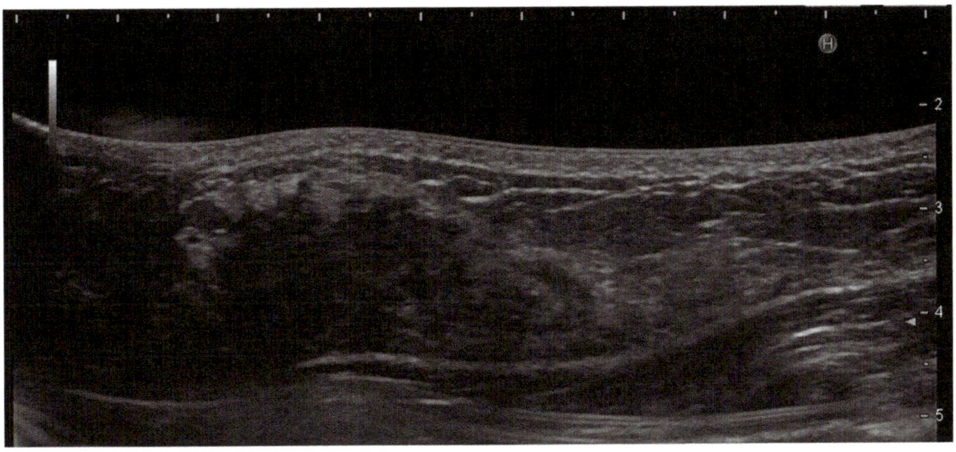

Fig. 4.23 Lobar glandular type

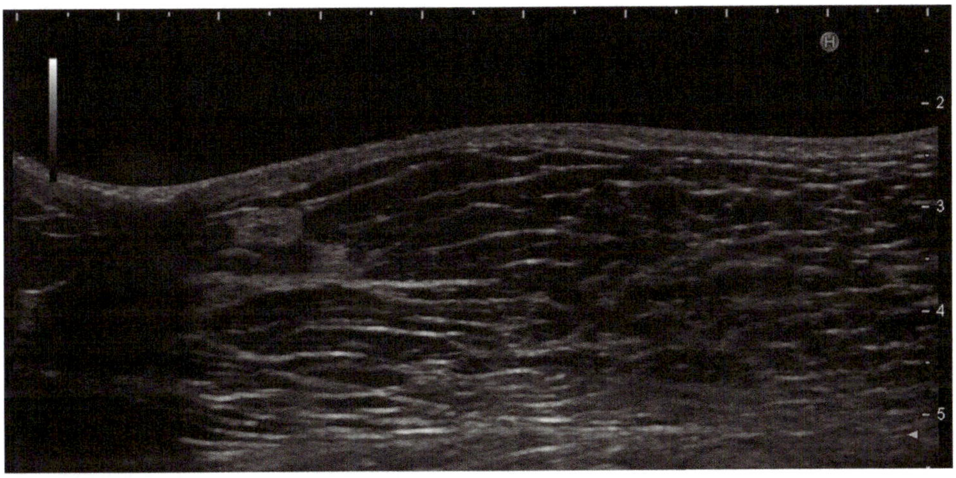

Fig. 4.24 Fatty lobar type

Classic involution successively characterized by:

- Reduction of the lower lobules and the lobules between Cooper's ligaments.
- Disappearance of superficial lobules and thinning out of the lobe.
- Reduction in the number of milk ducts and Cooper's ligaments.
- Complete disappearance of the ligaments together with a disappearance of the lobes reduced to a connective covering membrane does not always follow the accepted pattern.

1. In the case of early puberty, the premature development of the breast may occur without any anatomical modification attached to it.
2. Early pre-menopausal involution of the breasts can occur in younger women without any really identifiable specific reason or cause.

On the other hand, it is very frequent (between 20 and 30% of the cases) to note an absence of lobe involution after the menopause. Frequently, women aged between 70 and 80 retain perfectly preserved lobes, although they do not take any kind of treatment, and, in some cases, important signs of epithelial proliferation are to be noted. A complementary study of the biological parameters remains to be carried out for these patients (Figs. 4.25 and 4.26).

3. There also exist physiological variations linked to some treatments in general, but more specifically to hormonal treatments: prolonged hormone replacement therapy tends to stop involution.

Pregnancy and lactation deeply transform the appearance of the breast with an important distension of the lobes forming a compact hyper-echogenic mass within which ductal courses are visible at different degrees of swelling sometimes related to transitory cystic swellings. The compressed fatty tissue disappears entirely or is reduced to a thin strip in front of the lobes. Modifications also appear in cases of inflammation or of a trauma, after an operation, after radiotherapy, and after inserting implants. The whole range of benign as well as malignant pathology produces more localized alterations within the lobes (Fig. 4.27) [5].

The specific modifications are alluded to in further chapters.

There exists of course a major physiological variation linked to epithelial hyperplasia which deeply modifies the appearance and contents of the lobes. Given its importance and given also the fact that it has not been much described, that it is even completely overlooked in many books dealing with breast imaging and that it is essential to recall basic notions of anatomo-pathology, a whole chapter is devoted to epithelial hyperplasia.

To sum up this chapter on physiological variations, let us recall that there exist three morphological types of breasts, glandular, fibrous, and fatty:

– Glandular type: the lobes have a rather important hypo-echogenic appearance. It may be difficult, not to say impossible, to distinguish

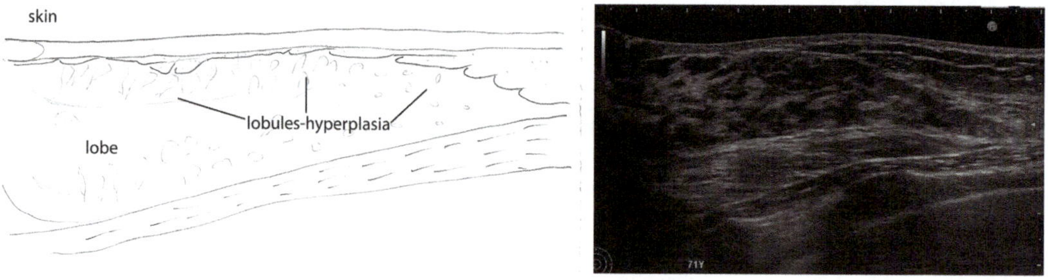

Fig. 4.25 (**a**, **b**) A typical lobar epithelial proliferation in an old woman, as present in 20–30% of the post menopausal women (here a 71 year old woman)

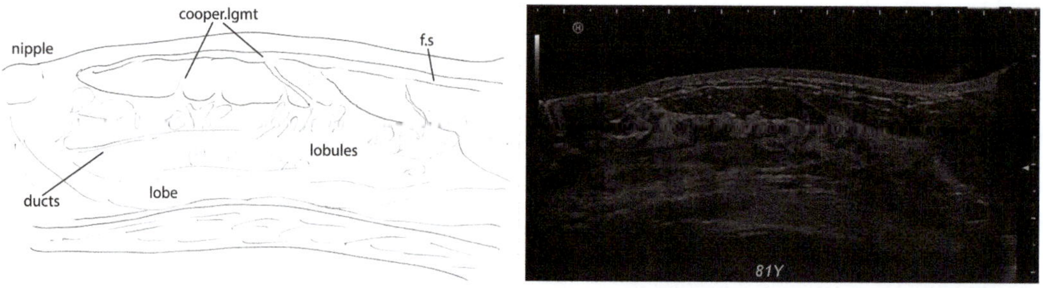

Fig. 4.26 (**a**, **b**) Post-menopausal lobar persistence in a 81 year old woman. Absence of lobe involution

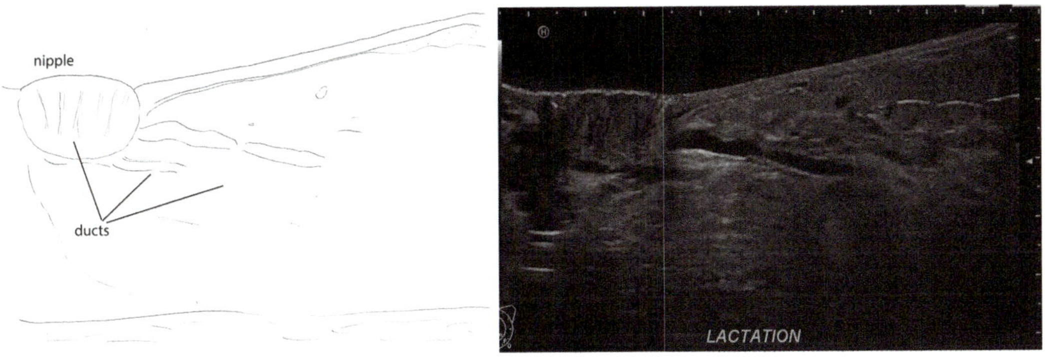

Fig. 4.27 (**a**, **b**) Typical pattern during lactation with some ductal dilatation associated with lobar remodelling and disappearance of the classic anatomy

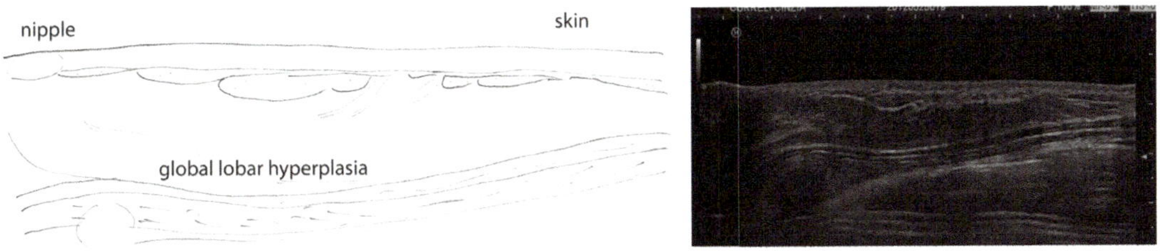

Fig. 4.28 (**a**, **b**) Glandular morphotype: the internal lobular anatomy is totally masked by a global hypertrophic hyperplasia (ductal and lobular)

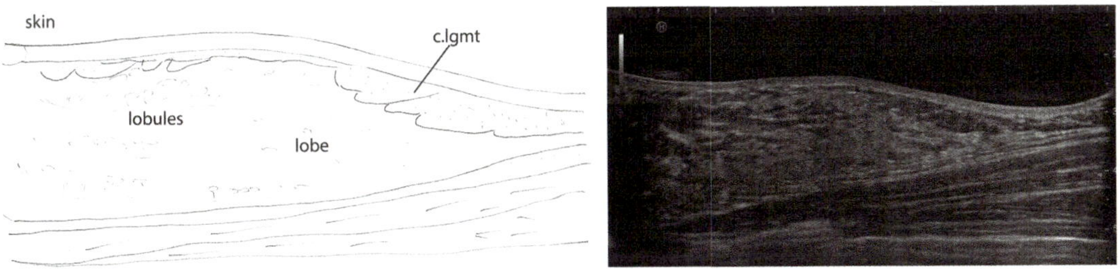

Fig. 4.29 (**a**, **b**) Fibrous type with predominant connective tissue concealing the epithelial structures

between the various lobes and ducts in some extreme cases.

- Fibrous type: hyper-echogenic lobes have clear predominantly fibrous contents concealing most of the hypo-echogenic epithelial structures.
- Fatty type: the connective and epithelial structures are swamped in a great mass of fatty tissue modifying the usual appearance of the lobes. The connective sheath around the ducts is distorted by very numerous small hypo-echogenic fatty compartments (Figs. 4.28, 4.29, 4.30).
- However, let it be said that the vast majority of lobar scanning does not relate to these extreme cases. Lobar scanning in general reveals hyper-echogenic lobes with their usual epithelial contents in accordance with a classic evolutionary process. The appearance of the lobes may correspond to one of these three morphological types, fatty, glandular or fibrous, but to a moderate extent only.
- If lobar echography may appear complex and difficult to interpret, one must constantly refer

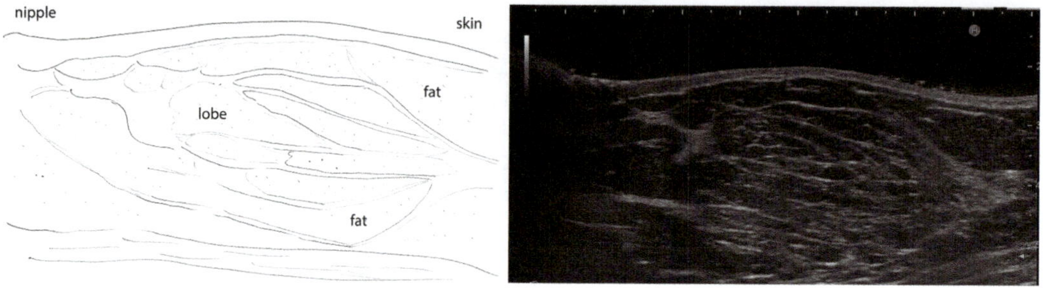

Fig. 4.30 (**a**, **b**) Fatty type: global fatty infiltration between the ductal axes (38 year old women)

oneself to lobar anatomy and use a strict technique with good mechanical equipment.

- In these conditions, the lobar concept achieves its full significance: from a precise anatomical study, from the analysis of the epithelial structures of the lobes, from the knowledge of their evolution and/or involution, and from the understanding of the variations, either physiological or in the wake of a treatment, it becomes much easier to detect the first pathological modifications of the breast. Thanks to the contribution of the "sick lobe theory" (Tot), the examination of the breast is becoming more thorough, it is becoming the essential basis for a better diagnosis and an earlier treatment better adapted to each patient.

References

1. Teboul M. Practical ductal echography, guide to intelligent and intelligible ultrasonic breast imaging. Madrid: Medgen SA; 2004. p. 240–340.
2. Teboul M. Advantages of ductal echography (DE) over conventional breast investigation: the requirement for an anatomically led breast ultrasonography. Med Ultrason. 2010;12:32–42.
3. Amy D. Lobar ultrasound of the breast. In: Tot T, editor. Breast cancer, a lobar disease. New York: Springer; 2011. p. 153–62.
4. Teboul M. A new concept in breast investigation: echohistological acino-ductal analysis or analytic echography. Biomed Pharmacother. 1988;42: 289–96.
5. Gallager S, Martin J. Early phases in the development of breast cancer. Cancer. 1969;24:1170–8.

Epithelial Hyperplasia

5

D. Amy, T. Tot, and G. Botta

Take-Home Messages

1. The impressive improvements in mammary ultrasound allow one to bring to light the modifications corresponding to epithelial proliferation.
2. At present, it is impossible to distinguish between the various stages of hyperplasia and in situ cancer through echography.
3. The benefit of the identification of hyperplasia lies on the fact that it allows to identify the women at risk (according to the clinical context) who should be given particular supervision involving all the techniques in breast Imaging.
4. It is a significant improvement to be able to distinguish a lobular modification from a ductal one.

Given the number of objections encountered, it may seem a challenge to devote a chapter to epithelial hyperplasia as visualized by echography.

D. Amy, M.D.
Centre du sein, Aix-en-Provence, France

T. Tot, M.D., Ph.D.
Department of Pathology and Clinical Cytology, Falun Central Hospital, Falun, Sweden

G. Botta, M.D. (✉)
Department of Pathology, Sant Anna Hospital, Torino, Italy
e-mail: giovanni.botta@unito.it

The first of these objections originally lies in the refusal by some of our peers to face the idea that ultrasound may be able to identify hyperplasia. For them, it is simply preposterous, since the diagnosis of hyperplasia purely belongs to the anatomopathological field, while ultrasound is merely a method of imaging.

The second objection comes from the fact that a large majority of colleagues admit, when questioned, that they cannot imagine delivering such a diagnosis since it has never been done before.

The third objection relates to the fact that 10 cm by 10 cm large anatomopathological slices allowing a global study of mammary structures are not in use, as our colleagues continue to work in their laboratories with small 2 cm by 2 cm preparations.

Lastly we can add that pathological classifications often are complex, and the relative lack of accuracy in distinguishing a "usual ductal hyperplasia" (UDH) from a "ductal carcinoma in situ" (DCIS) or from a small budding cancer dampens the enthusiasm of echographers.

And yet it is precisely these hurdles that make such a study stimulating, in the hope that future technical progress will make it possible to overcome all these difficulties. The opinions of Tot and Botta find certainly their place here (Fig. 5.1).

Let us indicate that the appearance of epithelial structures affected by hyperplasia is rather similar to fatty tissue around the lobes. It is

D. Amy (ed.), *Lobar Approach to Breast Ultrasound*, https://doi.org/10.1007/978-3-319-61681-0_5

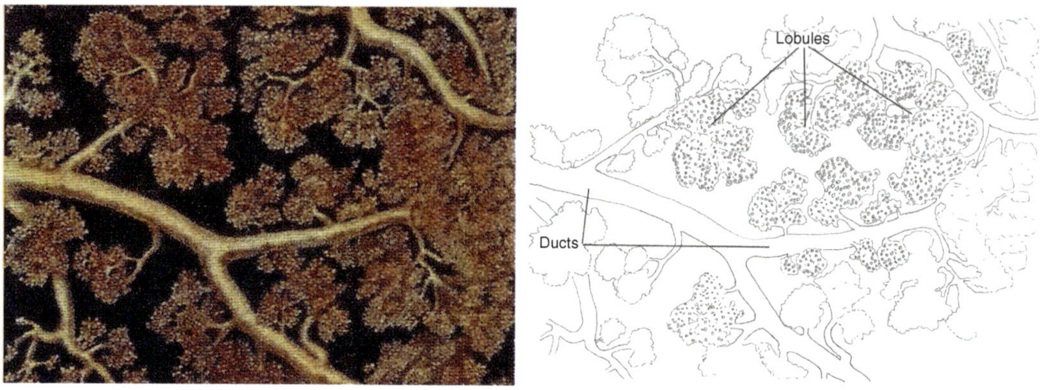

Fig. 5.1 Anatomopathologic preparation of lactating women with hypertrophic colorated lobules (Cooper A.P 1840: On the anatomy of the breast. Wellcome Institute library, London.)

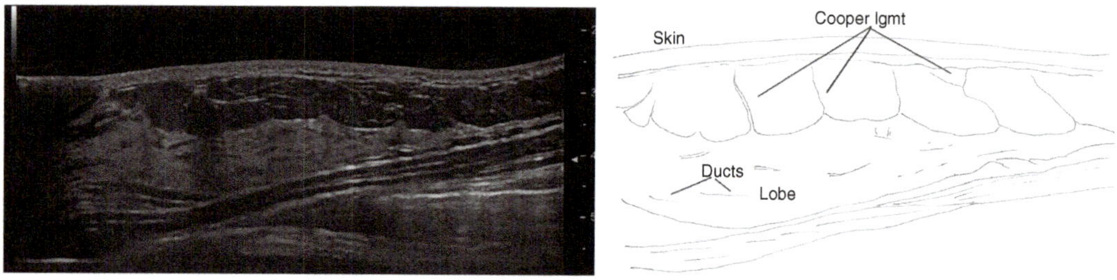

Fig. 5.2 The lobe is hyperechogenic with fibroconnective predominance. The ductal and/or lobular epithelial structures are not visible, their size below the millimeter not allowing ultrasound analysis

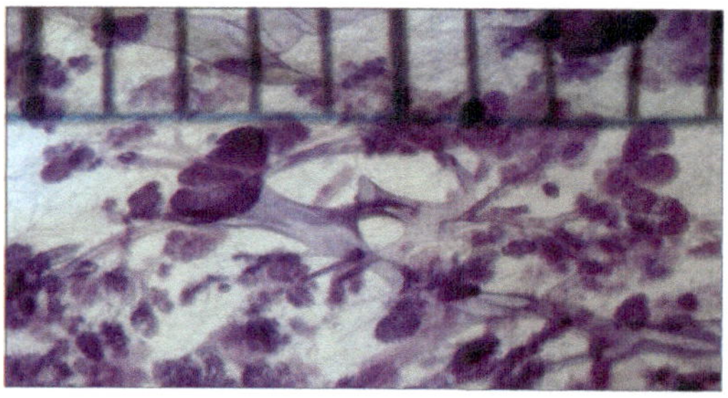

Fig. 5.3 Anatomopathologist section with termino-ducto-lobular units connected to different ducts (courtesy of Pr. T. TOT)

therefore absolutely necessary to distinguish clearly between what is intralobar epithelial tissue and what is around the lobes. Within the lobe, a zone in particular must be analyzed: it has been noted that a large number of lesions were localized at the level of the TDLUs at the root of Cooper's ligament and at the junction of the ligamentous and ductal axes (Fig. 5.2).

This makes the examination of the intralobar acini-ductal structures much easier: one just has to follow the ductal axis and focus on the meeting point of Cooper's ligaments.

What echographic changes are to be noted on the acinus-ductal axis affected by UDH?

If there is no epithelial proliferation, neither the ducts nor the lobules can be analyzed easily.

One notes a widening of the ductal and/or lobular structures which present a hypoechogenic "solid-like" appearance with fine internal echoes together with an occasional fine centro-ductal anechogenic liquid layer (Fig. 5.3).

According to the stage of evolution of UDH/ADH, the ductal axes or the lobules can be clearly visible and more or less well delineated at first. They appear like converging hypoechogenic blocks which are heterogeneous in the case of more advanced hyperplasia. The ductal axes have a more or less twisted or linear aspect; the lobules are egg-shaped, piriform, or bushy according to the stage of evolution. The big difference in acoustic impedance between the supportive tissue around the ducts or lobules and the contents of the ducts themselves allows us to identify UDH. The differentiation in the ductal or lobular epithelial structures allows us to assess better the origin of the lesions observed.

In the course of adolescence, the lobes display more or less important characteristic lobular and ductal distention. This transitory appearance is later modified according to the age in life. This echographic appearance may have been unduly described as "honeycomb" or "tiger skin" appearance, when in fact it is only a case of juvenile epithelial proliferation. Its analysis does not mean a loss of diagnostic sensitivity but, on the contrary, a precise understanding of the internal architectural modifications of the lobes which enclose thousands of lobules in each breast (Fig. 5.4).

In an adult woman, the appearance of lobes without proliferation is very hyperechogenic and homogeneous, with more or less visible fine ducto-lobular hypoechogenic structures.

In the case of UDH, the distention undergone by the epithelial structures preferably affects the lobules located along the upper ducts of the lobe in the zone close to the areola or at the back of it. The lower or distal ducts and lobules are less distorted and distended in a vast majority of cases (Figs. 5.5 and 5.6).

Lobules with ULH can be located on the Cooper's ligaments themselves, which causes their thickening. Cooper's ligaments are not mere connective, supportive structures; they also correspond to lobar extensions.

In the case of "atypical" development of the lobes at the level of axillary prolongations or occasionally some distance away (latero-sternal, laterothoracic, under clavicular zone, along Giraldes' ligament), there exist seemingly isolated "lobular islets" corresponding to exocentric opaque spots on the mammogram. At their level, the conjunction of UDH/ADH signs and fibro-microcystic dystrophy, adenosis, or adenosclerosis is not unusual. Ultrasound peripheral scanning of the upper part of the breast is therefore essen-

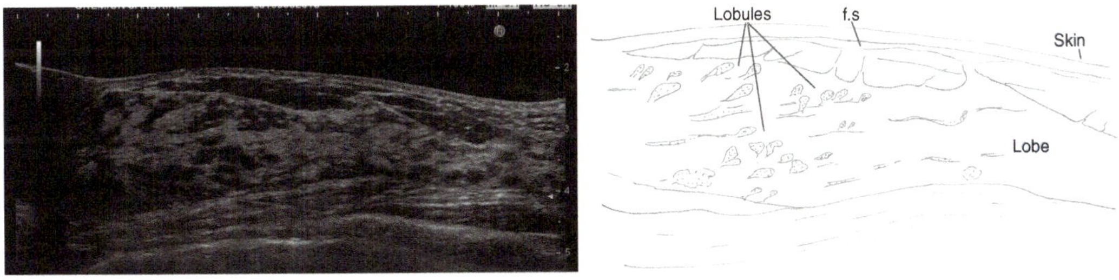

Fig. 5.4 Within the hyperechogenic lobe, some ductal or lobular epithelial structures display usual epithelial proliferation, UDH for the ducts and ULH for the lobules. As their size increases, their modified inner structures become echo-visible, thanks to the change in their acoustic impedance

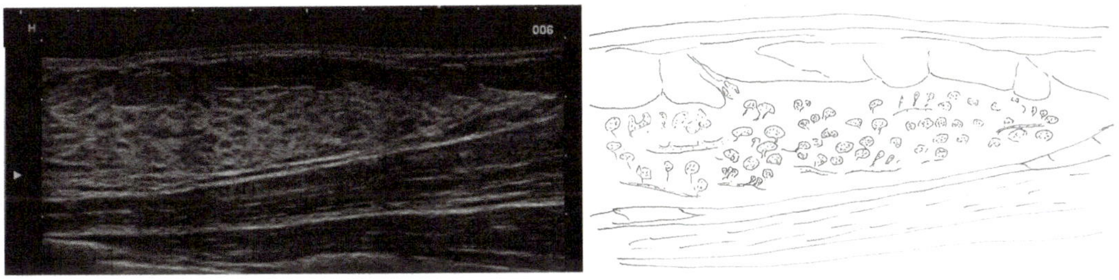

Fig. 5.5 Characteristic appearance of an adolescent girl or young woman with a lobe filled in, for the major part, with lobules and ducts distorted by transitory juvenile hyperplasia. The terms often used (modification of the fibroglandular tissue, of the mammary layer, of heterogeneous zones) betray shortcomings in the analysis; one must simply speak of signs of benign epithelial hyperplasia in the lobe of a young woman

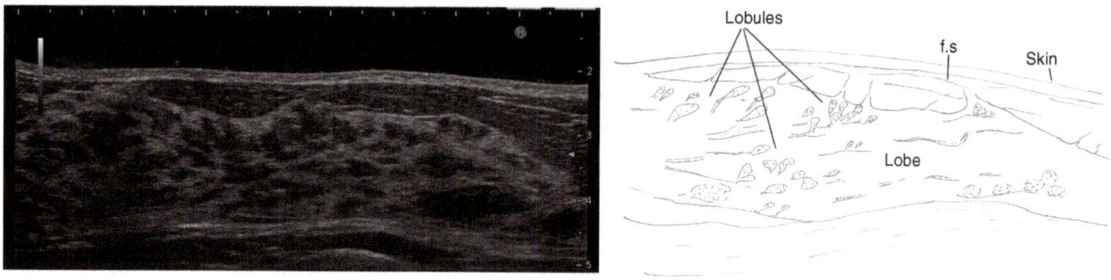

Fig. 5.6 Young female presenting an important ductal and lobular hyperplasia: hypoechogenic intralobar structures

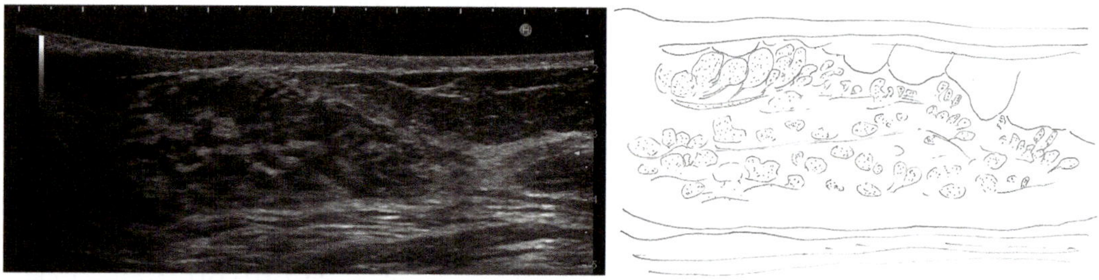

Fig. 5.7 The description is much more tricky with a very heterogeneous appearance of the contents of the lobes, a certain amount of anatomical anarchy, and a mixture of lobular and ductal distention, which makes the investigation problematic. The hypertrophic appearance of the lobules concealing the twisted, distended ductal axes within a messy organization shows the limitations of ultrasound exploration

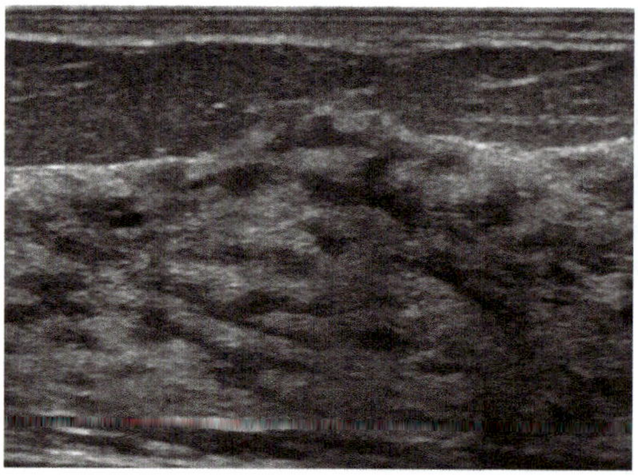

Fig. 5.8 Ductal dilatation of several ducts similar to Fig. 5.9: hypoechogenic pattern of the ductal lumen

tial so as not to overlook these anatomic variations.

UDH can regress spontaneously or persist over long periods without any evolution.

Gallager and Martin [1] and De Brux [2] have described hyperplasia as a stage in evolution which could anticipate the development of benign or malignant pathology.

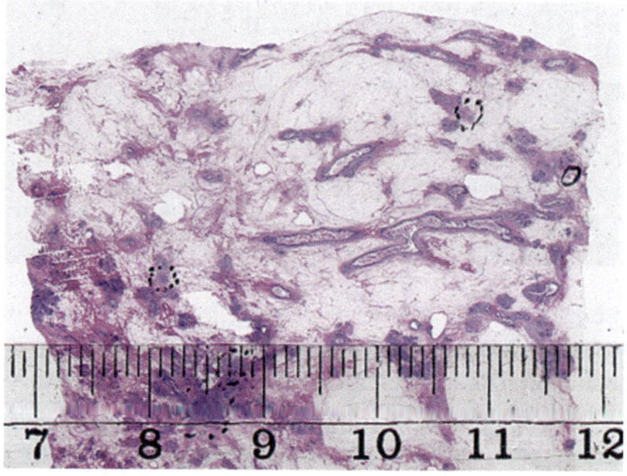

Fig. 5.9 Large anatomopathologic section with dilatation of different ducts full of epithelial cells (Courtesy of Pr. T. TOT)

The regular use of hormone treatment clearly increases the postmenopausal persistence of echographic signs of UDH/ADH (Figs. 5.7, 5.8, and 5.9).

However, in over 20% of the patients not receiving hormonal replacement therapy, the premenopausal aspect of the lobe (not or hardly involuted) persists after the menopause in combination with clear signs of epithelial proliferation.

In order to be able to assert the nature of modifications observed through ultrasound in the lobes, during the 1990s, we carried out numerous ultrasound-guided punctures in hypoechogenic intralobar zones. The anatomopathological results coincided exactly, asserting the presence of epithelial hyperplasia, which enabled us to describe the echographic signs of UDH/ULH. Of course, we now avoid unnecessary punctures in these specific areas.

Nevertheless, although echography is but one technique of imaging, it enables us to identify the patients at risk who have to remain under close scrutiny with very regular mammographic and echographic checkups. The combination of these two techniques is essential.

The understanding of the precise anatomy of the breast and the analysis of the physiological variations and in particular the identification of structures displaying epithelial proliferation mark an improvement and an essential step forward in the understanding of mammary pathology. Fortunately, in case of doubt, the combination of clinical and mammographic information with MRI if need be and the signs of evolutions should allow us to reduce diagnostic errors.

The term "hyperplastic breast disease" is often used to cover histologically similar lesions, such as usual ductal hyperplasia, atypical ductal hyperplasia, and columnar cell lesions with and without atypia (the last one often designated as flat epithelial atypia). The common histological feature of these lesions is presence of multiple cell layers in the epithelial cell compartment of the ducts, lobules, or both.

The normal ducts and lobules of the breast exhibit a single layer of the epithelial cells and myoepithelial cells.

In myoepithelial hyperplasia, more than one layer of myoepithelium is present around the ducts and acini. In epithelial hyperplasia, more than one layer of the epithelial cells is present, and the lumen of the ducts and lobules is partially filled and narrowed or totally filled and obliterated with the layers of epithelial cell. The lumen may also be dilated in some cases. The involved ducts are regularly thickened and the lobules are somewhat enlarged. This makes it easier to detect the hyperplastic ducts and lobules with radiological examination.

Usual ductal hyperplasia is a benign lesion, but it is associated with a slightly increased (1.5–2-fold) risk of subsequent development of breast carcinoma [3]. No consistent genetic changes were found associated to usual ductal hyperplasia. The histological hallmark of this lesion is intraluminal presence of a polymorphous small cell population. The cells are irregularly spaced and irregular slit-like spaces are seen at the periphery of the involved ducts. This cell population is heterogeneous regarding the phenotype of the cells which can be traced with staining for estrogen receptors and/or for cytokeratin 5/6.

Atypical ductal hyperplasia is a lesion different from usual ductal hyperplasia, despite the similarity of the names. Atypical ductal hyperplasia shows similarity to low-grade ductal carcinoma in situ in its histological appearance and phenotype. It is characterized by the presence of a monomorphic small cell population within the lumina of the lobules (rarely ducts), by diffuse intense estrogen receptor expression and the absence of expression of cytokeratin 5/6 [4]. Frequent genetic aberrations found in atypical hyperplasia are also identical to those in low-grade ductal cancer in situ. Atypical ductal hyperplasia is associated with a moderately increased (threefold to fivefold) risk of subsequent development of breast carcinoma [3].

Columnar cell change is a lesion characterized by one or several layers of tall cylindrical epithelial cells with cytoplasmic protrusions ("apical snouts") within the ducts and/or lobules. The single-layer variant is designated as columnar cell change, and the multilayered variant as columnar cell hyperplasia. The cells may or may not exhibit cellular and nuclear atypia. The atypical variant of columnar cell change and columnar cell hyperplasia is also referred as flat epithelial atypia, as mentioned above. Flat epithelial atypia is often associated with lobular neoplasia and low-grade invasive carcinomas.

In addition to hyperplasia, many other lesions may also lead to enlargement of the lobules. Such enlargement is frequently caused by adenosis, metaplastic processes, or microcystic dilatation of the acini. Adenosis also represents a proliferative lesion as hyperplasia, but in this lesion, the epithelial compartment of the acini remains single cell thick, although the number of the acini is increased. The many variants of adenosis, metaplasias, and cystic lesions are so often present that they are considered being normal constituents of breast tissue.

5.1 Intraductal/Lobular Proliferation

The lobule, together with its terminal duct, has been called the terminal duct lobular unit (TDLU). This represents the structural and functional unit of the breast (Fig. 5.10).

The normal lobule consists of a variable number of blind-ending terminal ductules, also called acini, each with its typical double cell layer. It consists of an inner (luminal) epithelial cell layer and an outer (basal) myoepithelial cell layer (Fig. 5.11).

Sometimes epithelial cells increase in number. This is called hyperplasia.

Hyperplasia can occur in the ducts (ductal hyperplasia) or the lobules (lobular hyperplasia).

Epithelial proliferations confined to the mammary ductal-lobular system are classically divided into five major categories based on their architectural and cytologic features:

1. Usual ductal hyperplasia (UDH),
2. Atypical ductal hyperplasia (ADH)
3. Ductal carcinoma in situ (DCIS)
4. Atypical lobular hyperplasia (ALH)
5. Lobular carcinoma in situ (LCIS)

The clinical importance of these lesions are the following:

- Relative common lesions in the "screening era" (in the "premammographic screening era," they were incidental finding)
- The natural history of these lesions is poorly understood (further studies will be necessary). Uniform classification and reporting of benign breast disease is needed to better delineate the relationship of specific benign breast disease pathologies and increased risk of breast cancer.
- Even if they are a non-obligate precursor to invasive breast cancer, we find an increased risk of developing a subsequent breast-invasive cancer (different risk for each group).

5.1.1 Usual Ductal Hyperplasia (UDH or Ductal Hyperplasia Without Atypia or Ductal Intraepithelial Neoplasia, DIN1A)

UDH is a benign epithelial proliferation of the cells lining the ducts. These cells show a trend to enlarge and modify the contour of the ducts, to create bridges within the lumen, causing fenestrations, and eventually to completely fill and distend the duct.

The cells are invariably benign, showing a disordered growth pattern, and their nuclei vary in size, shape, and orientation. The cells show no polarization neither a regular streaming. No or very few mitoses are present. In other words, in usual hyperplasia, the pattern of cells is very close to normal. No change in the surrounding stroma is present, such as elastosis or fibroblastic proliferation or reactive mononuclear cell infiltrates.

Rarely necrosis is observed. The rare presence of necrosis does not preclude a diagnosis of UDH if the architectural and cytologic features of the proliferation support that diagnosis.

In some cases, the proliferative epithelium of the terminal ductal-lobular units shows the so-called "columnar changes" characterized by a single or a double layer of columnar cells that are of regular size and shape with relatively bland nuclear features and which are arranged perpendicular to the basement membrane. The nuclei are uniform, typically ovoid, with finely dispersed chromatin. Cell luminal aspect shows apical snouts and blebs. Secretions and microcalcifications are often present in the duct lumen [5, 6] (Table 5.1) (Fig. 5.12).

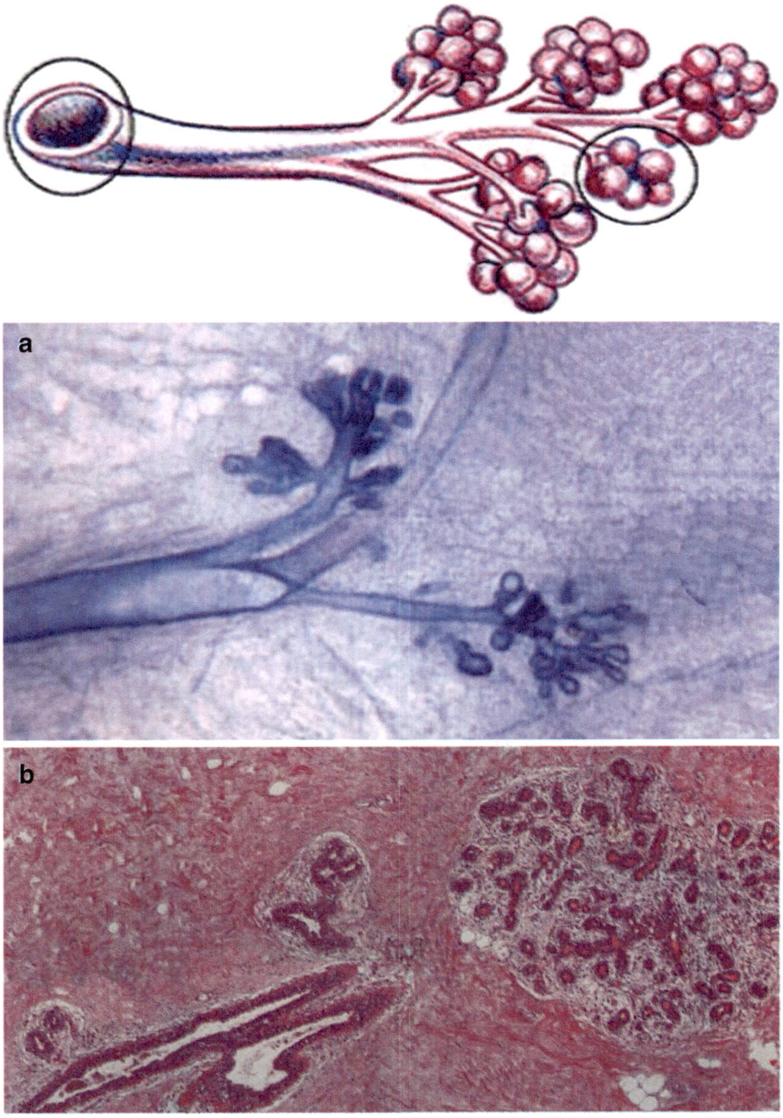

Fig. 5.10 Terminal ductal-lobular unit (TDLU) system: normal morphology in different woman life period (**a**, menopause; **b**, after puberty)

5.1.1.1 Size of Lesions

The extension of these lesions are quite different: from a few millimeters (if they involve one or few terminal ducts) to several centimeters (if they involve a whole lobe).

5.1.1.2 Immunophenotype and Genetics

The UDH cells show heterogeneous expression of estrogen receptor (ER). Some cells are strongly positive, others are more weakly positive, and others are negative (Fig. 5.13). All show a low proliferation rate (Ki67).

A mosaic pattern of expression of high-molecular-weight cytokeratins (CKs) as demonstrated with antibodies to CK5/6 is a characteristic feature.

5.1.1.3 Clinical Course and Prognosis

Hyperplasia doesn't cause any symptoms or pain or a lump that can be felt; it is usually suspected by chance on a screening mammogram.

Certain diagnosis is possible only by histology. Diagnosis is made by a fine needle aspiration or by a biopsy where cells or a piece of tissue is removed and checked under a microscope.

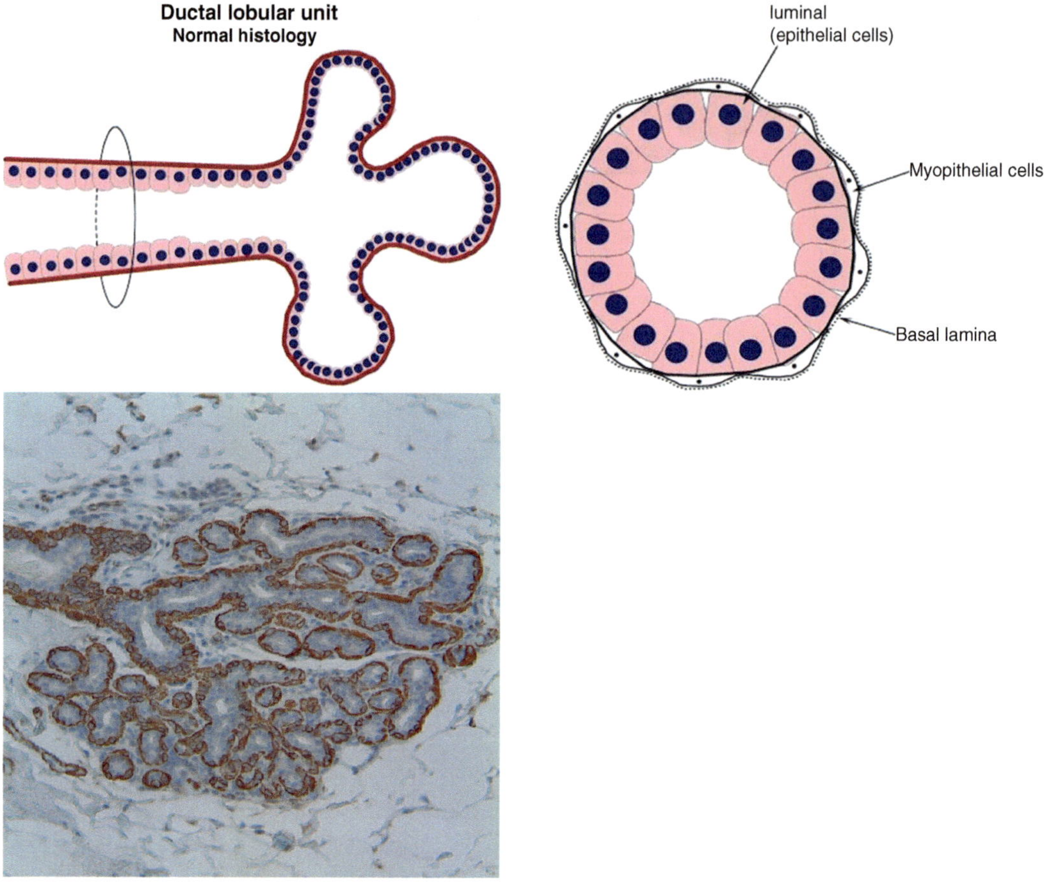

Fig. 5.11 Ductal-lobular unit. A single epithelial cell layer (A) surrounded by myoepithelial cells (B) laying on basal membrane (C) (modified by Modena 2006). Below: Either both the terminal ducts and the lobules are surrounded by myoepithelial cells (immunohistochemically marked by actin, brown-stained) (100×)

Table 5.1 Ductal hyperplasia without atypia

Cytologic features	Architectural features
Heterogeneous cell population in cell size, shape, and orientation	Solid, fenestrated, or micropapillary
Nuclei with variation in size, shape, and orientation of nuclei	Duct lumens irregular, variable in size and shape
Estrogen receptor (ER): heterogeneous expression	Special type: "columnar change" with microcalcifications
Proliferation index (Ki67): low	
High-molecular-weight cytokeratins (CKs): mosaic pattern	

Usual ductal hyperplasia (without atypia) faintly increase the risk for subsequent breast cancer (relative risk 1.27–1.88) unless a strong family history was present. UDH lesions do not represent direct cancer precursors but rather are markers of a generalized increase in breast cancer risk. A recent meta-analysis of retrospective and prospective observational studies published from 1972 to 2010 reports a summary risk estimate for breast cancer following proliferative disease without atypia 1.76 (95% CI 1.58–1.95). Women with benign proliferative breast disease should more closely adhere to an accurate annual screening.

At present, no prognostic factors or biomarkers permit to identify patients with UDH who

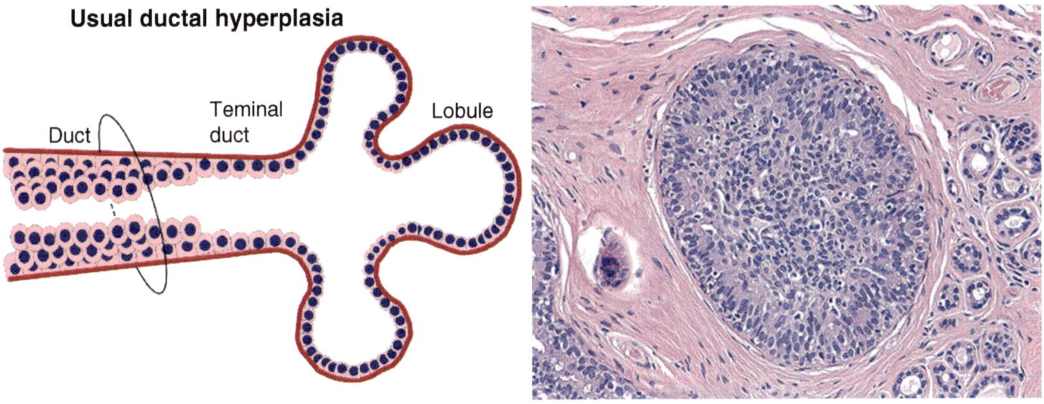

Fig. 5.12 Usual ductal hyperplasia (UDH): schematic drawing modified by Modena 2006 (left) and histological example (100×) (right)

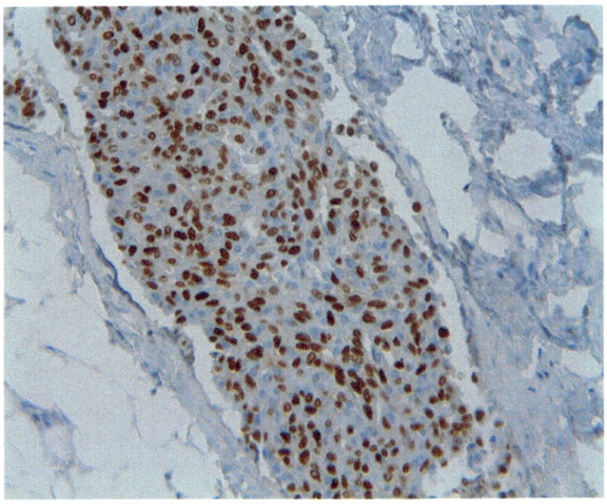

Fig. 5.13 Usual ductal hyperplasia (UDH) usually present heterogeneous expression of estrogen receptor (immunohistochemical for ER, brown-stained cells) (100×)

have higher risk to develop invasive breast cancer.

Uniform classification and reporting of benign breast disease are needed to better delineate the relationship of specific benign breast disease pathologies and increased risk of breast cancer [7, 8].

5.1.2 Atypical Ductal Hyperplasia (ADH or Ductal Intraepithelial Neoplasia 1B, DIN1B)

ADH is a very tiny epithelial proliferation confined to the mammary ductal-lobular system involving one or two ducts or two ductal spaces with an aggregate size of maximum 2 mm in diameter and is composed in part by usual duct hyperplasia or even normal epithelium, combined with neoplastic cell population similar to that seen in low-grade DCIS. Monomorphic cells with polarized nuclei growth in ductal lumen-shaping rigid bridges ("Roman bridges") characteristics of low-grade ductal epithelial neoplasia (Fig. 5.14). A special type show columnar epithelial change (Fig. 5.15).

In other words, there are quantitative and qualitative criteria for the diagnosis of atypical duct hyperplasia. Quantitatively, the lesion should not involve more than two ducts or be larger than 2 mm; qualitatively, in the same ducts, morphological features of usual duct hyperplasia and low-grade duct intraepithelial neoplasia coexist [9, 10].

The definition of atypical ductal hyperplasia (ADH) is derived from surgical resection specimens and relies on a combination of histological, morphological, and size extent criteria. For this reason, accurate diagnosis of ADH is not possible on core biopsy. The limited tissue sampling that can be achieved using core biopsy guns (often by stereotactic methods for foci of microcalcification) may provide insufficient material for the definitive diagnosis of atypical ductal hyperplasia [11] (Table 5.2) (Fig. 5.16).

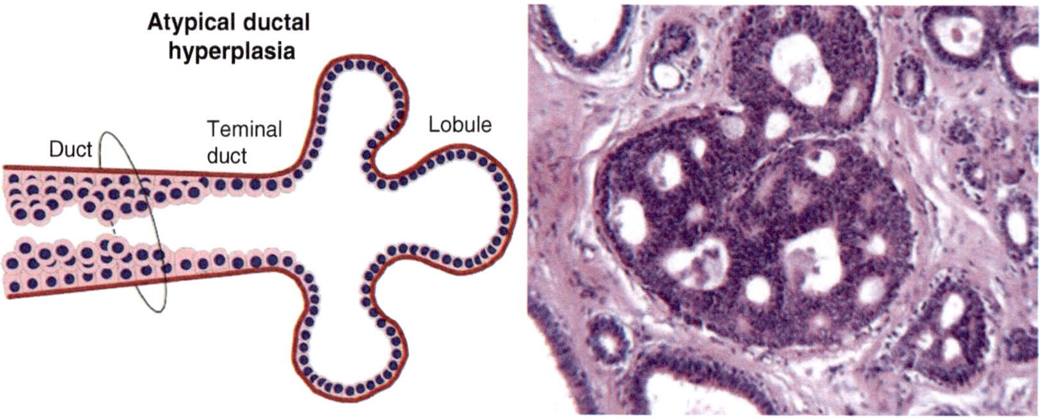

Fig. 5.14 Atypical ductal hyperplasia (ADH): schematic drawing modified by Modena 2006 (left) and histological example (100×) (right)

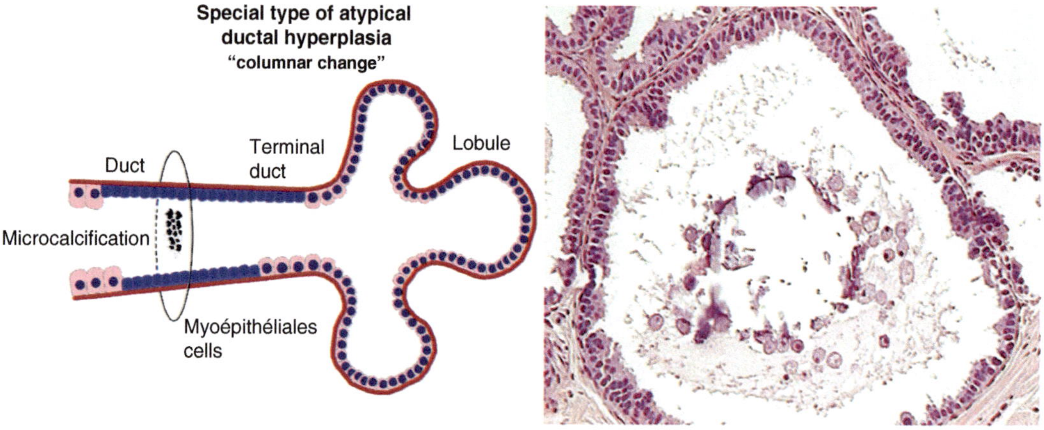

Fig. 5.15 Special type of atypical ductal hyperplasia (columnar change): schematic drawing modified by Modena 2006 (left) and histological example (100×) (right)

Table 5.2 Atypical ductal hyperplasia

Cytologic features	Architectural features
Two kinds of ductal cells: 1. Typical cells (normal or usual hyperplasia) 2. Atypical cells similar to that of low-grade ductal carcinoma in situ	Atypical cell proliferation with: – Roman bridges – Micropapillary pattern – Cribriform pattern – Solid pattern – Columnar change (Fig. 5.15)
Estrogen receptor (ER): high expression	Tiny lesion: involvement of less than two ductal spaces or 2 mm in extent
Proliferation index (Ki67): low	
High-molecular-weight cytokeratins (CKs): absent	

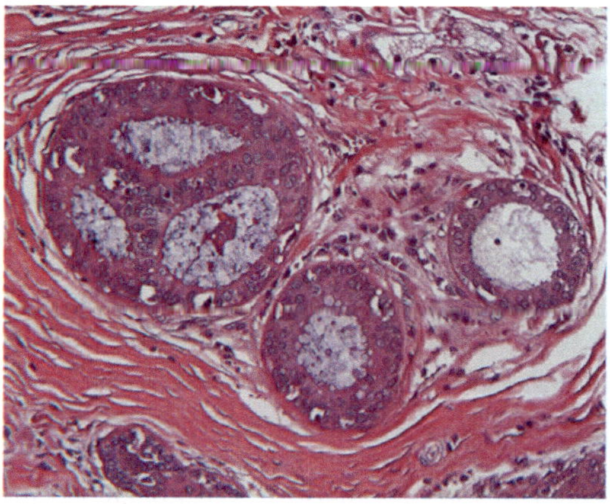

Fig. 5.16 A case of atypical ductal hyperplasia. The extension of the lesion is less than 2 mm by definition

5.1.2.1 Size of Lesions

For definition, ADH should not be larger than 2 mm (Fig. 5.16).

5.1.2.2 Immunophenotype and Genetics

Sometimes differentiating atypical duct hyperplasia from low-grade ductal carcinoma in situ is very difficult and may not be considered a well-reproducible diagnosis among pathologists.

Immunohistochemical stains help to differentiate florid examples of usual epithelial hyperplasia from subtle atypical duct hyperplasia or from low-grade ductal carcinoma.

The ADH cells typically show strong and uniform expression of ER and have a low proliferative rate (Ki 67). Expression of high-molecular-weight CKs by CK5/6 immunostaining is absent [12].

Genetic studies have identified several recurrent genomic alterations including losses at 16q and 17p and gains at 1q; these genetic abnormalities are similar to those seen in low-grade DCIS [13, 14] (Table 5.2).

5.1.2.3 Clinical Course and Prognosis

ADH is associated with an increased risk of subsequent breast cancer (3.5–5 times higher than that of a woman with no breast abnormalities). A recent meta-analysis of published studies evaluating the association of biopsy-proven benign breast disease with risk of developing breast cancer reports for ADH a summary risk estimate of 3.28 (95% CI 2.54–4.23). These cancers occur with approximately equal frequency in both breasts [8, 15–17].

This cancer risk range is partly caused by a collection of not homogenous lesions. Differentiating atypical duct hyperplasia from low-grade ductal carcinoma in situ is sometimes very difficult and may not be considered a well-reproducible diagnosis among pathologists.

ADH doesn't cause any symptoms or pain or a lump that can be felt; it is usually suspected by chance on a screening mammogram and confirmed histologically on core biopsy.

The clinical impact of such a diagnosis changes on the basis of the specimens.

Finding an atypical hyperplasia on a core biopsy is considered by many an indication to proceed with a surgical removal because in a limited sample it can not be excluded that hyperplasia could be associated with more severe lesions. The finding of ADH in large-excision specimens or quadrantectomy must be carefully histologically examined to choose the best clinical care (follow-up or endocrine therapy or subsequent radiotherapy if associated to DCIS). *Patients with ADH not associated to DCIS are most often managed by close follow-up.*

Anti-estrogen medications (tamoxifen and aromatase inhibitors) may also be used to reduce the risk of developing breast cancer. At present, no biomarkers can identify which patients with ADH are more likely to develop invasive breast cancer [15].

Several clinical factors such as young age of patient, family history, and dense breast increase the associated risk with ADH of developing breast cancer.

An assessment of an individual's risk based on multiple factors should be preferred before deciding on prevention strategies [18].

5.1.3 Ductal Carcinoma In Situ (DCIS or Ductal Intraepithelial Neoplasia, DIN1C)

Carcinoma in situ of ductal type (DCIS) is a heterogeneous group of lesions that have in common the presence of neoplastic epithelial cells confined to the mammary ductal-lobular unit without any invasion through the basal membrane. Sometimes the carcinoma cells spread backward along the duct (lobular cancerization) (Fig. 5.17). They differ in their clinical presentation, histological features, biomarker profile, genetic abnormalities, and biologic potential.

In most cases, DCIS involves the breast in a unicentric, lobar distribution; true multicentric disease is uncommon [19, 20].

One obstacle to progress in this area has been variability in how DCIS is reported by pathologists. Although the classification of ductal carcinoma in situ is not yet accepted worldwide, in our

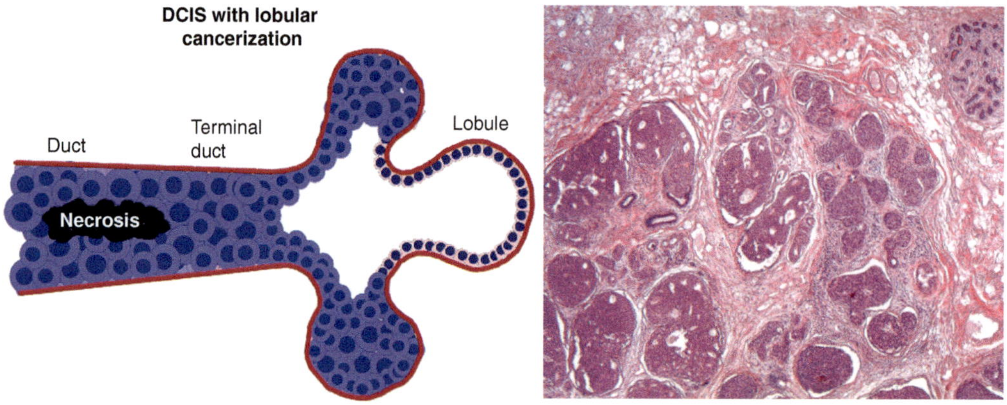

Fig. 5.17 DCIS carcinoma cells spread along the duct into the lobule (lobular cancerization). (Left, schematic drawing modified by Modena 2006: right, histological specimen, 100×)

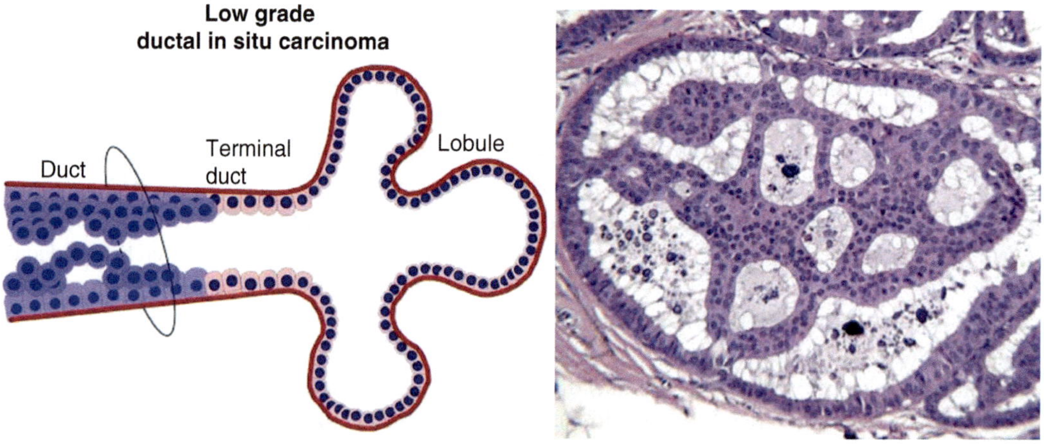

Fig. 5.18 Low-grade ductal carcinoma in situ (DCIS): schematic drawing modified by Modena 2006 (left) and histological example (100×) (right)

routine practice, we classify DCIS on the basis of two characteristics: the morphological pattern of growth (cribriform, papillary, micropapillary, solid, and comedocarcinoma) and the degree of differentiation (well, moderately, or poorly differentiated or G1, G2, or G3) based on nuclear morphology, mitosis index, and the presence of necrosis. The grade increases according to nuclear atypia and number of mitoses. According to the recommendations of the College of American Pathologists, we report the presence of necrosis as extensive (as in comedocarcinoma) or as focal [16].

Low-grade DCIS (G1) are characterized by *small cells with well-defined cell membranes that exhibit uniform size, shape, and placement* containing monomorphic, regular nuclei with small nucleoli and few mitotic figures. *Cell population of low-grade DCIS is similar to atypical duct hyperplasia, but the lesion involves more than two ducts (extension > 2 mm).* There is no perfect correlation between pattern of growth and grade of differentiation, but usually cribriform and micropapillary patterns are more often low-grade lesions (Fig. 5.18).

By contrast, *high-grade DCIS (G3)* is composed of cells with large, pleomorphic nuclei that have irregular chromatin and prominent nucleoli. Mitoses are frequent and may be atypical. Central, comedo-type necrosis is often present.

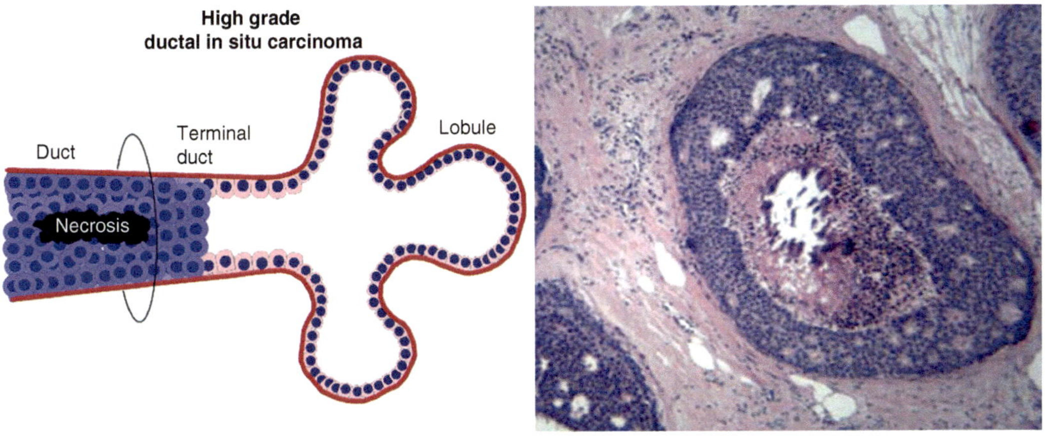

Fig. 5.19 High-grade ductal carcinoma in situ (DCIS): schematic drawing modified by Modena 2006 (left) and histological example (100×) (right)

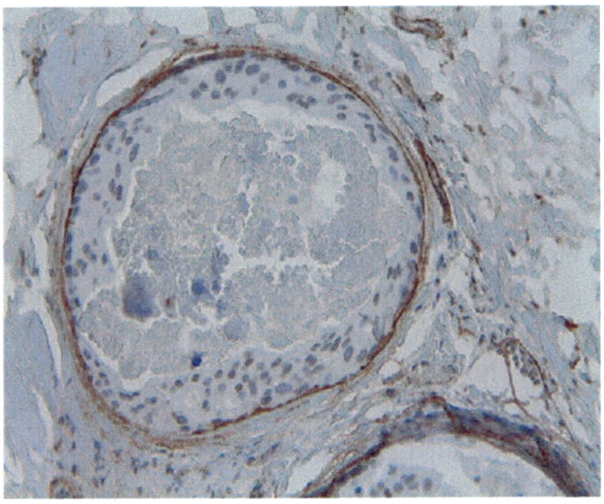

Fig. 5.20 High-grade DCIS: A layer of myoepithelial cells surround the enlarged duct (Immunohistochemical for actin, brown-stained) (100×)

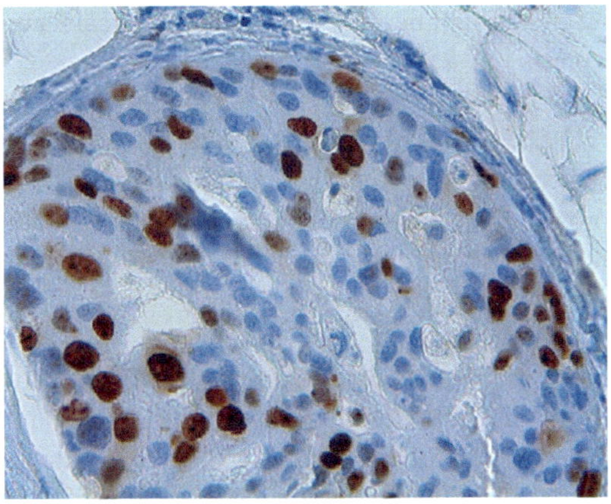

Fig. 5.21 High-grade DCIS: high proliferation index (Immunohistochemical for Ki67, brown-stained cells) (125×)

Solid and comedocarcinoma growing pattern are typical of high-grade DCIS.

Calcifications are often found within the central necrotic material and usually matches with a linear, branching, or casting pattern on mammography (Figs. 5.19, 5.20, and 5.21).

A diagnosis of *intermediate-grade DCIS* (G2) is formulated when the cells comprising the lesion do not fulfill the cytologic criteria for either low-grade or high-grade DCIS as described earlier. The growth pattern may be solid, cribriform, micropapillary, or papillary, or the cells may form arcades and bridges, can be difficult to classify, and tend to show less nuclear pleomorphism than high-grade lesions and cellular polarization. The presence of necrosis, even focal, assigns the lesion to at least a G2 grade.

Calcifications are common and, when present, are usually rounded and laminated (psammomatous) and deposited within intraluminal. These calcifications may be detected by mammography.

Fibroblastic proliferation with collagen deposition (desmoplastic reaction), chronic inflammation, and vascular proliferation (angiogenesis) is often seen in the stroma surrounding the involved spaces. These stromal modifications may be so prominent that it results in a palpable abnormality in the breast. Involvement of nipple (Paget disease) is almost invariably associated with high-grade DCIS.

Nuclear grade, the presence of necrosis, and distance from margins are generally agreed to be the most important determinants that correlate with local recurrence and are routinely reported by most pathologists. The extent (size) of DCIS is also important for predicting the risk of local recurrence because big size increases the risk to have involved margins or to miss area of invasion.

5.1.3.1 New Classification

On the basis of molecular studies that show common genetic mutation in UDH as in ADH/DCIS, Tavassoli have introduced a new terminology that replaces the term ductal carcinoma in situ and lobular carcinoma in situ, respectively, with ductal intraepithelial neoplasia (DIN) and lobular intraepithelial neoplasia (LIN). In this classification, DIN is graded into a three-tier scale (DIN1e3), and DIN1 is further divided into three classes: DIN1A, which corresponds to flat epithelial atypia; DIN1B, which corresponds to atypical ductal hyperplasia; and DIN1C, which corresponds to well-differentiated grade (grade 1) ductal carcinoma in situ. DIN2 corresponds to moderately differentiated (grade 2) ductal carcinoma in situ, and DIN3 to poorly differentiated (grade 3) ductal carcinoma in situ (Table 5.3).

DIN classification simplifies terminology of ductal and lobular lesions and is pleasing to surgeon and oncologist who require a simpler terminology without the word "carcinoma" to better explain the pathology report to the patient. The problem is that DIN/LIN terminology may imply an expected progression from low- to high-grade lesions, while this is probably untrue.

Table 5.3 Comparison between old and new ductal carcinoma in situ (DCIS) classification

Old terminology	New classification (according to Tavassoli [21])[a]
Flat epithelial atypia	DIN 1a
Atypical duct hyperplasia	DIN 1b
Low-grade (G1) ductal carcinoma in situ	DIN 1c
Intermediate-grade (G2) ductal carcinoma in situ	DIN 2
High-grade (G3) ductal carcinoma in situ	DIN 3

[a]Tavassoli FA. Mod Pathol. 1998;11(2):140–54

5.1.3.2 Size of Lesions

The extent of DCIS refers to the volume of breast tissue with ducts and lobules involved by DCIS. Extension of DCIS is very variable and can range from 0.1 cm to involvement of all 4 quadrants of the breast. Because the ductal system is a complex three-dimensional structure that rarely is grossly visible, a simple and precise method to measure extent is not available. Mammography compresses and distorts the ductal system. Ultrasound allows an accurate study of mammary lobe, but often DCIS and microcalcification are undetectable. Also breast specimens after surgical remotion usually flatten and may distort the ductal system. At present, the preferable method to determine DCIS extent is to serially section and completely submit the whole breast specimen.

A method accurate for assessing the extent of carcinoma in situ of the breast and feasible for routine diagnosis is to use large-format (10 × 8 cm) contiguous histology sections. This kind of histological approach enhances mammographic pathologic correlation, documents the lesion for adequate and reproducible analysis of the extent and distribution of the disease, and preserves the relation of the lesions to each other and to the circumferential surgical margin. This method allows pathologist to study the DCIS extension and clear margins, parameters that correlate significantly with the rate of local recurrences [22–25] (Fig. 5.22).

5.1.3.3 Clinical Presentation

Ductal carcinoma in situ (DCIS) was a rare diagnosis before the introduction of screening mammography, but now composes 20–30% of all breast cancers.

Clinically most DCIS is suspected by mammographic microcalcifications. However, up to 30% of DCIS lesions may present with other mammographic findings, such an area of architectural distortion (desmoplastic reaction).

Less commonly, DCIS presents as a palpable mass or associated to a pathologic nipple discharge

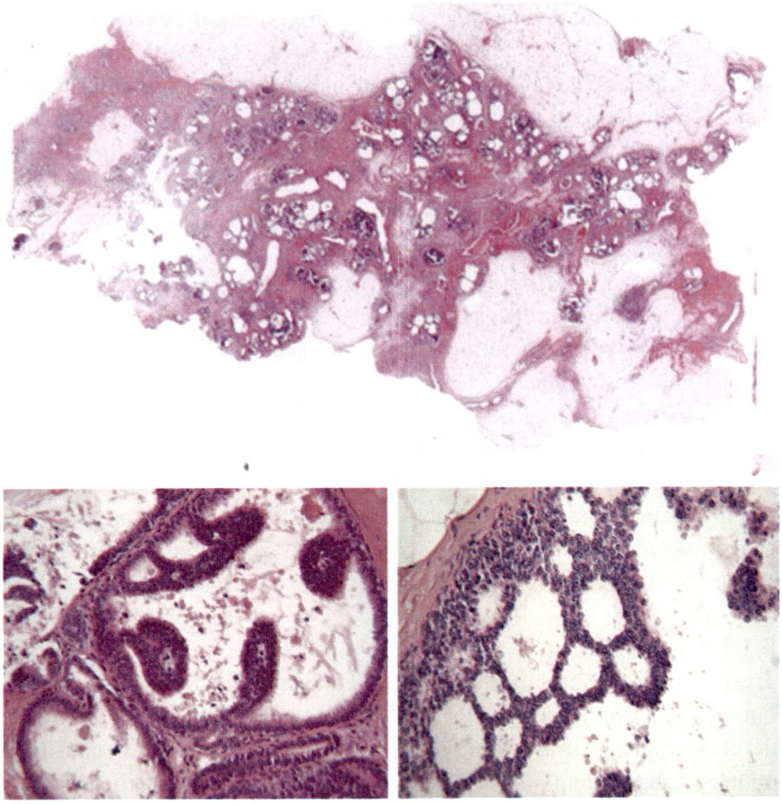

Fig. 5.22 An extensive DCIS involving the whole lobe studied with large-format histologic section. At the bottom: high magnification (125×) showing micropapillary type (left) and cribriform pattern (right)

(Paget disease of the nipple). Sometimes they are incidental microscopic finding in breast tissue removed because of another abnormality.

5.1.3.4 Biomarkers and Genetics

Low-grade DCIS lesions typically show diffuse and strong expression of ER and progesterone receptor (PR) and a low proliferation index and do not show HER2 protein overexpression or gene amplification.

In contrast, high-grade DCIS lesions may be ER and PR positive or negative, have a high proliferative rate, and frequently show HER2 protein overexpression and gene amplification.

The accumulation of p53 protein and p53 gene mutations is commonly seen in high-grade DCIS. Expression of high-molecular-weight CKs by CK5/6 immunostaining is absent in low-grade, intermediate-grade, and most high-grade DCIS except for a small proportion of high-grade DCIS. Tamoxifen has been shown to significantly reduce the risk of local recurrence in patients with ER-positive DCIS. Therefore, determination of the ER status of DCIS should be a routine part of the pathologic evaluation of these lesions [26].

Recent molecular studies have provided evidence that low-grade DCIS and high-grade DCIS are genetically distinct disorders. Low-grade lesions are characterized by chromosomal losses at 16q and 17p and gains at 1q, whereas high-grade lesions show losses at 11q, 14q, 8p, and 13q and gains at 17q, 8q, and 5p, among other alterations [13, 14, 27].

5.1.3.5 Natural History, Clinical Course, and Prognosis

DCIS is a non-obligate precursor to invasive breast cancer, but its natural history is poorly understood.

If no treatment is offered, about 14–46% of patients with DCIS will progress to invasive cancer within 10 years [5–7].

Following a diagnosis of ductal carcinoma in situ, the subsequent risk of developing an invasive carcinoma is almost tenfold, and recurrences may appear even after many years after the original diagnosis [26]. About 50% of the recurrences are again ductal carcinoma in situ, but half of them will be invasive carcinomas, despite there currently being no evidence for a direct evolution (Figs. 5.23 and 5.24).

Risk of recurrence after surgical treatment is strongly correlated with the grade of DCIS. The higher the grade of DCIS differentiation, the higner the risk of recurrence [28]. Nonetheless, a substantial risk of ipsilateral invasive recurrence is noted among all grades of DCIS, although low-risk lesions tend to progress to grade 1 invasive cancers with a more favorable prognosis. Subsequent development of invasive cancer in the ipsilateral breast will probably represent a new primary tumor, because phenotypic progression is uncommon in breast cancer [29].

5.1.3.6 Treatment

Treatment of DCIS is aimed at complete eradication of the lesion to prevent local recurrence or development of an invasive carcinoma. Treatment options range from mastectomy to breast-conserving therapy (i.e., excision and radiation therapy or excision alone) with or without anti estrogen therapy. Although mastectomy achieves cure rates approaching 100%, this represents overtreatment for many patients, especially those with small- or well-differentiated DCIS. In current clinical practice, mastectomy is generally reserved for those with extensive disease, and most patients with more limited DCIS are managed with breast-conserving therapy followed by radiation and/or hormonal therapy.

Patients with DCIS treated only by breast-conserving therapy are at risk for recurrence. The most important factors that influence that risk are margin of excision, patient age, and grade and size of DCIS. It is suggested to personalize treatment taking into account all these variables (The University of Southern California/Van Nuys Prognostic Index) [30].

The identification of biomarkers that might be helpful in determining which patients with DCIS are at high and low risk of progression to invasive breast cancer is an area of active investigation [2], but at the present time, no markers singly or in combination are sufficiently validated for routine clinical use. The only molecular marker in routine clinical use in the management of DCIS in the UK is the ER; ER-negative tumors are more likely to recur [8, 16, 17]. The human epidermal growth factor receptor 2 (HER2) is inversely related to ER receptor status in DCIS [18, 19], but its prognostic significance remains controversial.

Recently, a commercially available reverse transcription polymerase chain reaction-based assay has been introduced to help stratify the risk of local recurrence and subsequent invasive cancer in patients with DCIS, but the clinical utility of this assay remains to be determined [1].

Although there should theoretically be no risk of lymph node involvement or metastatic disease

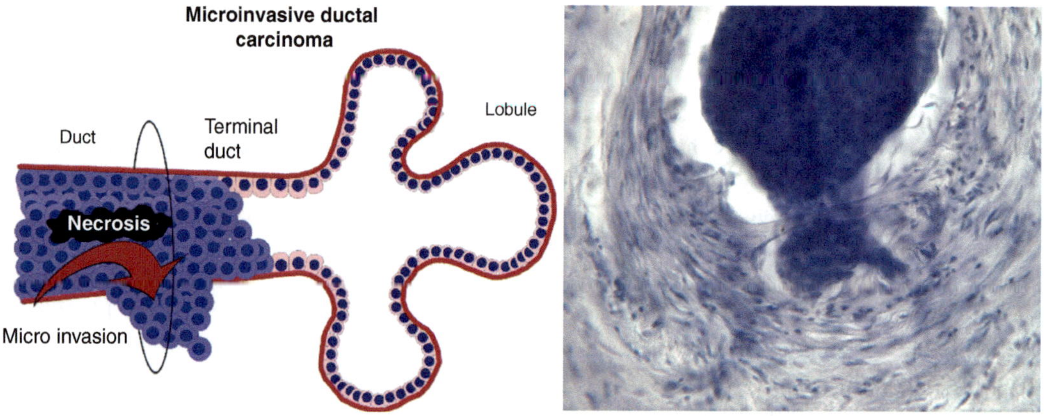

Fig. 5.23 Microinvasion in a ductal carcinoma in situ: schematic drawing modified by Modena 2006 (left) and histological example (100×) (right)

among patients with DCIS, a small proportion of these (between 1% and 2%) develop axillary nodal or distant metastases due to the presence of invasive carcinoma that was not sampled or not recognized (Figs. 5.23 and 5.24). This happens more often in high-grade lesions and very large DCIS. In these patients, it is suggested to biopsy the sentinel node.

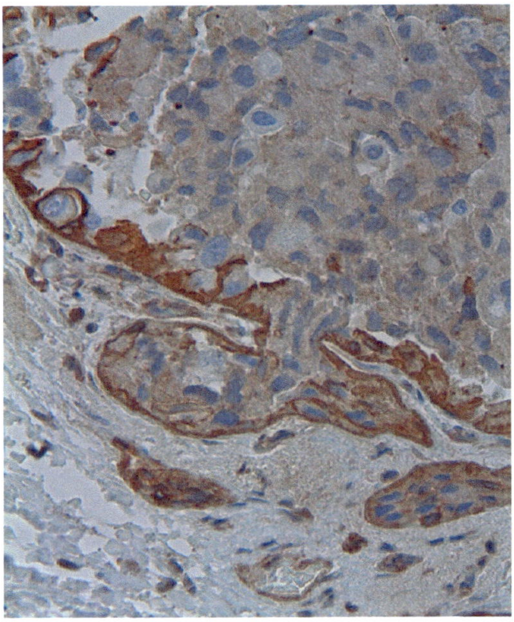

Fig. 5.24 Ductal carcinoma in situ with microinvasion. Myoepithelial cells (brown-stained) are present around DCIS and are partially missed around microinvasion focus

5.1.4 Lobular Neoplasia: Atypical Lobular Hyperplasia (ALH) and Lobular Carcinoma In Situ (LCIS) (LIN1, LIN2, and LIN3)

Lobular carcinoma in situ (LCIS) and atypical lobular hyperplasia (ALH) are related lesions most often characterized by a proliferation of small, loosely cohesive epithelial cells, with scant cytoplasm and a high nuclear/cytoplasm ratio and rare, if any, mitoses. Intracytoplasmic vacuoles are often present. This proliferation is localized within the terminal duct lobular units (TDLUs) involving and expanding lobules and ductules. Although there is no definite consensus on this issue, in our routine practice, the distinction between ALH and LCIS is made based on the percentage of acini in the affected terminal duct lobular unit distended by lobular proliferation (<50% for ALH and 50% for LCIS) and whether the abnormal cells completely fill at least one lobular unit [31] (Figs. 5.25 and 5.26).

In about three-quarters of the cases, the cells of LCIS involve the terminal ducts and/or extralobular ducts [7]. The growth of the cells within the ducts is called «pagetoid spread»

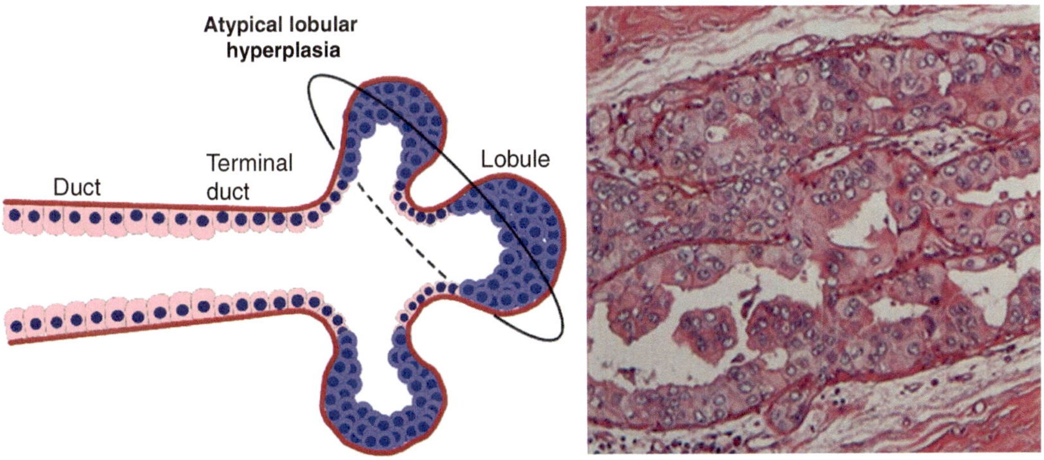

Fig. 5.25 Atypical lobular hyperplasia (ALH): schematic drawing modified by Modena 2006 (left) and histological specimen (right; 200×)

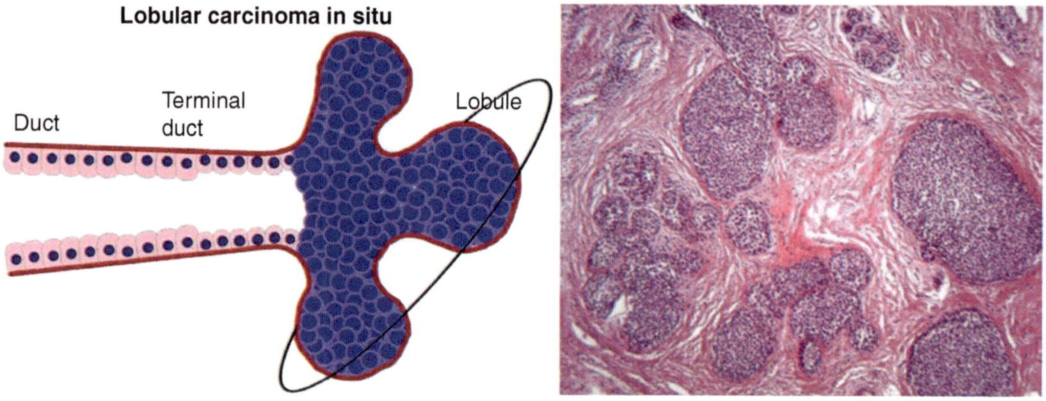

Fig. 5.26 Lobular carcinoma in situ (LCIS): schematic drawing modified by Modena 2006 (left) and histological example (100×) (right)

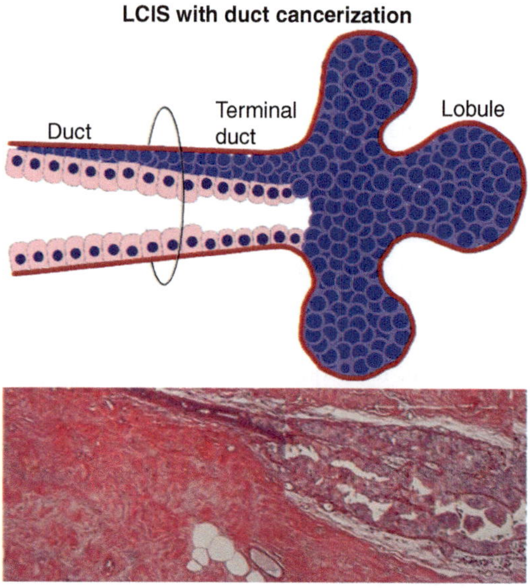

Fig. 5.27 Lobular neoplasia involving the TDLU duct: schematic drawing modified by Modena 2006 (above) and histological specimen (below, 100×)

(Fig. 5.27) which means growth of neoplastic cells between the myoepithelial cell layer and the luminal cells. In addition to involving lobular acini and ducts, LCIS may involve a variety of lesions including usual ductal hyperplasia, ductal carcinoma in situ (DCIS), fibroadenomas, intraductal papillomas, columnar cell lesions/flat epithelial atypia, and benign-sclerosing lesions.

Some authors have suggested to group ALH and LCIS together under the single term *lobular neoplasia*. (1) The term "lobular neoplasia" removes the word "carcinoma" from the diagnosis of an in situ lesion, and it eliminates the need to make the morphologic distinction between ALH and LCIS, which shows low reproducibility. However, the major disadvantage of this approach is that it combines into one category lesions that show different developing cancer risk. (2) Therefore, it remains clinically useful to continue to distinguish ALH from LCIS [32–34].

Likewise for DCIS, Tavassoli [35] suggests to classify these lesions as lobular intraepithelial neoplasia (LIN) grading in this manner:

LIN1 is characterized by delicate changes which consist in the partial or total replacement of normal acini epithelial cells by loosely cohesive, small, uniform, round cells which does not fill completely lobule lumina.

LIN2 is characterized by more evident changes which consist in larger distension of acini by small round cells filling and distending the lobule lumina with persistence of stroma between acini (Fig. 5.28).

LIN3 is divided into two further classes (A and B) according to the type of neoplastic cells. Type A is characterized by the same cells as LIN1 and LIN2, with a greater distension of acini without any intervening stroma between them; type B

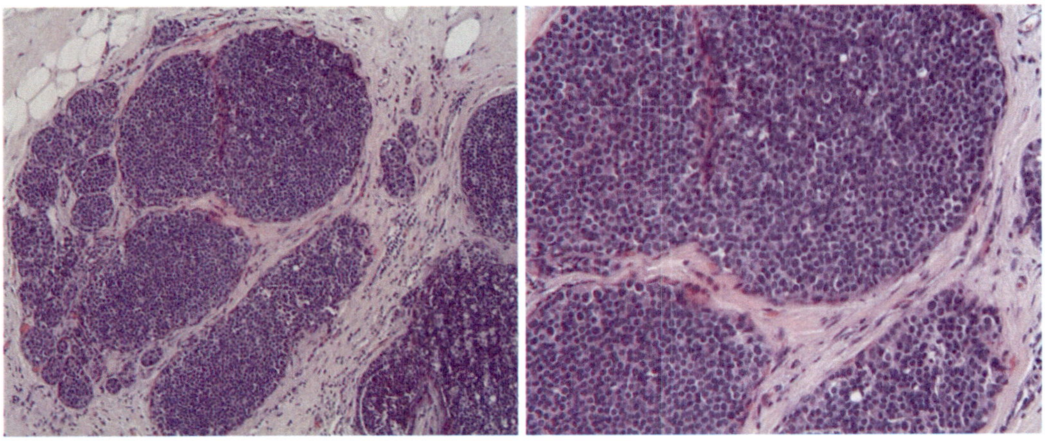

Fig. 5.28 Classic type (LIN2) of lobular carcinoma in situ (LCIS) histological specimen (left 100× and right 125×)

Table 5.4 Comparison between old and new lobular neoplasia classification

Old terminology	New classification (according to Tavassoli and Bratthauer [35])
Atypical lobular hyperplasia	LIN1
Classic type lobular carcinoma in situ	LIN 2
High-grade or pleomorphic lobular carcinoma in situ	LIN 3

Bratthauer GL, Tavassoli FA. Virchows Arch. 2002;440:134–8

is characterized by more atypical cells. This distinction (types A and B) is purely morphological, without any clinical implication, and sometimes the two types of cells coexist (Table 5.4).

5.1.4.1 Size of Lesions

Very variable: range from <1 mm to several centimeters.

5.1.4.2 Clinical Presentation

ALH and LCIS are always an incidental microscopic finding in breast tissue removed for another abnormality. It is more commonly seen in breast biopsies performed for mammographic microcalcifications than in those in which the indication for biopsy is a palpable mass.

Lobular neoplasia is usually not grossly identifiable. Even then, it is an infrequent finding, we find an estimated prevalence of 0.4–3.8% in women with otherwise benign breast biopsies.

5.1.4.3 Immunophenotype and Genetics

The cells of classical LCIS have a low proliferative rate, are typically strongly and diffusely estrogen receptor (ER)-positive, and does not show HER2 overexpression or gene amplification or p53 gene alterations. Lobular neoplasia is characterized by mutation in the CDH1 gene, also known as E-cadherin [36]. The immunohistochemical stain for E-cadherin is a very useful tool to distinguish lobular (E-cadherin-negative) from ductal (E-cadherin-positive) neoplasia with a dubious morphology [37]. Molecular techniques show the same genetic abnormalities in both atypical lobular hyperplasia and lobular carcinoma in situ, and this data suggest that lobular neoplasia group different steps in a continuum of progress [38, 39].

5.1.4.4 Natural History, Clinical Course, and Prognosis

Long-term follow-up studies of women diagnosed with ALH find a fourfold increased risk for breast cancer (invasive or in situ) [40, 41].

Women diagnosed with LCIS have a relative risk of subsequent breast cancer 8–10 times higher than the general population. LCIS in some patient may represent a breast cancer risk factor, while in others it behaves as a direct breast cancer precursor. Arguments supporting LCIS as a risk factor include the bilateral nature of the breast cancer risk and the fact that in most studies the majority of breast cancers that develop in women with LCIS are invasive ductal carcinomas of no special type. In other case, LCIS represents direct breast cancer precursors since coexistent LCIS and invasive lobular carcinomas frequently exhibit the same genetic alterations [27]. Besides, invasive lobular carcinomas are much more prevalent among patients with LCIS than in the general (Fig. 5.29) [11, 12, 27]. At the present time, however, it is not possible to determine which LCIS lesions are more likely to act as risk indicators and which are more likely to act as precursors. Therefore, the most appropriate management for patients with LCIS is close observation (with or without treatment with selective ER modulators, such as tamoxifen or raloxifene).

The management of patients with low-differentiated LCIS variants (LIN 3) is more problematic since the natural history of these lesions is poorly understood.

Some clinical features (a positive family history in women <40 years of age, maximal distension of involved spaces, a mixture of type A and B cells, >10 involved spaces, and focal E-cadherin staining) have all been reported to be associated with a greater risk of cancer development.

Lobular neoplasia is managed as a global relative risk factor since it is frequently multifocal and bilateral [42]. Treatment considerations include excisional biopsy, hormone therapy prophylaxis, and rarely bilateral mastectomy. After surgical removal of the lesion, clinical surveillance, such as yearly mammography and breast examinations, is recommended for women with lobular neoplasia. Patient involvement in the choice of management options is a key aspect of care. Women should receive adequate information regarding the implications of a diagnosis of LCIS and the risks and benefits of the different management options (Table 5.5) (see cancer.org/acs/groups/content/@editorial/documents/document/acspc-044552.pdf).

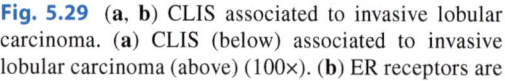

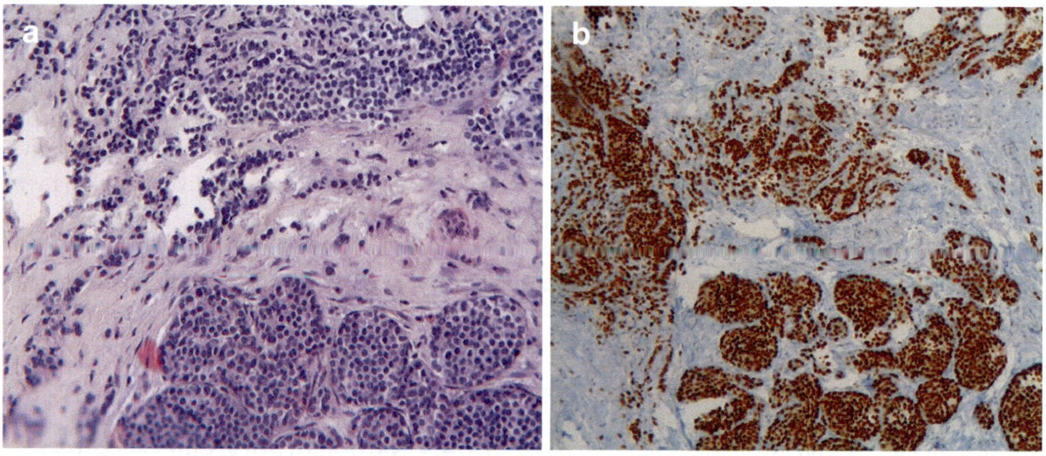

Fig. 5.29 (**a**, **b**) CLIS associated to invasive lobular carcinoma. (**a**) CLIS (below) associated to invasive lobular carcinoma (above) (100×). (**b**) ER receptors are evident either in situ carcinoma or in invasive carcinoma (immunohistochemical reaction for ER, brown-stained cells)

Table 5.5 Lobular neoplasia: key remarks

	Atypical lobular hyperplasia	Lobular carcinoma in situ
Risk of subsequent breast carcinoma	× 4–5	× 8–10
		Multicentricity in 60–80% of cases; bilaterality in 25–30%
Diagnosis by core biopsy	Excision is not mandatory but recommended	Excision should be performed
Treatment of choice[a]	Clinical surveillance[a]	Clinical surveillance/hormone therapy/mastectomy No evidence to support radiotherapy[a]

[a]Involve patients in the therapeutical choice

Conclusion

Despite progress in understanding the molecular and clinical heterogeneity of in situ breast cancers and efforts to better target treatments based on the risk of progression or recurrence, at present, many uncertainties for women affected by these lesions remain.

Is my lesion a carcinoma or not? My lesion has been removed completely, and why is the risk still high? High risk in both breasts? What a 5 times increased risk means? These are some of the most frequent questions asked by patients. In the era of "Internet pseudoculture," it is not easy to communicate diagnosis and prognosis to patient with a proliferative breast lesion. Only a right comprehension allows to involve patient in the complex choice of the best therapy for that woman.

Additional research will help to advance our understanding of molecular aspect of these lesions in order to identify new biomarkers that can predict new subtype of breast proliferation with different prognosis. As molecular and clinical research continues to select different prognostic subtypes and better therapies, there is a concurrent need for the development of more effective patient communication tools for in situ cancers, focusing on the nature of the disease, treatment options, and prognosis [30, 43–48].

Acknowledgment Thanks to Dr. Riccardo Arisio for the general support and to Silvia Botta for pathological drawings.

References

1. Gallager HS, Martin JE. Early phases in the development of breast cancer. Cancer. 1969;24:1170–8.
2. De Brux J. Histopathologie du sein. Paris: Masson; 1979.
3. Lakhani SR, Ellis IO, Schnitt SJ, Tan PH, van de Vijver M. WHO classification of tumours of the breast. Lyon: International Agency for Research on Cancer (IARC); 2012.
4. Tot T, Tabár L, Dean PB. Practical breast pathology. 2nd ed. Stuttgart, New York: Thieme; 2014.
5. Pinder SE, Reis-Filho JS. Non-operative breast pathology: columnar cell lesions. J Clin Pathol. 2007;60:1307–12.
6. Mastropasqua MG, Viale G. Clinical and pathological assessment of high-risk ductal and lobular breast lesions: What surgeons must know. Eur J Surg Oncol. 2017;43:278.
7. Hartmann LC, Sellers TA, Frost MH, et al. Benign breast disease and the risk of breast cancer. N Engl J Med. 2005;353(3):229–37.
8. Dyrstad SW, Yan Y, Fowler AM, et al. Breast cancer risk associated with benign breast disease: systematic review and meta-analysis. Breast Cancer Res Treat. 2015;149:569–75.
9. Page DL, Dupont WD, Rogers LW, Rados MS. Atypical hyperplastic lesions of the female breast. A long-term follow-up study. Cancer. 1985;55:2698–708.
10. Tavassoli FA, Norris HJ. A comparison of the results of long-term follow-up for atypical intraductal hyperplasia and intraductal hyperplasia of the breast. Cancer. 1990;65:518–29.
11. Ellis IO, Humphreys S, Michell M, et al. Guidelines for breast needle core biopsy handling and reporting in breast screening assessment. J Clin Pathol. 2004;57:897–902.
12. Otterbach F, Bankfalvi A, Bergner S, Decker T, Krech R, Boecker W. Cytokeratin 5/6 immunohistochemistry assists the differential diagnosis of

atypical proliferations of the breast. Histopathology. 2000;37(3):232–40.
13. Bombonati A, Sgroi DC. The molecular pathology of breast cancer progression. J Pathol. 2011;223(2):307–17.
14. Lopez-Garcia MA, Geyer FC, Lacroix-Triki M, Marchio C, Reis-Filho JS. Breast cancer precursors revisited: molecular features and progression pathways. Histopathology. 2010;57(2):171–92.
15. Collins LC, Baer HJ, Tamimi RM, Connolly JL, Colditz GA, Schnitt SJ. The influence of family history on breast cancer risk in women with biopsy-confirmed benign breast disease: results from the Nurses' Health Study. Cancer. 2006;107(6):1240–7.
16. Fitzgibbons PL, Henson DE, Hutter RV. Benign breast changes and the risk for subsequent breast cancer: an update of the 1985 consensus statement. Cancer Committee of the College of American Pathologists. Arch Pathol Lab Med. 1998;122(12):1053–5.
17. Schnitt SJ. Benign breast disease and breast cancer risk: morphology and beyond. Am J Surg Pathol. 2003;27(6):836–41.
18. Menes TS, Kerlikowske K, Lange J, Jaffer S, Rosenberg R, Miglioretti DL. Subsequent breast cancer risk following diagnosis of atypical ductal hyperplasia on needle biopsy. JAMA Oncol. 2017;3:36. https://doi.org/10.1001/jamaoncol.2016.3022.
19. Sanders ME, Schuyler PA, Simpson JF, Page DL, Dupont WD. Continued observation of the natural history of low-grade ductal carcinoma in situ reaffirms proclivity for local recurrence even after more than 30 years of follow-up. Mod Pathol. 2015;28:662–9.
20. Lester SC, Connolly JL, Amin MB. College of American pathologists protocol for the reporting of ductal carcinoma in situ. Arch Pathol Lab Med. 2009;133:13–4.
21. Tavassoli FA. Mod Pathol. 1998;11(2):140–54.
22. Tot T, Tabár L. Mammographic–pathologic correlation of ductal carcinoma in situ of the breast using two- and three-dimensional large histologic sections. Semin Breast Dis. 2005;8:144–51.
23. Foschini MP, Flamminio F, Miglio R, et al. The impact of large sections on study of in situ and invasive duct carcinoma of the breast. Hum Pathol. 2007;38(12):1736–43.
24. Biesemier KW, Alexander C. Enhancement of mammographic-pathologic correlation utilizing large format histology for malignant breast disease. Semin Breast Dis. 2005;8:152–62.
25. Tot T, Ibarra JA. Examination of specimens from patients with ductal carcinoma in situ of the breast using large-format histology sections. Arch Pathol Lab Med. 2009;133(9):1361.
26. Allred DC, Anderson SJ, Park S, et al. Adjuvant tamoxifen reduces subsequent breast cancer in women with estrogen receptor-positive ductal carcinoma in situ. A study based on NSABP Protocol B-24. J Clin Oncol. 2012;30:1267–73.
27. Simpson PT, Reis-Filho JS, Gale T, Lakhani SR. Molecular evolution of breast cancer. J Pathol. 2005;205(2):248–54.
28. Lagios MD, Margolin FR, Westdahl PR, et al. Mammographically detected ductal carcinoma in situ: frequency of local recurrence following tylectomy and prognostic effect of nuclear grade on local recurrence. Cancer. 1989;63:616–24.
29. Wallis MG, Clements K, Kearins O, et al. The effect of DCIS grade on rate, type and time of recurrence after 15 years of follow up of screen-detected DCIS. Br J Cancer. 2012;106:1611–7.
30. Silverstein MJ, Lagios MD. Choosing treatment for patients with ductal carcinoma in situ: fine tuning the University of Southern California/Van Nuys Prognostic Index. J Natl Cancer Inst Monogr. 2010;2010:193–6.
31. Page DL, Dupont WD, Rogers LW. Ductal involvement by cells of atypical lobular hyperplasia in the breast: a long-term follow-up study of cancer risk. Hum Pathol. 1988;19:201–7.
32. Page DL, Kidd TE Jr, Dupont WD, Simpson JF, Rogers LW. Lobular neoplasia of the breast: higher risk for subsequent invasive cancer predicted by more extensive disease. Hum Pathol. 1991;22(12):1232–9.
33. Lakhani SR, Schnitt S, O'Malley F, van de Vijver M, Simpson PT, Palacios J. Lobular neoplasia. In: Lakhani SR, Ellis IO, Schnitt SJ, Tan PH, van de Vijver MJ, editors. WHO classification of tumours of the breast. Lyon: IARC Press; 2012. p. 78–80.
34. Schnitt SJ, Morrow M. Lobular carcinoma in situ: current concepts and controversies. Semin Diagn Pathol. 1999;16(3):209–23.
35. Bratthauer GL, Tavassoli FA. Lobular intraepithelial neoplasia: previously unexplored aspects assessed in 775 cases and their clinical implications. Virchows Arch. 2002;440:134–8.
36. Collins LC, Aroner SA, Connolly JL, Colditz GA, Schnitt SJ, Tamimi RM. Breast cancer risk by extent and type of atypical hyperplasia: an update from the nurses' health studies. Cancer. 2016;15(122):515–20.
37. Vos CB, Cleton-Jansen AM, Berx G, et al. E-cadherin inactivation in lobular carcinoma in situ of the breast: an early event in tumorigenesis. Br J Cancer. 1997;76:1131–3.
38. Lu YJ, Osin P, Lakhani SR, Di Palma S, Gusterson BA, Shipley JM. Comparative genomic hybridization analysis of lobular carcinoma in situ and atypical lobular hyperplasia and potential roles for gains and losses of genetic material in breast neoplasia. Cancer Res. 1998;58:4721–7.
39. Lakhani SR, Audretsch W, Cleton-Jensen AM, et al. on behalf of Eusoma. The management of lobular carcinoma in situ (LCIS). Is LCIS the same as ductal carcinoma in situ (DCIS). Eur J Cancer. 2006;42:2205.
40. Hartmann LC, Degnim AC, Santen RJ, Dupont WD, Ghosh K. Atypical hyperplasia of the breast—risk assessment and management options. N Engl J Med. 2015;372:78–89.
41. Hartmann LC, Radisky DC, Frost MH, et al. Understanding the premalignant potential of atypical hyperplasia through its natural history: a longitudinal cohort study. Cancer Prev Res (Phila). 2014;7:211–7.

42. Benson JR, Jatoi I, Toi M. Treatment of low-risk ductal carcinoma in situ: is nothing better than something? Lancet Oncol. 2016 Oct;17(10): e442-e451.
43. Ward EM, DeSantis CE, Chieh Lin C, et al. Cancer statistics: breast cancer in situ. CA Cancer J Clin. 2015;65:481–95.
44. de Mascarel I, Brouste V, Asad-Syed M, Hurtevent G, MacGrogan G. All atypia diagnosed at stereotactic vacuum-assisted breast biopsy do not need surgical excision. Mod Pathol. 2011;24:1198–206.
45. McGhan LJ, Pockaj BA, Wasif N, Giurescu ME, McCullough AE, Gray RJ. Atypical ductal hyperplasia on core biopsy: an automatic trigger for excisional biopsy? Ann Surg Oncol. 2012;19:3264–9.
46. Rudolf U, Jacks LS, Goldberg JI, et al. Nomogram for predicting the risk of local recurrence after breast-conserving surgery for ductal carcinoma in situ. J Clin Oncol. 2010;28:3762–9.
47. Miyake T, Shimazu K, Ohashi H, et al. Indication for sentinel lymph node biopsy for breast cancer when core biopsy shows ductal carcinoma in situ. Am J Surg. 2011;202:59–65.
48. Williams KE, Barnes NL, Cramer A, et al. Molecular phenotypes of DCIS predict overall and invasive recurrence. Ann Oncol. 2015;26:1019–25.

Text Recommended

Schnitt SJ, Collins LC. Biopsy interpretation of the breast. Philadelphia, PA: Wolters-Kluwer/Lippincott-Wilkins and Williams; 2013.
Hoda SA, Koerner FC, Brogi E, Rosen PP. Rosen's breast pathology. Philadelphia, PA: Lippincott Williams & Wilkins; 2014.
Modena S. Trattato di senologia. Padova: Piccin; 2006.

Benign and Malignant Ultrasound Semiology

6

Norran Hussein Said and Ashraf Selim

6.1 Cystic Abnormalities

Ultrasound is the method of choice to differentiate cystic from solid masses seen by mammography and evaluate palpable lumps in women under the age of 30. The simple breast cyst is the most common benign abnormality. Breast cysts are either simple, complicated or complex [1, 2]; refer to Table 6.1. A cyst is a fluid-filled cavity that is associated with terminal duct dilation. The clinical value of documenting a mammographic density by US as cystic alleviates the need for biopsy or aspiration and reduces the BIRADS score from 3 to 2.

Table 6.1 Characteristics of cysts

Simple	Complicated	Complex
– Anechoic nature – Well-circumscribed margins – Thin uniform echogenic capsule – Posterior acoustic enhancement – Thin edge shadows – Devoid of any Doppler signal – Becomes indented on compression	– Mobile internal echoes – Layered mobile fluid – No septa or mural nodules or other criteria of complex cysts	– Thick isoechoic septations – Mural nodules – Presence of a fibrovascular stalk – Microlobulated outline – Clustered microcysts

6.1.1 Simple Cyst

As in any body organ, a simple cyst will be a well-defined, round or oval anechoic mass with smooth borders and posterior acoustic enhancement. It will be devoid of any Doppler signal and may have edge shadows. Simple cysts are easily compressible, apart from those under tension which may not be compressed. US has an accuracy of 96–100% in evaluation of the internal matrix of masses seen on mammography [3, 4]. In certain cases when cysts exhibit angulated margins, they are usually surrounded by fibrous tissue. Scanning in two orthogonal planes is important to eliminate any suspicion of artefacts that may resemble septa or solid components, e.g., reverberation artefacts (Fig. 6.1), volume averaging or side lobe artefacts. Another common artefact is by inadequate gain which may cause false positives when gain is too high, making a cyst resemble a solid mass with ill-defined margins, and false negatives when gain is too low causing the reverse.

N.H. Said, M.D., F.R.C.R. (✉)
Breast Imaging Consultant, Egyptian National Breast Screening Program, Cairo; Nasser Institute, Cairo, Egypt
e-mail: norranhussein@yahoo.com

A. Selim, M.D.
Radiology Department, Cairo University, Cairo, Egypt
e-mail: a_selim@yahoo.com

D. Amy (ed.), *Lobar Approach to Breast Ultrasound*, https://doi.org/10.1007/978-3-319-61681-0_6

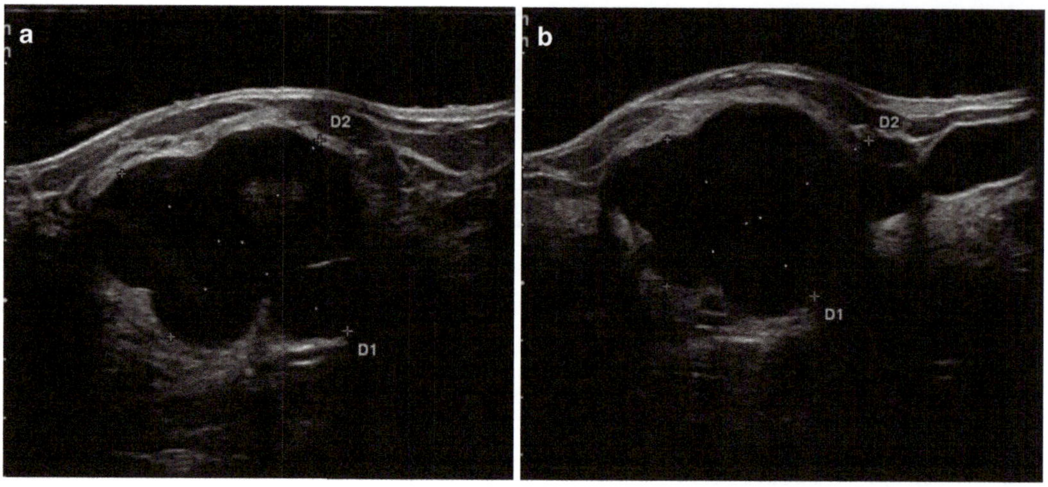

Fig. 6.1 (**a**) Simple cyst showing a reverberation artefact and (**b**) same cyst using different probe angulation without artefact

6.1.2 Complicated Cyst

A complicated cyst contains mobile internal echoes that may be layered and could shift with different patient positioning. Lack of mobility of these echoes may confuse with a solid mass. Biopsy is advisable only if the cyst is enlarging. The risk of malignancy among complicated breast cysts is less than 2%; these cysts generally can be managed with short-interval follow-up or aspiration. It is usually a proteinacous/haemorrhagic cyst or an abscess [1, 2, 5].

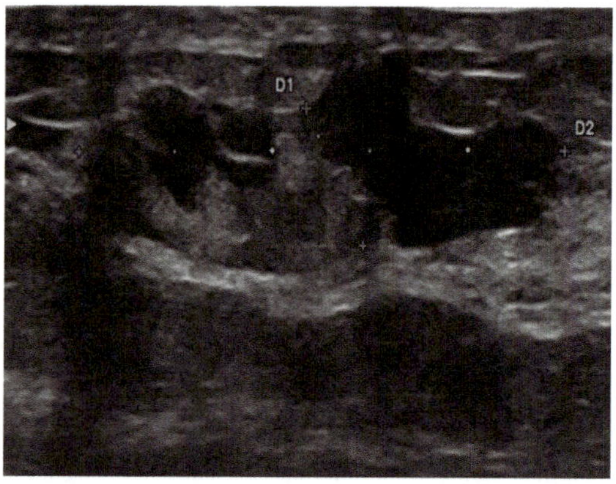

Fig. 6.2 A complex cyst with mixed anechoic and echogenic components

6.1.3 Complex Cyst

A complex cyst will contain anechoic (cystic) and echogenic (solid) components (Fig. 6.2). The most common cause of a complex cyst is the early stage of fibrocystic disease. The terminal ductal lobular unit or TDLU usually appears isoechoic and is formed of the terminal duct, the ductules and the intralobular stroma. Although these structures are all difficult to differentiate by US, in the setting of early-stage fibrocystic disease, cystic changes may predominate in one part, while fibrosis may predominate in another part. In late stages of fibrocystic disease, cystic changes predominate and their diagnosis is simple [1, 6]. However, complex cystic breast masses have a substantial chance of being malignant [7]; malignancy was reported in 23 and 31% of cases in two series [1, 5, 8]. Recognizing specific criteria of malignancy as thick isoechoic septations (Fig. 6.3), fibrovascular stalk or microlobulated outline is essential for diagnosis (Table 6.1).

Septations (Fig. 6.2) may be thick or thin, and echogenicity may vary, appearing iso- or hyperechoic. Thick isoechoic septations are suspicious for intracystic papillomas or carcinomas. Intracystic mural nodules are isoechoic internal projections extending from the cyst wall. They mainly represent papillary apocrine metaplasia (PAM) in fibrocystic disease (Fig. 6.4); never-

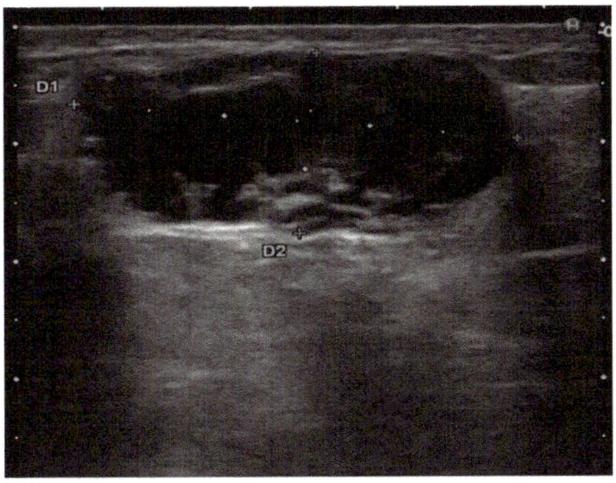

Fig. 6.3 A complex cyst with some thick isoechoic septations

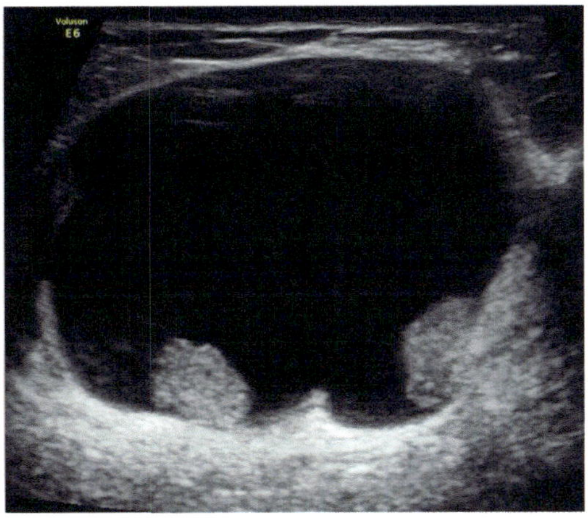

Fig. 6.4 This large cyst with multiple mural nodules, proved to be PAM

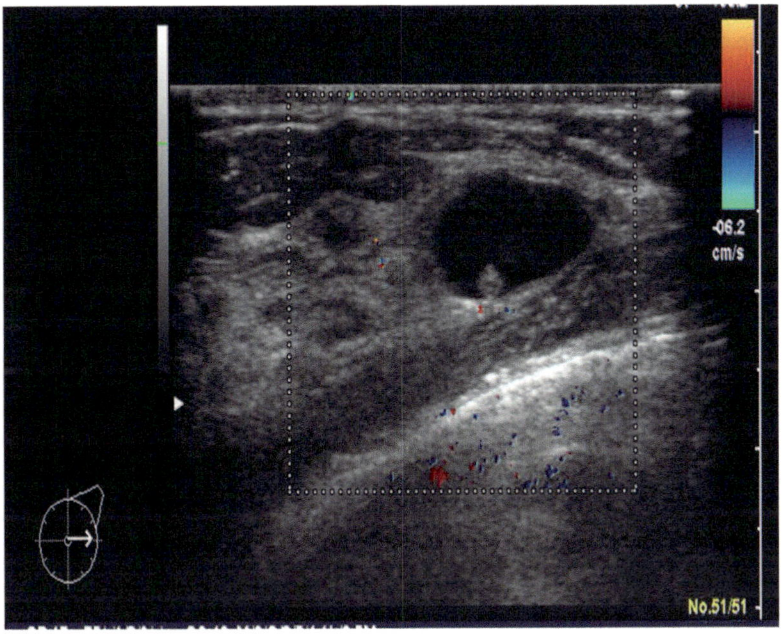

Fig. 6.5 A complex cyst with a mural nodule, that proved to be cancerous (courtesy of Dr. D Amy)

theless intracystic papilloma and carcinomas (Fig. 6.5) can't be ruled out. The main difference is their growth pattern; nodules of PAM would evolve within an already formed cyst, while nodules of a carcinoma/papilloma will grow within a duct, which later forms a cyst. In most cases, PAM does not have a fibrovascular stalk visible by colour Doppler. However, the presence of arterial flow within a mural nodule is suspicious for an intracystic neoplasm and requires biopsy. Microlobulated outline has also been associated with malignancy [6, 9]. Occasionally a cluster of microcysts can be associated with malignancy. This is a group of tiny anechoic foci that measure no more than 5–7 mm, with thin linear intervening septa. They occur in the lobular portion of the TDLU and are usually fibrocystic disease or apocrine metaplasia (Fig. 6.6).

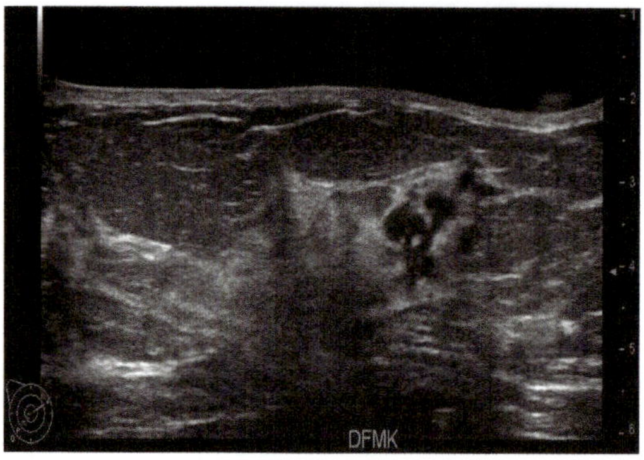

Fig. 6.6 Showing a cluster of microcysts (Courtesy of Dr. D Amy)

6.1.4 Specific Lesions

Galactocele: An avascular cyst with well-defined margins that appears during or shortly after lactation and contains milk. It results from obstruction of one or more lactiferous ducts with inspissation of milk products. It may have low-level internal echoes sometimes moving on compression due to the echogenic milky contents with posterior acoustic enhancement. A cyst with a fat-fluid level is a pathognomonic yet uncommon finding of a galactocele. It appears as a wavy line that separates the upper anechoic fatty liquid from the lower echogenic proteinaceous material.

Abscess: A hypoechoic mass with mobile fluid contents and usually well-defined margins yet may present with ill-defined outline. Its margins are thick and echogenic, will have posterior acoustic enhancement and may show a sinus tract (Fig. 6.7). It is usually tender on examination and often has Doppler flow only at its periphery.

Mastitis: Whether puerperal or nonpuerperal mastitis, it will appear as a diffuse or focal skin thickening along with subcutaneous increased fat echogenicity (Fig. 6.8) showing tubular and reticular anechoic structures suggestive of dilated lymphatics (interstitial oedema).

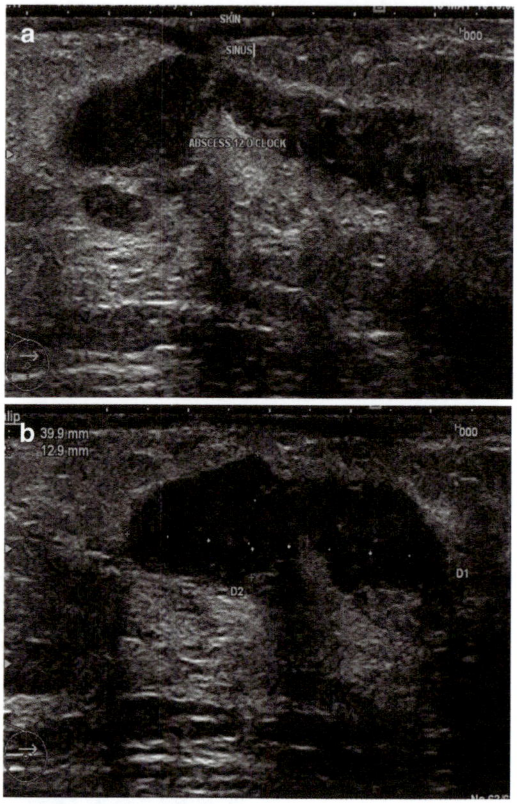

Fig. 6.7 (**a**, **b**) Showing a breast abscess. Note the sinus tract in (a) extending from the thickened dermis

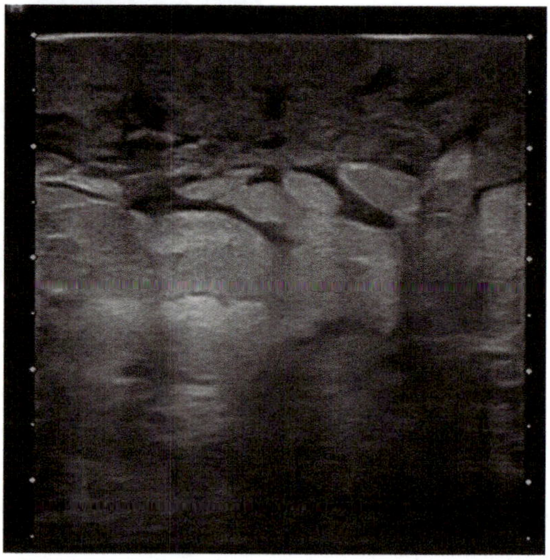

Fig. 6.8 A case of mastitis with skin thickening, subcutaneous oedema with diffuse echogenic texture

6.2 Solid Masses

The main goal of ultrasound is differentiating benign from malignant breast disease. This task although difficult has become more feasible with the advanced high resolution of equipment, operator experience and standardized interpretation criteria using the BIRADS lexicon. Nevertheless, there is still an overlap in analysis between some benign and malignant masses, where biopsy becomes advisable for final diagnosis.

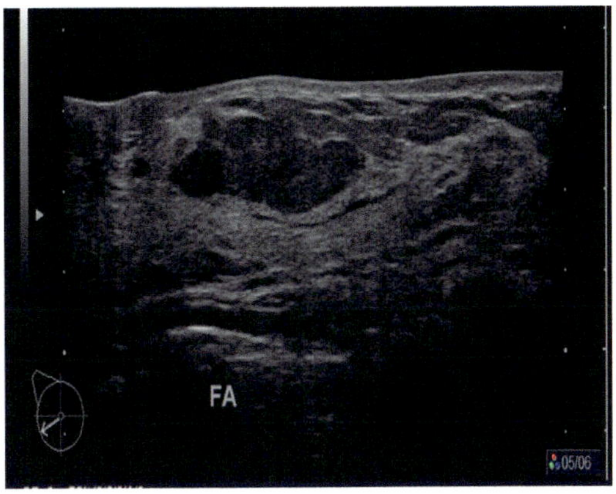

Fig. 6.10 A lobulated hypoechoic solid fibroadenoma. Note the linear duct nicely demonstrated below (courtesy of Dr. D Amy)

6.2.1 Benign Solid Masses

Benign solid nodule findings include hyperechoic texture/homogenous hypoechoic texture, sharply defined margin, wider than tall shape, minimal lobulations and a circumferential marginal capsule. These would be categorized as a BIRADS three finding, with a less than 2% risk of malignancy.

6.2.1.1 Fibroadenoma

Fibroadenomas are the most common solid breast mass in girls under 20 years of age. They are elliptical in shape, with minimal lobulations and with their longer axis aligned parallel to the chest wall. They are slightly hypoechoic to isoechoic texture to fat (Figs. 6.9 and 6.10). This depends on the variability of their stromal and epithelial elements. The more cellular components, the more hypoechoic nature of the mass. Those with acellular stroma can be almost isoechoic. Technical developments with harmonic imaging are beneficial in distinguishing isoechoic fibroadenomas from fat, by making them more hypoechoic. Usually fibroadenomas are homogenous in texture, with only 21% appearing heterogenous, which may be due to calcifications or internal echogenic septa. Its echogenic capsule actually represents a pseudocapsule composed of compressed breast tissue. This is unlike a cyst, whose capsule is formed of a duct or lobule wall. The presence of a capsule confirms that the edges of a mass are displacing rather than infiltrating the surrounding tissue. Sound transmission of fibroadenomas depends on their cellular content. Masses with high epithelial contents have enhanced sound transmission with posterior enhancement, while those with calcifications cause posterior shadowing. Most fibroadenomas have minimal epithelial content and normal sound transmission. During scanning, most fibroadenomas should appear mobile apart from those that have undergone infarction and become adherent to adjacent tissues. Most are mildly compressible; the greater the epithelial contents, the more compressible the fibroadenoma. Fibroadenomas that have undergone secretory changes due to pregnancy, lactation or birth control pills will be more mobile and more compressible than others. Only 40–50% of fibroadenomas have the classic findings of an elliptical or gently lobulated shape, wider than tall dimensions and a complete thin capsule [9, 10].

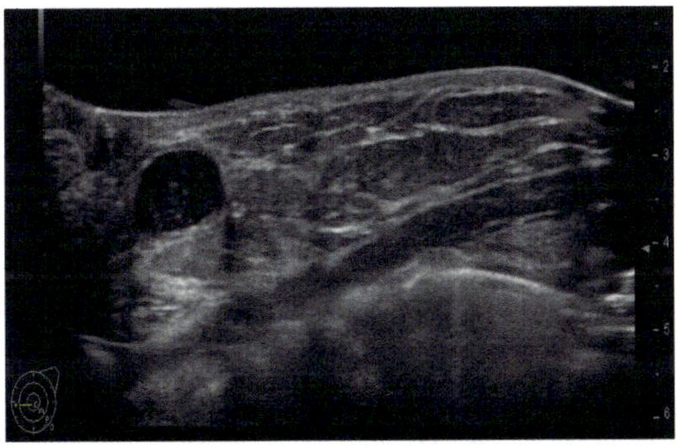

Fig. 6.9 A well-defined oval-shaped hypoechoic fibroadenoma (courtesy of Dr. D Amy)

6.2.1.2 Giant Fibroadenomas

These are large masses, often in young women (sometimes referred to as juvenile fibroadenoma), over 5–10 cm in diameter. Often, they appear lobulated and fill the entire viewing screen. They have well-circumscribed borders and are homogenous, yet some may show occasional septa and intermediate echogenicity. Slight posterior acoustic enhancement may be visible.

6.2.1.3 Papilloma

This benign mass will appear as a well-circumscribed lobulated hypoechoic/echogenic intraductal mass (Fig. 6.11). Occasionally it may show some vascularity on colour Doppler. Typically it will be retroareolar or central in location. Multiple papillomata (papillomatosis) will be mostly seen peripheral in location (Fig. 6.12) and are associated with duct ectasia.

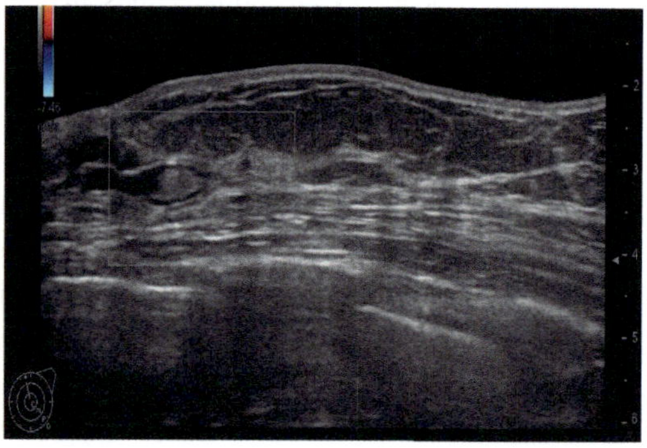

Fig. 6.11 A dilated duct with a single intraductal echogenic papilloma (courtesy of Dr. D Amy)

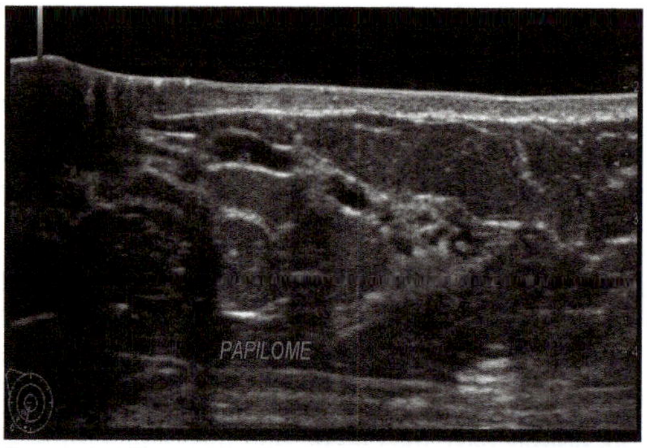

Fig. 6.12 Multiple echogenic papillomata within a dilated duct (Courtesy of Dr. D Amy)

6.2.1.4 Hamartomas

A circumscribed mass containing a heterogenous mixture of fat and fibroglandular tissue echo patterns surrounded by a pseudocapsule. Occasionally they may contain cysts. Compressibility and through transmission will vary according to its predominant components.

6.2.1.5 Lipomas

Homogenous well-circumscribed mass of isoechoic or hyperechoic texture to fat, causing no disruption of surrounding tissues and no posterior acoustic changes. They are compressible in most cases.

6.2.1.6 Haemangiomas

Hyper- or isoechoic mass with heterogenous echogenicity and strong vascularity on colour Doppler, yet no surrounding tissue disruption. No posterior acoustic changes. A hypoechoic area within may represent vessel thrombosis.

6.2.1.7 Focal Fibrosis

This is a benign stromal proliferation with obliteration of milk ducts and acini. US appearance has no definite characteristics, yet the area in question usually appears slightly more echogenic.

6.2.1.8 Diabetic Mastopathy (DM)

It usually presents in premenopausal diabetic women, 20 years after onset of type 1 diabetes. US findings are suspicious and may show angular margins, ill-defined edges and posterior shadowing. Multifocal and bilateral findings may be present. Colour Doppler will probably be negative, as DM is avascular.

6.2.1.9 Pseudoangiomatous Stromal Hyperplasia (PASH)

A benign focal overgrowth of stromal tissue that is usually similar to normal fibroglandular tissue by US. However, sometimes it may appear similar to a fibroadenoma as a focal hypoechoic mass or to a carcinoma with ill-defined edges and angular microlobulated margins.

6.2.1.10 Adenosis

This represents proliferation of glandular tissue (small duct segments and acini) with increase in periductal and perilobular tissue. Sclerosing adenosis implies periductal sclerosis and constriction of lobular lumina. US findings are only microcystic changes. Microcalcifications visible on mammography will be difficult to visualize by US.

6.2.1.11 Atypical Ductal/Lobular Hyperplasia

Benign abnormalities that have no specific US features.

6.2.1.12 Fat Necrosis

Usually appears as an irregular hypoechoic mass with posterior shadowing in the early stage. Late-stage fat necrosis may form an oil cyst with hypoechoic/echogenic texture and calcified margins. It is typically associated with trauma and postoperative scarring.

6.2.2 Malignant Solid Masses

According to Tibor Tot in 2005, a hypothesis that breast carcinoma is a lobar disease from the start correlates with finding simultaneous or asynchronous foci that develop within a single sick lobe. More than one sick lobe may also be present in the same woman on the rare occasion of multicentric or bilateral cancers. Because the malignant transformation may appear at any locus of the sick lobe, its timing will determine the focality of the disease [11–13]. Three patterns are seen most often; if most of the potentially malignant cells within the sick lobe are transformed into malignant clones simultaneously, the entire lobe will become cancerous causing an extensive tumour, which is easily recognized on US [14]. The 2nd pattern is when only a segment of the lobe is affected, making the tumour burden relatively limited. The 3rd pattern is the peripheral type which involves the lobules usually without the segmental and lactiferous ducts. The tumour burden is low but may be extensive because the involved lobules may be distant from each other in a large sick lobe. Typical examples of this form are LCIS and DCIS. Low-grade lesions tend to be localized within the terminal ducts and lobules where high-grade lesions often involve the larger ducts [15].

There are various sonographic findings that are suspicious for malignancy. However, in 2004, Stavros divided suspicious findings into hard, soft and mixed. Hard findings have a higher PPV and are associated with invasive malignancy. They include spiculations, angular margins and acoustic shadowing (Figs. 6.13 and 6.14). Soft findings include duct extension, branch pattern and calcifications and are associated with DCIS. Mixed findings such as microlobulations, taller than wide shape, and hypoechogenicity can be seen in both invasive Ca and DCIS. Sound transmission is typically enhanced in medullary and colloid carcinomas and elicits shadowing in invasive ductal and tubular cancers [9, 16]. Characterizing small less than 5 mm cancers is the most challenging US task, especially if their shape is oval, with difficulty identifying other criteria (Figs. 6.15 and 6.16).

With the theory of the sick lobe in mind, the issue of multifocality/multicentricity is always a diagnostic challenge, especially in evaluating the dense breast by mammography. Multifocal tumours are described as multiple tumours within the same quadrant of the breast (Figs. 6.17, 6.18, 6.19). Multicentricity implies multiple tumours in different quadrants of the breast or separated by 5 cm or more. The subareolar region is the most common site for additional foci of invasive disease. Tot and Tabar in 2005 found that only one third of cancers were unifocal, one third multifocal

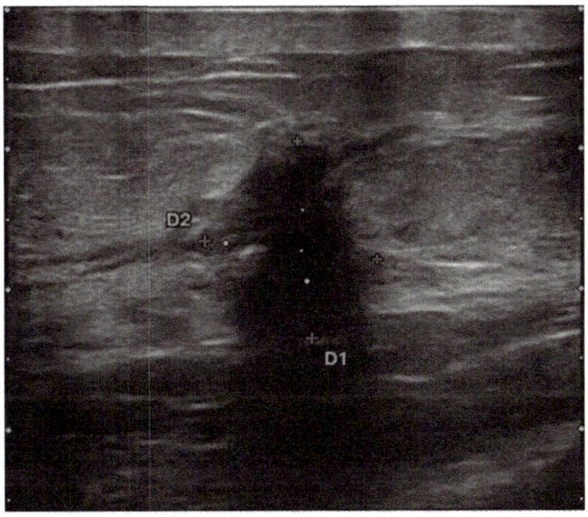

Fig. 6.13 A classical hypoechoic malignant mass is seen with spiculated borders and taller than wide dimensions, as well as posterior shadowing

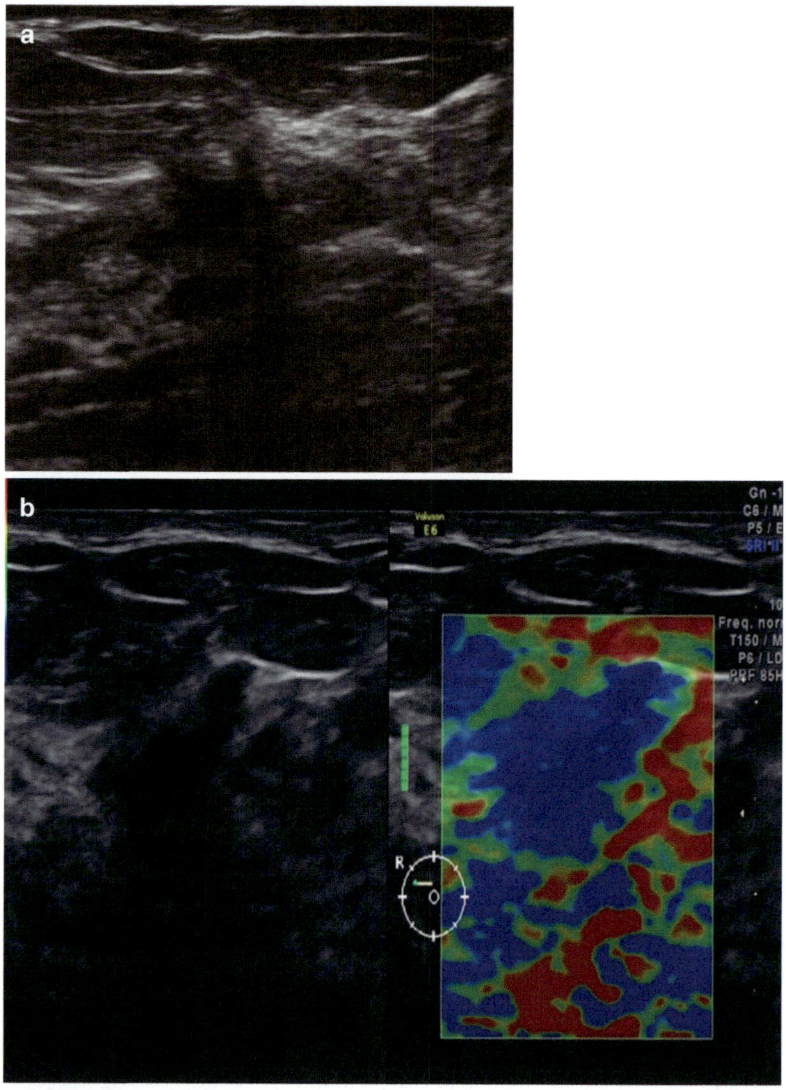

Fig. 6.14 (**a**) A focal hypoechoic cancerous mass is seen provoking the surrounding glandular tissue and (**b**) showing its hard suspicious findings on elastography

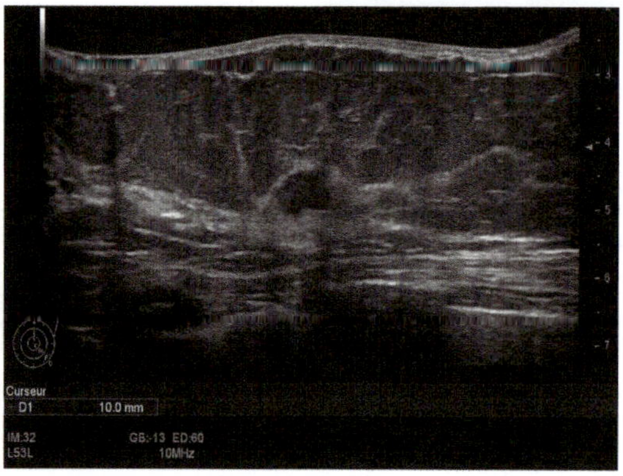

Fig. 6.15 A small 10 mm rather oval cancer with irregular margins and echogenic halo (courtesy of Dr. D Amy)

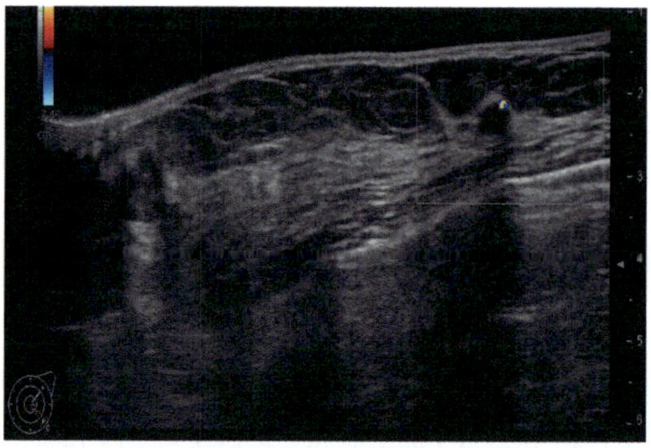

Fig. 6.16 A focal marginal vascularity in a small 5 mm oval-shaped cancer (courtesy of Dr. D Amy)

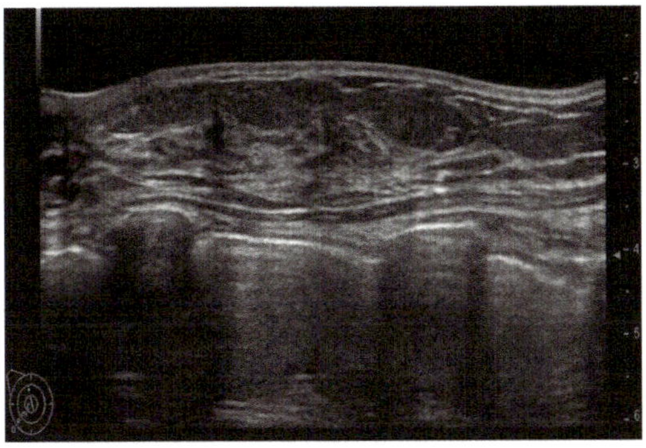

Fig. 6.17 Two tiny hypoechoic foci of cancer are seen along the same plane within the same sick lobe (courtesy of Dr. D Amy)

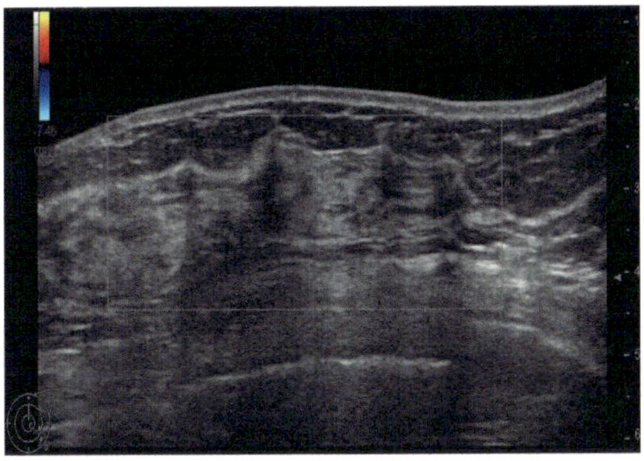

Fig. 6.18 Four cancerous foci are seen arranged in a linear consecutive pattern within the same sick lobe (courtesy of Dr. D Amy)

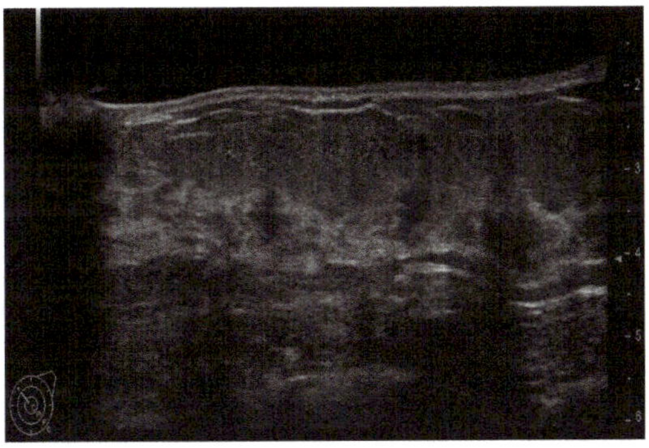

Fig. 6.19 Three multifocal cancerous foci (courtesy of Dr. D Amy)

in situ components and one third multifocal invasive components. Breast cancer is not necessarily small at its earliest stages of development; on the contrary, it is widespread and multifocal in the majority of cases [15].

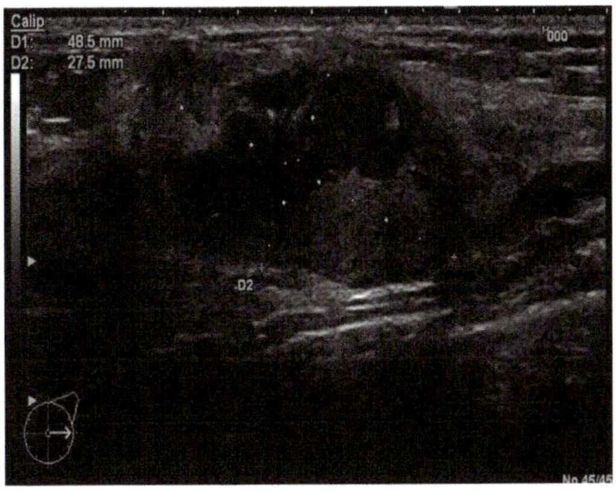

Fig. 6.20 A large malignant mass with central necrotic breakdown

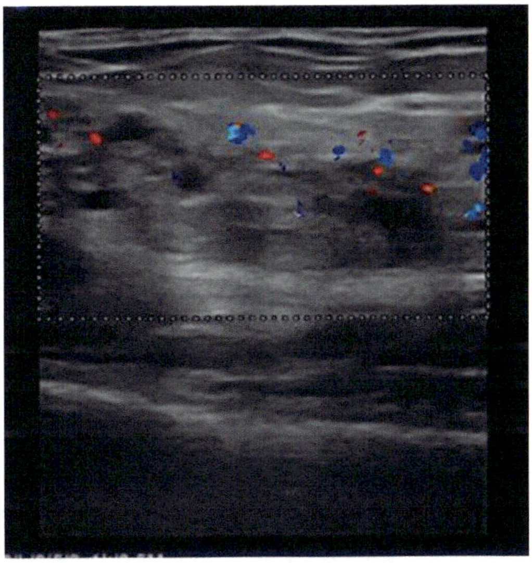

Fig. 6.21 Intraductal spread from an invasive duct carcinoma is demonstrated by linear nodularity along a ductal plane with scattered vascularity on color doppler

High-grade cancers are usually associated with necrosis that worsens its prognosis. These cancers are usually soft and well defined (Fig. 6.20). Both blood flow and oxygen levels are reduced in necrosis preventing immunologic and chemotherapeutic agents from reaching them. Necrosis may be liquifactive, haemorrhagic or fibrotic. Intraductal spread is also associated with higher tumour grade and its site of origin (Fig. 6.21). The more central the tumour, the more extensive the intraductal spread [16].

One of the paths of least resistance for invasion is along Cooper's ligaments toward the skin. This causes flattening and dimpling of the skin. Lymph vessel invasion is difficult to be detected by imaging studies, except in certain cases where we find the interstitial oedema that suggests lymphatic obstruction by malignant spread. It is associated with a higher risk of axillary lymph node metastases, which implies more aggressive disease.

6.2.2.1 DCIS

If an in situ carcinoma is present behind the nipple, it almost always involves only one lactiferous duct. This finding confirms the theory of the sick lobe, because otherwise multiple ducts are expected to be involved. However, DCIS usually has no specific US characteristics. Sometimes a dilated duct may be seen and very rarely a solid intraductal mass.

6.2.2.2 Invasive Ductal Carcinoma (IDC)

The pattern of intraductal carcinoma spread within the breast has a pyramid-like shape with apex at the nipple [13, 17]. This cancer invades the ductal basement membrane. It forms an irregular indistinct mass hypo- or isoechoic, rarely hyperechoic, with an echogenic halo, posterior shadowing, taller and wide and with spiculations disrupting the surrounding glandular tissue.

6.2.2.3 Invasive Lobular Carcinoma (ILC)

This tumour may appear as a hypo- or isoechoic mass in the nodular form and as an area of distortion in the diffuse form. It may cause focal disruption of the surroundings and subtle posterior shadowing. The mass type may confuse with invasive duct carcinoma. The diffuse type is difficult to detect (Fig. 6.22).

6.2.2.4 Invasive Papillary Carcinoma

This tumour develops from a benign papilloma and therefore appears as an oval or lobulated mass, rarely irregular shaped. It should be distinguished from intracystic papillary cancer which is a mural nodule within a well-defined cyst (Fig. 6.23).

6.2.2.5 Medullary and Mucinous Carcinoma

Imaging findings of these two tumours are very similar, usually a well-circumscribed tumour with microlobulations (Fig. 6.24). They can appear iso- or hypoechoic with enhanced sound transmission.

6.2.2.6 Tubular Carcinoma

This cancer is indistinguishable by imaging from IDC.

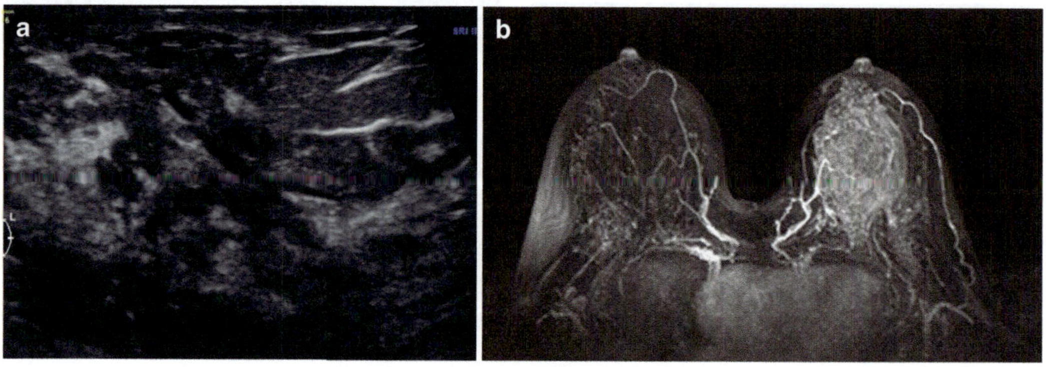

Fig. 6.22 (**a**) US showing a left para-areolar area of architectural distortion and altered texture. (**b**) MRI showing an enhancing mass on maximum intensity projection of the same case. Pathology: ILC

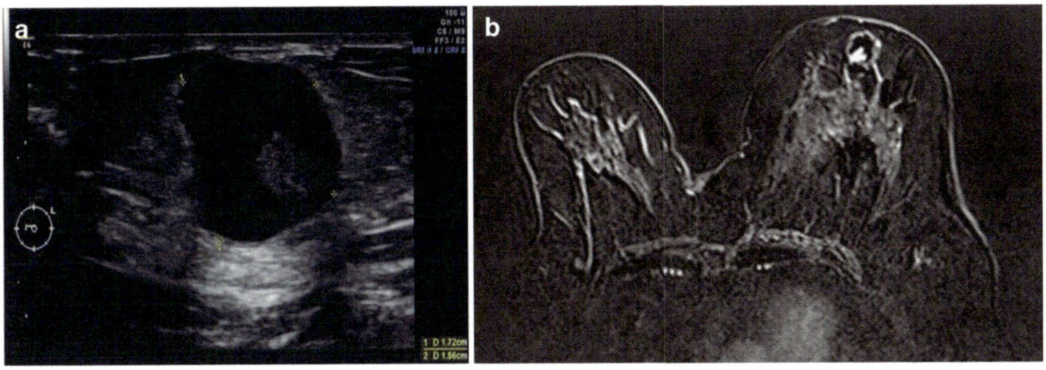

Fig. 6.23 (**a**) Showing a cyst with internal mural nodule in the LT retroareolar region. b) Axial subtraction MRI showing marginal enhancement of the cyst wall and enhancement of the mural nodule. Pathology: intracystic papillary carcinoma

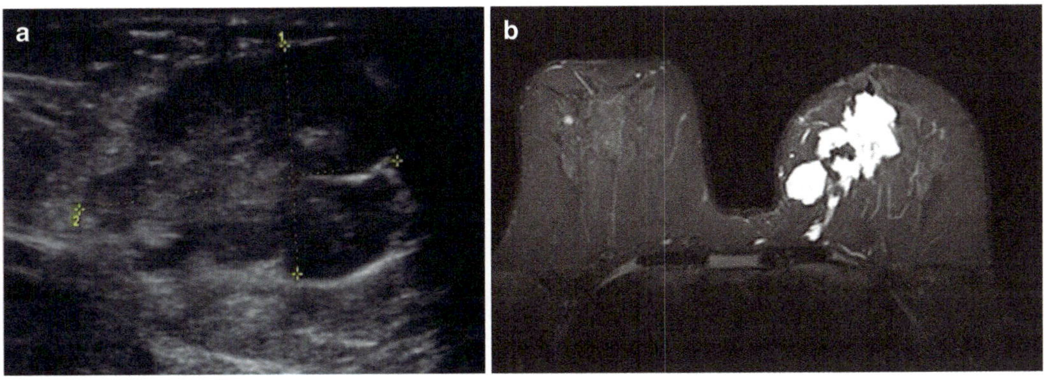

Fig. 6.24 (**a**) Showing a lobulated solid mass. (**b**) Axial T2 IR image showing bright signal intensity of the same mass on MRI (classical sign of medullary and mucinous carcinoma). Pathology: mucinous carcinoma

6.2.2.7 Inflammatory Breast Cancer

Asymmetric diffuse skin thickening is seen with oedematous changes of subcutaneous tissues in the form of increased fat echogenicity with tubular and reticular anechoic structures suggestive of dilated lymphatics (interstitial oedema). A mass may be present but often no focal mass is identified. The presence of diffuse vascularity by power Doppler is occasionally seen.

6.2.2.8 Paget's Disease

A rare form of DCIS involving the nipple that causes its erosion. US may show skin thickening around the areola, with possible retroareolar duct dilatation. Late-stage Paget's carcinoma will show the classical reviewed findings of a malignant mass.

6.2.2.9 Phyllodes Tumour

Usually hypoechoic to surrounding fat with a firm echogenic capsule. Differentiation between benign and malignant phyllodes is challenging, yet malignant phyllodes may have angular margins. There is a lack of desmoplastic reaction, with evidence of enhanced sound transmission in most cases. Sometimes it is associated with internal calcifications and small 3 mm cysts. Lesions that are larger than 8 cm in size, or which contain cysts larger than 3 mm, are mostly malignant.

6.2.2.10 Lymphoma

Non-Hodgkin's lymphoma is more common than Hodgkin's disease. Usually there is a secondary involvement through systemic disease, with bilateral axillary lymphadenopathy. The mass is well defined and hypoechoic with enhanced sound transmission and homogenous texture. The sonographic appearance is that of a highly cellular lesion with low desmoplastic reaction.

6.2.2.11 Sarcoma

It is typically heterogenous with high vascularity on colour Doppler and elicits normal to enhanced through transmission (Fig. 6.25). Sarcomas may arise from a phyllodes tumour. They can be circumscribed or spiculated.

6.2.2.12 Metastases

Characteristics of metastases are usually according to the primary cancer. Usually they are highly cellular and so don't create a desmoplastic reaction (Fig. 6.26). Nodules are usually oval shaped and well defined with hypoechoic texture and without an echogenic halo as their desmoplastic reaction is minimal. However, sometimes, they may cause an inflammatory reaction with an ill-defined area of increased echogenicity. On colour Doppler, most metastases are highly vascular; this is attributed to their haematogenous route of spread.

6.2.2.13 Recurrent Cancer

As reviewed in earlier chapters, the theory of the sick lobe implies that it is already malconstructed from its initialization, and the carcinoma develops after several decades of postnatal life necessary for the accumulation of genetic alterations. Thus the biological timing may be valid for a very long period of time. Consequently breast

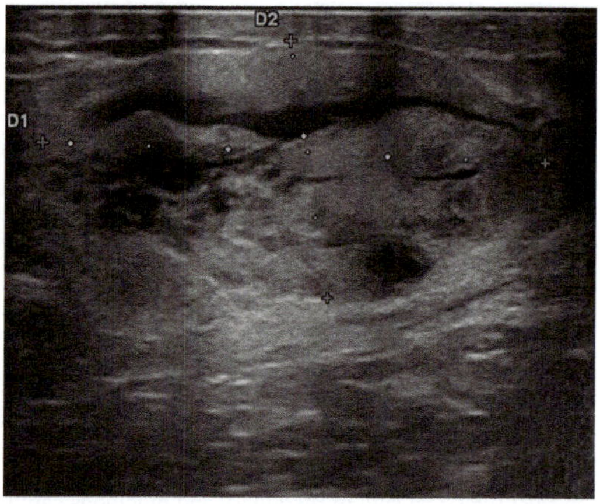

Fig. 6.25 US of a well-defined mass with mixed isoechoic and linear hypoechoic areas, proved to be a sarcoma

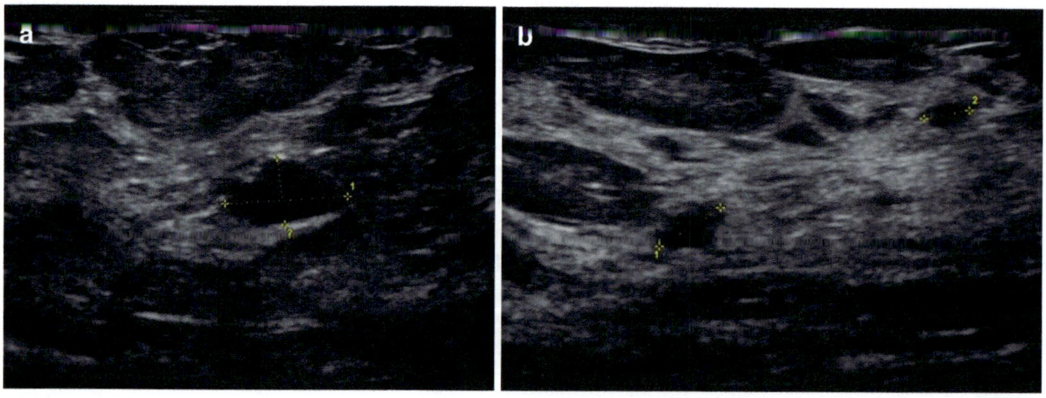

Fig. 6.26 (**a**, **b**) showing multiple metastatic deposits

carcinoma is a lifelong disease that can be interrupted only by the elimination or destruction of the sick lobe. The vast majority of local recurrences appear in the area adjacent to the surgical scar, indicating that they have developed in part of the surgically removed sick lobe [13]. By US, recurrent cancer is difficult to differentiate from postoperative scarring, unless the case is advanced. Findings would be similar to invasive cancer with an irregular spiculated mass, posterior shadowing and colour Doppler vascularity. In these cases, contrast studies by mammography or MRI would be advisable.

References

1. Berg WA, Campassi CI, Loffe OB. Cystic lesions of the breast: sonographic-pathologic correlation. Radiology. 2003;227(1):183–191.2.
2. Mendelson EB, Berg WA, Merritt CR. Towards a standardized breast ultrasound lexicon, BI-RADS: ultrasound. Semin Roentgenol. 2001;36(3):217–25.
3. Hilton SV, Leopold GR, Olson LK, Willson SA. Real time breast ultrasonography: application in 300 consequetive patients. AJR. 1986;147:479–86.
4. Jellins J, Kossof G, Reeve TS. Detection and classification of liquid filled masses in the breast by gray scale echography. Radiology. 1977;125:205–12.
5. Doshi DJ, March DE, Crisi MG, Coughlin BF. Complex cystic breast masses: diagnostic approach and imaging pathologic correlation. Radiographics. 2007;27:S53–64.
6. Stavros AT. Sonographic evaluation of breast cysts. In: Breast ultrasound. Philadelphia, PA: Lippincott Williams & Wilkins; 2004. p. 276–350.
7. Venta LA, Kim JP, Pelloski CE, Morrow M. Management of complex breast cysts. AJR Am J Roentgenol. 1999;173(5):1331–6.
8. Doshi DJ, March DE, Coughlin BF, Crisi GM. Accuracy of ultrasound-guided percutaneous biopsy of complex cystic breast masses. In: Radiological Society of North America scientific assembly and annual meeting program. Oak Brook, Ill: Radiological Society of North 1- Radiological Society of North America 655; 2006.
9. Rahbar G, Sie AC, Hansen GC, Prince JS, Melany ML, Reynolds HE, Jackson VP, Sayre JW, Bassett LW. Benign versus malignant solid breast masses: US differentiation. Radiology. 1999;213(3):889–94.
10. Stavros AT. Benign solid nodules; specific pathologic diagnosis. In: Breast ultrasound. Philadelphia, PA: Lippincott Williams & Wilkins; 2004. p. 529–96.
11. Tot T. DCIS, cytokeratins, and the theory of the sick lobe. Virchows Arch. 2005;447:1–8.
12. Tot T. The theory of the sick breast lobe and the possible consequences. Int J Surg Pathol. 2007;15:369–75.
13. Tot T. The theory of the sick lobe. Breast Cancer. 2011:1–17. https://doi.org/10.1007/978-1-84996-314-5_1.
14. Tabar L, Chen HT, Yen MFA, Tot T, Tung TH, Chen LS, Chiu YH, Duffy SW, Smith RA. Mammographic features can predict long term outcomes reliably in women with 1-14mm invasive carcinoma. Cancer. 2004;101:1745–59.
15. Tot T, Tabar L. Radiologic-pathologic correlation of ductal carcinoma insitu of the breast using 2 and 3 dimensional large histologic sections. Semin Breast Dis. 2005;8:144–51.
16. Stavros AT. Malignant solid nodules; specific types. In: Breast ultrasound. Philadelphia, PA: Lippincott Williams & Wilkins; 2004. p. 597–688.
17. Mai KT, Yazdi HM, Burns BF, Perkins DG. Pattern of distribution of intraductal and infiltrating ductal carcinoma: three dimensional study using serial coronal giant sections of the breast. Hum Pathol. 2000;31:464–74.

Breast Elastography

7

Dominique Amy, Jeremy Bercoff, and Ellison Bibby

7.1 Introduction

With more than a decade's experience of practising elastography, and after carrying out a large number of examinations using both techniques (strain and shear wave) and taking part in numerous work and research groups, in particular the one of the WFUMB to lay down guidelines in breast ultrasound in 2015 (WFUMB guidelines and recommendations on the clinical use of ultrasound elastography: Ultrasound Med. and Biol: 41(5):1126–47 March 2015), we are faced with specific remarks, which calls for some comments:

1. The first cause of error is linked to a wrong positioning of the patient and of the probe: one cannot carry out an elastographic examination with a probe held obliquely from the breast, as for B-mode imaging, in strain or SWE (see Chap. 3). It is absolutely essential that the patient should be in an internally oblique position for the examination of the external part of the breast and in an externally oblique position for the internal zone of the breast. The probe will be perfectly horizontal and strictly perpendicular to the skin (with addition of a footplate for the strain elastography) and held by the fingertips without any excessive compression. That way, the perfect immobility required in SWE will be easy to maintain.
2. The second cause of error which is often noted lies in the excessive pressure on the breast. Many echographers follow the rule of compressing the breast in order to flatten it and thus increase the resolution, which is true for general echography but is best avoided in breast ultrasound (see Chaps. 3 and 4). Furthermore, as one compresses the breast, the elasticity of its components changes and the elastographic results are distorted. Confusion also arises from the use of the term 'compression' in the strain technique. Elastography is a technique of electronic palpation exercising ad hoc minimal pressure but requiring an inversion of pressure for superficial lesions. For these little minute shallow superficial lesions, the strain technique has to be modified. One must produce an inversion of pressure in the breast, which causes an extension of the lesion (we call this technique the 'Parkinson-vibrating technique'). This technique must be coupled with superficial,

D. Amy, M.D. (✉)
Centre du sein, Aix-en-Provence, France
e-mail: domamy@wanadoo.fr

J. Bercoff, Ph.D.
R&D Ultrasound Dept, SSI SupersonicImagine, Aix-en-Provence, France
e-mail: jeremy.bercoff@supersonicimagine.fr

E. Bibby, M.Sc.
Hitachi Medical Systems UK, Wellingborough, UK
e-mail: e.bibby@hitachi-medical-systems.com.uk

D. Amy (ed.), *Lobar Approach to Breast Ultrasound*, https://doi.org/10.1007/978-3-319-61681-0_7

rapid vibrations (unlike the slow compression advised for deeper lesions). The combination of vibration and inversion of pressure is ideal for any anomaly located in the superficial part of the breast. To summarise we will use three types of different compression/vibration: no manual compression, minimal vibration and significant compression.

As concerns the SWE technique, some authors have criticised the method as they obtained inaccurate results for small benign lesions. These anomalies concern fatty breast of older women with a very high degree of involution and a poor amount of connective structures. The radiologist having at his disposal this characteristic mammogram knows that, in this specific case, he has to precompress the breast lightly in order to achieve a satisfactory result. This problem does not occur with younger women whose lobes are perfectly shaped. Elastography is an essential complementary examination in senology, but it has to be adapted to the various morphological types of breasts.

3. The third cause of error is due to the size and difficult positioning of the regions of interest (ROI) in the calculations of the ratio (fat/lesion ratio F/LR), that is, the ratio of elasticity between the softest and the stiffest tissues. The first ROI must necessarily be located on the lesion itself and the second at the level of the subcutaneous fat. Various locations have been suggested by the users (same depth as the lesion itself, at the level of the underlying muscle, etc.), but none of these is satisfactory because they contradict the very definition of the F/L ratio.
4. Elastography is not a screening technique, but it must be considered as a method of analysis for a lesion already uncovered in B-mode and for which complementary information is desirable. Referring ourselves to the enclosed bibliography, let us simply recall that the use of elastography has in particular made it possible to reduce by 50% the number of unnecessary punctures concerning either benign lesions or confirmed physiological variations. This figure can in itself vindicate the good practice of echography/elastography and convince the users that minimum basic training in this technique is desirable.
5. The elastography is an ideal complementary exam for minimal breast cancer (from 4 to 15 mm) not useful for big lesions and for liquid collections (haematoma, cyst, lymphocele, abscess ectasia aneurysm with the specific blue-green-red sign in strain elastography or blind area with SWE). Elastography has been proving a good accuracy in the characterisation of benign or suspicious lesion as a complementary technique of B-mode imaging and improved accuracy in interventional ultrasound (puncture of millimetric cancer or a non-mass lesion). Elastography has a great potential to evaluate the management of neoadjuvant chemotherapy treatment and lastly for the evaluation of histologic informations and of the lesion aggressiveness.

7.2 Real-Time Tissue Elastography RTE

7.2.1 Background

Palpation is a diagnostic technique that has been used for millennia and is still considered valuable today, both by clinicians and for patient self-examination, especially in the detection of breast tumours where most focal cancers have a high stiffness contrast compared to both the normal breast and many benign lesions. Real-time tissue elastography (RTE) is a non-invasive method for creating images of tissue stiffness and so offers the potential of early-stage differentiation of benign and malignant tissue whilst overcoming some of the significant limitations of palpation: that of the skill and experience required of the examiner, as well as the ability to detect small, less superficial lesions.

7.2.2 Technical Principles of RTE

Real-time tissue elastography (RTE) is a strain imaging technique where the transducer is used to apply repetitive minimal compression/vibration to the tissues. The subsequent tissue displacement is tracked between pairs of RF-echo frames and the strain calculated from the axial gradient of the displacements. The ratio of stress/strain is called Young's or elastic modulus. Under an equal amount of stress, a stiff region strains less than surrounding soft tissue, so a display of the strain distribution provides an image of relative tissue stiffness. Using a colour map to code different magnitudes of strain, the two-dimensional strain image can be translucently superimposed on the conventional B-mode image, allowing easier interpretation of the spatial relationship between the strain data and the morphology (Fig. 7.1).

Real-time tissue elastography is easily implemented into conventional ultrasound platforms without the need for specialised hardware. RTE is an elasticity imaging method that uses the standard imaging transducer with freehand manipulation it produces images covering the full field of view at real-time frame rates, with a spatial resolution similar to the conventional B-mode ultrasound; and has the ability to generate sufficient contrast resolution to display small differences in tissue stiffness (has a wide dynamic range for strain estimation) [1].

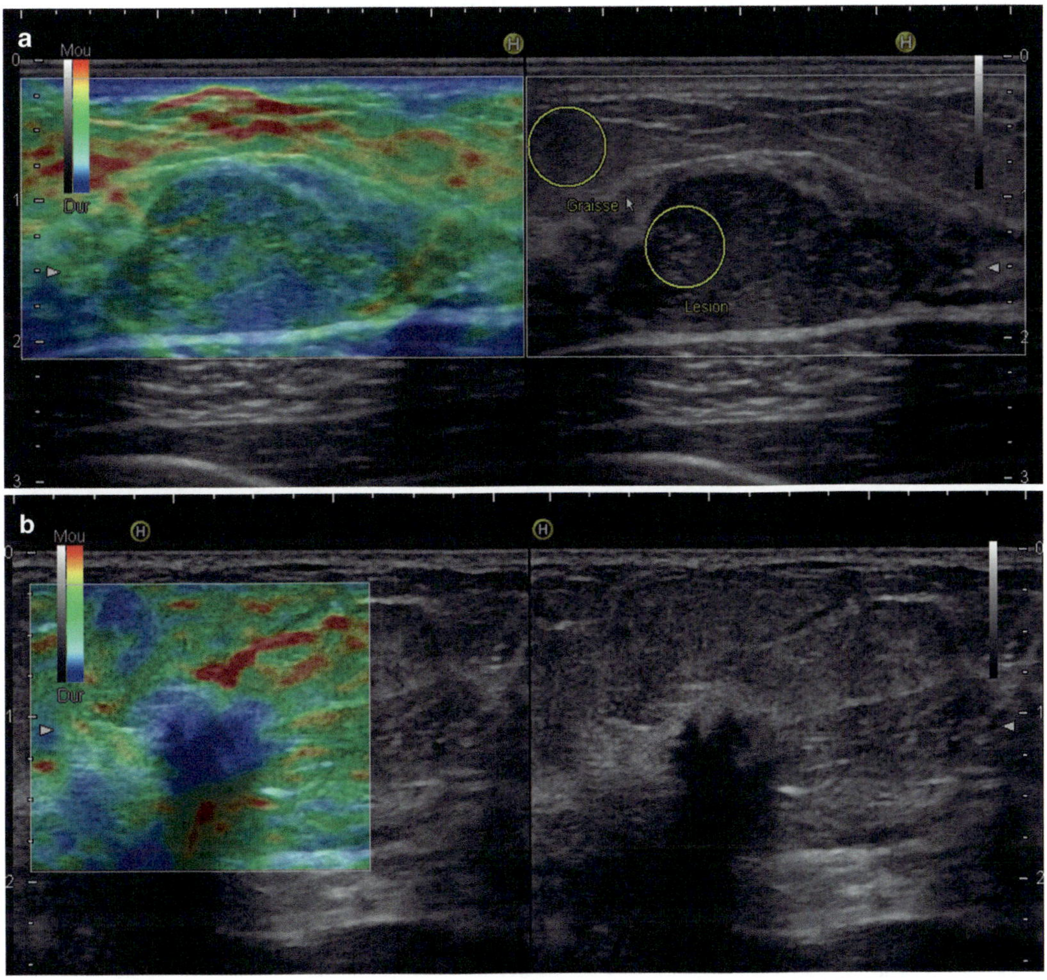

Fig. 7.1 (**a**) Example of a benign (soft) and (**b**) a malignant (hard) breast lesion. The translucent display of the strain image superimposed on the conventional B-mode does not hide the tumour architecture seen in the B-mode image

7.2.3 Practical Application

Strain elastograms generated by palpation with the imaging transducer provide a natural extension of the B-mode imaging examination, but as with all new imaging methods, practice of the technique and adherence to some basic principles are required.

7.2.3.1 Selection of Transducer

The transducer frequency should be chosen as for B-mode imaging: lower frequencies will allow assessment of deeper lesions and higher frequencies offer better spatial resolution. A range of frequencies between 5 and 18 MHz is available. The attenuation can be assessed from the B-mode image: a good quality B-mode image with adequate penetration to the pectoralis muscle is a pre-requisite to obtaining a good quality elastogram. Another consideration for transducer selection is the size and shape of the active face that is in contact with the patient. Linear transducers with an active length of 40, 50 and 92 mm are available for breast scanning. For proper assessment of large tumours, or for evaluation of multifocal lesions that develop along the ductal axis, the wider field of view offered by a long linear transducer is recommended (Fig. 7.2).

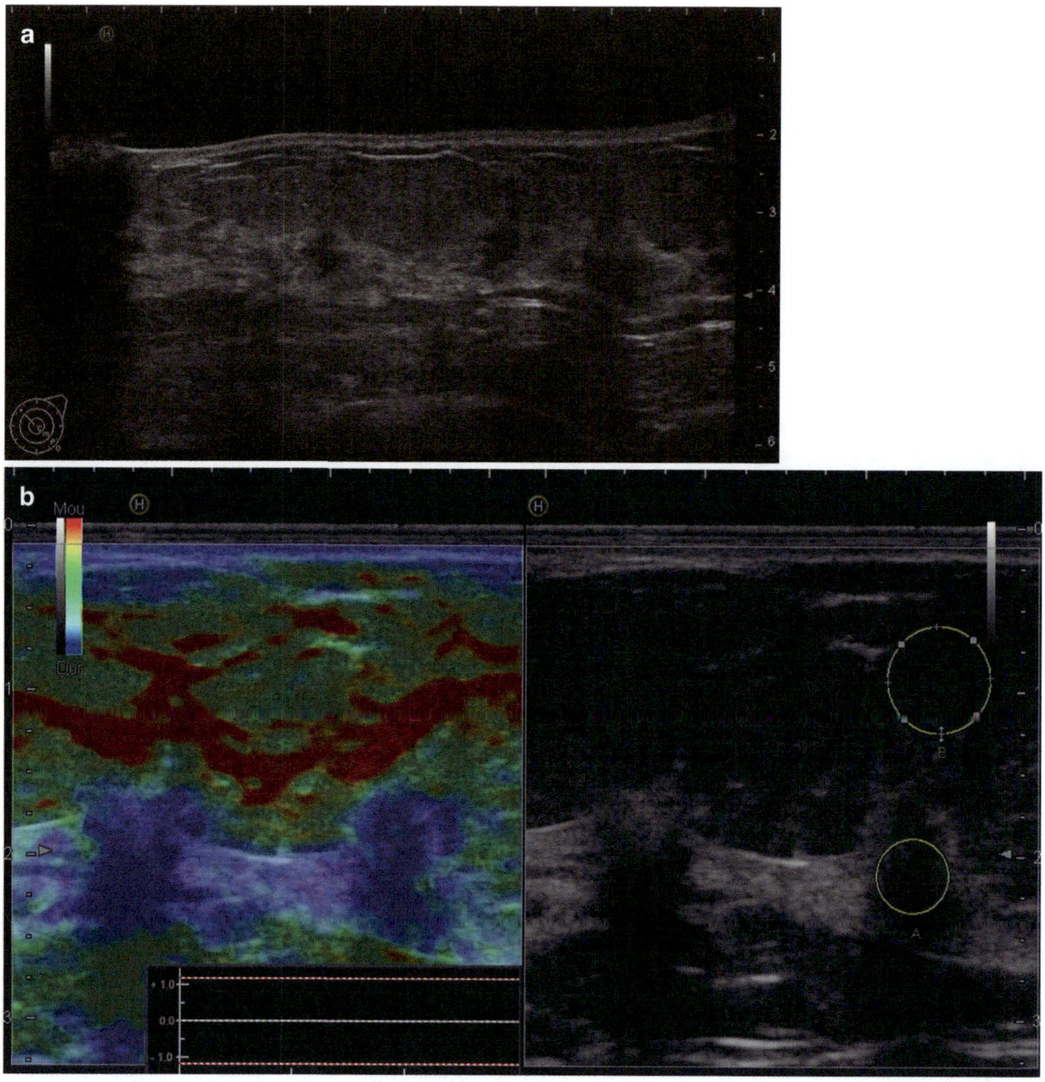

Fig. 7.2 (a) B-mode example of a multifocal cancer using the 92 mm linear array transducer. (b) Transducer with 50 mm footprint used to show bifocal cancer using RTE

7.2.3.2 Applying Compression/Use of Footplate Extenders

Real-time tissue elastography is accurate for a wide range of compression speeds and amplitude of movement and therefore well suited to a free-hand compression/vibration technique. The most likely cause of failure to achieve consistent, reproducible elastograms is the use of too strong precompression. Firm pressure is often used in conventional B-mode imaging, creating a strong depression of the skin. This is not the case for elasticity imaging. Applying sufficient gel between the probe and the skin will ensure that good contact is made with minimal pressure so that no precompression (depression) of the tissues is made. The transducer should be held parallel to the skin surface, and from that start position, small repetitive displacements of 1–2 mm will achieve the strain values of around 1% that are necessary to allow estimation of stiffness. It is recommended to focus on the elastogram in the dual screen during the examination as focusing on the B-mode results in a tendency to push too hard with the probe, which can produce false-negative elastography images.

The speed of movement is not important; however it should be matched to the frame rate. A lower frame rate should be used with a slower rate of transducer movement in order to get sufficient displacement between frames. A rate of around 2 Hz with a high frame rate setting has been shown in practice to give the best quality elastograms in phantom experiments [2].

An alternative to transducer palpation is to hold the transducer still and allow the internal physiological pulsations from cardiac, respiratory or muscle contractions to generate the strain image. The system can be preset for either technique, minimal compression or no compression. However, since displacements are measured only in an axial direction, better results are generally obtained when slight uniaxial stress is applied.

Manual probe manipulation can result in large transducer displacements, out-of-plane movement, in-plane lateral movements and rotational probe motion. To minimise these undesired movements and to constrain movement to an axial plane, the use of a 'footprint extender' is recommended for linear transducers (Fig. 7.3). The footplate extender can improve the uniformity of the applied stress and maximise the depth of stress penetration.

7.2.3.3 ROI Size/Position (Region of Interest)

The RTE image displays relative stiffness of tissue, so it is important to include sufficient normal

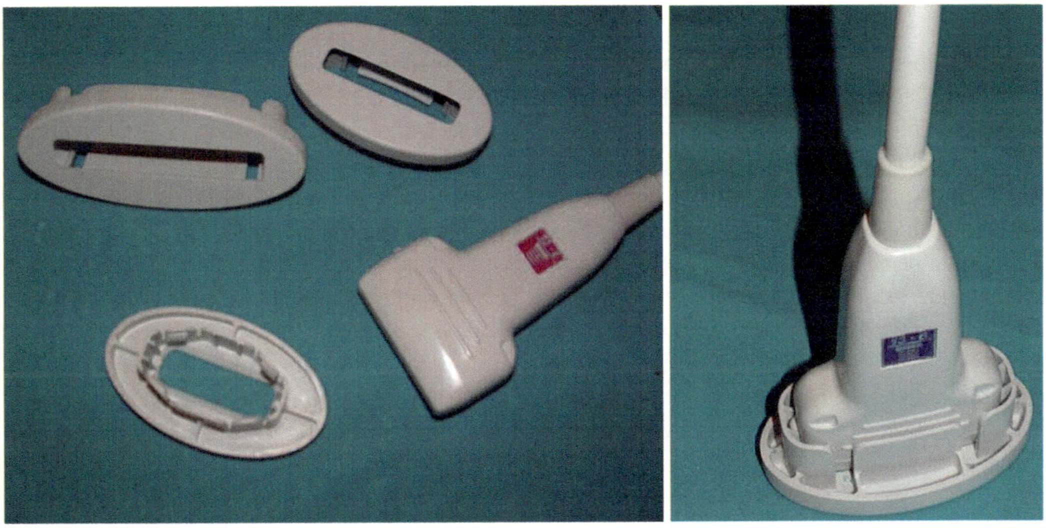

Fig. 7.3 Footplate extender minimises out-of-plane or rotational probe movements, and as a result, the stress field is transmitted more uniformly

or reference tissue surrounding the lesion of interest. The best image quality was recorded in phantom experiments when the 'lesion' of interest covered 25–50% of the ROI [2].

For breast imaging, the lesion should be centred in the ROI which should extend anterio-posteriorly from the subcutaneous fat tissue to the pectoralis muscle but excluding the thoracic cage and the width adjusted to keep the lesion of interest within 25% of the ROI width [3]. In the case of a large lesion, the ROI can be placed towards the edge of the lesion, so that surrounding normal tissue is included in the evaluation (Fig. 7.4b).

7.2.3.4 Colour Maps

Greyscale, hues of a single colour and rainbow colour maps amongst others are offered to display the different strain values in the image. Some users prefer to denote red as stiff (representing danger or alarm) and blue as soft, whereas others have chosen the reverse (blue is thought to give better transparency enabling the colour overlay of the region of stiffness to be compared to the morphology of the lesion depicted by the B-mode display), so careful investigation of the labelling of the displayed colour bar is necessary for correct interpretation of the elastogram (Fig. 7.4c).

7.2.3.5 Quality Parameters (Strain Graph)

In order to check the quality and reproducibility of the elastography image, freeze the image and review the stored cine loop frame by frame. A consistent colour pattern obtained in a number of consecutive frames indicates a good reliable technique.

The strain graph (Fig. 7.5a) displays the mean strain (as a percentage) in the ROI over time and can provide feedback to the user on the degree and uniformity of his/her compression technique. The scale of the display can be chosen and the amplitude and speed of movement adjusted so that the induced strain remains between the recommended values 0.5 and 1.0%.

Information given by the strain graph can improve operator technique. Once in freeze mode, the strain graph can be used to guide selection of the 'optimum' frame for analysis, during the 'release' or 'relaxation' phase (Fig. 7.5b).

7.2.3.6 Additional Tools Which Aid Workflow in Breast Examinations

Selecting Good Quality Frames for Assessment

Auto frame select is a function that automatically picks out the most appropriate frame for measurement from the multiple frames in the cine store on freeze (based on consideration of the balance of the strain values in the image and its consistency over time) (Fig. 7.6). This function reduces examination time, offers improved accuracy and removes operator bias from the frame selection.

Frame averaging is a temporal averaging technique which removes noise and improves accuracy for measurement (Fig. 7.7).

7.2.4 Methods of Assessment/Quantification

7.2.4.1 Tsukuba Score

A five-point scale, the Tsukuba score, has been described to classify elasticity images based on a visual assessment of the colour pattern in the suspected lesion relative to the subcutaneous fat and surrounding breast tissue (Fig. 7.8). With a cut-off point between 3 and 4, Itoh [3] showed similar performance for breast lesion diagnosis to conventional ultrasound for real-time tissue elastography using this classification system, with easier interpretation. Schwab [4] reported near-perfect intra-observer agreement and moderate to substantial interobserver agreement with respect to BI-RADS classification and Tsukuba score.

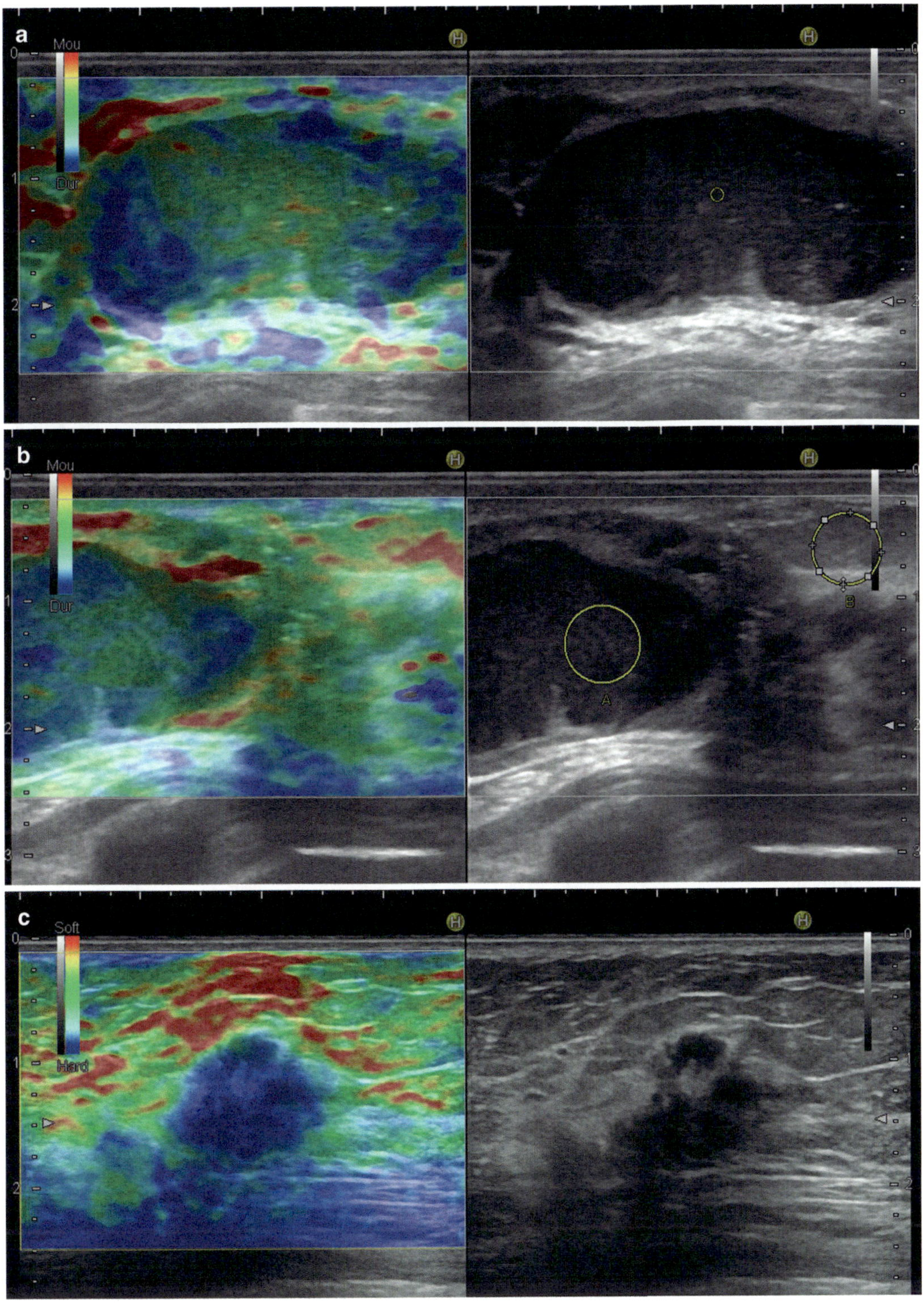

Fig. 7.4 (**a**) Large lesion which occupies more than 50% of the ROI. (**b**) Lesion placed on the edge of the ROI so that sufficient normal tissue is included in the ROI. (**c**) Ideal position. The lesion is centred in the ROI which extends anterio-posteriorly from the subcutaneous fat tissue to the pectoralis muscle but excludes the thoracic cage, and the width is adjusted to keep the lesion within 25% of the ROI width. Note the labelling of the colour bar, *red* indicating softer tissues and *blue* stiffer tissues

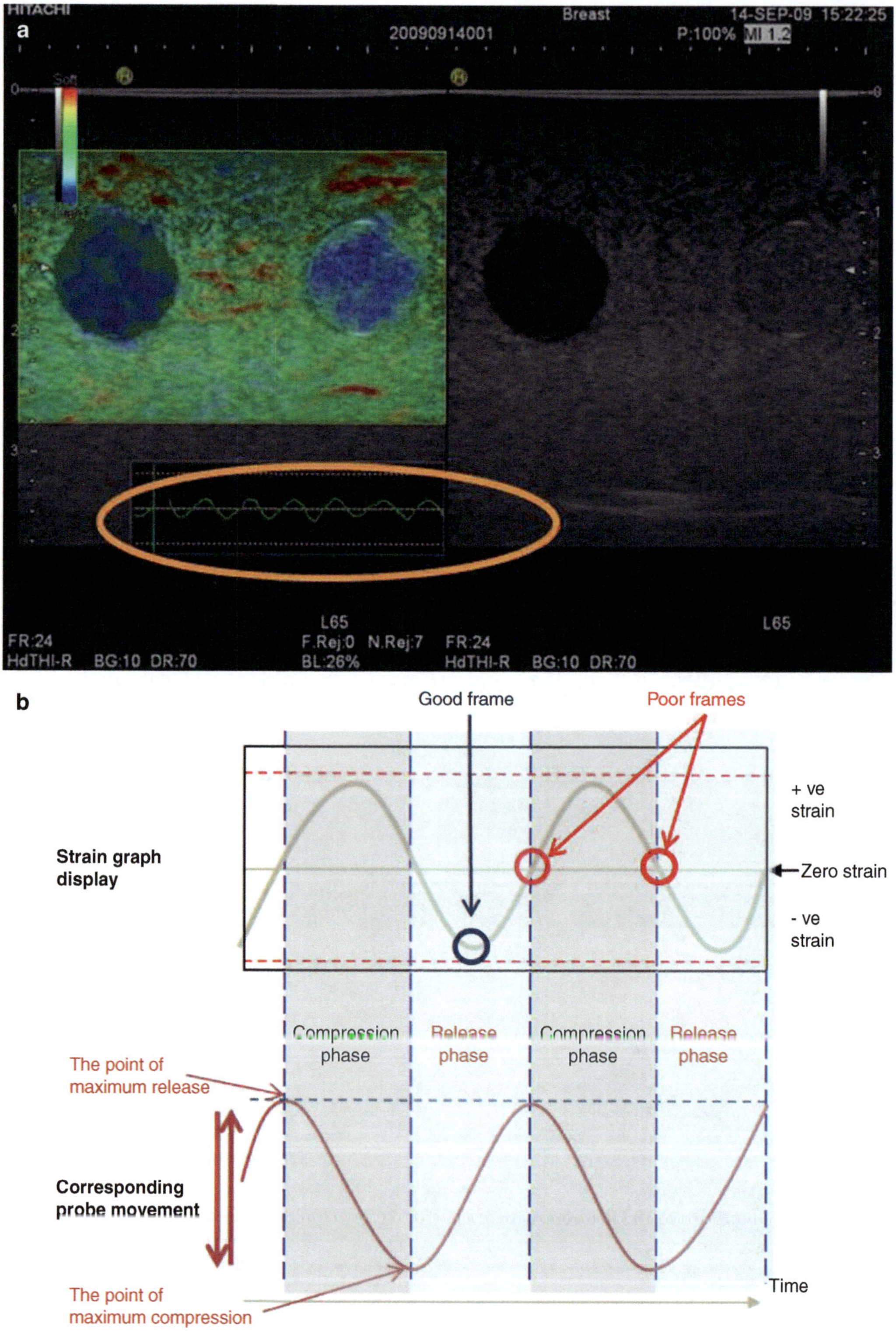

Fig. 7.5 Strain graph display (**a**). Interpretation of strain graph (**b**)

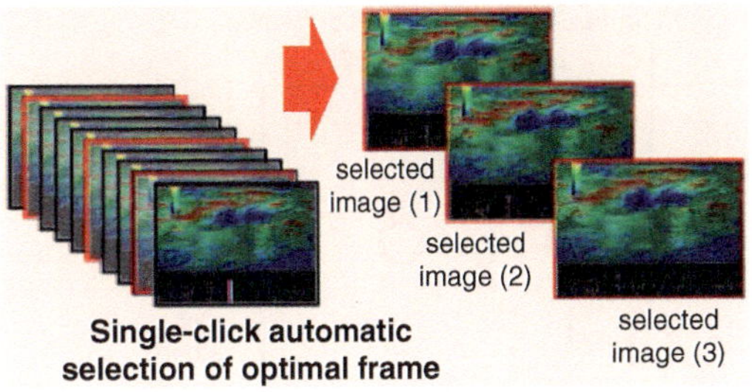

Fig. 7.6 Auto frame select function

7.2.4.2 Fat Lesion Ratio: Assist Strain Ratio

The strain ratio is a simple on-line tool that can be used for quantifying the tissue stiffness within the suspicious area relative to the subcutaneous fat. This semi-quantitative measurement is also known as the fat lesion ratio. An ROI that best circumscribes the inside of the lesion is selected and a second ROI is placed in adjacent reference tissue (Figs. 7.9 and 7.10).

$$\text{Fat Lesion ratio is calculated: } \quad \text{FLR}\left(\text{B}/\text{A}\right)=\frac{\text{Mean strain of fat}\left(\text{B}\right)}{\text{Mean strain in lesion}\left(\text{A}\right)}$$

Havre showed that the strain ratio can provide reliable and reproducible results in a phantom and that best results were obtained when the reference tissue was at a similar depth from the transducer to the region of interest but was independent of the relative size of the reference area. However, in practice in breast applications, the subcutaneous fat tissue should be selected as the reference tissue. Compared to the visual scoring of lesions, the strain ratio removes some of the subjectivity in interpretation of the elastogram and allows greater sensitivity to changes in stiffness. Thomas and Zhi both reported more reliable diagnostic results using strain ratio over visual scoring [6, 7].

Further technical developments have led to the implementation of a semi-automatic fat lesion ratio measurement, where the operator places a cursor within the breast lesion; the software algorithm detects the tumour boundary as displayed on the B-mode image and places an ROI that inscribes its margins. A second reference ROI is placed in adjacent tissue using probability distribution analysis to identify the fat layer. Early study has shown that the semi-automatic ratio measurement is similar to that of the strain ratio values determined with the conventional manual method, with the advantage that it can improve the reproducibility, remove operator bias and shorten the measurement time [8, 9].

7.2.5 4D Real-Time Tissue Elastography

As in other clinical applications, notably in obstetrics, acquiring and storing a 3D volume of ultrasound data can provide opportunity for further processing (Fig. 7.11). Multiplanar reconstruction allows the display of tissue architecture in planes not achievable with conventional 2D ultrasound, and 3D rendering can provide an image more easy to interpret by those not familiar with ultrasound imaging. In the same way, 3D/4D elastograms can be helpful both to aid diagnosis and to offer the surgeon a pre-procedural overview.

7.2.6 RTE Conclusion

Real-time tissue elastography is an additional tool for the breast sonographer that when added to other ultrasound modalities (B-mode, colour Doppler) can increase diagnostic confidence in the differentiation between benign and malignant diseases without adding significantly to the length of the examination. As with all ultrasound imaging, there is a short learning curve to acquire the necessary skills for acquisition and interpretation of the elastograms, but with technology advances already implemented since its first commercial introduction, and developments continuing into the future, the operator dependence has been significantly reduced and clinical results continue to validate its accuracy and reproducibility.

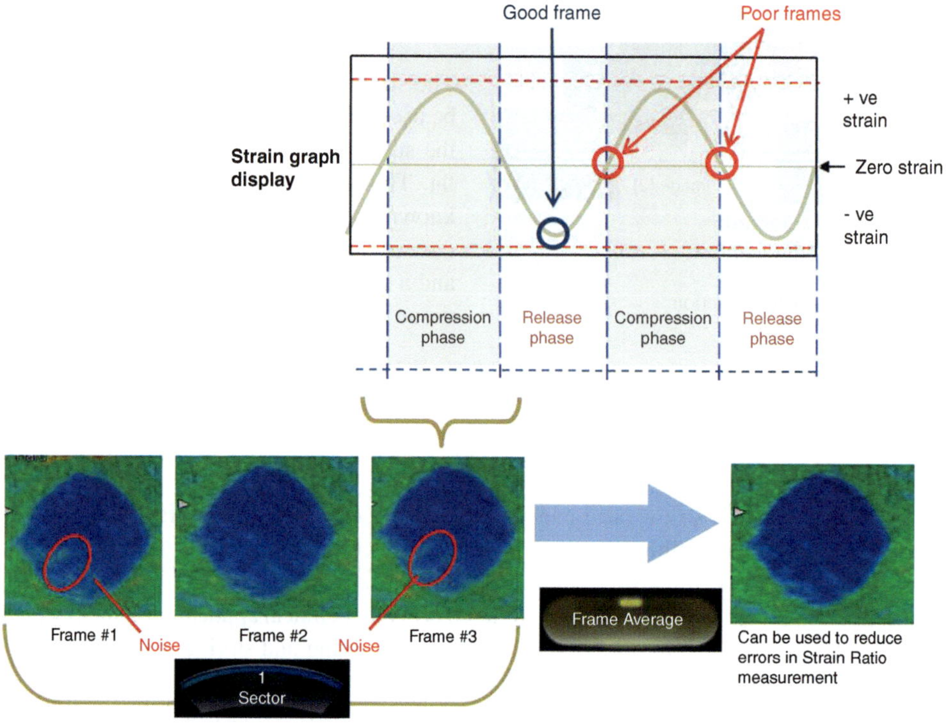

Fig. 7.7 Frame averaging improves the accuracy for measurement

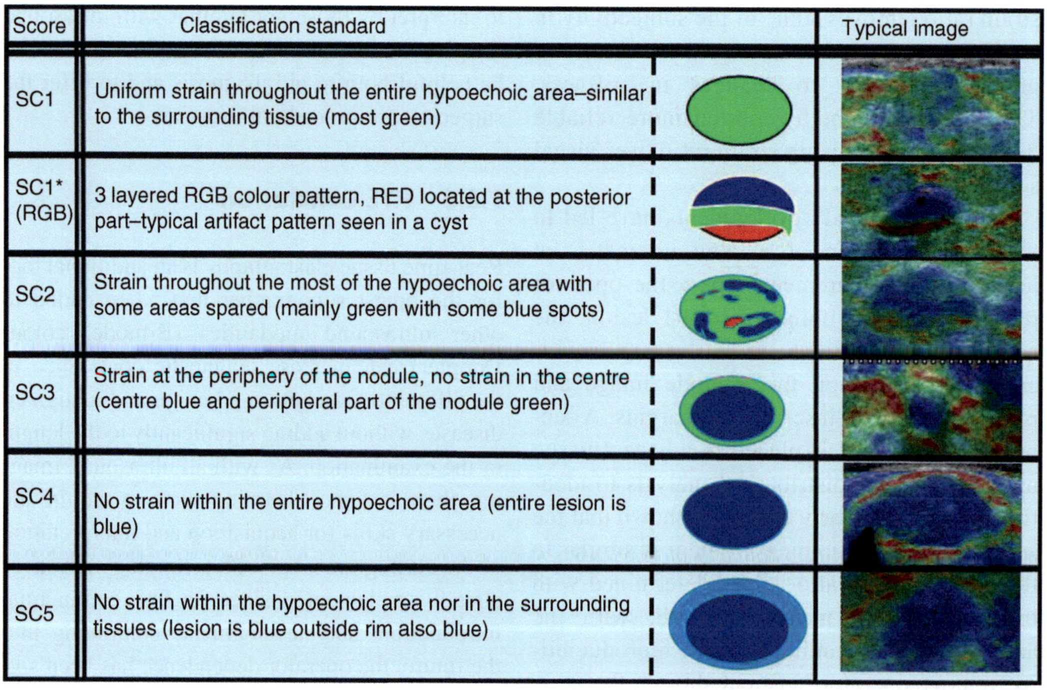

Score	Classification standard	Typical image
SC1	Uniform strain throughout the entire hypoechoic area–similar to the surrounding tissue (most green)	
SC1* (RGB)	3 layered RGB colour pattern, RED located at the posterior part–typical artifact pattern seen in a cyst	
SC2	Strain throughout the most of the hypoechoic area with some areas spared (mainly green with some blue spots)	
SC3	Strain at the periphery of the nodule, no strain in the centre (centre blue and peripheral part of the nodule green)	
SC4	No strain within the entire hypoechoic area (entire lesion is blue)	
SC5	No strain within the hypoechoic area nor in the surrounding tissues (lesion is blue outside rim also blue)	

Fig. 7.8 Tsukuba score (Adapted from score published: ref. [3]). *The initial classification has been subsequently modified to add the BGR (blue-green-red) score, an artefactual pattern characteristic of many cystic nodules, including those with internal echoes, and has been reported as a useful diagnostic sign [5]

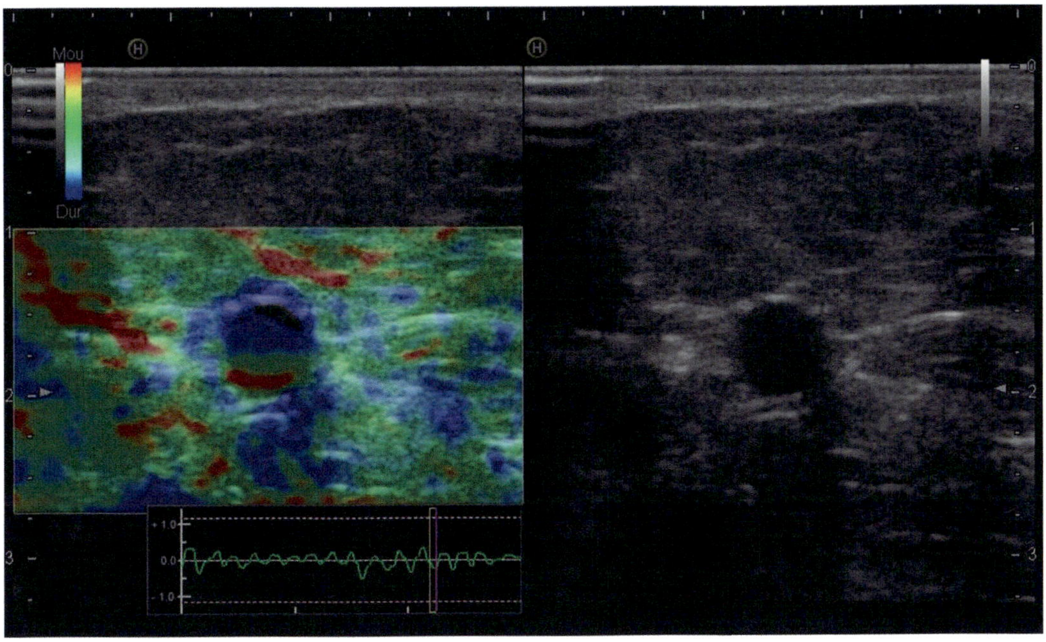

Fig. 7.9 Example of a small breast cyst demonstrating the three-layer blue-green-red (BGR) sign

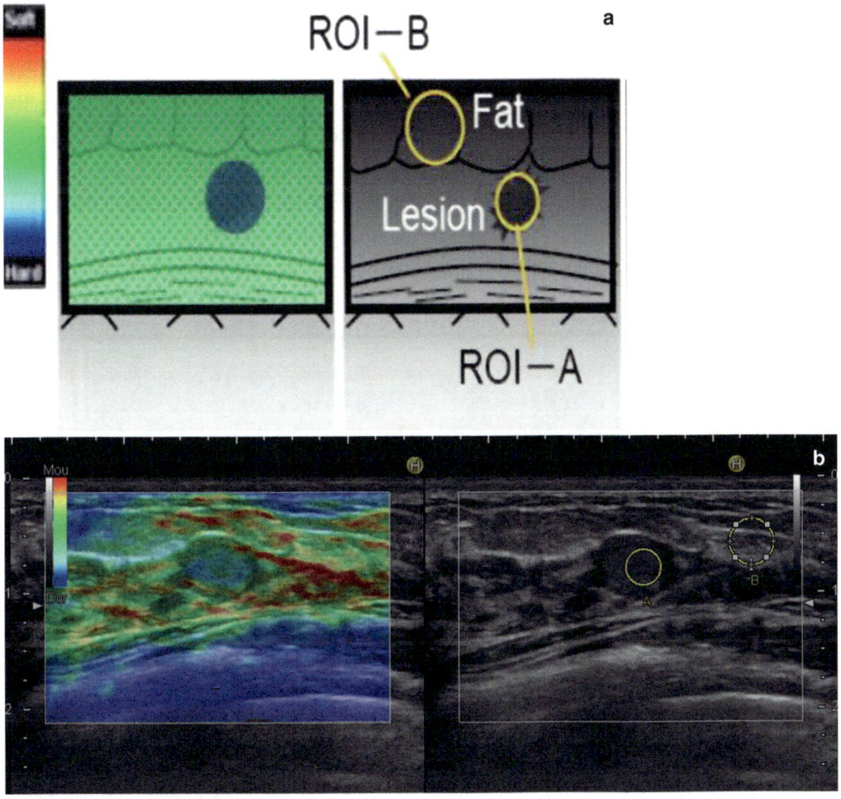

Fig. 7.10 (**a**) Fat lesion ratio measurement. ROI A is placed within the breast mass and ROI B in the subcutaneous fat layer. Fat lesion ratio = B/A. (**b**) Example of FLR measurement in benign breast lesion (FLR = 2.9)

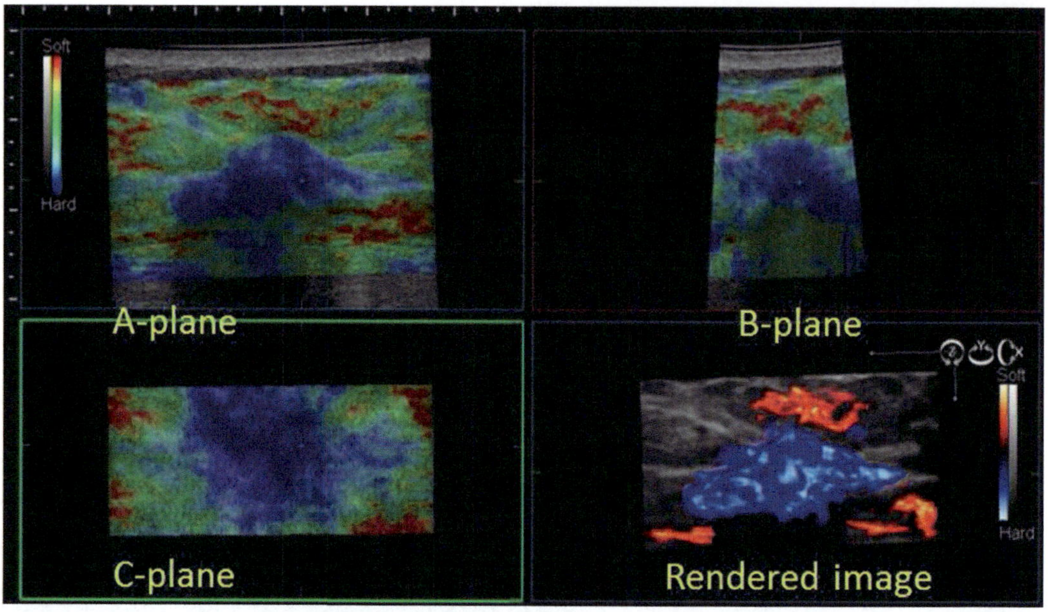

Fig. 7.11 4D RTE. Spread of invasion is clearly visualised in the C-plane and the 3D volume of stiffness portrayed in the rendered image

7.3 Shear Wave Elastography (SWE)

7.3.1 Overview

Ultrasound imaging provides both morphological (grayscale images) and functional (flow imaging) imaging of soft tissue. Using advanced technologies, a third dimension can be added to ultrasound: physio-pathological information through the assessment of tissue elasticity.

ShearWave™ Elastography (SWE) is an ultrasound imaging mode providing tissue elasticity maps of human organs. SWE has the specificity to be real time, user independent and quantitative. Elasticity is measured in (kilo)Pascal and displayed in real time in a colour-coded map as illustrated in the figure below.

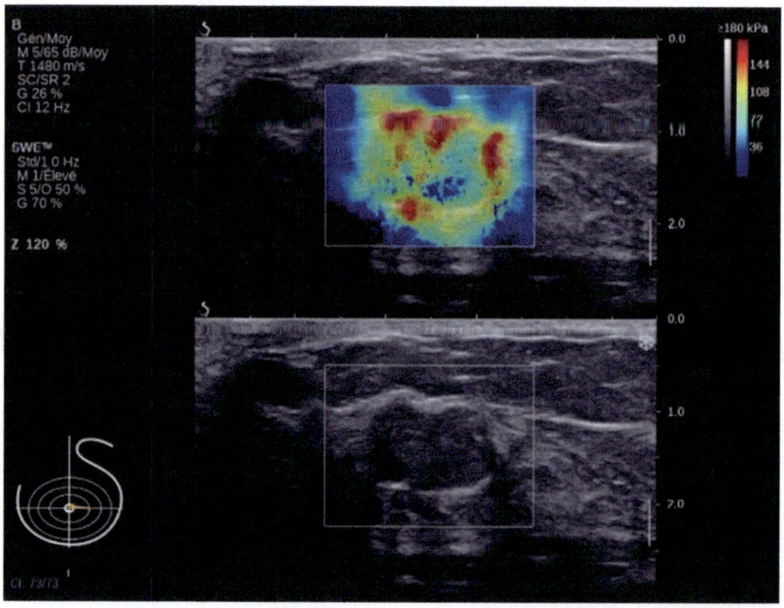

SWE is available on all transducers and most clinical applications available on SuperSonic Imagine's Aixplorer® system (all except OB and vascular) and has proven its benefits in many clinical challenges. For breast imaging, SWE perfectly complements classical B-mode ultrasound imaging, offering ease of use, improved diagnostic and better management of breast cancer.

7.3.2 Physics of Tissue Elasticity

Two kinds of mechanical waves propagate in the human body: compressional waves and shear waves. Compressional waves travel significantly faster than shear waves in soft tissue: typical values are 1500 m/s for compressional waves compared to 1–10 m/s for shear waves. Ultrasound waves used in ultrasonography are compressional waves in the MHz frequency range. Shear waves have not been used on ultrasound machines until recently. Unlike compressional waves, they have the specificity to reflect tissue elastic properties: Shear waves propagate faster in hard tissue than in soft tissue. This is illustrated in Fig. 7.12 where shear waves are shown in media containing either a hard inclusion or a soft inclusion and compared with a homogeneous medium.

In heterogeneous media, the shear wave front is distorted (slowed down in soft tissue or accelerated in hard tissue) demonstrating its sensitiveness to tissue stiffness. Under some specific assumptions (the medium is isotropic and purely elastic), the tissue elasticity can be directly linked to the shear wave propagation speed through the following formula: $E = 3\rho c^2$. Measuring tissue elasticity can therefore be achieved by a three-step methodology:

(a) Inducing shear waves in the body
(b) Measuring their propagation speed at each pixel of an area of interest
(c) Displaying the resulting speed or elasticity on an image

7.3.3 Principles of SWE

ShearWave™ Elastography combines innovative ultrasound technologies (Bercoff et al.) to induce and image shear waves with the goal to provide the user maximal ease of use and reliability.

7.3.3.1 Automatic Shear Wave Generation

The generation of shear waves in the body is performed using any ultrasound probe available on the system. The probe sends special ultrasound focused beams that act as virtual fingers remotely palpating organs. This phenomenon, known in physics as the radiation force of ultrasound waves, is illustrated in Fig. 7.13.

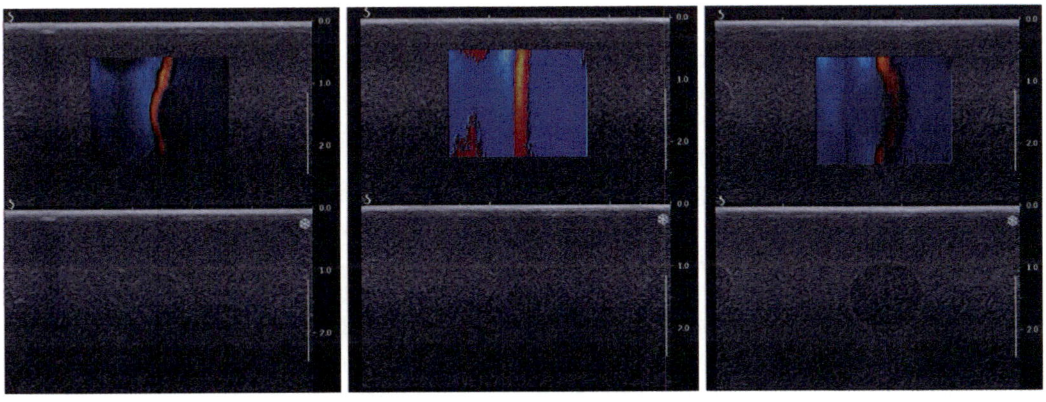

Fig. 7.12 Shear waves propagating in a soft inclusion (*left*), in a homogeneous tissue (*middle*) and a hard inclusion (*right*)

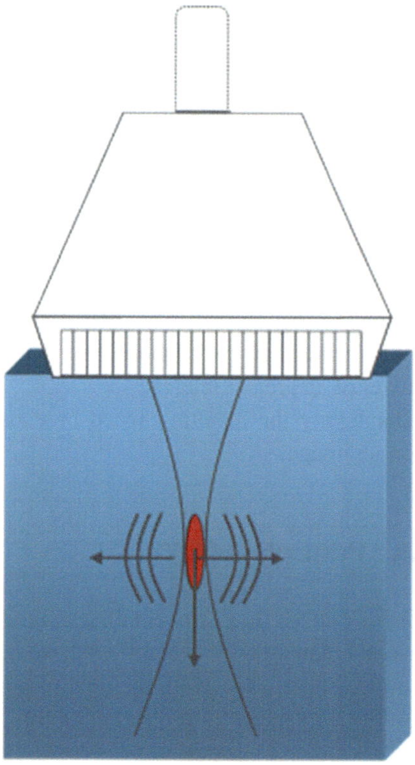

Fig. 7.13 At focus, ultrasound waves act as a virtual finger pushing the tissue in the direction of their propagation

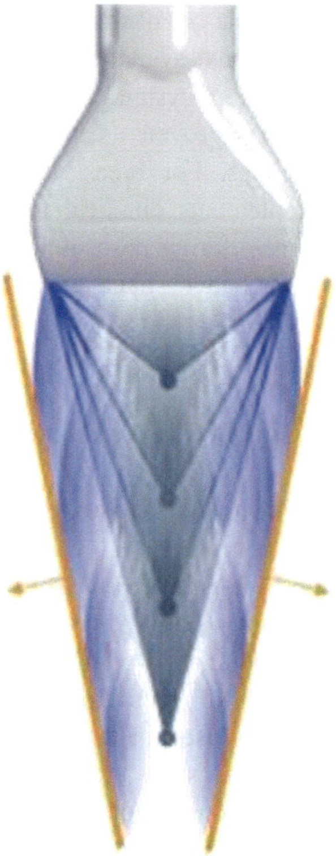

Fig. 7.14 Supersonic shear wave generation

Thanks to this technology, shear waves can be automatically generated in tissue without any action from the users. One drawback of the method is the small amplitude of the shear waves and their resulting fast attenuation. To compensate for the shear wave weakness, Aixplorer uses a specific technology based on the generation of supersonic source. The focused beam (or virtual palpating finger) is moved in the medium at a supersonic speed (i.e. faster than the induced shear waves) and creates a shear bang (like the sonic bang of supersonic airplanes) where the shear waves are confined along a Mach cone. This is illustrated in Fig. 7.14.

The supersonic bang generates high amplitude shear waves without significantly increasing the local acoustic power delivered in the body. Such waves are of enough amplitudes to propagate in soft tissue through several centimetres. The supersonic generation of shear waves is a key contributor of the robustness and reliability of SWE.

7.3.3.2 Ultrafast Imaging of Shear Waves

Shear wave frequencies vary between 20 and 2000 Hz in the body. To correctly analyse shear wave propagation and calculate their speed (without bias or artefacts), they should be imaged at frame rates at least twice higher than their maximum frequency (Nyquist sampling rule), typically 4000–5000 images/s. This is way faster than the current capabilities of ultrasound systems (capable of reaching 50–100 images/s). Aixplorer® uses its unique ultrafast imaging capabilities to capture shear waves and measure their propagation speed. Aixplorer® is capable of imaging the body at frame rates up to 20,000 images/s.

Figure 7.15 shows a shear wave propagation captured by Aixplorer® ultrafast camera.

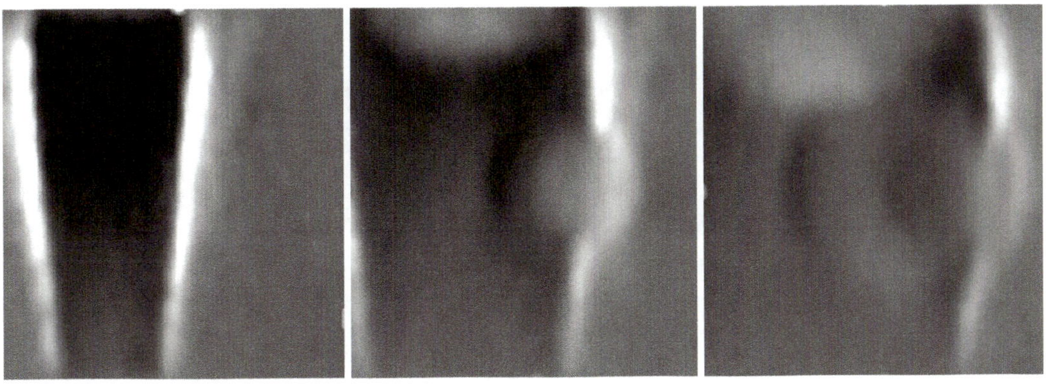

Fig. 7.15 Mach cone of shear waves propagating laterally in a tissue containing a hard inclusion. The propagation of the shear wave over the whole area lasts a few tens of milliseconds

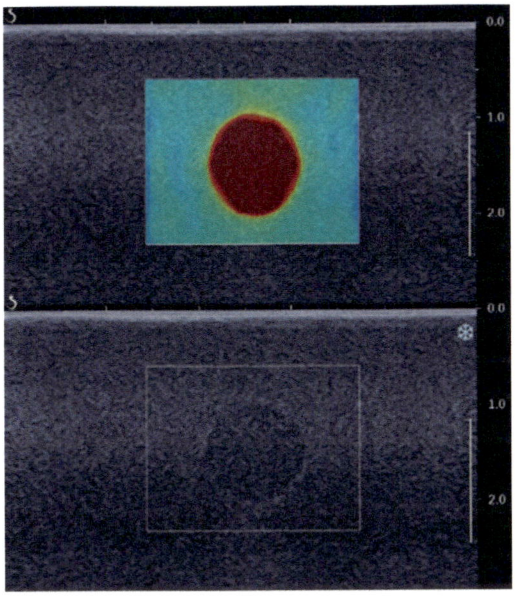

Fig. 7.16 Elasticity map perfectly displaying the harder inclusion (that can be barely seen on the ultrasound image)

From the propagation movie, the system calculates the shear wave speed at each pixel and displays an elasticity map as illustrated in Fig. 7.16.

As the elasticity map is acquired and displayed in a few hundreds of milliseconds, the information is refreshed in real time on the screen, providing a truly real-time elasticity imaging mode.

7.3.4 Using SWE

Thanks to its real-time capabilities and advanced technologies, ShearWave™ Elastography can be performed in a similar manner to any other ultrasound imaging mode. There are no additional tools or setup and no special scanning protocols, just the ultrasound probe itself used in the same way than in conventional B-mode. A typical workflow of SWE for breast imaging is described below.

7.3.4.1 Scanning

The user should first localise the region of interest in standard B-mode, adjust settings to have the best B-mode image and then switch on the SWE mode.

Once in SWE, some recommendations for optimal results are suggested:

- Reduce the compression applied on the organ as much as possible.
- Scan softly and slowly. SWE frame rates are lower as conventional B-mode frame rates. Make sure the SWE image is stable in time (over 1/2 s) to ensure optimal measurements.

It is important to know that soft tissues tends to become harder when compressed hard. This is a natural and normal phenomenon and the SWE mode is sensitive to it. This is illustrated in Fig. 7.17 where two SWE images are acquired on

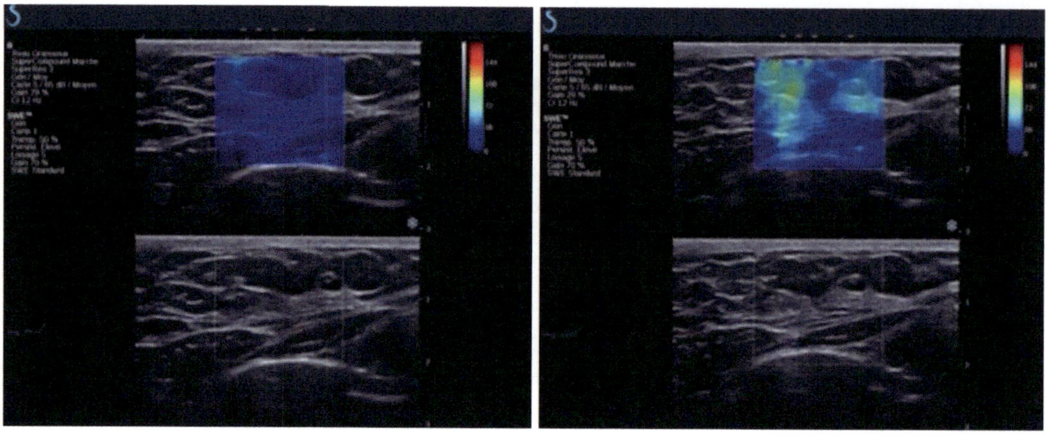

Fig. 7.17 *Left*: gentle compression (good practice). *Right*: hard compression

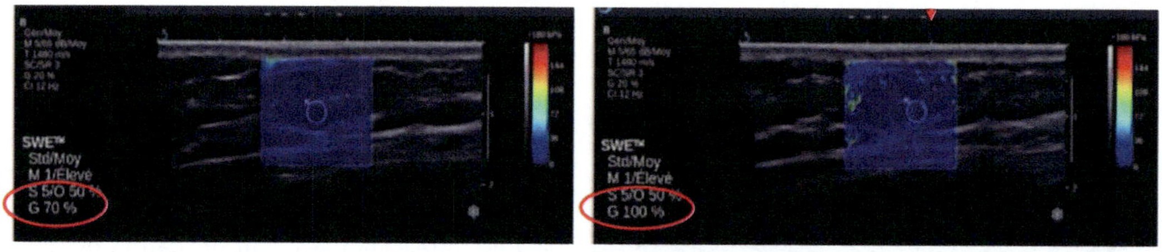

Fig. 7.18 *Left*: good gain level—the box is filled and no noise appears. *Right*: Too much gain. Noisy pixels are visible on the image

normal breast tissue, one with gentle compression and the second with hard compression.

The SWE map clearly shows the stiffening of the breast tissue under compression (cyan and yellow areas are of higher stiffness). To ensure consistent results, it is necessary to apply a gentle compression, as low as achievable whilst keeping a good image quality. A good way to check the good level of compression is to make sure the SWE shows a uniform deep blue map on normal breast tissue (and not cyan or yellow areas) as illustrated on Fig. 7.17, left.

7.3.4.2 Optimising the SWE Image

Whilst scanning in real time using SWE, a few settings are available to optimise the quality of the map.

- Box size: SWE default box size is adapted to cover most breast lesions. For some specific very large lesions, the box can be enlarged. There will be a very subtle reduction of frame rate and image quality but no change in measured elasticity values.
- Gain: SWE should be adjusted to the highest value that does not show pixel noise, as illustrated in Fig. 7.18.
- Res/pen setting

This is an important setting of SWE mode as it sets the trade-off between resolution and penetration of the mode. Three levels are available: resolution, standard and penetration. Standard is the default value and is adapted to most of the clinical cases. Switch to resolution should be done when the lesion is small and shallow. It will provide better spatial resolution and less temporal persistence. Switch to penetration mode should be considered when there is a lack of signal in the SWE box. This typically happens in large, hypoechoic and irregular lesions. Penetration mode improves signal-to-noise ratio at the expense of spatial resolution and is better suited to measure very high stiffness values (this is usually the case for the kind of lesions considered).

In some cases, typically in very hypoechoic lesions, even in penetration mode, there could be some areas where there is a lack of SWE signal. This means that the system is not able to catch the shear wave propagation due to the lack of ultrasound signals in strongly hypoechoic areas. This is a limitation of the mode, but it does not impact its clinical value as it only concerns limited areas of the maps. This is illustrated on the example below of a breast cancer (BI-RADS® 5) (Fig. 7.19).

The two red circles show areas where there is a lack of SWE signal. They correspond to strongly hypoechoic regions. This does not prevent from measuring elasticity of the lesion and demonstrate that this lesion is significantly stiff [around 190 kPa for the max value].

- SWE scale

The SWE scale adjusts the image dynamics. It can be moved from 10 to 300 kPa in the breast application. The default scale [0–180] kPa is well adapted for most of the breast lesion cases. However, this scale can be changed to improve the visibility of the SWE map, as illustrated on the image below where the same inclusion is displayed with four different scales (Fig. 7.20).

Measured elasticity values are absolute and are fully independent of the chosen scale.

7.3.4.3 Quantification

Once the SWE images acquired, quantification can be performed in frozen mode using the Q-Box™ tool. A Q-Box™ can be positioned anywhere on the SWE map as illustrated in the

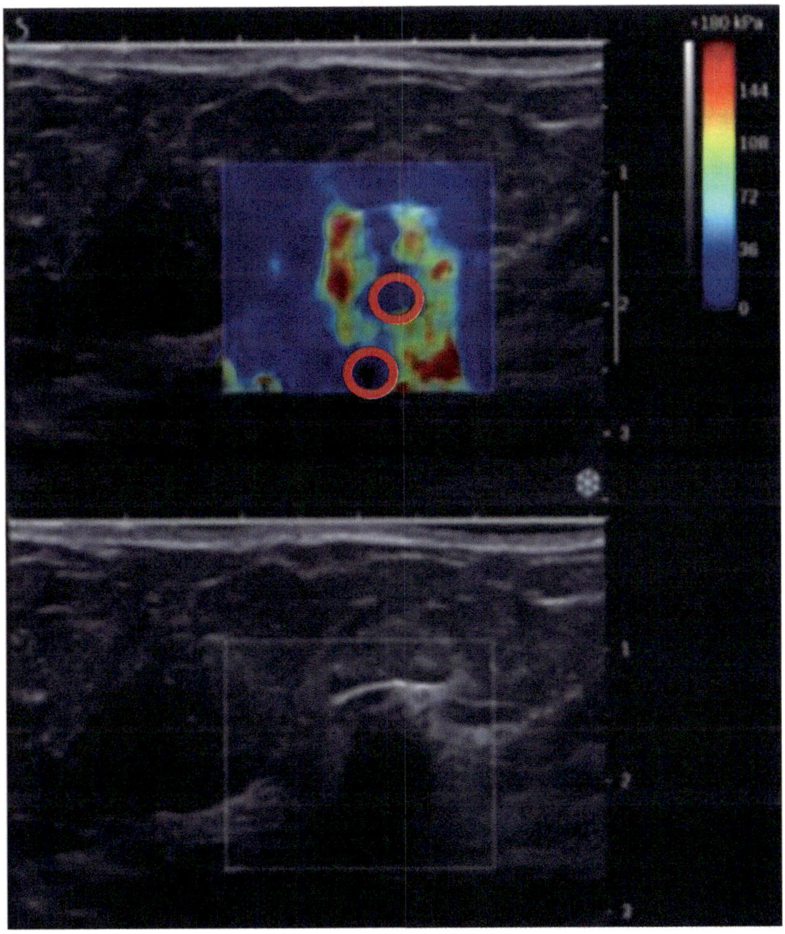

Fig. 7.19 SWE image of a hard breast lesion with some strongly hypoechoic lesions

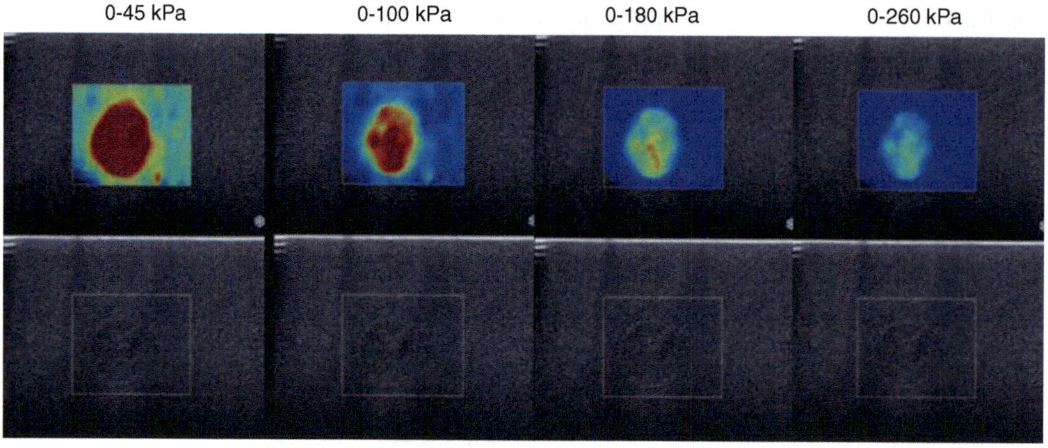

Fig. 7.20 Image of a hard inclusion under different scale values

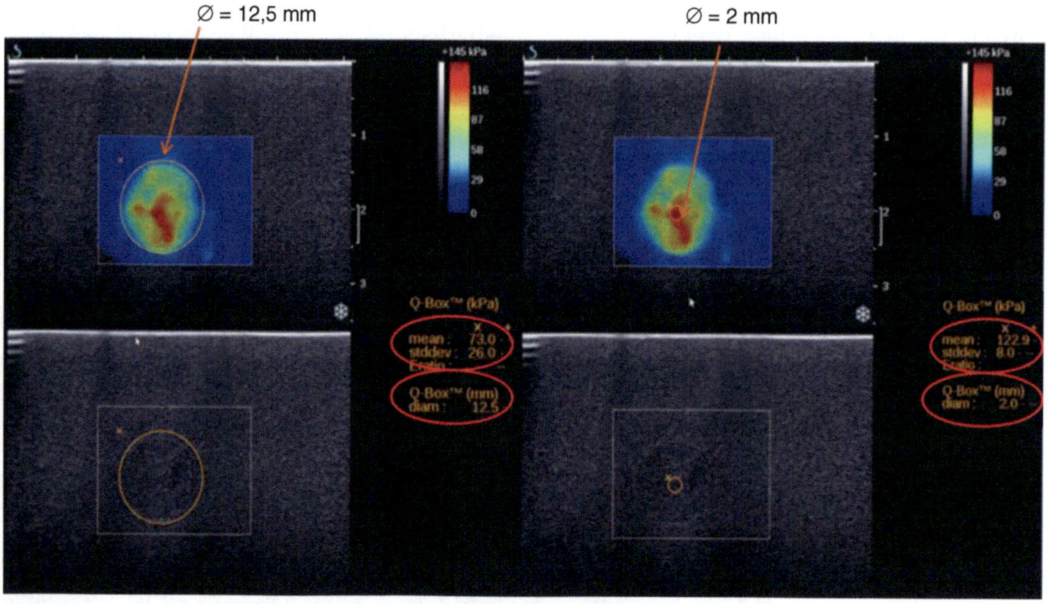

Fig. 7.21 Q-box tool of different sizes on the same lesion

image below. Its size can be adjusted by the user (Fig. 7.21).

Mean and standard deviation are provided for each Q-Box™ in kPa. The user can also switch the measurement unit to metres per seconds (m/s), representing the local speed of shear wave. Multiple Q-Box™ tools can be performed on the same SWE map. Ratio or averages can be derived from these quantitative measurements. On breast lesions, the ratio between the maximal lesion elasticity and fat tissue is a relevant parameter for lesion characterisation as it will be illustrated in the next paragraph.

7.3.5 Clinical Impact of SWE in Breast

Ultrasound imaging, when used for lesion characterisation, provides excellent sensitivity (above 90%) but moderate specificity. Forty to 50% of biopsies triggered by an ultrasound exam are negative. Also, around 2% of lesions considered as benign (BI-RADS 3) are malignant. The high number of false positives remains also a serious issue for the establishment of ultrasound imaging as a recognised screening tool. SWE, with its real-time capability, its ease of use and its ability to measure locally and quantitatively tissue stiffness, is able to very nicely complement classical ultrasound imaging and strengthen significantly the clinical value of the ultrasound exam in general. Below are reviewed some benefits of SWE in clinical framework of breast imaging.

7.3.5.1 SWE Is Almost Perfectly Reproducible

In a clinical study involving more than 750 breast lesions, Cosgrove et al. demonstrated that using three successive acquisitions, the results were similar in 88% of the cases and fully dissimilar in only 1% of the cases. The reproducibility of the quantitiveness of SWE has been also evaluated showing an intraclass correlation coefficient (ICC) of 0.87 for the mean elasticity value within the Q-box. Concerning the interobserver reproducibility, many studies have demonstrated higher scores for quantitativeness SWE (weighed on the max value within the Q-box) than for the classical BI-RADS assessment of lesions (Cosgrove et al., Lee et al., Tozaki et al., Gweon et al.). Moreover, by analysing SWE results on 24 publications, there is a good consistency over the studies between mean stiffness values found in benign lesions and mean stiffness values found in malignant lesions. This is illustrated in Fig. 7.22.

SWE helps the reduction of false positives in ultrasound imaging

Many studies have demonstrated the ability of SWE to increase specificity and the positive predictive value of the biopsy recommendation in the framework of breast lesion characterisation, as illustrated in Fig. 7.23.

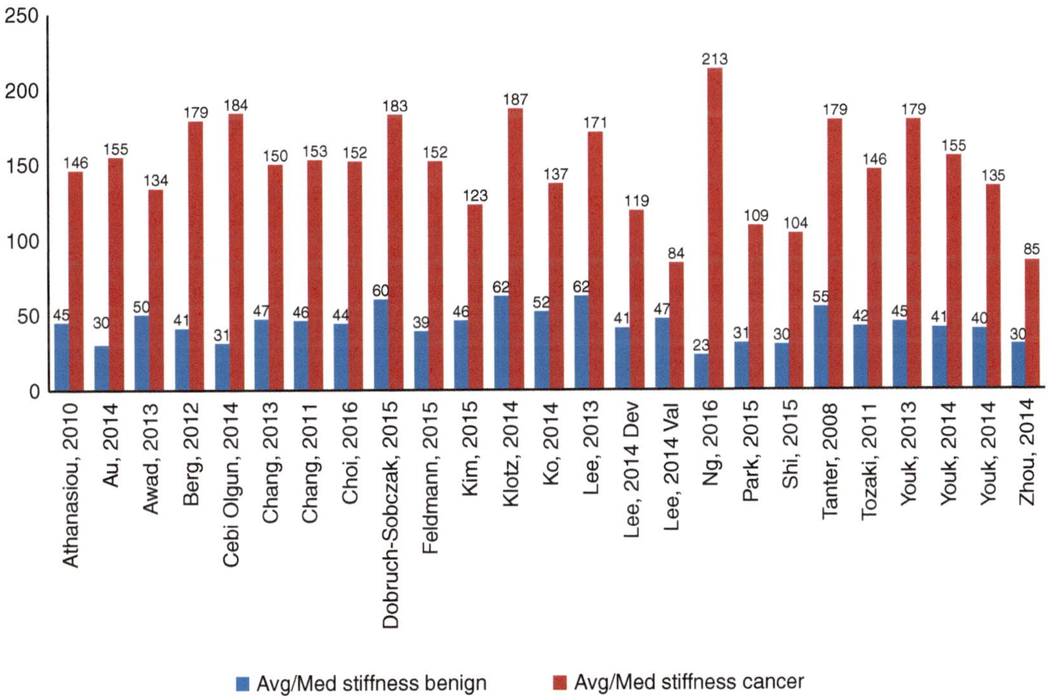

Fig. 7.22 Twenty-four peer-reviewed publications reported average SWE™ stiffness of benign and malignant masses. Malignant masses were always reported to be on average 2–3 times significantly stiffer than benign masses

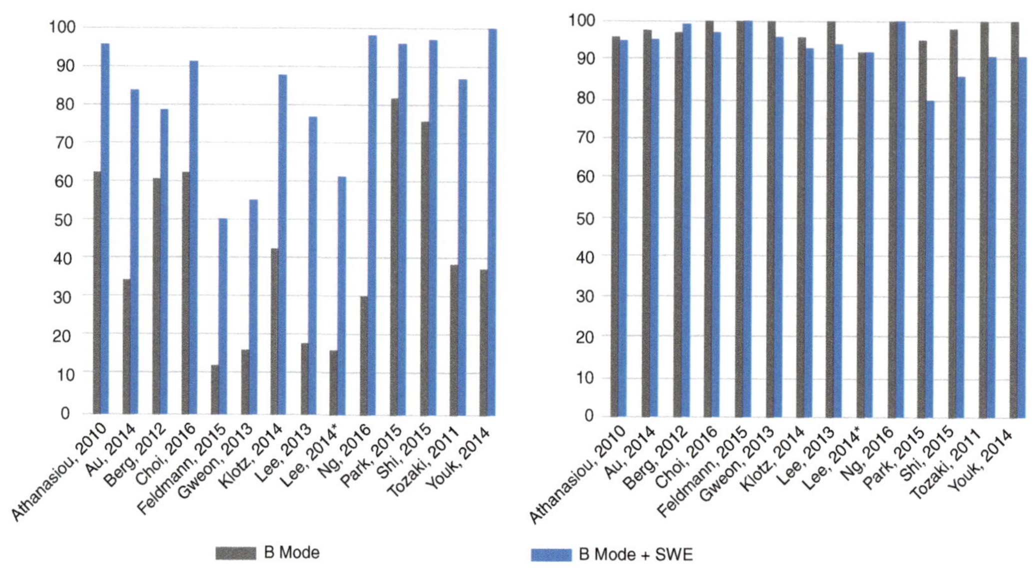

Fig. 7.23 Increased specificity (*left*). Preserved sensitivity (*right*)

They are summarised by the recommendation published in 2014 by the Korean Society of Ultrasound in Medicine (KSUM, Lee et al. 3):

Lesions classified BI-RADS 4a that are negative in SWE should not be biopsied but followed up.

- Lesions classified BI-RADS 3 that are positive in SWE should be biopsied.
- Adjust the follow-up period of BI-RADS 3 lesions that are negative in SWE to a BI-RADS 2 follow-up.

In addition, in the framework of breast screening, it has been demonstrated that the specificity of the ultrasound exam has been increased by 17.4% using SWE without any degradation of sensitivity [Lee et al. 2].

7.3.5.2 SWE Contributes to Better Sensitivity of the Ultrasound Exam

Evans et al. [Evans et al.] demonstrated 100% sensitivity and 100% negative predictive value when biopsying lesions that have mean elasticities above 50 kPa. Also, in the framework of an ultrasound exam following an MRI, SWE allowed sensitivity increase of 29% of the ultrasound exam [Plecha et al.].

7.3.5.3 SWE Helps Therapy Planning and Monitoring of Breast Lesions

Studies have shown interesting correlation between SWE signatures and lesion characteristics that may help therapy planning. First, the lesion size in SWE seems much better correlated to the histological size than the size on the measured ultrasound image [Mullen et al.]. Second, the maximum value of elasticity seems correlated with cancer severity [Berg et al. 2] and aggressiveness [Evans et al. 2]. Finally, on patients having neoadjuvant chemotherapy, stiffness using 3D SWE seems to be a very relevant parameter to assess treatment efficacy.

7.3.6 SWE Conclusion

Thanks to its ease of use, reliability and quantitativeness, SWE improves the clinical value of ultrasound at all stages from breast cancer screening to lesion characterisation and to therapy monitoring. The number and quality of publications demonstrating its benefits are growing daily, and it appears more and more as a key modality in the framework of breast cancer imaging.

References

1. Yamakawa M, Shiina T. Strain estimation using the extended combined autocorrelation method. Jpn J Appl Phys. 2001;40:3872–6.
2. Havre RF, Elde E, Gilja OH, Odegaard S, Eide GE, Matre K, Nesje LB. Freehand real-time elastography: impact of scanning parameters on image quality and in vitro intra- and interobserver validations. Ultrasound Med Biol. 2008;34:1638–50.
3. Toh A, Ueno E, Tohno E, Kamma H, Takahashi H, Shiina T, Yamakawa M, et al. Breast disease: clinical application of US elastography for diagnosis. Radiology. 2006;239:341–50.
4. Schwab F, Redling K, Siebert M, Schötzau A, Schoenenberger CA, Zanetti-Dällenbach R. Inter- and intra-observer agreement in ultrasound BI-RADS classification and real-time elastography Tsukuba score assessment of breast lesions. Ultrasound Med Biol. 2016;42(11):2622–9.
5. Cho N, Moon WK, Chang JM, Kim SJ, Lyou CY, Choi HY. Aliasing artifact depicted on ultrasound (US)-elastography for breast cystic lesions mimicking solid masses. Acta Radiol. 2011;52(1):3–7.
6. Thomas A, Degenhardt F, Farrokh A, Wojcinski S, Slowinski T, Fischer T. Significant differentiation of focal breast lesions: calculation of strain ratio in breast sonoelastography. Acad Radiol. 2010;17(5):558–63.
7. Zhi H, Xiao XY, Yang HY, Ou B, Wen YL, Luo BM. Ultrasonic elastography in breast cancer diagnosis: strain ratio vs 5-point scale. Acad Radiol. 2010;17(10):1227–33.
8. Baba H, Waki K, Murayama N, Iimura T, Miyauchi Y. Development of the FLR assistance for the strain ratio measurement in breast elastography. Medix. 2013;58:42–5.
9. Ueno E, Tohno E, Morishima I, Umemoto T, Waki K. A preliminary prospective study to compare the diagnostic performance of assist strain ratio versus manual strain ratio. J Med Ultrason (2001). 2015;42(4):521–31.
10. Youk JH, Son EJ, Gweon HM, Kim H, Park YJ, Kim JA. Comparison of strain and shear wave elastography for the differentiation of benign from malignant breast lesions, combined with B-mode ultrasonography: qualitative and quantitative assessments. Ultrasound Med Biol. 2014;40(10):2336–44.
11. Xiao Y, Yu Y, Niu L, Qian M, Deng Z, Qiu W, Zheng H. Quantitative evaluation of peripheral tissue elasticity for ultrasound-detected breast lesions. Clin Radiol. 2016;71(9):896–904.
12. Jing H, Cheng W, Li ZY, Ying L, Wang QC, Wu T, Tian JW. Early evaluation of relative changes in tumor stiffness by shear wave elastography predicts the response to neoadjuvant chemotherapy in patients with breast cancer. J Ultrasound Med. 2016;35(8):1619–27.
13. Evans A, Purdie CA, Jordan L, Macaskill EJ, Flynn J, Vinnicombe S. Stiffness at shear-wave elastography and patient presentation predicts upgrade at surgery following an ultrasound-guided core biopsy diagnosis of ductal carcinoma in situ. Clin Radiol. 2016. pii: S0009-9260(16)30267-7. https://doi.org/10.1016/j.crad.2016.07.004.
14. Paczkowska K, Rzymski P, Kubasik M, Opala T. Sonoelastography in the evaluation of capsule formation after breast augmentation - preliminary results from a follow-up study. Arch Med Sci. 2016;12(4):793–8.
15. Giannotti E, Vinnicombe S, Thomson K, McLean D, Purdie C, Jordan L, Evans A. Shear-wave elastography and greyscale assessment of palpable probably benign masses: is biopsy always required? Br J Radiol. 2016;89(1062):20150865.
16. Cha YJ, Youk JH, Kim BG, Jung WH, Cho NH. Lymphangiogenesis in breast cancer correlates with matrix stiffness on shear-wave elastography. Yonsei Med J. 2016;57(3):599–605.
17. Evans A, Sim YT, Thomson K, Jordan L, Purdie C, Vinnicombe SJ. Shear wave elastography of breast cancer: sensitivity according to histological type in a large cohort. Breast. 2016;26:115–8.
18. Liu B, Zheng Y, Huang G, Lin M, Shan Q, Lu Y, Tian W, Xie X. Breast lesions: quantitative diagnosis using ultrasound shear wave elastography - a systematic review and meta-analysis. Ultrasound Med Biol. 2016;42(4):835–47.
19. Chamming's F, Le-Frère-Belda MA, Latorre-Ossa H, Fitoussi V, Redheuil A, Assayag F, Pidial L, Gennisson JL, Tanter M, Cuénod CA, Fournier LS. Supersonic shear wave elastography of response to anti-cancer therapy in a xenograft tumor model. Ultrasound Med Biol. 2016;42(4):924–30.
20. Bae JS, Chang JM, Lee SH, Shin SU, Moon WK. Prediction of invasive breast cancer using shear-wave elastography in patients with biopsy-confirmed ductal carcinoma in situ. Eur Radiol. 2017;27(1):7–15.
21. Džoić Dominković M, Ivanac G, Kelava T, Brkljačić B. Elastographic features of triple negative breast cancers. Eur Radiol. 2016;26(4):1090–7.
22. Ng WL, Rahmat K, Fadzli F, Rozalli FI, Mohd-Shah MN, Chandran PA, Westerhout CJ, Vijayananthan A, Abdul Aziz YF. Shearwave elastography increases diagnostic accuracy in characterization of breast lesions. Medicine (Baltimore). 2016;95(12):e3146.
23. Lee S, Jung Y, Bae Y. Clinical application of a color map pattern on shear-wave elastography for invasive breast cancer. Surg Oncol. 2016;25(1):44–8.
24. Kilic F, Velidedeoglu M, Ozturk T, Kandemirli SG, Dikici AS, Er ME, Aydogan F, Kantarci F, Yilmaz MH. Ex vivo assessment of sentinel lymph nodes in breast cancer using shear wave elastography. J Ultrasound Med. 2016;35(2):271–7.
25. Choi JS, Han BK, Ko EY, Ko ES, Shin JH, Kim GR. Additional diagnostic value of shear-wave elastography and color Doppler US for evaluation of breast non-mass lesions detected at B-mode US. Eur Radiol. 2016;26(10):3542–9.

26. Skerl K, Vinnicombe S, Thomson K, Mclean D, Giannotti E, Evans A. Anisotropy of solid breast lesions in 2D shear wave elastography is an indicator of malignancy. Acad Radiol. 2016;23(1):53–61.
27. Elseedawy M, Whelehan P, Vinnicombe S, Thomson K, Evans A. Factors influencing the stiffness of fibroadenomas at shear wave elastography. Clin Radiol. 2016;71(1):92–5.
28. Bernal M, Chammings F, Couade M, Bercoff J, Tanter M, Gennisson JL. In vivo quantification of the nonlinear shear modulus in breast lesions: feasibility study. IEEE Trans Ultrason Ferroelectr Freq Control. 2016;63(1):101–9.

References: SWE

Athanasiou A, et al. Radiology. 2010;256(1):297–303.
Au FW, et al. AJR Am J Roentgenol. 2014; 203(3):W328–36.
Awad FT. Egypt J Rad Nuc Med. 2013;44(3):681–5.
Bercoff J, et al. IEEE Trans Ultrason Ferroelect Freq Contr. 2004;51(4):396–408.
Berg WA, et al. Radiology. 2012;262(2):435–49.
Berg WA, et al. AJR Am J Roentgenol. 2015;205(2): 448–55.
Çebi Olgun D, et al. Diagn Interv Radiol. 2014;20(3): 239–44.
Chang JM, et al. AJR Am J Roentgenol. 2013;201(2): W347–56.
Chang JM, et al. Breast Cancer Res Treat. 2011; 129(1):89–97.
Choi JS, et al. Eur Radiol. 2016;26(10):3542–9.
Cosgrove DO, et al. Eur Radiol. 2012;22(5):1023–32.
Dobruch-Sobczak K, et al. Ultrasound Med Biol. 2015;41(2):366–74.
Evans A, et al. Br J Cancer. 2012 Jul 10;107(2):224–9.
Evans A, et al. Breast Cancer Res Treat. 2014 Jan;143(1): 153–7.
Feldmann A, et al. Ultrasound Med Biol. 2015;41(10): 2594–604.
Gweon HM, et al. Eur Radiol. 2013 Nov;82(11):680–5.
Kim SJ, et al. Medicine (Baltimore). 2015 Oct; 94(42):e1540.
Klotz T, et al. Diagn Interv Imaging. 2014;95(9): 813–24.
Ko KH, et al. Eur Radiol. 2014;24(2):305–11.
Lee SH, et al. Eur Radiol. 2013;23(4):1015–26.
Lee SH, et al. Radiology. 2014;273(1):61–9.
Lee SH, et al. Practice guideline for the performance of breast ultrasound elastography. Ultrasonography. 2014;33(1):3–10.
Mullen, et al. Clin Radiol. 2004;69(12):1259–63.
Ng WL, et al. Medicine (Baltimore). 2016 Mar;95(12):e3146.
Park J, et al. Eur J Radiol. 2015;84(10):1943–8.
Plecha DM, et al. Radiology. 2014 Sep;272(3):657–64.
Shi XQ, et al. Ultrasound Med Biol. 2015;41(4):960–6.
Tanter M, et al. Ultrasound Med Biol. 2008;34(9):1373–86.
Tozaki M, Fukuma E. Acta Radiol. 2011;52(10): 1069–75.
Youk JH, et al. Eur Radiol. 2013;23(10):2695–704.
Youk JH, et al. Ultrasonography. 2014;33(1):34–9.
Youk JH, et al. PLoS One. 2015;10(9):e0138074.
Zhou J, et al. Radiology. 2014 Jul;272(1):63–72.

8 Differential Diagnosis of Breast Cancer by Doppler and Sonoelastography Applied to the Lobar Ultrasonography

Aristida Colan-Georges

8.1 The Differential Diagnosis of the Breast Diseases in the Classical Radiological and Imaging Techniques in Use

The differential diagnosis in the radiological and imaging diagnosis of breast diseases was less performing and with low significance; that was due to the less specific descriptors of the breast findings, by one hand, and to the non-anatomical scanning and interpreting of the pathological findings, neglecting the normal radial lobar architecture of the breast, by the other hand. None of the individual or grouped well-known descriptors of the breast masses in US (upon Stavros [1], and after that included and developed in the US BI-RADS assessment, since 2003 up to 2013 in the fifth edition) have enough specificity in the characterization of a breast malignancy, to avoid the mandatory biopsy in any suspect lesion. No isolated ultrasonographic descriptor, such as shape, orientation, contour, internal structure, and posterior effects, included in the US BI-RADS assessment, can accurately predict a benign or malignant lesion. Mammography cannot differentiate the solid from the fluid lesions, and the microcalcifications used as indirect sign for the positive and the differential diagnosis of breast cancer have low specificity, while their absence cannot completely exclude a breast malignancy.

The most valuable demonstration of the mammographic limits is revealed by the comparative studies including the old screen-film mammography, the newest digital mammography, and the sectional imaging techniques (US, MRI, tomosynthesis). Most comparisons between the two mammographic techniques, including a large study of Sala and col. of a total of 242,838 mammograms (171,191 screen-film mammography group and 71,647 digital mammography group), have demonstrated a false-positive rate higher for the screen film than for the digital mammography (7.6% and 5.7%, respectively; $P < 0.001$) [2]; in addition, the false-negative results are less illustrated.

Digital mammography seems to improve the detection of the breast cancer with 27% in women under 50 years old, compared with the analogue technique, according to the American College of Radiology Imaging Network (ACRIN) that conducted a large Digital Mammographic Imaging Screening Trial (DMIST) in the United States concerning 49,528 women [3]. However, all screening methods are intended in the diagnosis of a cancer as early as possible, neglecting the benign or premalignant lesions; thus the incidence of the breast cancer rested unchanged; moreover,

A. Colan-Georges, M.D., Ph.D.
Imaging Center Prima Medical,
County Clinical Emergency Hospital,
Craiova, Romania
e-mail: aristida_georgescu@yahoo.com;
acgeorges.radiology@gmail.com

D. Amy (ed.), *Lobar Approach to Breast Ultrasound*, https://doi.org/10.1007/978-3-319-61681-0_8

the last recommendation for the breast cancer screening is neglecting the importance of the lesions assessed in the second category of the US BI-RADS. In the meantime, there are not equivalent assessments to the screening US BI-RADS for the symptomatic patients, which are examined without standardized protocols, with some complementary imaging techniques used before the final biopsy because of lack of differential diagnosis.

The classical US was used as a complementary technique of examination in differentiating the solid from the fluid lesions depicted on the mammography; there were used some suggestive descriptors for the benign, indeterminate, and malignant masses upon Stavros. In the classical US, the role of the vascular assessment was underevaluated, limited to the number of poles, size, and course (over three poles for malignant lesions upon 2003 US BI-RADS, with enlargement of the vessels and tortuous course). The sonoelastography was developed the latest, practically after 2003 with the aim to improve the differential diagnosis; it was initially criticized due to the various manufacturers and different scoring or quantitative assessments, and the 2013 US BI-RADS recommends it "with prudency, only if positive results."

The development of the automated breast volume scanning (ABVS) was intended to be used as screening test that is exploring the whole breast, more objective, and with possibilities of computed aided diagnosis (CAD). However, the orthogonal planes remain non-anatomical related to the lobar architecture, the normal breast parenchyma represented by ducts and lobules is neglected, and the coronal plane (plane C) has not a proved relationship with the nipple. Some encouraging studies revealed the value of the ABVS, such as the analysis of Brem and col. [4], which reported for a total of 15,318 women presented to screening mammogram and complementary ABVS, a number of 112 women detected with breast cancer (0.73%): 82 with screening mammography from which 17 were not detected by ABVS and an additional 30 detected with ABVS alone. They concluded the combined techniques were more performing, but that implies double screening techniques, raised costs, and no useful irradiation to 99.27% of women without cancer.

MRI sensibility is superior to any classical method in use, especially in detecting the multiple breast cancer (Fig. 8.1), without possibility to differentiate the multifocal from the multicentric lesions (arbitrarily considered multifocal in the same quadrant and multicentric in different quadrants or at least 5 cm interval). Because of lack of specific descriptors useful in the differential diagnosis, the specificity of the breast MRI is lower, even using the contrast-enhancing curves; thus the number of biopsies is still increased (Figs. 8.1 and 8.2); moreover, the higher costs and the limited availability restrain its use for specific indications [5].

The absence of a pathognomonic descriptor or of an association of descriptors with high accuracy for the positive and the differential diagnosis determined in practice the use of multiple complementariness techniques, with unsatisfactory results. A comprehensive study of Berg and col. from 2012 [5] concerning a total of 2662 women that underwent 7473 mammogram and ultrasound screenings, which detected 111 breast cancer events, illustrated the inconsistency of each technique: 33 cancers were detected by mammography only, 32 by ultrasound only that illustrates the non-concordant diagnosis, just 26 by both techniques, and 9 by MRI after false-negative mammography plus ultrasound; however 11 cancers were not detected by any imaging screening. By conclusion a combined examination with the main techniques in use failed in detection of 9.9% of cases. The sensitivity for mammography plus US was 0.76 (95% CI, 0.65–0.85) and the specificity 0.84 (95% CI, 0.83–0.85). The best sensitivity had MRI and mammography plus US of 1.00 (95% CI, 0.79–1.00), but the specificity decreased to 0.65 (95% CI, 0.61–0.69). The authors concluded the addition of screening US or MRI to mammography in women at increased risk of breast cancer

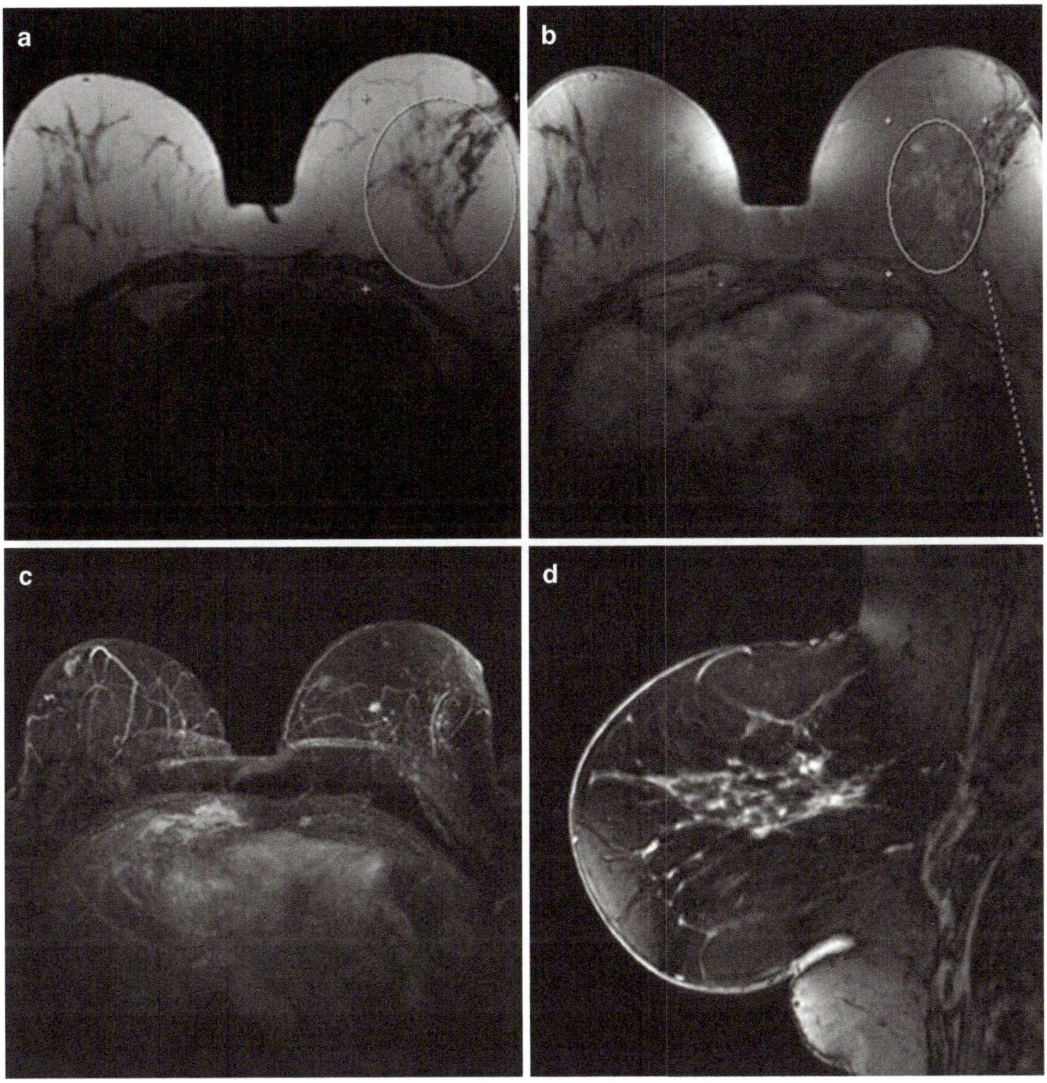

Fig. 8.1 Multiple cancer with small foci in the inner quadrants of the L breast in a 72-year-old patient with previous cancer present the R breast treated conservatory; the lesions present hyposignal T1, with enhancing contrast agent. It is difficult to localize and to precise their multifocal or multicentric type, even using 3D reformatting acquisition or complementary scanning planes (**a**, axial T1WI; **b**, axial T1 Fat-Sat contrast WI; **c**, axial 3D T1 Fat-Sat contrast reformatting image; **d**, sagittal T1 Fat-Sat contrast MPR)

resulted in not only a higher cancer detection yield but also an increase in false-positive findings.

We may conclude the low specificity in the breast cancer detection with isolated or combined radiological and imaging techniques of diagnosis in use is conditioned not only by the inherent technical limits but also by the non-anatomical scanning in arbitrary sagittal, coronal, or oblique plans, in the non-anatomical interpreting of the findings using artificial descriptors mostly borrowed from the mammographic lexicon ("dense" breast, "fibro-glandular tissue," "architectural distortion," etc.).

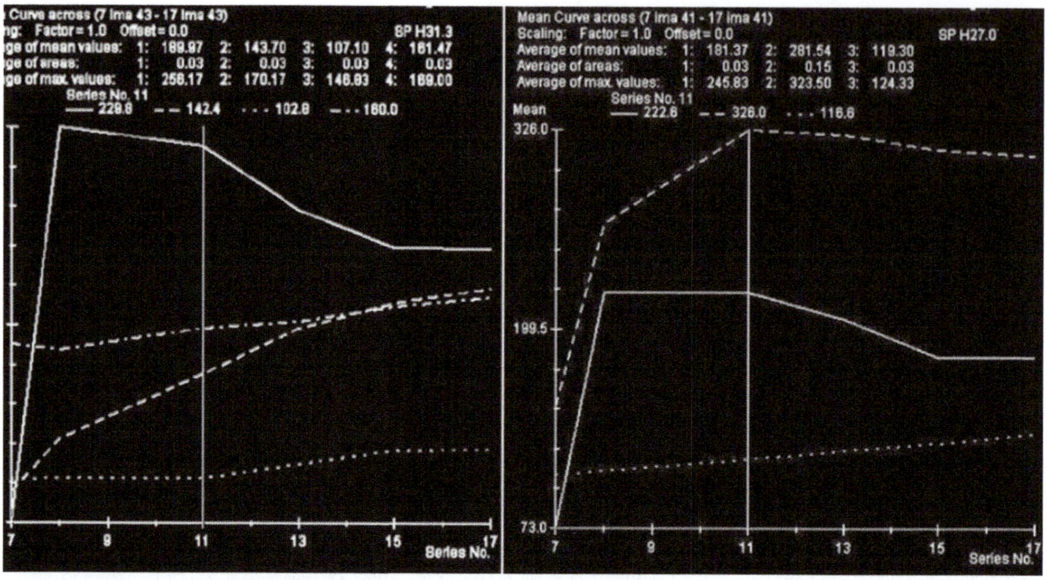

Fig. 8.2 The same case: the specificity of MRI is low, and the contrast-enhancing curves are dependent on the subjective choice of the region of interest (ROI) and on the lesion size; for the smallest, the partial volume artifact is conducting to false-negative diagnosis (*left* image), and for the 5–10 mm lesions, the enhancing curve is suggesting moderate suspect lesion; in conclusion, the global extension of the disease is underestimated

8.2 Significant Descriptors of the Breast Cancer in the New Concept of the Full-Breast Ultrasonography Related to the US BI-RADS Assessment

Last years, more practitioners adopted the anatomical technique of breast ultrasound based on the radial scanning with interpreting of the lobar architecture promoted by Teboul and Halliwell since 1995 [6] and largely spread after 2003 [7]; the lobar view of the breast US corresponding to the gross section of Tot and col. [8] was consequently promoted in all the world by Amy [9, 10], which also had contributions in the conceiving by manufacturers of the long linear probe provided with a water-bag, for a larger radial section without breast deformation and with better visualization of the nipple and superficial layers. These achievements completed with the Doppler examination and the real-time sonoelastography were defined under the concept of "full-breast ultrasonography" (FBU) [11], which allows a comprehensive noninvasive characterization of the breast anatomy and pathology, with better differentiation of the benign from the malignant lesions and with differentiation of some premalignant ductal-lobular changes, unapparent in the other techniques.

FBU realizes a whole-breast mapping using the well-known descriptors used by Stavros and US BI-RADS lexicon but related to the lobar anatomy centered by the ductal-lobular tree. The standardization of the technique made possible the reproducibility and the operator-independent scanning, with better follow-up characterization (Fig. 8.3).

The differential diagnosis of the abnormal findings is more accurate, avoiding unnecessary irradiation and biopsies or other more expansive additional techniques of examinations, and is

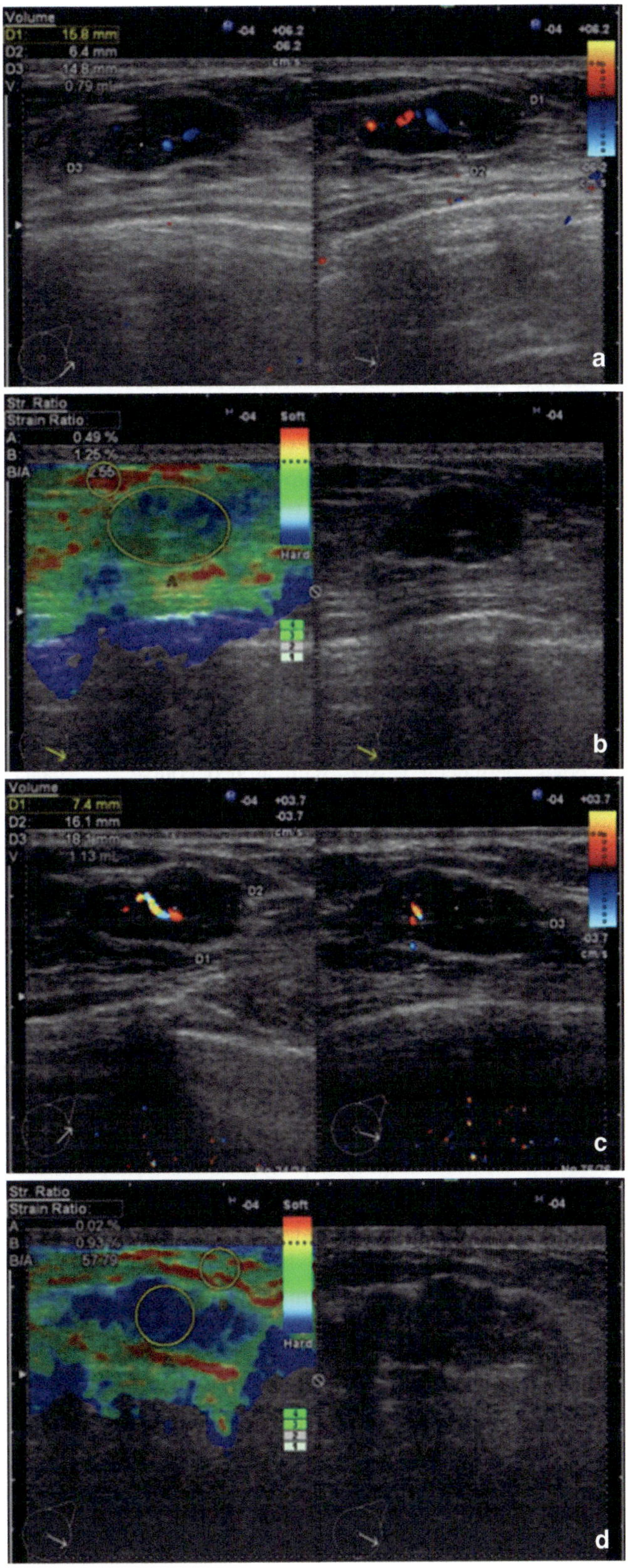

Fig. 8.3 Follow-up examination after 6 months interval of a peripheral lump at L 4:00 locations in a 38-year-old woman demonstrates an increasing volume from 0.79 ml (**a**) to 1.13 ml (**c**), a small increasing of the internal vasculature, increasing of the lobulations on the contour, and a higher stiffness from the score 2 Ueno with the strain ratio up to 2.55 (**b**) to a score 3 Ueno with the strain ratio up to 57.79 (**d**). The lesion assessed by US BI-RADS 4b was referred to conservatory surgery with extemporaneous pathological examination

based on a group of three descriptors: *the ductal connection (present or absent), the vascular characterization by Doppler, and the strain evaluation by sonoelastography.*

1. *The ductal connection* is mandatory in the characterizing of the anatomical appurtenance of a lesion: no hypoechoic mass will be suspect of breast cancer without ductal connection. The differential diagnosis includes other malignancies (breast lymphoma, sarcomas) or benign lesions (lipoma encompassed in and buttressed by surrounding dense hyperechoic fibrous tissue, fibrous tissue, others).
2. *Doppler characterization* with new evaluation in the FBU. The 2013 US BI-RADS assessment [12] stated a better role of the techniques of Doppler (absent, peripheral, internal) and SE, but with some limits. Doppler assessment is used for the evaluation of the new formations of vessels in solid tumors, allowing the differentiation of the benign from the malignant masses: for the benign lesions less than three vascular poles, peripheral vessels with arched course, "in basket orientation," with few, thin internal branches or without salient Doppler signal are suggesting; for the malignant masses, more vascular poles, concordant with the tumor size, the enlargement of the vessel diameter compared with those in the normal breast area, and the intratumoral arteriovenous shunts that give rise to flow detected as high-velocity signals, with aliasing similar to other cancers (thyroid, primary hepatocellular, and renal cancer [13–15]) were demonstrated. The intratumoral microvessel density is an important prognostic marker of survival in breast cancer [16, 17]. The use of contrast-enhanced US (CEUS) increased the sensitivity and specificity to 100% in the differential diagnosis of benign/malignant primary breast lesions according to Kedar [18]; moreover, CEUS of the breast had high accuracy for the assessment within 2 mm of pathologic tumor size according to Van Esser [19].

   In our experience, all these vascular descriptors are useful in FBU in the differential diagnosis of benign/malignant breast lesion; in addition, the anatomical scanning uses the vascular assessment especially in demonstrating the multifocal ductal carcinoma with intralobar distribution by intraductal spreading following the lowest pressure; the number of salient vessels and their size and velocity is proportional with the main tumor size and decreases as the size of the secondary (the nearest) or tertiary (distant) malignant foci increases. Moreover, all descriptors of the new formation vasculature used in the US BI-RADS lexicon are more or less subjective and should be completed by one of the most important, objective, and with pathognomonic value in the differential diagnosis: the incident angle of the plunging artery described by Kujiraoka et al. [20]. Any cancer type focal, multifocal, or multicentric will be found with at least one vascular pole with incident angle of the plunging artery; thus the scanning in the radial and antiradial plane is mandatory (Fig. 8.4); except for the diffuse increased vasculature in the lobar or the diffuse cancer (inflammatory breast cancer), and for the lactating breast, which can be differentiated adding the SE. (Figs. 8.5 and 8.6).
3. *The breast SE*, despite the EFSUMB guidelines, is still unstandardized, because of different manufacturers and of various scoring systems; this is the reason two follow-up SE performed with different systems may be impossible to evaluate for any benign or malignant evolution of a breast lesion. However, the real-time SE upon the Ueno (Tsukuba) scoring is best correlated with the US BI-RADS assessment (Fig. 8.7).

The sensibility of the SE is quite high for the differential diagnosis of the infracentimetric cancers that do not demonstrate malignant descriptors, the sentinel satellite lymph nodes, the local recidivism, and the malignant scars. SE in malignant less vascularized lesions is more sensitive than breast contrast MRI (Fig. 8.8); however, the diagnostic value of the SE alone must not be overestimated, because of the low specificity for

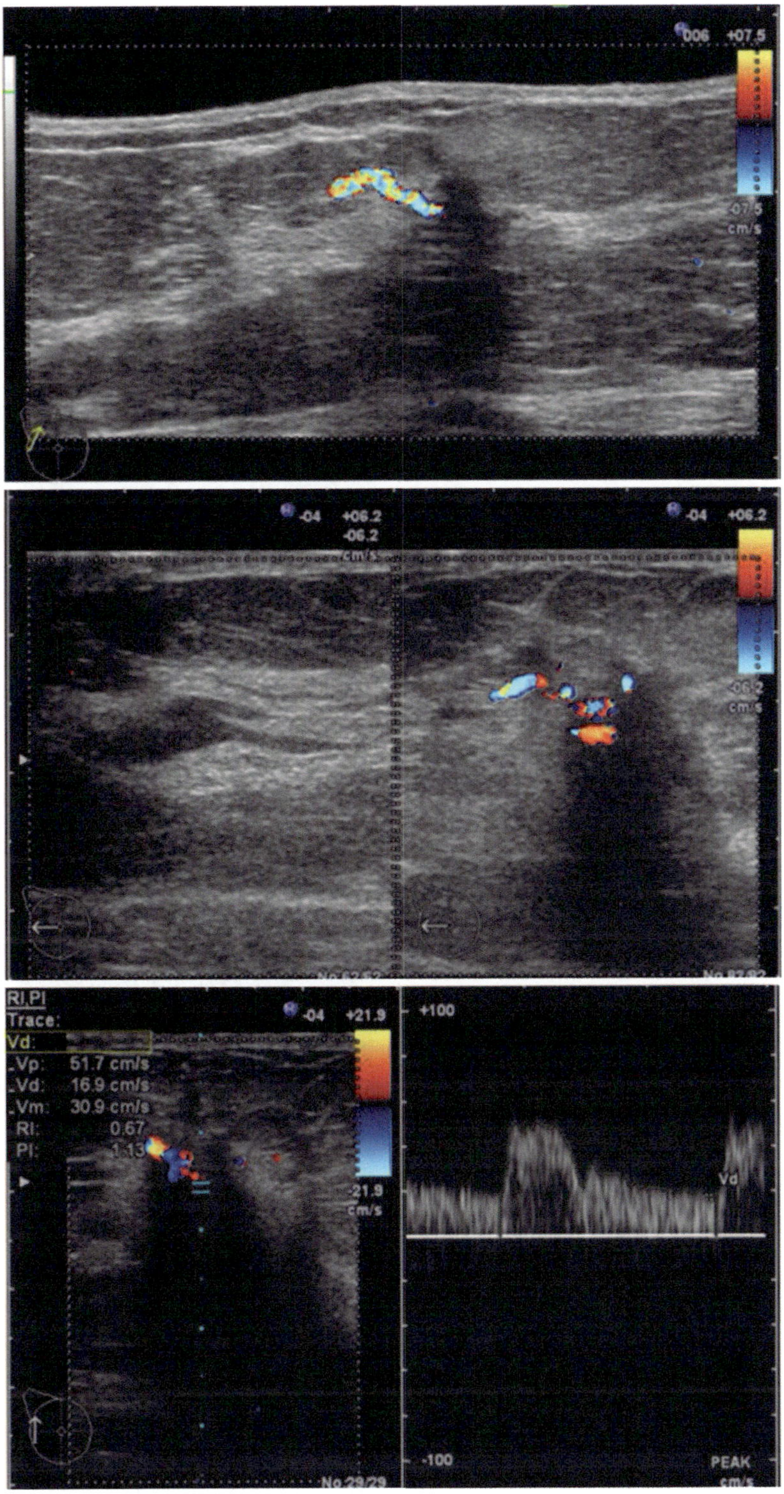

Fig. 8.4 Malignant type of new formation vasculature in ductal echography: the hypoechoic lesion with ductal connection demonstrates large, tortuous vessels, with aliasing and an incidental angle of the plunging artery after Kujiraoka et al. [20]

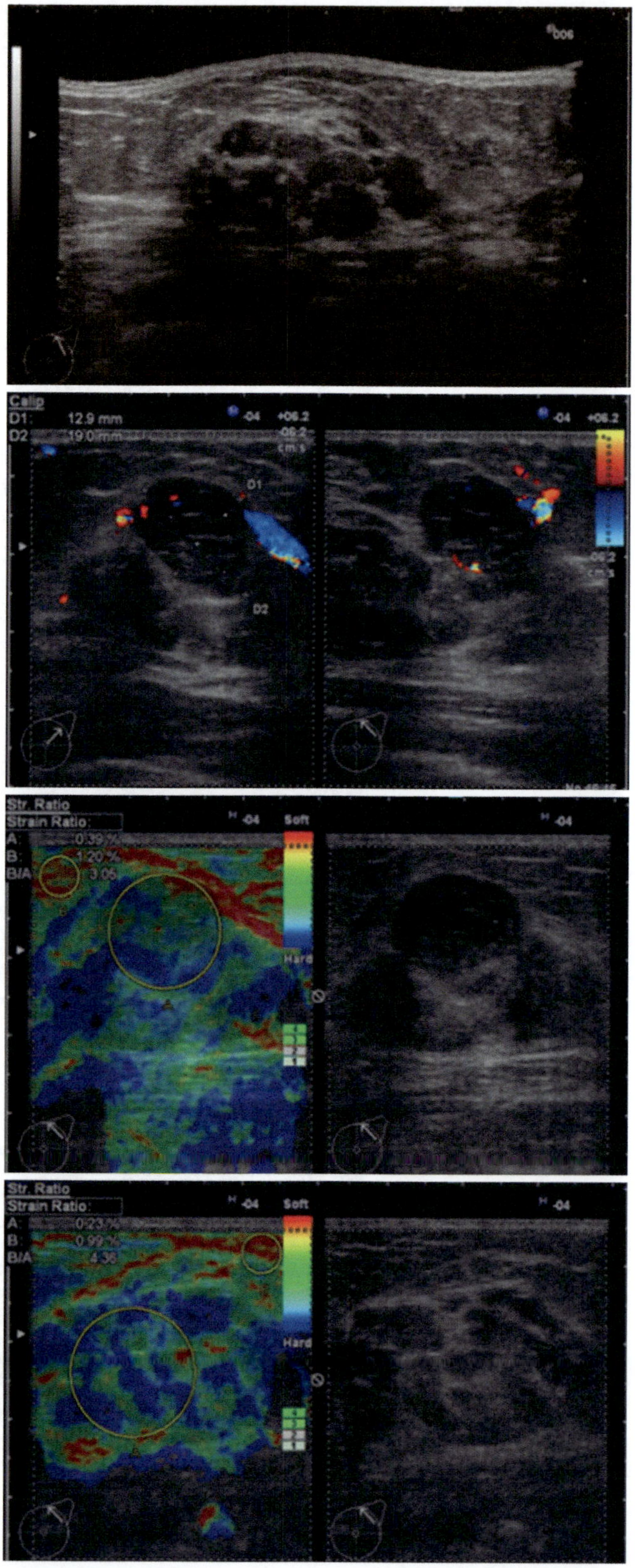

Fig. 8.5 FBU demonstrates a multifocal cancer type ILC, in a 59-year-old patient: the hypoechoic masses with ductal connection of various size and shape are grouped in the left axillary glandular prolongation, with pathological new formation vasculature and high strain

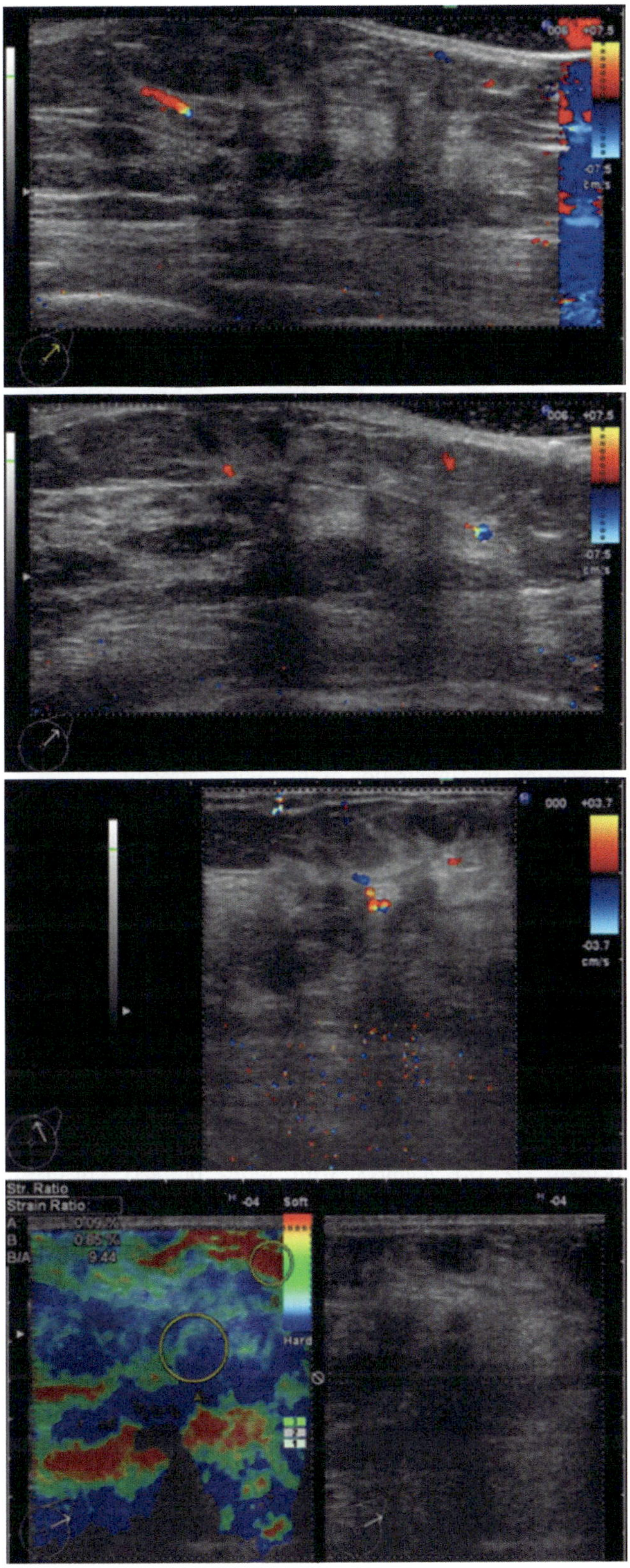

Fig. 8.6 Comparative FBU demonstrates a lobar type of an IDC in a 68-year-old patient: the small hypoechoic lesions with acoustic shadowing, new formation vasculature, and high strain are connected by the ductal tree and distributed in a lobar volume (radial and antiradial scans), suggesting the intraductal spreading way of the malignancy (multifocal breast cancer)

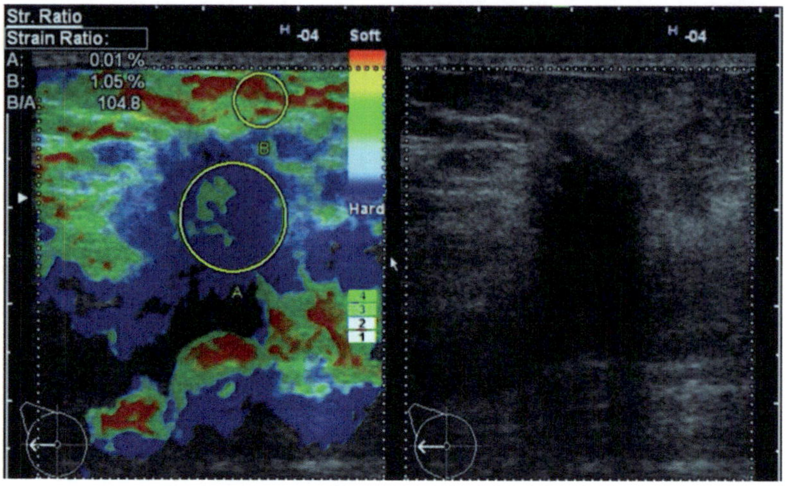

Fig. 8.7 The SE aspect of an IDC with halo in 2D US and acoustic intense shadowing demonstrates a score 5 Ueno and high strain with FLR over 100.0, with posterior artifact, concordant with the malignant microcalcifications visualized on the mammography—BI-RADS 5 category

the score 4–5 Ueno, found in malignant lesions as well as in benign ones (scars, sclerosing adenosis, suture granulomas, etc.), which will be further detailed.

FBU improves the differential diagnosis of the breast cancer because of integration of the anatomical view with the vascular findings and the SE scoring; this integration of the SE was already recommended by users of the classical US, for avoiding some false-positive and false-negative diagnosis [21]. In the anatomical radial scanning, SE was proved the best tool in the differential diagnosis of the inspissated duct or cyst that may mimic solid lesions in 2D US but illustrate a BGR or summation-BGR score [22].

Some solid findings such as a nonvascularized fibroadenoma with hypoechoic aspect may have a score 2 or 3 Ueno, while an atypical mucinous, medullary, or papillary carcinoma type illustrates benign 2D US features with more or less increased new formation vasculature and a score 4 Ueno.

FBU may diagnose not only the nodular type of breast cancer but also the lobar and the diffuse cancer, based on the illustration of the pathological ductal lobar tree; the pathological correspondence of the FBU findings is superior, the radial scanning allowing the differential diagnosis of the multifocal cancer (in the same lobe, possible in different quadrants) from the multicentric cancer (in different mammary lobes, possible in the same quadrant), being proved the lobes may overlap, but they have no ductal interconnections.

8.3 Differential Diagnosis of the False-Positive Cancers Using the FBU: Breast Cancer and Pseudo-malignant Lesions

There are two types of errors reported in the diagnosis of the breast cancer in the classical US: the false-positive and the false-negative findings [23].

The false-positive findings result in falsely high BI-RADS category assignment such as lipoma encompassed in and buttressed by surrounding dense hyperechoic fibrous tissue, fibrous tissue and scar with acoustic shadow, inspissated echogenic ductal secretions, ducts with fluid-debris level or fat-fluid level, fibro-microcystic dysplasia, etc.

It is generally assumed the fatty breast is easier to examine by mammography, but it is difficult to diagnose in US, because both fatty layers and malignant lesions are hypoechoic, and some benign lesions could mimic malignancies in the 2D US in the arbitrary transverse and sagittal scans. The false-positive results published by the classical US were determined by the non-anatomical scanning and interpreting of the breast images and by the inconsistent use of the

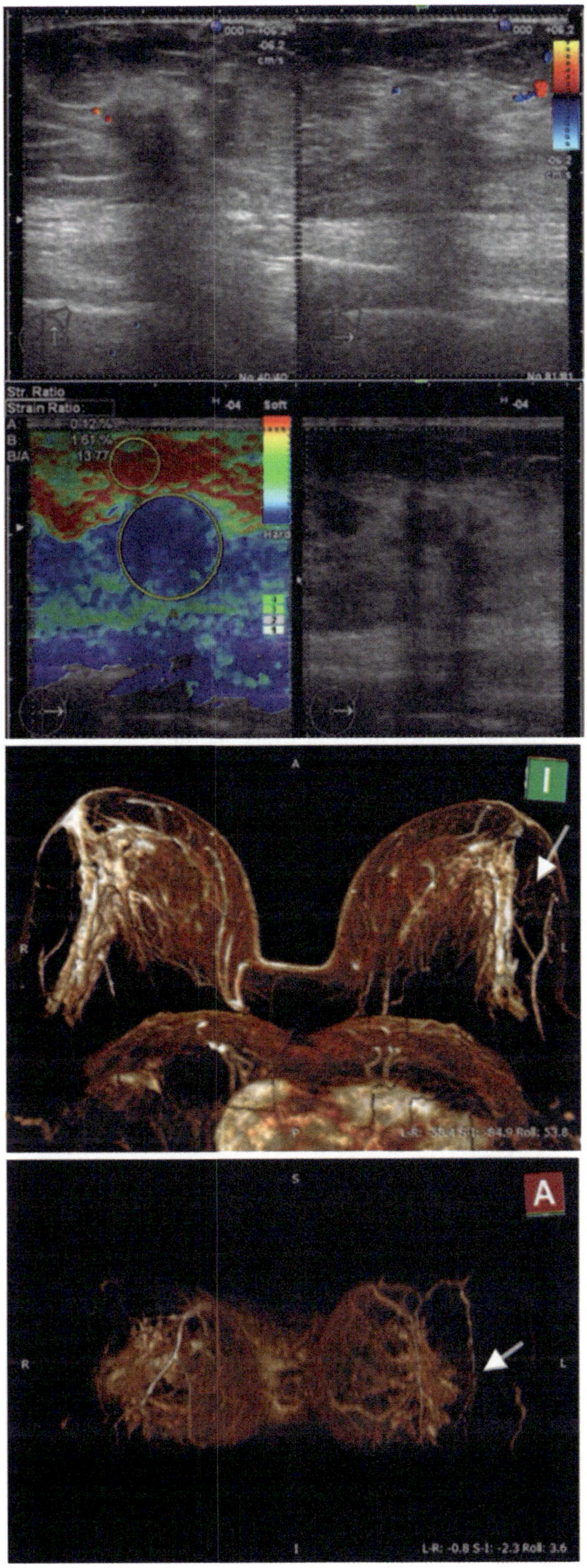

Fig. 8.8 Atypical findings in a 57-year-old patient, which presented a lump in L 3:00, with mammographical assessment BI-RADS 0 and inconsistent findings in 2D US (isoechoic aspect but with acoustic shadowing, thin peripheral new formation vasculature but with incident angle of the plunging arteries) and without pathological significant lesions or enhancement curves in MRI examination (not shown); the SE demonstrates a score 5 Ueno, and a second look of the MRI with 3D reconstruction of the T1 contrast-WI confirms an asymmetrical discrete enhancement in the same area (arrows in the axial and frontal views). The US-guided biopsy confirmed breast malignancy

Doppler characterization; the unsatisfactory results published about SE were related to its use as an independent method of examination that was compared with the 2D US alone. By consequence, it is assumed SE cannot differentiate the benign scars, the fibro-microcystic dysplasia (FMCD), and the calcified fibroadenoma from malignant lesions, all of them presenting low elasticity.

The radial scanning used in FBU allows a better differential diagnosis by illustrating the ductal connection of the breast cancer, while the lipomas are located either in the pre- or retromammary fatty tissue or between some branches of the ductal tree. Moreover, all hypoechoic findings with acoustic shadow which may have increased stiffness at SE, such as scars, diabetic fibrous mastopathy, and fibro-microcystic dysplasia, do not illustrate new formation vasculature with suspect descriptors (incident angle of the plunging artery, tortuous enlarged vessels, high velocity with aliasing).

The inspissated ducts or cysts and other segmental ductal abnormalities (ducts with fluid-debris level or fat-fluid level) have benign findings in FBU, with absence of suspect vasculature and a benign score at SE, type score 2, 3, BGR, or complex BGR.

Better results of the SE in the differential diagnosis are related to some recommendations for the technique of acquisitions:

- For the real-time SE, we should avoid a strong compression (range 5–6) that would determine false-positive images, most tissues looking hard.
- A small area of the surrounding tissues do not allow a good evaluation of the lesion stiffness, but a large region of interest (ROI) from the skin to the ribs offer a large scale of elasticity from the softest (fat) to the hardest (bone).
- The evaluation of the stiffness of a pathological finding must not be resumed to a unique measurement, but we should note an average of 3–4 qualitative and quantitative (FLR) sonoelastographic evaluation for each lesion, in radial and antiradial scans; the quantitative results may be expressed in strain ratio for the Hitachi devices and in kilopascal (kPa) or m/s for the shear wave elastography.
- In characterizing the benign lesions, it is useful to determine the highest strain ratio (FLR) or stiffness measured as pressure units (kPa), expressed in the report as "high elasticity/low strain of up to…," rather than the mentioning of a unique precise value; similarly, for the malignant assessment, it would be suitable to mention the lowest value of the quantitative measurements, to reassure the surpassing of the cutoff value: "low elasticity/high strain of FLR over…" or "low elasticity of over …kPa."

As illustrated, we mention an analyze of a series of 810 FBU, including randomly symptomatic and screening patients, which identified 149 cancers in 132 patients; from all, we had three false-positive cases of breast cancer, all of them in the beginning of this series, determined by the insufficient training; the diagnosis was based mainly on the DE with the presence of the malignant BI-RADS descriptors reinforced by the overestimated diagnostic value of the real-time SE of scored 4 or 5 Ueno but neglecting the Doppler less salient signal; in two cases, the surgical biopsy was performed, and the pathological result précised fibro-microcystic dysplasia, and the third case presented a chronic over infected deep hematoma, confirmed by FNA biopsy. The secondary analize of the images noted absent/reduced vasculature of suspect lesions, with benign acute angle of the plunging vessels, and a complex SE with increased stiffness areas combined with a summation/complex BGR score [24].

Fibro-microcystic dysplasia represents a pseudotumoral form of the cystic disease, considered by some authors as a premalignant lesion, but of lower risk for developing malignancy upon others (0.3% according to Venta et al. [25]), comparing with the ductal and lobular atypical hyperplasia; its importance in the differential diagnosis is done by the similar findings with many breast cancers on mammography, classical breast US, SE alone, and MRI. The fibro-microcystic dysplasia appears in the DE as a pseudo-malignant mass with hypoechoic aspect, connected to the ducts, with irregular/spiculated borders, acoustic shadowing, but without significant new vasculature on Doppler. Sometimes such small nodules are found in the site of the terminal ductal-lobular specific units (TDLU), considered as the initial site for the developing of any mammary lesion, either benign or malignant [26]. In our experience, there were no cases of breast cancer (without chemotherapeutic or radiotherapeutic treatment) without Doppler salient abnormal signal. Moreover, fibro-microcystic dysplasia presented a summation-blue-green-red (BGR) score at real-time SE, similar to the fluid structures over 4 mm diameter, with a low to medium FLR concordant with the benign lesions (Figs. 8.9, 8.10, and 8.11). The fibro-microcystic dysplasia represents the key in the differential diagnosis for the SE, but it was not well interpreted in the literature, even by the promoters of the real-time SE, which did not describe the summation-BGR score (we have chosen this term because the strain of the sum of the cluster of immeasurable cysts was similar to those of a unique cyst of appropriate volume).

The strain ratio of the fibro-microcystic dysplasia is not characteristic, according to the "hard" ROI selected inside the lesion; the selection of the whole area of BGR complex or summation type generally presented a strain ratio

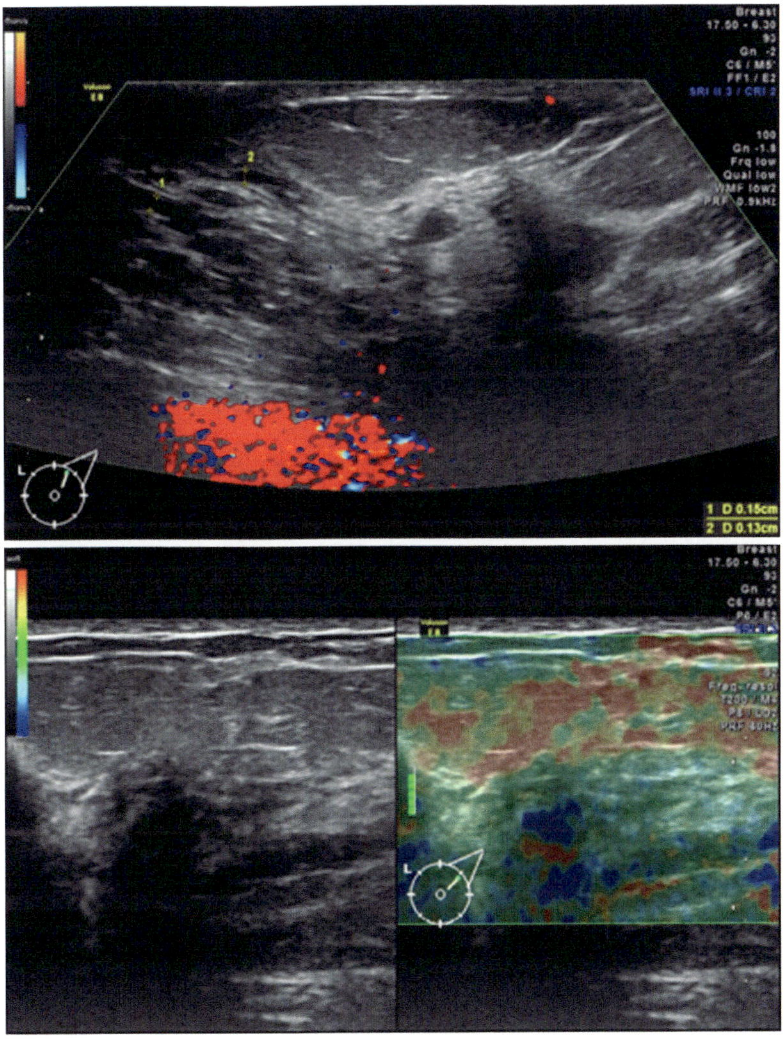

Fig. 8.9 FBU in a 56-year-old patient illustrates central ectasia and a pseudo-malignant peripheral lesion with ductal connection, with ill-defined, hypoechoic, and spiculated borders, with acoustic shadowing and taller than wide; the negative Doppler and the BGR-type score made the differential diagnosis in this fibro-microcystic dysplasia

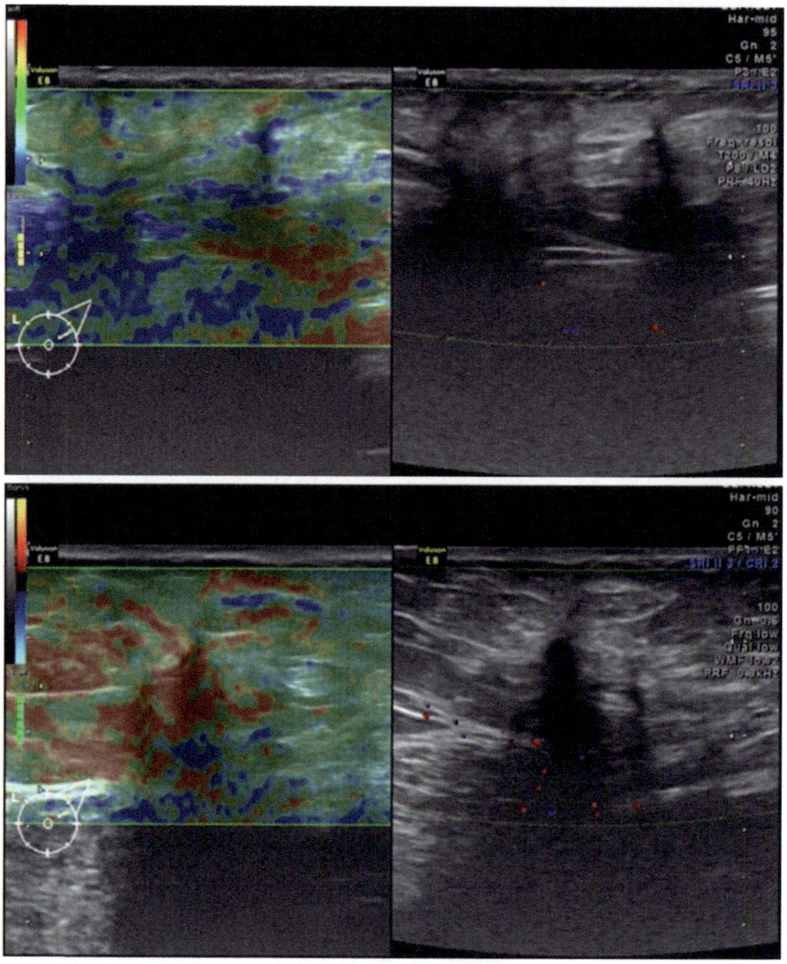

Fig. 8.10 FBU in a 69-year-old patient with lobar malignant findings both at mammography and 2D US; the negative Doppler and the BGR-type score suggest a fibro-microcystic disease, concordant with the biopsy

(FLR) of <4.70 considered for the cutoff value [22] and conducted to the final diagnosis as a benign lesion with low risk to develop cancer, assessed by US BI-RADS 3 category.

Fibrocystic dysplasia is a frequent finding, considered by some authors as a form of the "sick lobe" [27, 28]; it is easy to diagnose in the limited phenotype, with few measurable transonic cysts, or in the diffuse phenotype of the Reclus disease, but the diagnosis is more difficult in the inspissated cysts and in the nodular fibro-microcystic lesions (Fig. 8.12). In a series of 819 patients, we found 282 (34.43%) cases with fibrocystic dysplasia, of which 79 (9.6%) cases included the nodular type presenting a clinical pseudotumoral more or less painful aspect [22]; FBU illustrated unique or multiple lesions with multicentric or multifocal distribution, sized between 0.5 and 3 cm. There were frequently associated (macro) cysts, ductal ectasia, in few cases ductal papilloma, benign nodular hyperplasia (fibroadenoma), or diffuse ductal or lobular hyperplasia but rarely was present a breast cancer (Fig. 8.13).

Ductal ectasia in non-breastfeeding women is present in many painful breasts, both in benign and malignant diseases. Nipple discharge and especially bloody nipple discharge is considered having a benign etiology in 80% of cases (duct papilloma, duct ectasia) and rarely may be malignant (duct carcinoma). The usual radiological and imaging differential diagnosis is difficult due to many factors:

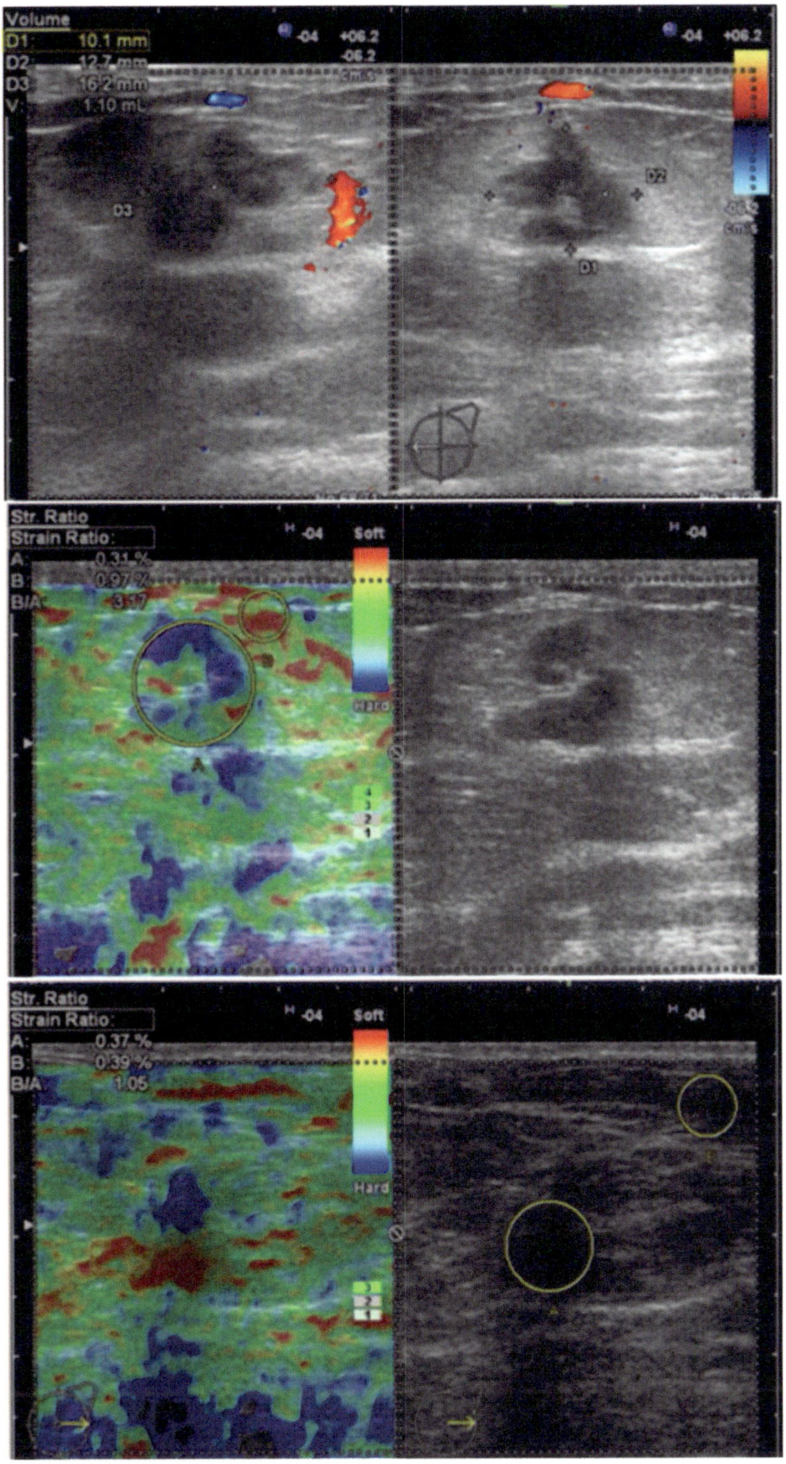

Fig. 8.11 FBU in a 60-year-old patient with pseudo-nodular infracentimetric findings grouped in a TDLU location; there are some peripheral salient vessels in Doppler examination; the hypoechoic structure and the irregular shape with variant orientation are unspecific, but the BGR score of the SE is suggesting for the nodular fibro-microcystic dysplasia

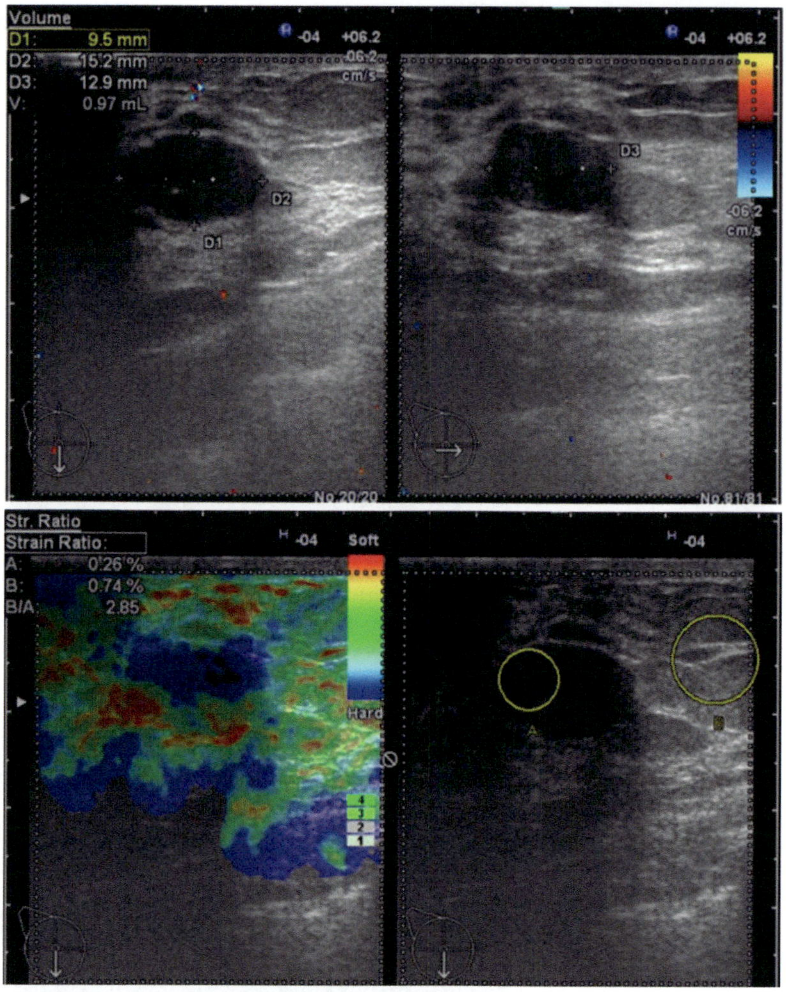

Fig. 8.12 Inspissated cyst, the differential diagnosis with a solid mass: the absence of any Doppler signal together with a BGR score, whatever the protein content of the cystic fluid

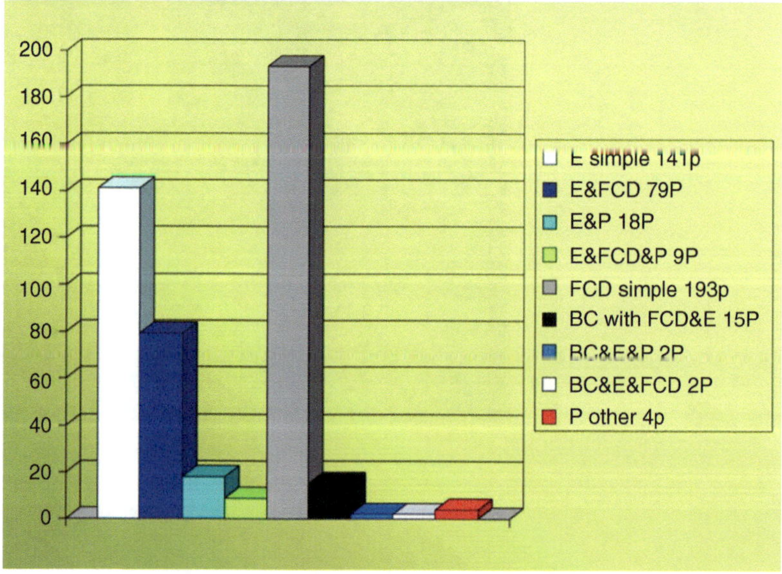

Fig. 8.13 Distribution of the secretory changes: E simple = ductal ectasia without other abnormalities; FCD = Fibrocystic dysplasia, including FMCD; P = papilloma; BC = breast cancer (upon [22])

- The mammography and the tomosynthesis cannot visualize the normal and abnormal ductal walls, but sometimes the intraductal microcalcifications localize and orientate the diagnosis.
- Mammography may demonstrate intraductal calcifications in bloody nipple discharge both in chronic galactophoritis and in comedo DCIS; frequently the mammography underestimates the extension of DCIS because it cannot detect the ductal walls without microcalcifications [29].
- The radiological galactography is an invasive technique, with uncertain results.
- The classical US does not explore the ductal tree.
- The ABVS and MRI, despite their multiplanar techniques, have low resolution and may incidentally illustrate segments of thickened ducts.

FBU differentiates the chronic galactophoritis inside the group of ductal ectasia and demonstrates the absence of a pathological periductal vasculature in the presence of a chronic infection with various types of staphylococcus (*S. aureus*, *S. albus*, *S. epidermidis*, and so on), *E. coli*, proteus, and *Candida albicans* (sometimes found equally in acute mastitis of lactating women) [30] (Fig. 8.14). The differential diagnosis of the chronic galactophoritis is made with the physiologic (breastfeeding) or pathological hyperprolactinemia (galactorrhea) that demonstrates a diffuse increased breast vasculature or hyperemia (Fig. 8.15) and with segmental ectasia with localized (peri-)ductal vasculature associated with papilloma or breast cancer.

In addition, the real-time SE is useful in the differential diagnosis of duct ectasia whatever the fluid density, presenting in thin and middle ductal ectasia the score 1 Ueno-like (green walls with red lumen) and in large, pseudo-cystic ducts the BGR score; the ductal papilloma and DCIS may demonstrate the score 2 and 3 Ueno (Fig. 8.16).

The chronic no puerperal breast infections are frequent but rarely diagnosed and treated; usually the nipple discharge or the fine-needle aspirate is intended only for the cytological tests, but the diagnosis of these infections is important because they represent the main cause of the painful breast without skin changes that could be treated; moreover, galactophoritis is frequently associated in the florid stage with ductal hyperplasia and in the final stage with ductal atrophy and nipple retraction, mimicking carcinoma or Paget disease [22]. These chronic infections may lead to the disfigurement of the breast secondary to repeated operations and to an empiric anti-staphylococcal treatment [30]. Their differential diagnosis by FBU allows conservative treatment avoiding unnecessary biopsies or the surgical procedures.

Ductal thickening differential diagnosis implies specific descriptors for different etiologies. Ductal hyperplasia may be either diffuse or segmental; the diameter of the ducts is increased, but this thickening must be correlated with the patient age and the individual breast ductal pattern: in the young woman, 1.5–2.5 mm is considered normal ductal thickness, while in the postmenopausal woman, the normal ducts are ranged <1.0 mm. The differential diagnosis is made by the preserving of the central hyperechoic line representing the virtual lumen in duct hyperplasia, while in intraductal papilloma, the thickening of the ducts is done by a central mass surrounded by thin walls. Ductal hyperplasia has a score 1 or 2 Ueno-like (Fig. 8.17), duct papilloma has a score 2 or 3 and low FLR, while DCIS appears with loss of the ductal central line sign, increased thickness, hypoechoic walls sometimes with hyperechoic granular echoes (without certitude of microcalcifications in the absence of the mammography), with at least a score 3 Ueno and salient vasculature (Fig. 8.18).

Lobular hyperplasia may appear as isoechoic micronodules connected to the ducts, usually in a TDLU location; the size of few millimeters must be interpreted according to the age and the physiological condition; there are not salient local Doppler signal, and the SE demonstrates a score 2 Ueno for the glandular area (terminal ductal-lobular structures and glandular stroma). FBU allows the differential diagnosis with the <5 mm breast cancer, which has always a ductal connection, and can

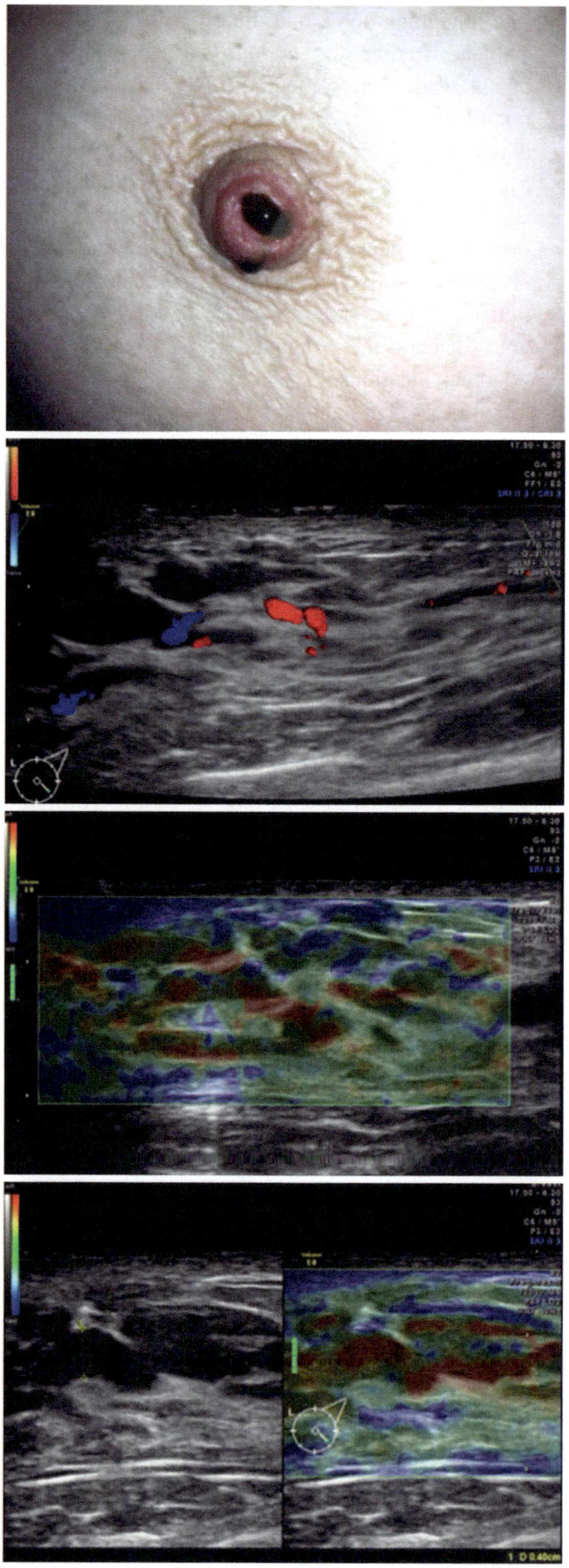

Fig. 8.14 Bloody discharge in a 35-year-old patient with duct ectasia overinfected with *Staphylococcus haemolyticus*; the color of the secretion may be different in the same breast, there are no skin changes, and the ductal content may be hypoechoic or with fluid-fluid level; the SE demonstrates a score 1 Ueno for the thin ecstasies or BGR for the largest ones

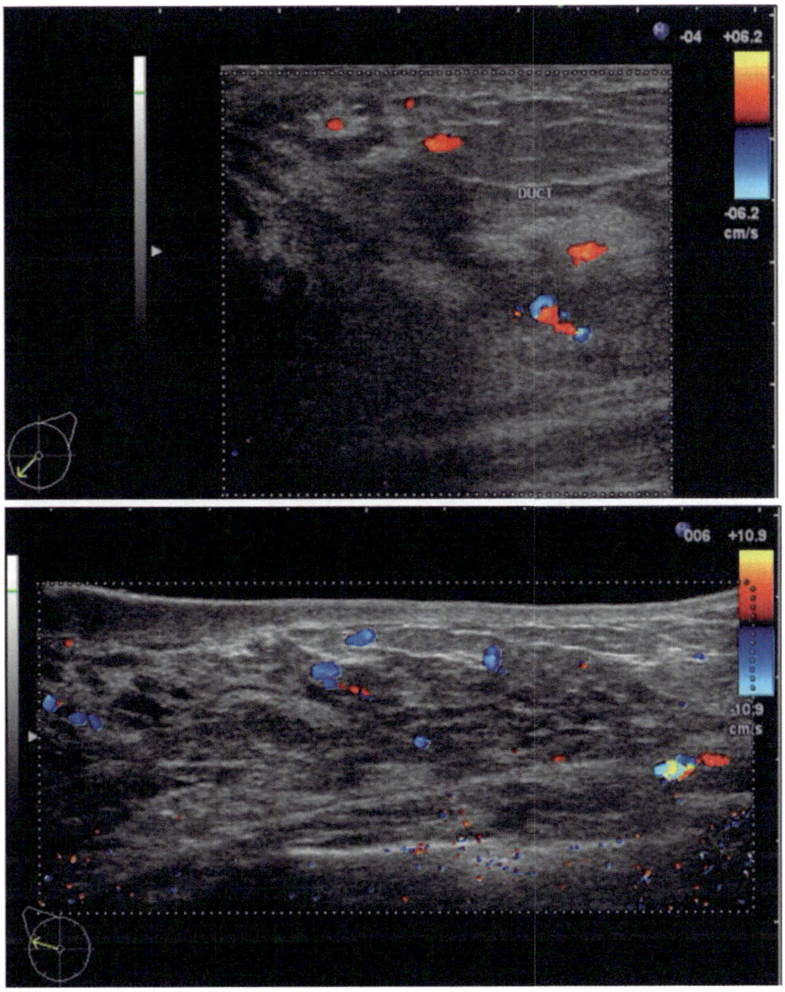

Fig. 8.15 Hyperprolactinemia (*upper* image) and lactating breast (*lower* image): reduced pre- and retromammary fatty tissue, dense parenchyma with small duct ectasia, and the pathognomonic increased diffuse breast vasculature; no breast edema or skin thickening found in acute mastitis

miss the acoustic shadow; the shape and the borders may be confusing of benign type, but usually there is a salient new formation vasculature which represents the most important tool in the differential diagnosis; the SE shows a score 3 or 4 Ueno for the small cancers, and its value is just complementary.

Suspect lesions <5 mm are not palpable and they are difficult to locate and characterize by mammography or breast MRI; a short-time US follow-up may be useful before the decision of biopsy. In our experience, a suspect lesion of 3.5 mm diameter with unipolar new formation vasculature doubled the dimensions and reached new vessels in 2-month interval, and the pathological report confirmed a DCIS. In other cases, a peripheral lobular hyperplasia in a postmenopausal woman, more hypoechoic than the surrounding parenchymal structures, with blurred stroma, without Doppler signal and with medium

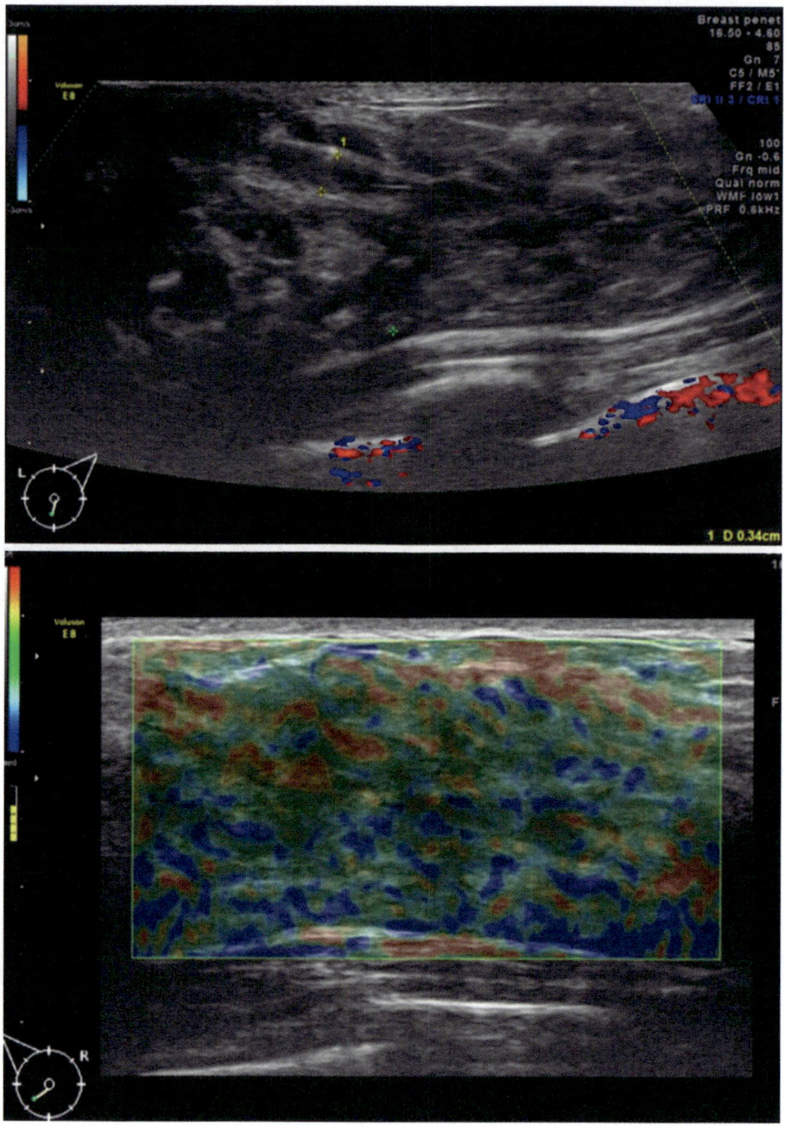

Fig. 8.16 Ductal hyperplasia in a 22-year-old patient with mastodynia: ductal thickness up to 3.5 mm associated with loss of the central line sign, without Doppler signal, and the SE with a global score 2 Ueno

FLR values, developed in a 9-month interval a multifocal lobular carcinoma with salient new formation vasculature and a score 5 Ueno for the glandular area.

The false-positive diagnosis of the benign hyperplastic scar as a local recidivate can be overruled in the FBU by the analysis of the duality vasculature and strain: in the early postoperative follow-up, the benign scars may illustrate thin peripheral reparatory vessels without important fibrosis, while in a late stage, there are no more vessels, and the strain is increased.

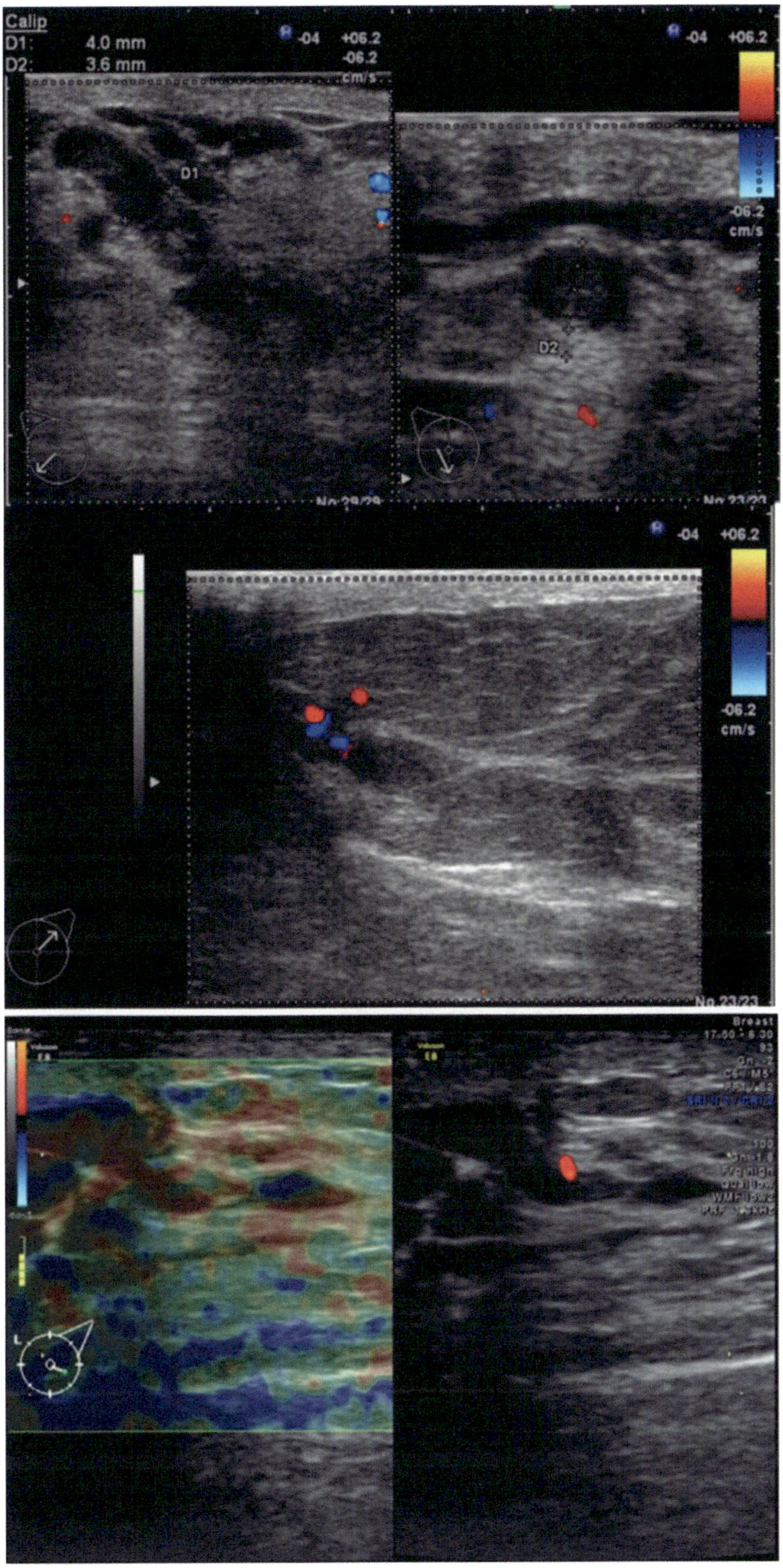

Fig. 8.17 Ductal papillomas

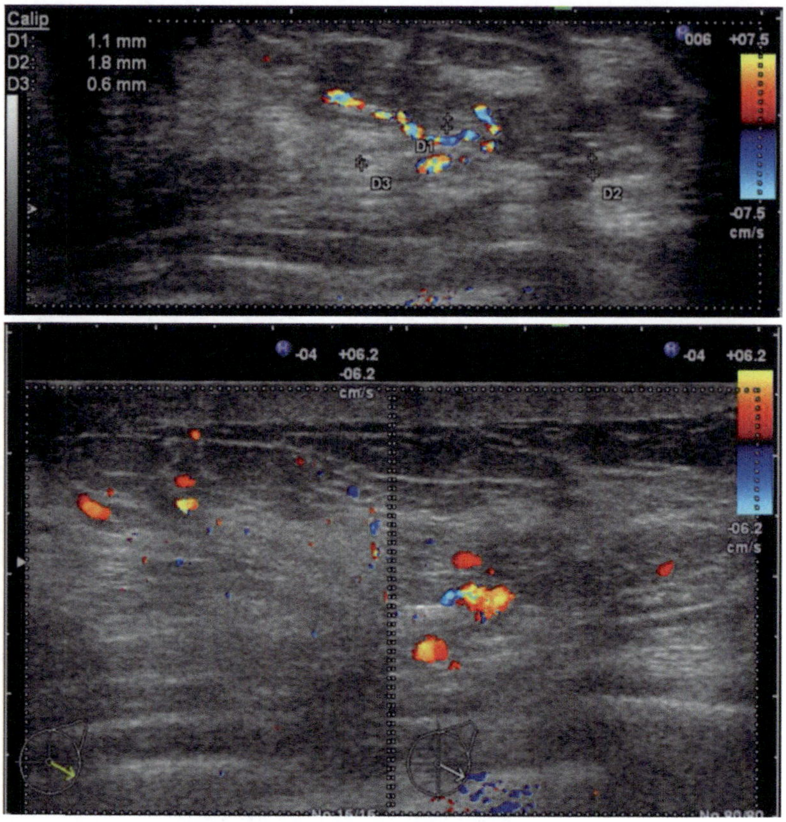

Fig. 8.18 Relapse of a DCIS in L 4:00 after conservative surgery a year before followed by radiotherapy; skin thickening and increased vasculature in the areas with inhomogeneous ductal thickening, illustrated using a long linear transducer (*upper* image) and a short high-frequency transducer (*lower* image) with composed double screen

8.4 Differential Diagnosis of the False-Negative Cancers Using the FBU: Breast Cancer with Pseudo-benign Appearances

The group of *false-negative findings* results in a false BI-RADS category assignment falsely too low, missing the diagnosis of the breast cancer. There are many different causes of false-negative diagnosis invocated in the classical US:

- Technical reasons: volume averaging in the near and in the far field, gain too low, time-gain curve too flat, and isoechoic nodules without high-frequency coded harmonics
- Some pathological specific conditions:
  - Lack of the posterior effects of colloid nodules with incomplete volume characterization
  - Papillary, medullary, and mucinous carcinomas with pseudo-benign features
  - Impossible visualization in US of the most malignant microcalcifications
  - Small carcinomas that lack specific suspicious features
  - DCIS with extensive necrosis
  - Diffusely infiltrative lesions such as classic infiltrating lobular carcinoma
  - Intracystic carcinoma

These reasons are correct, but they are applied to an incomplete US breast examination, limited to the possibilities of the 2D US, without mentioning of the Doppler and SE more specific aspects; some technical limits may be improved, but the sensibility of the US exam will not increase, and the false-negative diagnosis will persist because of the orthogonal axial and sagittal scanning, with risk of missed regions to the examination.

FBU aspect of the pseudo-benign findings in the gray-scale examination, such as colloid nodules and papillary, medullary, and mucinous carcinomas, will demonstrate the ductal connection of a mass and a salient new formation vasculature with suspect descriptors: incident angle of the plunging artery, tortuous course, enlarged lesional vessels, and higher velocity of the tumoral vessels with aliasing as compared with the normal flow in the rest of breast vasculature; complementary SE will add information about the strain alteration.

The differential diagnosis with other findings presenting salient abnormal vasculature includes the real benign lesions: some infected cysts with pericystic inflammation, the abscesses, infected hematomas, or ruptured implants demonstrate vascular changes; in these cases, SE offers a differential diagnosis presenting benign scores. Breastfeeding diffuse hyper-vasculature may be easily differentiated by SE from the acute mastitis and the malignant mastitis: the strain of the subcutaneous fatty tissue and of the mammary lobes is normal in hyperprolactinemia, the fatty tissue is inversely more stiff than the glandular structures in benign mastitis, and the stiffness is significantly increased for the glandular lobes in malignant mastitis [11]. These differential descriptors were neglected in the classical US because of lack of correlation of US available tools with the breast physiology and the lobar anatomy.

There are other cancers without microcalcifications or without stromal reaction with its characteristic spicules, with false-negative diagnosis in mammography and MRI. In these cases, the presence of the malignant new formation vasculature with increased flow and possible arterial-venous shunts may be characterized by Doppler and it corresponds to the MRI dynamic contrast curves, which are suspect for malignancy when depict rapid enhancing (pick) with plateau (done by new vessels with enlarged diameters) or wash-out (arterial-venous shunts).

Other differential diagnoses for pseudo-benign findings, such as diffuse infiltrating lobular carcinoma, DCIS, small carcinomas without acoustic shadow, peritumoral halo, or spiculated borders, are easy to perform using the mentioned three elements: the ductal-lesion connection inside the mammary lobe, the Doppler with malignant aspect, and SE with increased strain.

In the cases with previous mammography and important diagnosis discordances, a targeted short-term control FBU seems reasonable instead of a painful biopsy that has high risk of false diagnosis up to 25% in the literature [31–33]; a dynamic volume measurement of the suspect lesion (radial × antiradial × anterior-posterior diameter) with vascular and elastographic comparative characterization is more useful for the differential diagnosis than the hypoechogenicity, the long-axis/short-axis ratio, the posterior effects, or the stromal reaction (Figs. 8.19 and 8.20). The differential diagnosis in cases of simultaneous multiple lesions or of atypical cancers with discordances between the radiological and imaging techniques is based on the duality new vasculature-low elasticity with a score 4 or 5 Ueno and a high strain ratio (with the cutoff value of 4.7 for the Hitachi devices) (Figs. 8.21, 8.22, and 8.23).

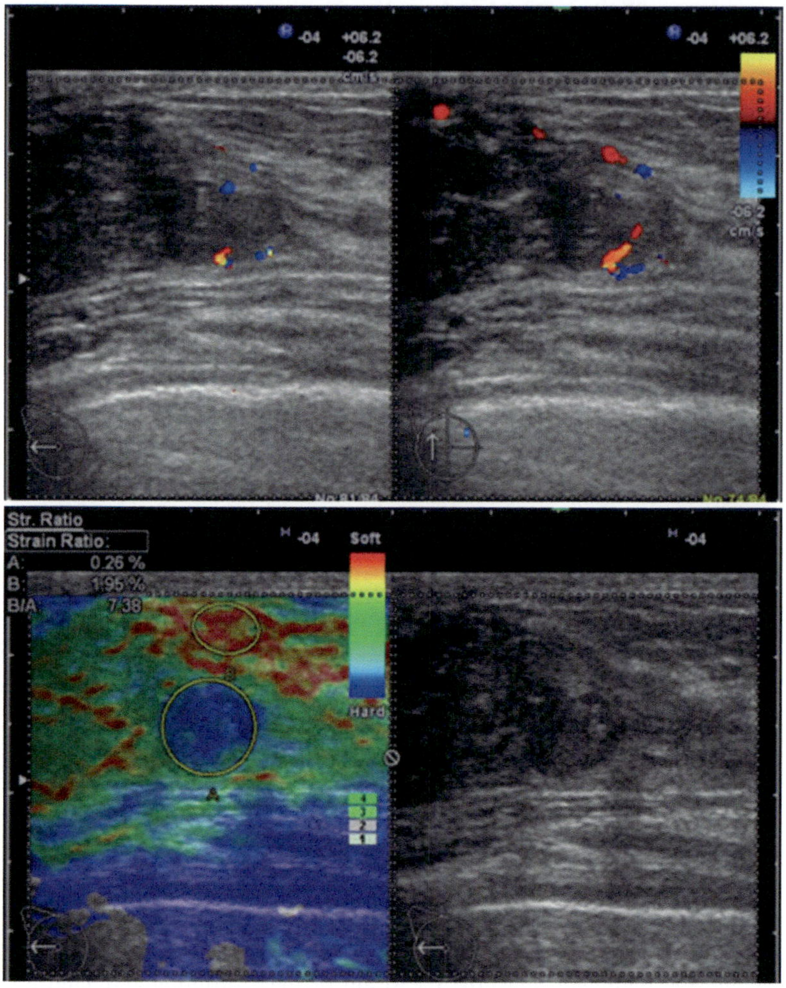

Fig. 8.19 Infracentimetric breast cancer at R 9:00, in a 37-year-old woman masked in 2D US by the dense breast parenchyma; the new formation vasculature and the score 4 Ueno with FLR over 7.00 make the differential diagnosis

8.5 Differential Diagnosis of Breast Scars

The differential diagnosis of the breast scars is possible by FBU not only in the conservative surgery but in cases with radical surgery-type mammectomy or mastectomy and breast cosmetic surgery (mastopexia, breast reduction, and breast reconstruction).

The scars may appear in US as linear or irregular hypoechoic area related with the skin scar, with more or less acoustic shadowing. The benign scars usually do not illustrate suspect vasculature, and the SE is unspecific with various strains, according to the etiology and the time of evolution; some cases illustrate suture granuloma with pseudo-nodular lesions, seroma and hematoma with BGR score, and architectural distortion in conservative treatments but with low strain, sometimes associated with nearby benign breast lesions (cysts, ductal ectasia or hyperplasia, fibroadenoma) (Figs. 8.24 and 8.25).

The radial scars are not related to surgical scarring and are rather a constructed image on the mammography, which illustrates a volumic projection in a plane, than a true pathological

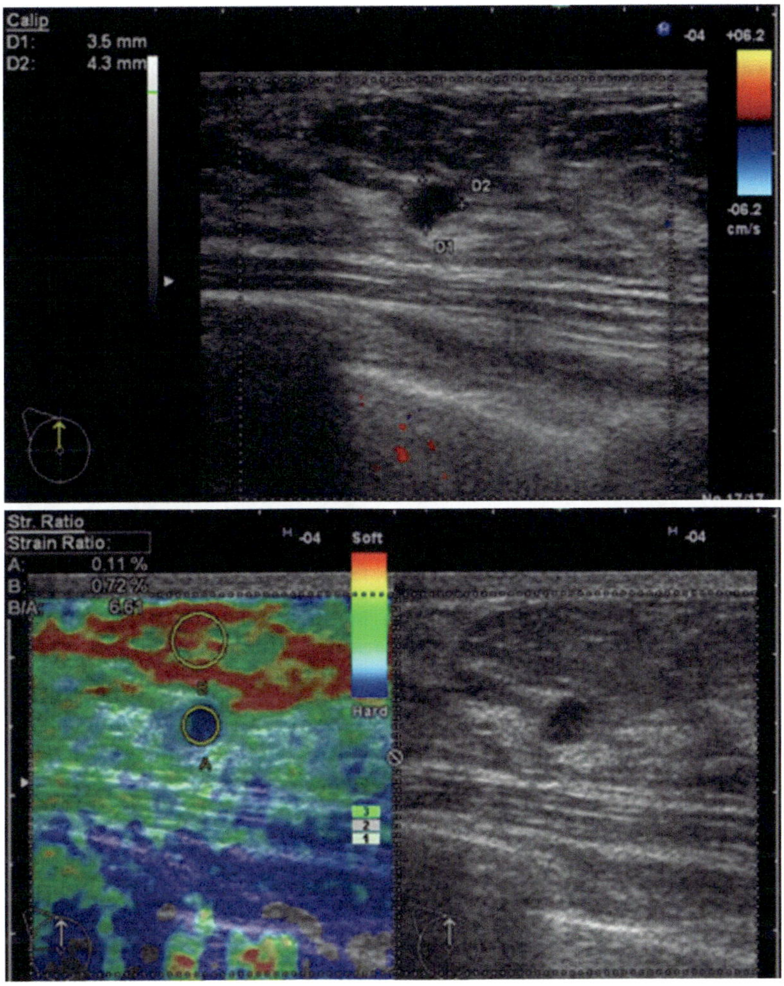

Fig. 8.20 Less than 5 mm breast cancer misdiagnosed in Doppler 2D US as cluster of microcysts; SE with a score 4 Ueno and FLR up to 6.60 recommended a short-time follow-up, with doubled lesion size and proven DCIS after 3 months; this case may explain some "interval" cancers

mass; in the classical US, they were described somewhere different characters, such as disturbed architecture of the surrounding breast parenchyma, ill- or well-defined mass with round or oval shape, acoustic shadowing, etc. Despite its fibrous core and a score 3 or 4 Ueno, there are no suspect new formation vasculatures in the so-called radial scar examined by FBU, and the benign aspect does not justify the recommendation for biopsy. The histopathological aspect confirms a benign lesion that contains hyperplastic tissue cells and a central fibrous core, with radial extension of tubular structures that have two rows of cells, epithelial and myoepithelial, justifying the spiculated peripheral borders. The radial scar is not palpable, and radiologically it is mimicking infiltrating carcinoma; some authors consider the risk of developing malignancy two times greater than in the normal population, but others affirm there is not a higher risk of radial scars than of fibrocystic disease, and there are no differences in the frequency of radial scars in women with and without breast cancer [34].

The "malignant scar" is a recent term used for the local recurrence of a breast cancer in the area of the surgical scar, to differentiate it from other local recurrences of the disease in the same

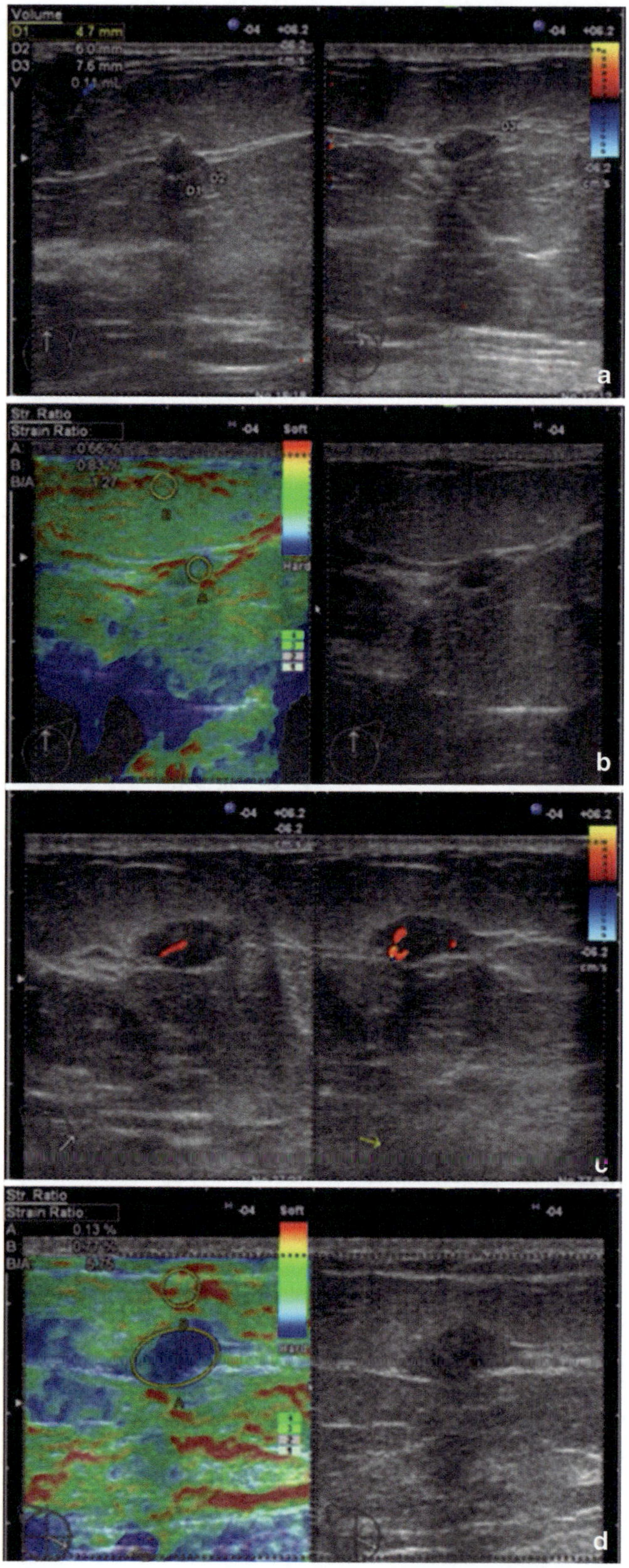

Fig. 8.21 Differential diagnosis of a benign infracentimetric nodule in L 12:00 (**a** and **b**), with a similar size breast cancer in R 4:00 (**c** and **d**), in a 42-year-old patient; the ductal connection and the 2D US findings are similar with benign descriptors upon Stavros and ACR BI-RADS assessment, but there are significant differences in Doppler signal and strain evaluation; the discrepancy between the 2D benign and the final FBU diagnosis is suggesting for atypical breast cancer of mucinous or medullary type

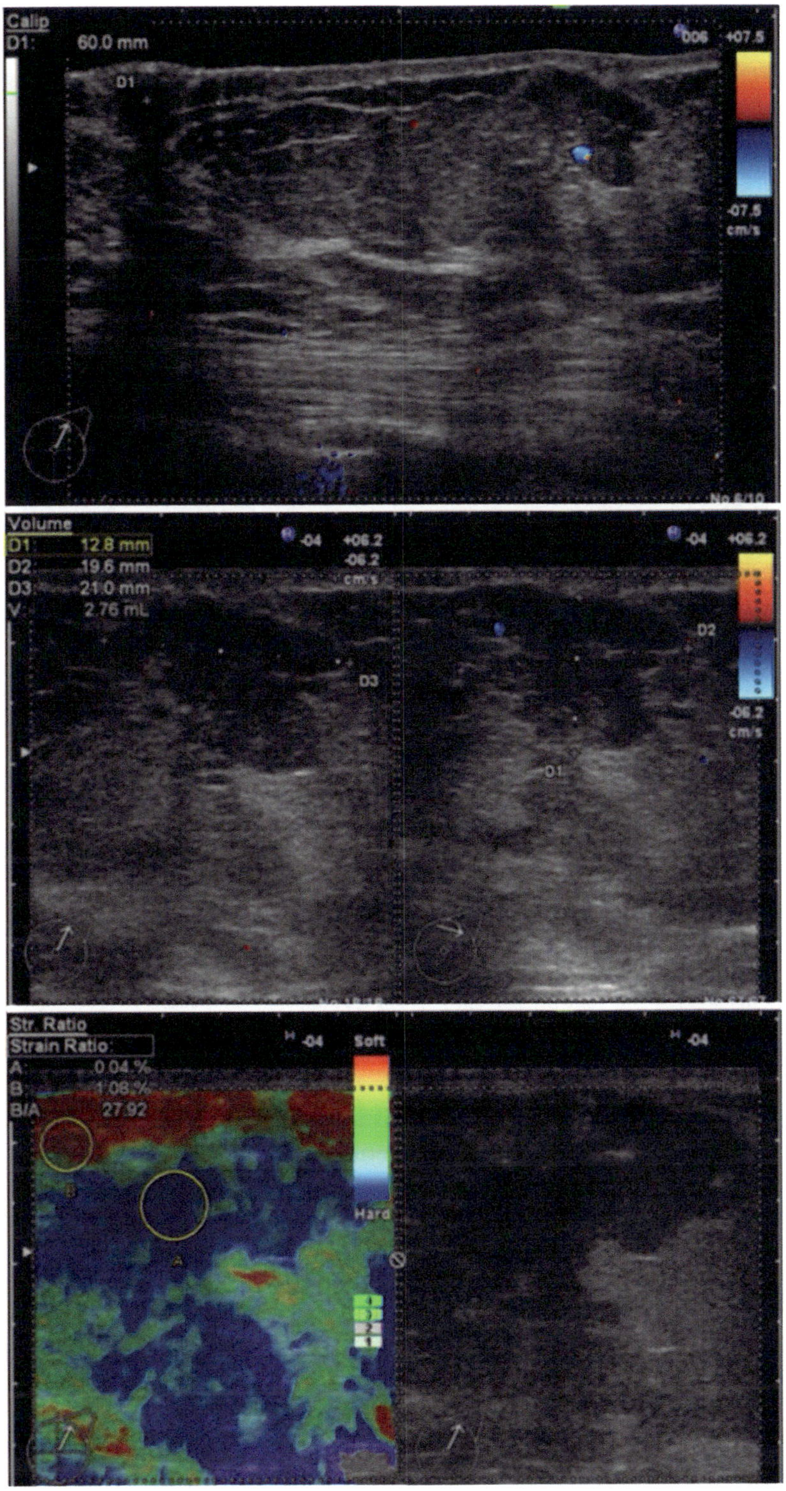

Fig. 8.22 FBU in an atypical breast cancer with 4 years evolution in L 1:00, in an 87-year-old patient: benign features (posterior acoustic enhancement, wider-than-tall and low-but-salient Doppler signal) and malignant descriptors (multi-lobulated borders, eccentric shadow, low elasticity with a score 5 Ueno, and FLR up to 27.92). The differential diagnosis should include fibro-microcystic dysplasia (SE summation-BGR score), trauma-contusion, hematoma (history, normal skin, complex BGR score), diabetic mastopathy (history, biological tests), lymphoma, etc. The pathological report confirmed mucinous cancer, not very rare in elderly women

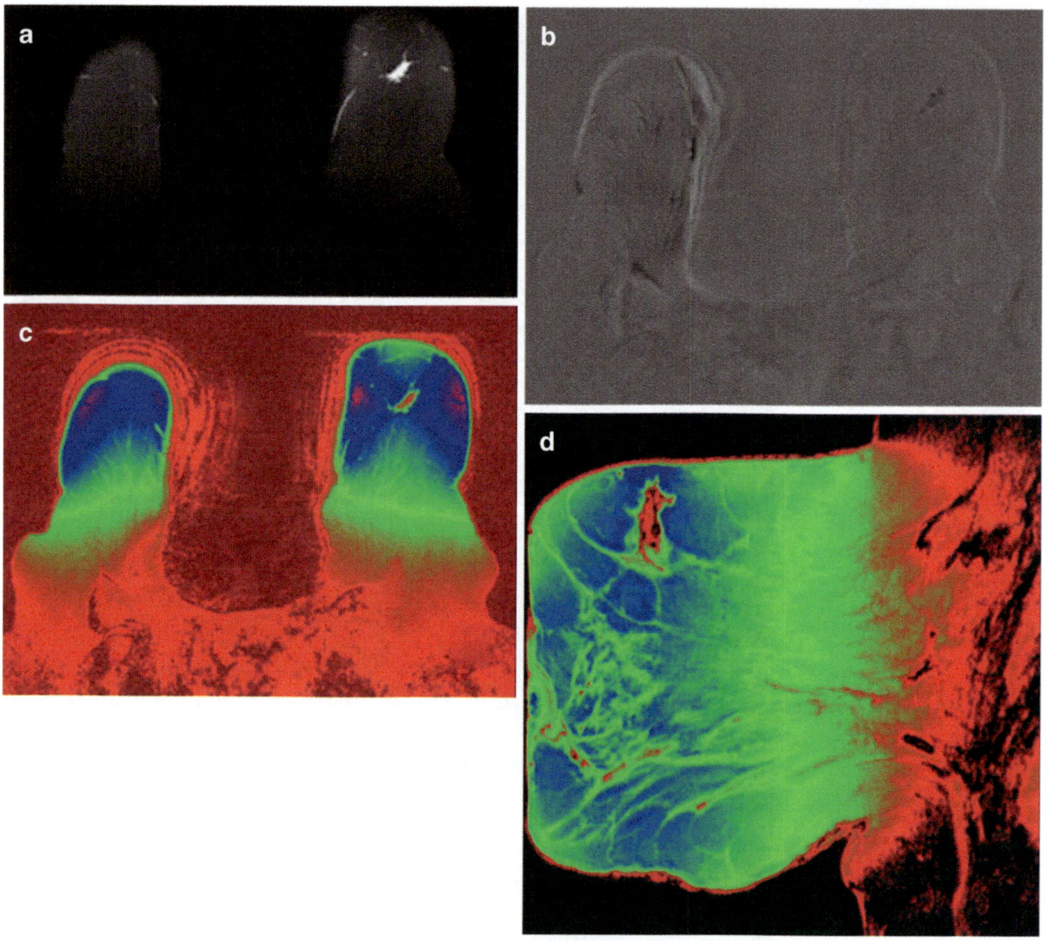

Fig. 8.23 Atypical breast cancer—the same case: MRI examination has a false-negative diagnosis, with hypersignal T2 Fat-Sat WI (**a**) and without contrast pathological enhancement (**b**) T1 Fat-Sat contrast subtraction WI; however, the retrospective color mapping of the contrast sequences (**c**—axial and **d**—sagittal views) was more useful in the characterization of the pathological mass, proving a reduced contrast enhancement undetected by the usual protocols

breast after conservative surgery, or distant from the scar in the small parts of the anterior hemi thorax after radical treatment, which can be considered as local metastases [35]. The earlier diagnosis of a malignant scar by the follow-up care during the complex treatment of the breast cancer is possible by US completed with Doppler and SE each 6 months during the first 3 (5) years and once a year after that (Fig. 8.26); in special cases, further imaging examinations for detection of distant metastases (CT, MRI, PET-CT) will be performed after individualized schedule.

The secondary malignancies closed to the surgical scar in the conservative treatment or in the ipsilateral breast are not rare, between 10% and 15% in the literature [36], and may be explained by the non-anatomical technique of excision-type lumpectomy or segmentectomy with arbitrary limits or even by incomplete excision of the mammary lobe containing the tumor, with possibility of missing some intraductal secondary foci of tumor dissemination. Because at least in the initial stages breast cancer develops inside a lobar structure, due to the complete distinction between the lobar ductal trees, the whole lobe must be excised according to the "sick lobe theory" [27, 28]; thus a new technique of conservative surgery was developed beginning with 1988 and perfected by Enzo Durante [10], with developments by Giancarlo Dolphin and others, which begin with the dissection of the sentinel lymph node, continue by mobilization of the nipple-areola complex for reducing scar formation, and finish with the

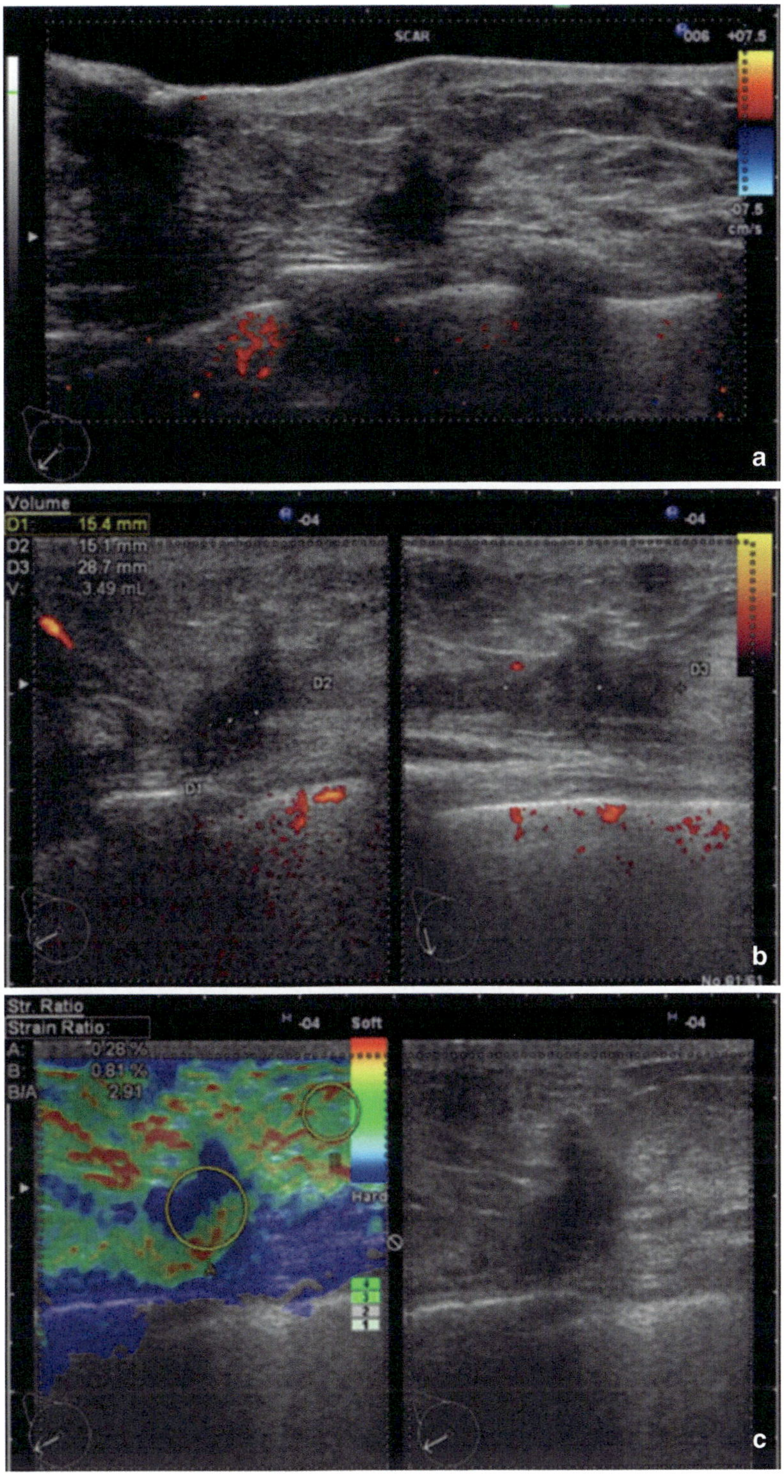

Fig. 8.24 Pseudo-malignant aspect of a chronic seroma after conservative surgery of breast cancer in a 58-year-old woman; seromas are frequent findings after a classical "segmentectomy," which does not respect the lobar anatomy

complete excision of a single affected lobe up to the nipple [37]. The removed lobe is then examined by US in the surgical room, and the presence of the tumor inside is verified. As results there are less 0.3% cancer relapses after Dolphin with conservative surgery of minimal but complete excision of the sick lobe; because the vascular supply is related to the

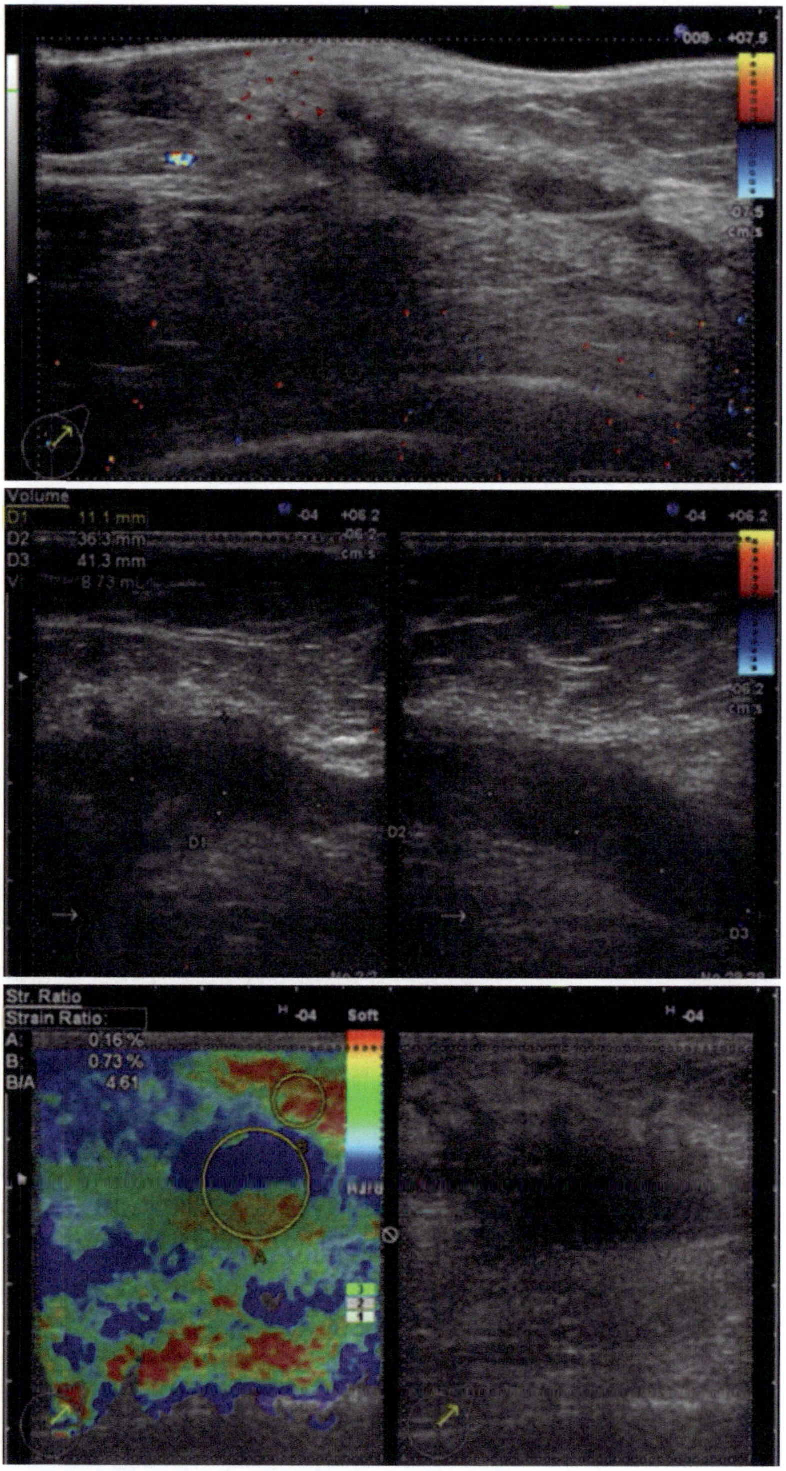

Fig. 8.25 Benign scar in a 38-year-old patient with conservatory surgery for breast cancer: the absence of a salient suspect vasculature (**a** and **b**) and the BGR score (**c**) are the most significant findings for the differential diagnosis with a malignancy, suggested by the hypoechoic mass with ductal connection and spiculated shape

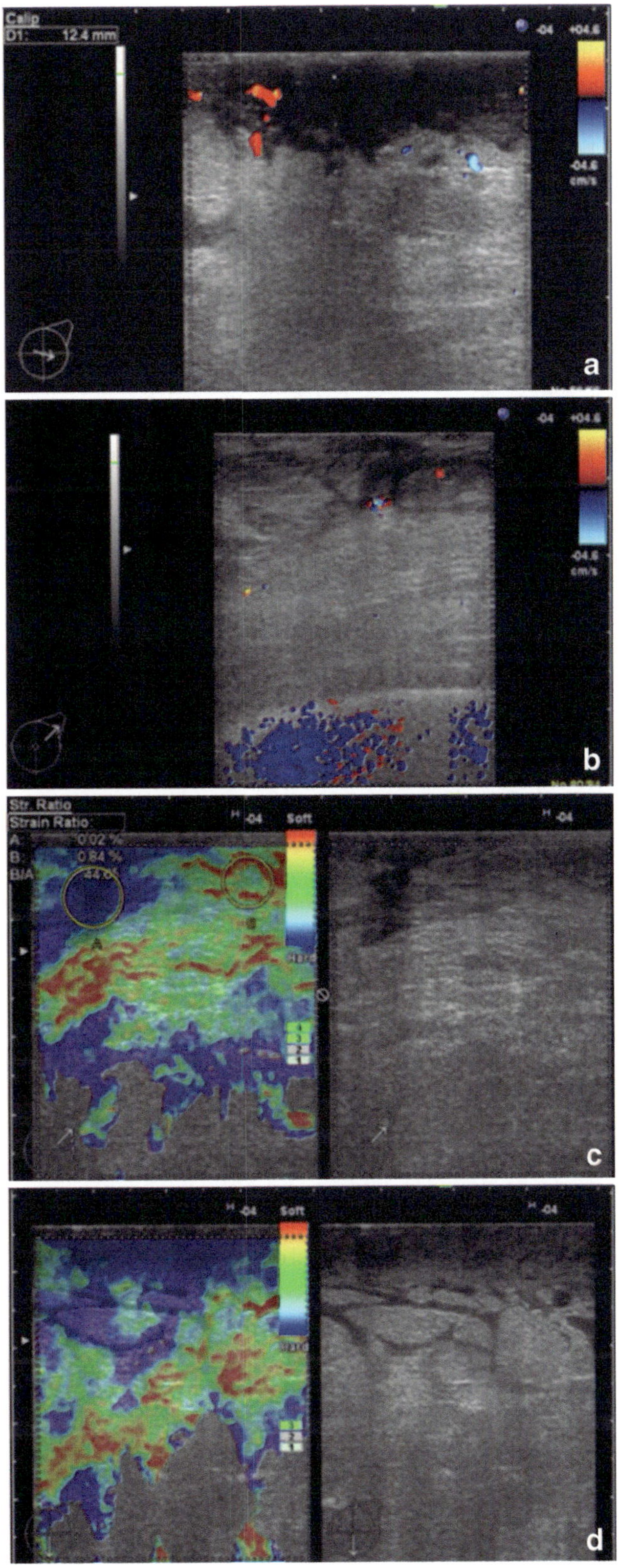

Fig. 8.26 Malignant breast scar in the left upper-outer quadrant with proliferative extension to the nipple-areolar complex in a 62-year-old patient: superficial mass with accentuate hypoechogenicity and multipolar new formation vasculature (**a** and **b**); the high strain with score 5 Ueno and FLR up to 44.65 (**c**) and lymphedema in the lower quadrants demonstrates increased hardness (**d**)

anatomical-functional unit of the mammary lobe, its complete excision reduces to minimal the risk of surgical seroma or hematoma, with esthetical and psychological best results (see the chapters about new surgical treatment of the breast cancer).

8.6 Differential Diagnosis of the Satellite Lymph Node Appearances

The study of the satellite lymph nodes by FBU is useful in all breast examinations, even in cases of normal breast findings, because there are other etiologies for abnormal lymph nodes, either systemic inflammatory processes (sarcoidosis), infectious diseases (bacterial lymphadenitis, tuberculosis, borreliosis), or malignancies (lymphoma, malignant melanoma, or lung, stomach, ovarian carcinomas). In some cases, there are other masses in the satellite areas, which must be differentiated from a metastatic lymph node: lipoma, sarcoma, seroma, aneurism, venous thrombosis, collagen vascular diseases, and miscellaneous (silicone implants, tattooing).

Mammography was the first technique of examination that visualized better in the MLO view the normal axillary lymph nodes (small, with oval shape and central lucency due to the fatty hilum/medullary) and the abnormal lymph nodes characterized by higher density, reduced or absent hilar fat, and a round, irregular, ill-defined shape with or without intra-nodal calcifications. Mammography may demonstrate abnormal axillary findings in cases without breast suspect findings, the so-called negative mammograms [38]; the breast cancer cannot be excluded, because the occult cancer to the radiological examination (missed cancers by mammography) may be found in screening mammograms about one in five breast cases, either in dense breasts or in small lesions, without microcalcification and stromal desmoplastic reaction [39]. However, the specificity of mammography for the axillary lymph nodes is low, and the sensibility is limited by the anatomical location, only the lowest axillary lymph nodes being accessible to the radiological examination, while the deeper ones and other stations (sub- and supraclavicular, internal mammary nodes) cannot be explored. The lymphadenography performed 24 h after injection of oil-soluble iodinated contrast agent or dynamic acquisition after water-soluble contrast is an invasive technique, with low accuracy for the completely invaded nodes, practically abandoned after US and CT development. A supplementary advantage has the FDG-PET as a noninvasive procedure that allows, within a single examination, the biological characterization of breast cancer and viewing of the entire body; however, FDG-PET has a lower sensibility than the sentinel lymph node biopsy in detecting the micro-metastasis [40].

MRI should be the best method of examination, because all satellite nodal stations can be visualized and characterized; however, the specificity of the MRI remains unsatisfactory, and the number of biopsies increased. The accuracy of MRI is not adequate to obviate either the pretherapeutic or the post-neoadjuvant chemotherapy status of the axillary lymph nodes [41] and could not replace the sentinel node biopsy.

US is able to detect all satellite stations: axillary, sub- and supraclavicular, internal mammary, thoracic lateral chain, and lateral cervical and spinal chains. A normal lymph node demonstrates at US scanning a thin hypoechogenic cortex in the periphery interrupted by the hyperechogenic fatty hilum that continues with the central nodal area or the medullary zone; Doppler signal may be absent, or few vessels (artery and veins) may be demonstrated in the hilum with centrifugal orientation, but without extension to the normal cortex. The lymphatic vessels are not salient in mammography or imaging techniques, because of their thin structure and of the low velocity of the lymph; anatomically the afferent lymphatic vessels penetrate the node cortex, and the efferent enlarged vessel leaves the node by hilum.

US completed with Doppler and SE, as an equivalent to the FBU, is useful in the differential diagnosis of the benign from the malignant nodes: the largest size is not significant, but the ratio transverse to longitudinal diameter is normally under 0.50; the main diameter with role in the differential diagnosis is the transverse one (short axes) that has <10 mm for the axillary benign nodes. Focal thickening with more hypoechoic texture of the node cortex is suspect of micro-metastases by the way of the afferent lymphatic vessels, and the presence of new formation cortical vessels with increased focal stiffness has great accuracy. The differential diagnosis with the benign adenomegaly includes the longer axis development; thin cortex even with undulated, microlobulated contour; large medullary area even with central hypoechoic aspect in benign reactive hystiocitosis (Fig. 8.27); reduced vasculature exclusively in the hilum; and a normal strain of score 1 or 2 Ueno or cortical BGR score significant for lymphedema. The axillary node hystiocitosis is usually present in chronic galactophoritis and is frequently described associated with breast cancers.

The abnormal malignant nodes tend to become more round because of the cortical thickening (Fig. 8.28), with increasing of the intracapsular pressure; this determines the obliteration of the central medullary area (hilar replacement) before increasing of the longitudinal axis of the involved node (Fig. 8.29); other descriptors mentioned in the literature such as unclear margins, node matting, and perinodal edema [42] are very rare, even in large, multiple metastases of the breast cancer. The peripheral flow and the transcapsular vessels seen on color Doppler represent one of the most significant descriptors for malignancy, but they are reduced or absent in necrotic nodes and after neoadjuvant chemotherapy or radiotherapy (Fig. 8.30); for an accurate diagnosis, the most authors recommend needle aspiration or biopsy

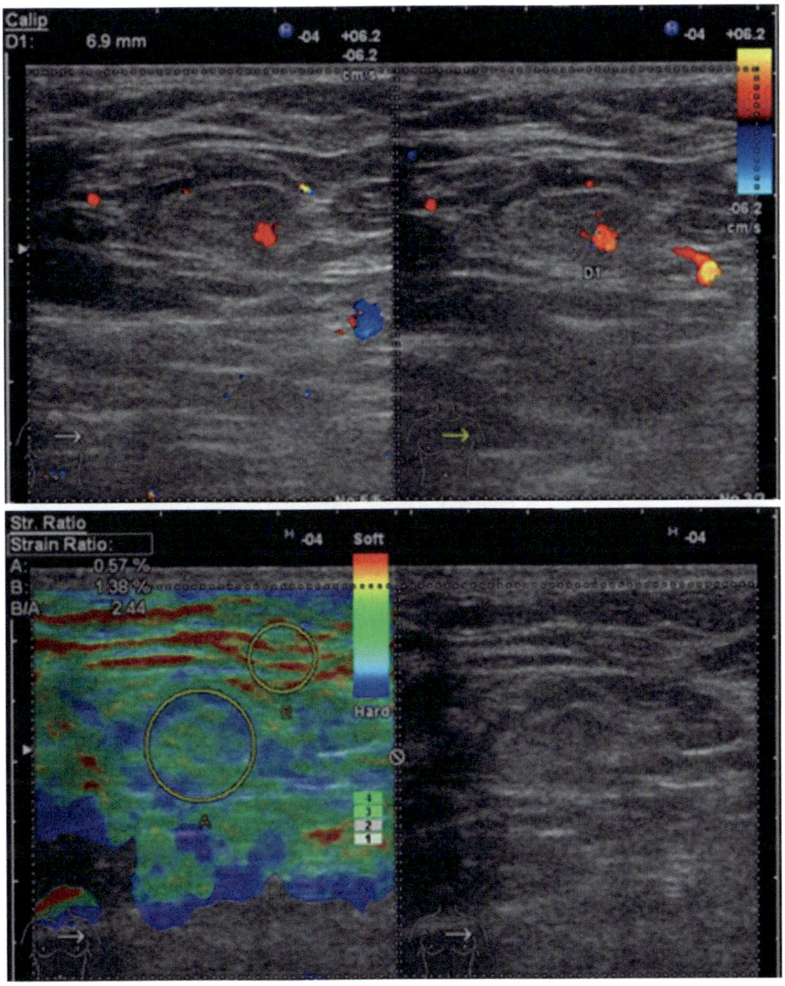

Fig. 8.27 Chronic lymphadenitis-type benign reactive histiocytosis: thin cortex, normal bloody vessels in the hilum, and moderate hypoechoic central area of the medullary (*upper* image); complementary benign SE type score 2 Ueno is reinforcing the diagnosis (*lower* image)

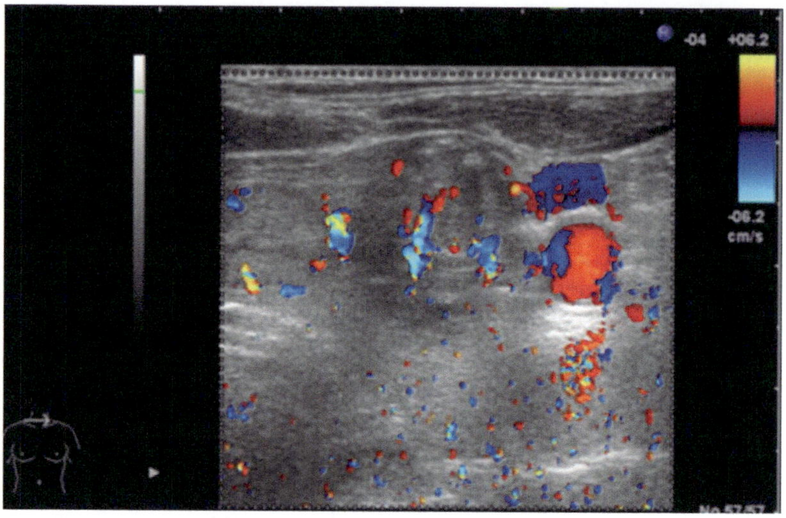

Fig. 8.28 Malignant left supraclavicular lymph node in a 58-year-old patient with left breast cancer; differential diagnosis with other metastasis (Virchow-Troisier sign), other tumors

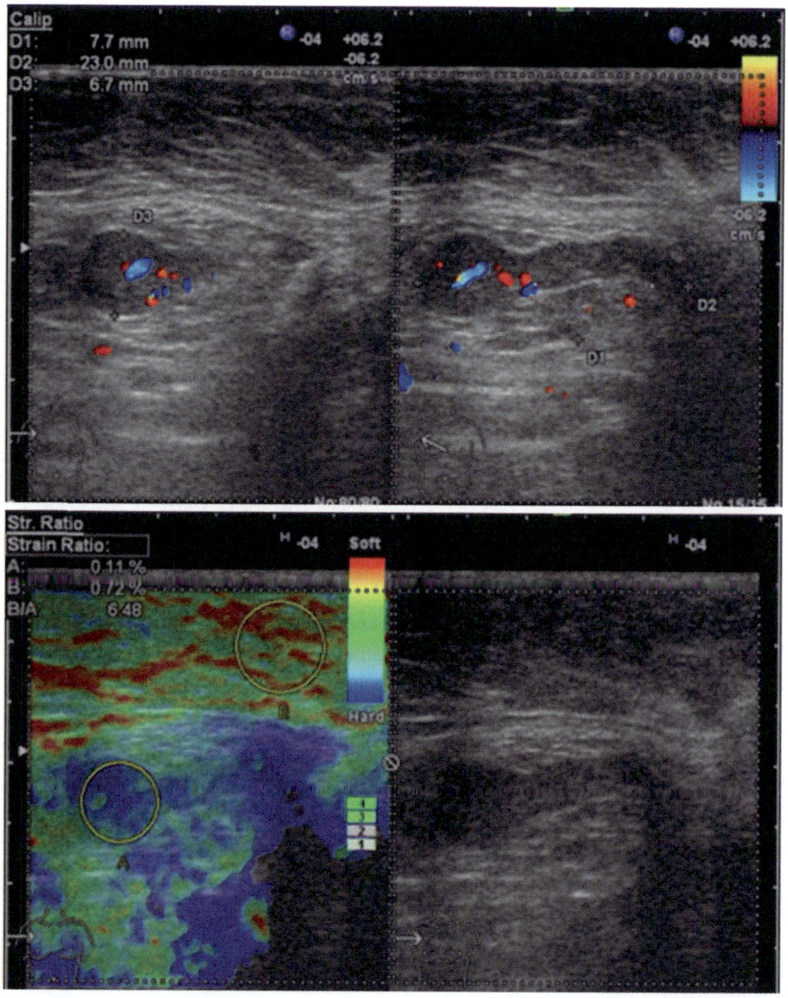

Fig. 8.29 Remnant lymph node with partial metastasis in a 65-year-old patient, with late recurrence 1 year after complex treatment, demonstrates cortical vasculature concordant with the focal thickening and increased strain

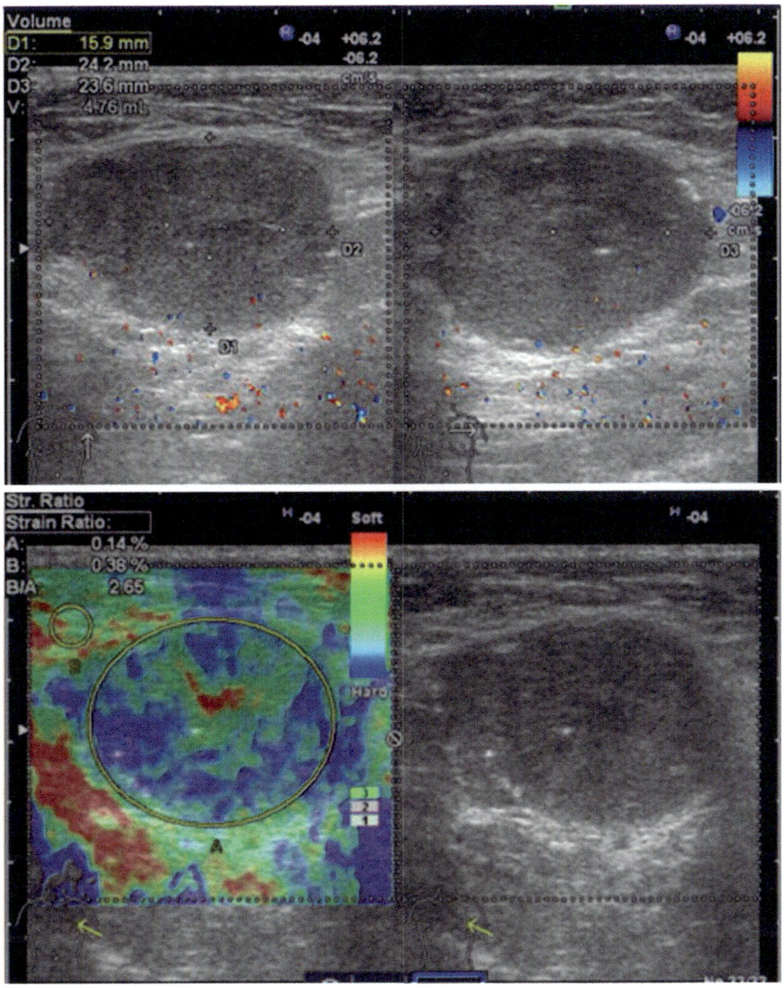

Fig. 8.30 Malignant left axillary lymph node after radiotherapy: the absence of pathological vasculature and the score 2 Ueno with FLR up to 2.65 are significant for the therapeutical response. Differential diagnosis with any benign findings

performed under US guidance. The Doppler examination is however a good tool of evaluation of the response to the therapy; when adding the SE, the accuracy is over 95% [35], because even in micro-metastases or in necrotic nodes, it presents a focal/global increasing of the SE score (3, 4, or 5 Ueno), with proportional increasing of the FLR; by opposite, the inflammatory nodes demonstrate the score 2 Ueno or BGR in the cases with edema or benign necrosis, associated with increased hilar vasculature. Some cancers with extensive microcalcifications determine calcifications in the node metastases, with very high FLR value, concordant with the CT aspect.

These descriptors of lymphadenopathy on FBU based on the vasculature and SE are more specific than the size, shape, internal architecture, or posterior effects and have an overall accuracy superior than those demonstrated by mammography, MRI, or FDG-PET, with reduced cost-benefit ratio. When present on FBU, the suspect axillary lymph nodes are correlated with the CA 15-3 level and the pathological reports; however, in practice usually a smaller number of suspect lymph nodes than the pathological report are found, which means not all micro-metastases could yet be diagnosed by noninvasive methods.

FBU is useful in the follow-up of treated cancers especially in detecting of the remnant ipsilateral axillary lymph nodes that could demonstrate late salient metastases and of the contralateral malignant lymph nodes that may appear after several years.

The differential diagnosis with other masses in the satellite areas of the breast cancer is based on the shape, size, anatomical reports, internal structure, vasculature, and strain; before any biopsy, the imaging diagnosis for particular cases could be completed with MRI or MDCT for the characterization of the local extension and the analysis of the bone integrity.

References

1. Stavros AT, Thickman D, Rapp CL, Dennis MA, Parker SH, Sisney GA. Solid breast nodules: use of sonography to distinguish between benign and malignant lesions. Radiology. 1995;196: 123–34.
2. Sala M, Salas D, Belvis F, et al. Reduction in false-positive results after introduction of digital mammography: analysis from four population-based breast cancer screening programs in Spain. Radiology. 2011;258(2):388–95. https://doi.org/10.1148/radiol.10100874.
3. Pisano ED, Gatsonis C, Hendrick E, et al. Diagnostic performance of digital versus film mammography for breast-cancer screening. N Engl J Med. 2005;353:1773–83.
4. Brem RF, Tabár L, Duffy SW, et al. Assessing improvement in detection of breast cancer with three-dimensional automated breast us in women with dense breast tissue: the SomoInsight study. Radiology. 2015;274(3):663–73. https://doi.org/10.1148/radiol.14132832.
5. Berg WA, Zhang Z, Lehrer D, et al. Detection of breast cancer with addition of annual screening ultrasound or a single screening MRI to mammography in women with elevated breast cancer risk. JAMA. 2012;307(13):1394–404. (ISSN: 1538-3598).
6. Teboul M, Halliwell M. Atlas of ultrasound and ductal echography of the breast (Relié). London: Blackwell Science Inc; 1995.
7. Teboul M. Practical ductal echography: guide to intelligent and intelligible Ultrasound imaging of the breast. Madrid: Saned Editors; 2003.
8. Tot T. Subgross morphology, the sick lobe hypothesis, and the success of breast conservation. Int J Breast Cancer. 2011;2011:634021 . 8 p. https://doi.org/10.4061/2011/634021.
9. Amy D. Lobar ultrasound of the breast. In: Tot T, editor. Breast cancer. London: Springer; 2010. https://doi.org/10.1007/978-1-84996-314-5_8.
10. Amy D, Durante E, Tot T. The lobar approach to breast ultrasound imaging and surgery. J Med Ultrasonics. 2015;42:331. https://doi.org/10.1007/s10396-015-0625-5.
11. Colan-Georges A. Atlas of full breast ultrasonography. New York, NY: Springer; 2016.
12. D'Orsi CJ, Sickles EA, Mendelson EB, Morvis EA, et al. ACR BI-RADS ® Atlas, breast imaging reporting and data system. Reston, VA: American College of Radiology; 2013.
13. Bamber JC, Sambrook M, Minassian H, Hill CR. Doppler studies of blood flow in breast cancer. In: Jellins J, Kobayashi T, editors. Ultrasonic examination of the breast. Chichester: John Wiley & Sons; 1983. p. 371–8.
14. Ramos IM, Taylor KJW, Kier R, Burns PN, Snower DP, Carter D. Tumor vascular signals in renal masses: detection with Doppler US. Radiology. 1988;168:633–7.
15. Shimamoto K, Sakuma S, Ishigaki T, Ishiguchi T, Itoh S, Fukatsu H. Hepatocellular carcinoma: evaluation with color Doppler US and MR imaging. Radiology. 1992;182:149–53.
16. Gasparini G, Weidner N, Bevilacqua P, et al. Tumor microvessel density, p53 expression, tumor size, and peritumoral lymphatic vessel invasion are relevant prognostic markers in node-negative breast carcinoma. J Clin Oncol. 1994;12:454–66.
17. Yang WT, Tse GMK, Lam PKW, et al. Correlation between color power Doppler sonographic measurement of breast tumor vasculature and immunohistochemical analysis of microvessel density for the quantitation of angiogenesis. J Ultrasound Med. 2002;21(11):1227–35.
18. Kedar RP, Cosgrove D, McCready VR, Bamber JC, Carter ER. Microbubble contrast agent for color Doppler US: effect on breast masses: work in progress. Radiology. 1996;198:679–86.
19. Van Esser S, Veldhuis WB, van Hillegersberg R, et al. Accuracy of contrast-enhanced breast ultrasound for pre-operative tumor size assessment in patients diagnosed with invasive ductal carcinoma of the breast. Cancer Imaging. 2007;7(1):63–8. https://doi.org/10.1102/1470-7330.2007.0012.
20. Kujiraoka Y, Ueno E, Yohno E, Morishima I, Tsunoda-Shimizu H. Incident angle of the plunging artery of breast tumors. In: Research and development in breast ultrasound. Tokyo: Springer; 2005. p. 72–5.
21. Christopher C. Ultrasound elastography of breast lesions. Ultrasound Clin. 2011;6:407–15. https://doi.org/10.1016/j.cult.2011.05.004.
22. Georgescu A, Bondari S, Manda A, Andrei E-M. The differential diagnosis between breast cancer and fibro-micro-cystic dysplasia by full breast ultrasonography-a new approach. Vienna: ECR; 2012. https://doi.org/10.1594/ecr2012/C-0167. EPOS™.
23. Stavros AT, Rapp LC, Parker HS. Breast ultrasound. Philadelphia, PA: Lippincott Williams & Wilkins; 2004.
24. Georgescu A, Enachescu V, Bondari A, et al. A new concept: the full breast ultrasound in avoiding false negative and false-positive sonographic errors. Vienna: ECR; 2011. https://doi.org/10.1594/ecr2011/C-0449.
25. Venta LA, Kim JP, Pelloski CE, et al. Management of complex breast cysts. Am J Roentgenol. 1999;173:1331–6.
26. Teboul M. Advantages of ductal echography (DE) over conventional breast investigation in the diagnosis of breast malignancies. Med Ultrason. 2010;12(1):32–42.

27. Tot T. The theory of the sick breast lobe and the possible consequences. Int J Surg Pathol. 2007;15(4):369–75. https://doi.org/10.1177/1066896907302225.
28. Tot T. The theory of the sick lobe. In: Tot T, editor. Breast cancer: a lobar disease. London: Springer; 2011. p. 1–18.
29. Holland R, Hendriks JH. Microcalcifications associated with ductal carcinoma in situ: mammographic-pathologic correlation. Semin Diagn Pathol. 1994;11(3):181–92.
30. Edmiston CE Jr, Walker AP, Krepel CJ, Gohr C. The nonpuerperal breast infection: aerobic and anaerobic microbial recovery from acute and chronic disease. J Infect Dis. 1990;162:695–9.
31. Graf O, Helbich TH, Hopf G, Graf C, Sickles EA. Probably benign breast masses at US: is follow-up an acceptable alternative to biopsy? Radiology. 2007;244:87–93.
32. Hertl K, Marolt-Musik M, Kocijancic I, et al. Haematomas after percutaneous vacuum assisted breast biopsy. Ultraschall Med. 2007;30:33–6.
33. Jackman RJ, Nowels KW, Rodriguez-Soto J, et al. Stereo-tactic, automated, large core needle biopsy of nonpalpable breast lesions: false-negative and histologic underestimation rates after long-term follow-up. Radiology. 1999;210:799–805.
34. Nielsen M, Christensen L, Andersen J. Radial scars in women with breast cancer. Cancer. 1987;59(5):1019–25.
35. Georgescu AC, Andrei ME. Full breast ultrasonography as follow-up examination after a complex treatment of breast cancer. Vienna: ECR; 2015. https://doi.org/10.1594/ecr2015/C-0266.
36. Freedman GM, Fowble BL. Local recurrence after mastectomy or breast-conserving surgery and radiation. Oncology. 2000;14(11):1561–81. discussion 1581-2, 1582-4.
37. Dolphin G. The surgical approach to the "sick lobe". In: Francescatti DS, Silverstein MJ, editors. Breast cancer: a new era in management. New York, NY: Springer; 2014. p. 113–32.
38. Görkem SB, O'Connell AM. Abnormal axillary lymph nodes on negative mammograms: causes other than breast cancer. Diagn Interv Radiol. 2012;18: 473–9.
39. American Cancer Society. Mammograms and other breast imaging tests. 2014. Last Medical Review: 12/8/2014 Last Revised: 4/25/2016; 2014 Copyright American Cancer Society.
40. Crippa F, Gerali A, Alessi A, Agresti R, Bombardieri E. FDG-PET for axillary lymph node staging in primary breast cancer. Eur J Nucl Med Mol Imaging. 2004;31(Suppl 1):S97–102.
41. Javid S, Segara D, Lotfi P, Raza S, Golshan M. Can breast MRI predict axillary lymph node metastasis in women undergoing neoadjuvant chemotherapy. Ann Surg Oncol. 2010;17(7):1841–6. https://doi.org/10.1245/s10434-010-0934-2.
42. Misselt PN, Glazebrook KN, Reynolds C, et al. Predictive value of sonographic features of extranodal extension in axillary lymph nodes. J Ultrasound Med. 2010;29:1705–9.

9 Lobar Ultrasonography in the Diagnosis of the Benign and Malignant Lesions of the Male Breast

Aristida Colan-Georges

9.1 New Anatomical Scanning and Interpreting of the US in Gynecomastia

9.1.1 Definition and Etiology of Gynecomastia

Gynecomastia is defined as benign proliferation of male breast glandular tissue, of various pathogenesis [1]. In pathology the gynecomastia is described as an enlargement of the male breast due to benign ductal and stromal proliferation; the lobules are rarely present in men, especially in estrogen-secreting tumors (testicular feminizing tumors, adrenal adenoma [2], adrenal carcinoma, hepatoma, lung cancer, pituitary adenoma). Three histological forms were described: florid, intermediate, and fibrotic, but no radiological imaging techniques of diagnosis in worldwide use were able to correlate their findings with these pathological types.

There are confusions of terms between physiological and asymptomatic gynecomastia, most authors considering them the same condition; thus the prevalence of asymptomatic gynecomastia is evaluated of 60–90% in neonates, 50–60% in adolescents, and up to 70% in men aged 50–69 years, upon Johnson and Murad citation of papers from 1981 up to 2008 [3], which reported various methods of diagnosis and analysis [4–7].

The real incidence of gynecomastia is practically unknown, because there was no technique of diagnosis available for all patients without irradiation risk and acceptable cost; moreover, the incidence is age influenced, the physiological type being usually unexplored mostly in young patients. Most reports of male breast pathology are referring to the mammographic incidence of breast diseases, such as a review of all mammograms for men for a 5-year interval at Mayo Clinic in Jacksonville, Florida, which found an incidence of gynecomastia of 62%; from all mammograms, the breast cancer represented only 1% of cases, and the rest included various benign masses or disorders such as lipomas, dermoid cysts, sebaceous cysts, lymphoplasmacytic inflammation, ductal ectasia, hematomas, and fat necrosis [8]. This analysis demonstrates the low incidence of male breast cancer in symptomatic patients, by one hand, and the unjustified irradiation for the large majority of 99% cases, with low risk, by the other hand.

We assume the *physiological gynecomastia* is usually symptomatic, because it determines a painful breast increasing volume; at least in neonate, it can develop milky nipple surge, due either to the transplacental maternal hormonal transfer such as prolactin or, possible, due to the hormonal ingestion by breastfeeding or by bottle-feeding cow milk,

A. Colan-Georges, M.D., Ph.D.
Imaging Center Prima Medical, County Clinical Emergency Hospital, Craiova, Romania
e-mail: aristida_georgescu@yahoo.com, acgeorges.radiology@gmail.com

D. Amy (ed.), *Lobar Approach to Breast Ultrasound*, https://doi.org/10.1007/978-3-319-61681-0_9

which contains either exogenous recombinant bovine growth hormone and insulin-like growth factor-1 (IGF-1) or estrogens, progesterone, and testosterone from milked cows throughout their pregnancy [9]; by consequence, in the last case, the human gonadotropin secretion is suppressed, and then the testosterone secretion decreases, and that results a disturbance of the sexual maturation of prepubertal children [10]. As evolution, in neonate and puberty, the gynecomastia is reversible, with spontaneous resorption; in elderly men, the physiological gynecomastia is irreversible but less developed than the pathological types.

Pathological gynecomastia represents the real disease of male breast enlargement and occurs in children at various ages besides neonate and puberty and in adulthood; it has an indeterminate prevalence, because there is usually an inadequate diagnosis protocol, based mainly on the clinical examination, eventually completed with mammography; the classical US is rarely used as a complementary tool for the differential diagnosis of breast masses, but not as basic method in the positive and differential diagnosis of male breast anatomy. Indeed, the variation in reported prevalence across studies was attributed according to Johnson and Murad [3] either to variations in the size of the palpable breast tissue (at least 0.5 cm to 2.0 cm diameter upon different authors) or to population characteristics such as age and setting of treatment (primary care versus referral clinics). Even in physiological gynecomastia, many patients are referred for painful breast and significant enlargement that determine anxiety and esthetical complaints; in such cases, the new ultrasound technique named *the Full Breast US* (FBU) is suitable.

The etiology of gynecomastia is undoubtedly endocrine, an imbalance between androgens and female hormones, especially estrogens, but sometimes prolactin, rarely progesterone, thyroxin and triiodothyronine, growth hormone, etc. Elevated estrogens are rarely related to an adrenal or gonadal neoplasm (feminizing tumors) but more commonly to the action of the tissue aromatase which determines the extragonadal conversion of androgens to estrogens in fatty tissues; however, not all obese male patients develop gynecomastia, but the most of cases illustrate pseudo-gynecomastia, with development of the fatty mammary layer around a small glandular mammary bud. Gonadal failure, primary or secondary, may determine a pathological or physiological gynecomastia; other conditions, such as medication (spironolactone), chronic hepatic insufficiency, and hyperthyroidism, may action by the sex hormone-binding globulin. Despite the less documented studies concerning large population and long-term survey, it seems reasonable to incriminate the effect of the certain medication or environmental exposures, mainly food estrogen-like contaminants, which activate the estrogen receptors. The use of medication is usually neglected in the patient history, because of the large spectrum of drugs that determine breast hypertrophy, such as hormones, antibiotics, antacids, cardiovascular regulators, chemotherapeutics, psychoactive agents, and others [3]. In our experience, the environmental exposures are the most important factors, because they action in the same way in the determinism of the precocious thelarche of girls, in many cases issued in the same family, as well as familial gynecomastia in various stages affecting father and son; in addition, the level and duration of the exposure are correlated with the severity of the clinical complaints (size of gynecomastia, pain) and with the pathologic aspect, from the simply enlarged mammary bud to branching ducts, duct hyperplasia, rarely duct ectasia fulfilled with milky secretion, and very seldom lobular development. In addition, once the exposure of the estrogen-like environmental contaminants or of the tumor-secreting hormones is removed, the gynecomastia may be partial or completely regressed.

9.1.2 Classical Diagnosis of Gynecomastia and New Full-Breast US

The diagnosis of gynecomastia in the classical approach is mainly based on the clinical examination, sometimes completed with mammography and rarely with basic US; any doubt leads to puncture diagnosis.

The clinical examination is subjective, but some information may be useful both in the initial diagnosis and in the follow-up examination. The inspection may detect a breast enlargement with increasing of the areolar size and pigmentation, usually asymmetrical; the Tanner stages applied to the male breast development are less characteristic than in girls; usually the breast appears as Tanner stages I, II, and III and rarely stage IV (Fig. 9.1). The palpation reveals a mammary mound of tissues firmer than the surrounding fatty layer, located centrally under the nipple-areolar complex, usually mobile against the pectoral fascia, tender or even painful in some cases. Because the small male nipples have hypoplastic ductules and pores, we may notice very seldom some milky fluid discharge.

The clinical differential diagnosis is made with the pseudo-gynecomastia, which appears as a breast enlargement without palpable retroareolar lump and without other eccentric breast tumors.

The main paraclinical test in use in the classical approach is represented by mammography, which is thought accurate for differentiating the true gynecomastia from a suspect mass that requires further tissue sampling. This approach seems to be anachronism, because it chooses as first intention a method that adds the risk of exposure to X-rays, and thus it is not valuable for all male patients of all ages; furthermore it must be completed with a complementary invasive technique represented by breast puncture. Some adepts of the mammography found this method

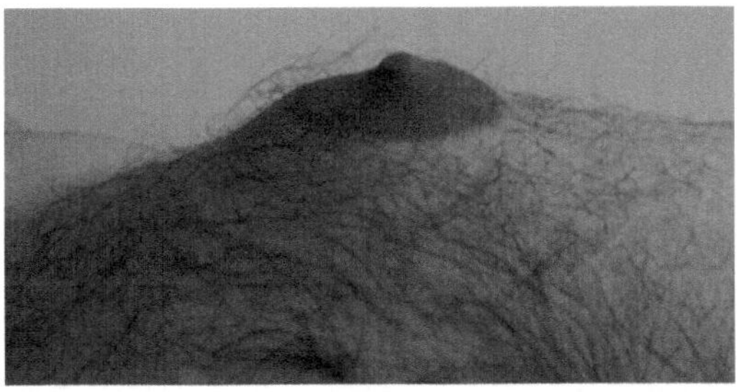

Fig. 9.1 Clinical appearance of gynecomastia, similar to the Tanner stage III/IV, with areola and nipple forming a secondary mound projecting from the contour of the surrounding breast [11]

to be fairly accurate in distinguishing malignant from benign male breast diseases, with a sensitivity and specificity over 90%; however, the positive predictive value for malignant conditions was low (55%), with inacceptable explanation of the low prevalence of malignancy in patients presenting with gynecomastia [12].

For the classical approach, breast male ultrasound is optional or rarely performed. There were described various types of US appearances of gynecomastia, without any referral to the anatomical or physiological real substrate:

- *Focal gynecomastia* can variably appear as a retroareolar, triangular, hypoechoic mass.
- *Early nodular gynecomastia* illustrates a subareolar fan or disc-shaped hypoechoic nodule surrounded by normal fatty tissue.
- *Diffuse glandular gynecomastia* has both nodular and dendritic features surrounded by diffuse hyperechoic fibrous breast tissue.
- *Chronic dendritic gynecomastia* appears as a subareolar hypoechoic lesion with an anechoic star-shaped posterior border, described in the literature as "fingerlike projection" or "spider legs" insinuating into the surrounding echogenic fibrous breast tissue.

In fact, the retroareolar *hypoechoic mass*, with or without *dendritic features*, *fingerlike projections*, or *spider legs*, represents the mammary bud with or without branching ducts, and the *hyperechoic fibrous breast tissue* is corresponding to mammary glandular specific stroma. In the classical US, there are no relationships with the breast salient vasculature in Doppler examination nor information about the SE; thus in doubtful cases, the breast biopsy is mandatory.

The most complete noninvasive technique of diagnosis is represented by the concept of the *Full Breast US (FBU)* [13], a new approach that uses the anatomical technique of the radial ductal US promoted by Teboul and col. [14, 15], completed with Doppler assessment and in some cases with SE. This technique is available for all, from the newborn boys to infants and elder men without risk of irradiation or other contraindications; the technique is applied to the lobar anatomy, similar to the woman breast, and may illustrate the various aspects of gynecomastia, allowing the differential diagnosis with pseudo-gynecomastia and breast tumors. FBU is useful in the early diagnosis of gynecomastia, conducting to the detection of some etiological factors (endocrine, metabolic, neoplastic, genetic, and toxic exogenous), which should be cured to prevent the late complementary disorders (metastases, infertility, and psychological disorders); moreover, the follow-up exams can be adapted to the patient age, postoperative changes, and any particular type or evolution of the disease.

The appearance in FBU of the normal male breast is represented by:

- The small mammary bud with hypoechoic aspect, of <1 cm diameter in the coronal plan and few millimeter thickness in the anterior-posterior diameter, located retroareolar, symmetrical, with more or less regular contour, but without any branching ducts.
- A thin linear hyperechoic interface between the mammary bud and the surrounding fatty tissue equivalent to the minimal glandular stroma.
- The absence of any vascular signal in Doppler examination related to the breast glandular bud.
- The surrounding fatty tissue more or less developed, but without significant enlargement of the male breast such as in pseudo-gynecomastia; its aspect is hypoechoic too, but with specific architecture at the examination with high-frequency transducers that illustrate internal thin discontinuous fibrous "septae"; SE allows a better delineation of the mammary bud from the fat.

The normal mammary bud must be illustrated in pseudo-gynecomastia, or as a contralateral reference image for a unilateral gynecomastia, or in ipsilateral eccentrically male breast mass, usually malignant (Figs. 9.2, 9.3, 9.4, 9.5 and 9.6).

Pseudo-gynecomastia presents a periglandular hypertrophy of the fatty tissue with good delineation of the *fascia superficialis corporis* and without development of the hyperechoic glandular stroma; there is no significant Doppler signal, and the SE demonstrates a low strain (Fig. 9.5).

The true gynecomastia gradually develops a male lobar mammary structure: from the pseudo-nodular parenchyma represented by the mammary bud, the ductal tree is progressively developed simultaneously with specific glandular stroma and new formation breast vasculature.

Stroma is wrongly described in the basic Senology as a "fibrous structure," and the breast itself is described as a vague "fibro-glandular tissue"; in fact, stroma is a tissue itself, the microenvironment that surrounds the breast epithelium

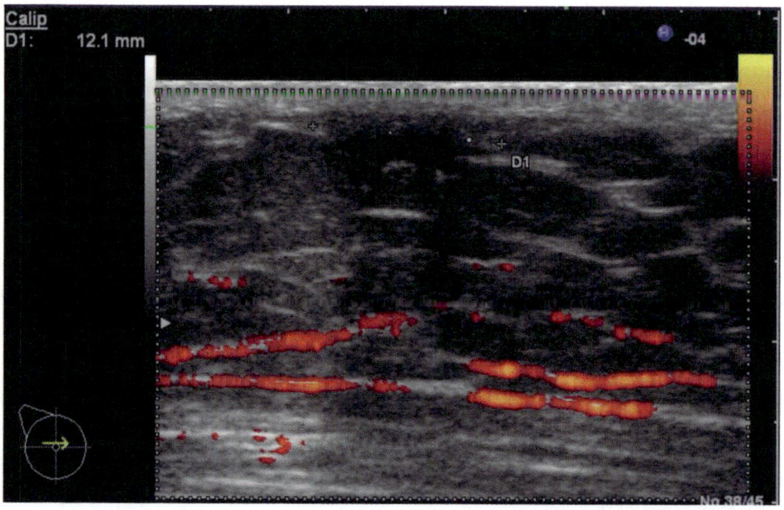

Fig. 9.2 Normal mammary bud in man

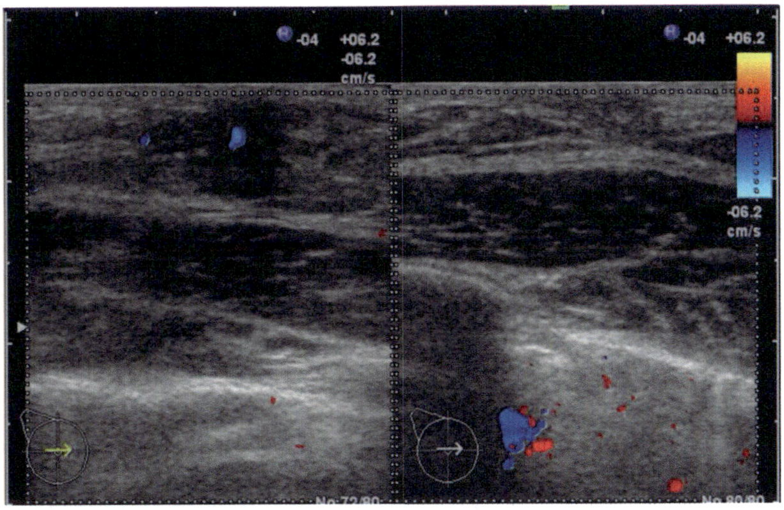

Fig. 9.3 Normal mammary bud in male (*left*) compared with nodular type of gynecomastia (*right*) in a 13-year-old boy

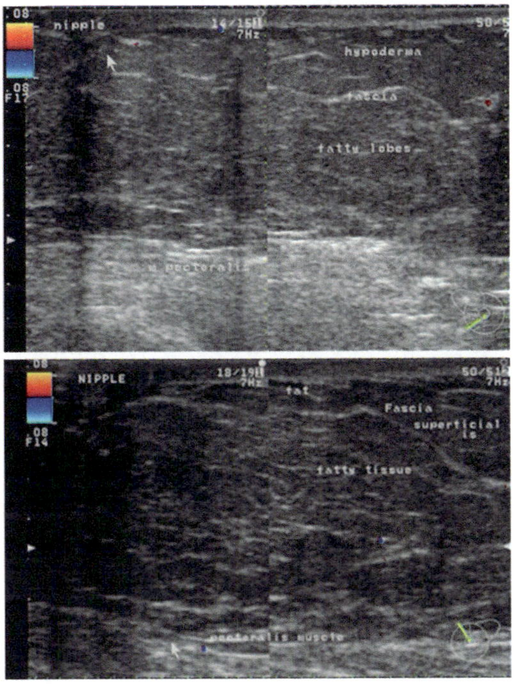

Fig. 9.4 Pseudo-gynecomastia in a 41-year-old man with esthetical complaints

(parenchyma) and that is composed of extracellular and cellular tissue network represented by fibroblasts, myofibroblasts, endothelial cells, adipocytes, and various immune cells. The normal glandular stroma has a nourishing role for the epithelium, but also it has the function of tissue hormonal secretion and tumoral growth regulator. Some stromal cells such as macrophages, mast cells, neutrophils, and lymphocytes are thought to be recruited by the primary tumor cells to increase tumor cell migration, angiogenesis, and invasion [16]. The development of the normal breast epithelium (parenchyma), the breast specific tissue with function in the milk secretion, is parallel with the development of the stroma, both in females (girls and pregnant women) and males of any age or type of gynecomastia; inversely, the involution of the breast epithelium, in menopausal woman and in the physiological gynecomastia, is accompanied by stromal atrophy. The same relationship was demonstrated the last years in breast cancer: the ductal and lobular carcinoma do not just brake and invade the surrounding stroma, but the stromal components change their morphology and properties, playing active roles in breast cancer metastasis, by a collaborative work between tumor microenvironment and neoplastic cells at the site of local invasion and vascular intravasation [17].

The limits of the mammography in the anatomical illustration of the female and male breast, due to the planar projection of a volumic organ with various tissues, some of them without radiological appearance (mammary epithelium and fat), are added to the limits of the all basic sectional imaging techniques that are neglecting the breast radial architecture, resulting a misunderstanding of the breast development, function, and

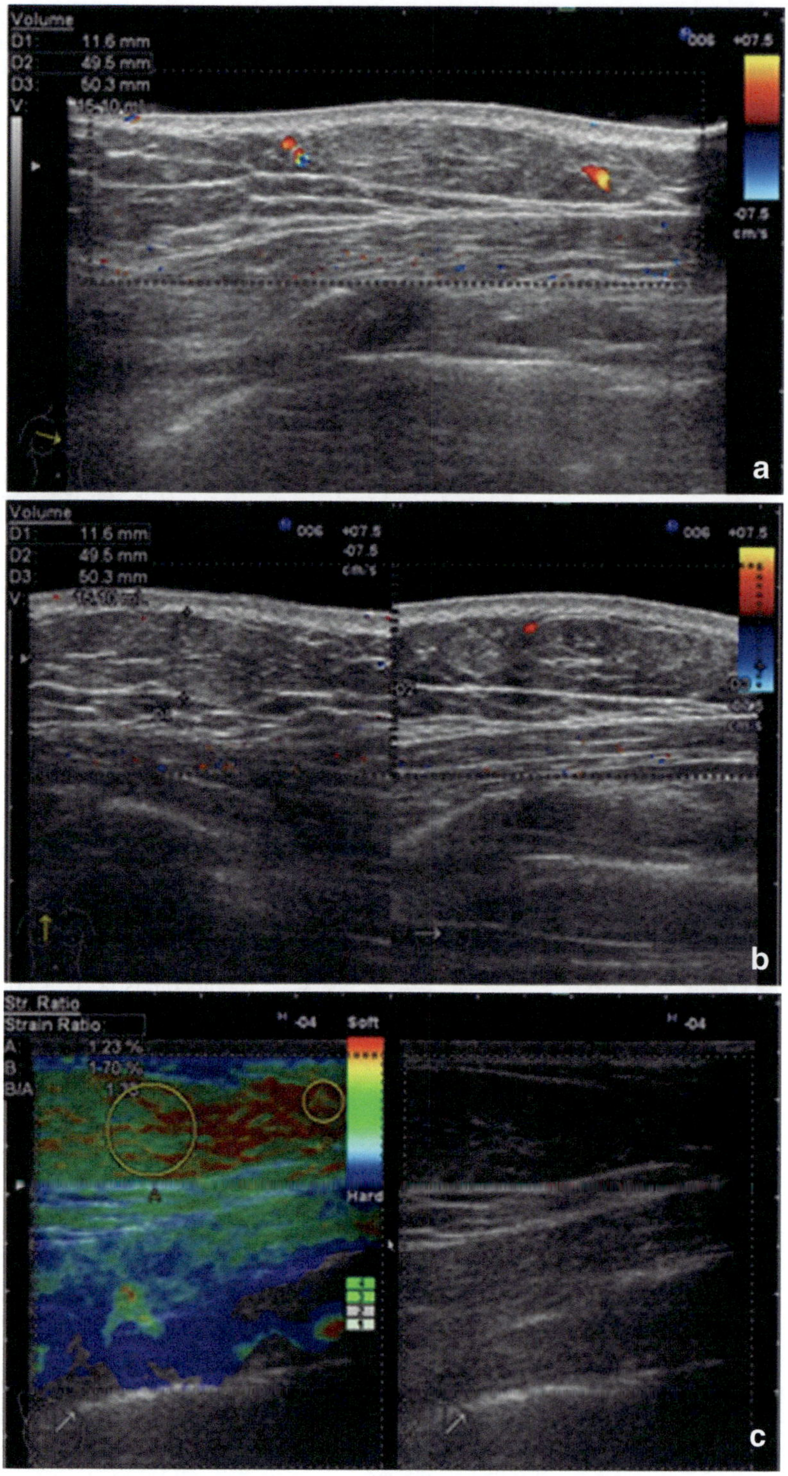

Fig. 9.5 Pseudo-gynecomastia aspect in FBU: eccentric mass in the upper-inner quadrant (**a**), with isoechoic heterogeneous internal structure, between the superficial fascia and the pectoral muscle (**b**), with reduced vasculature and score 1 Ueno (**c**), suggestive for a lipoma

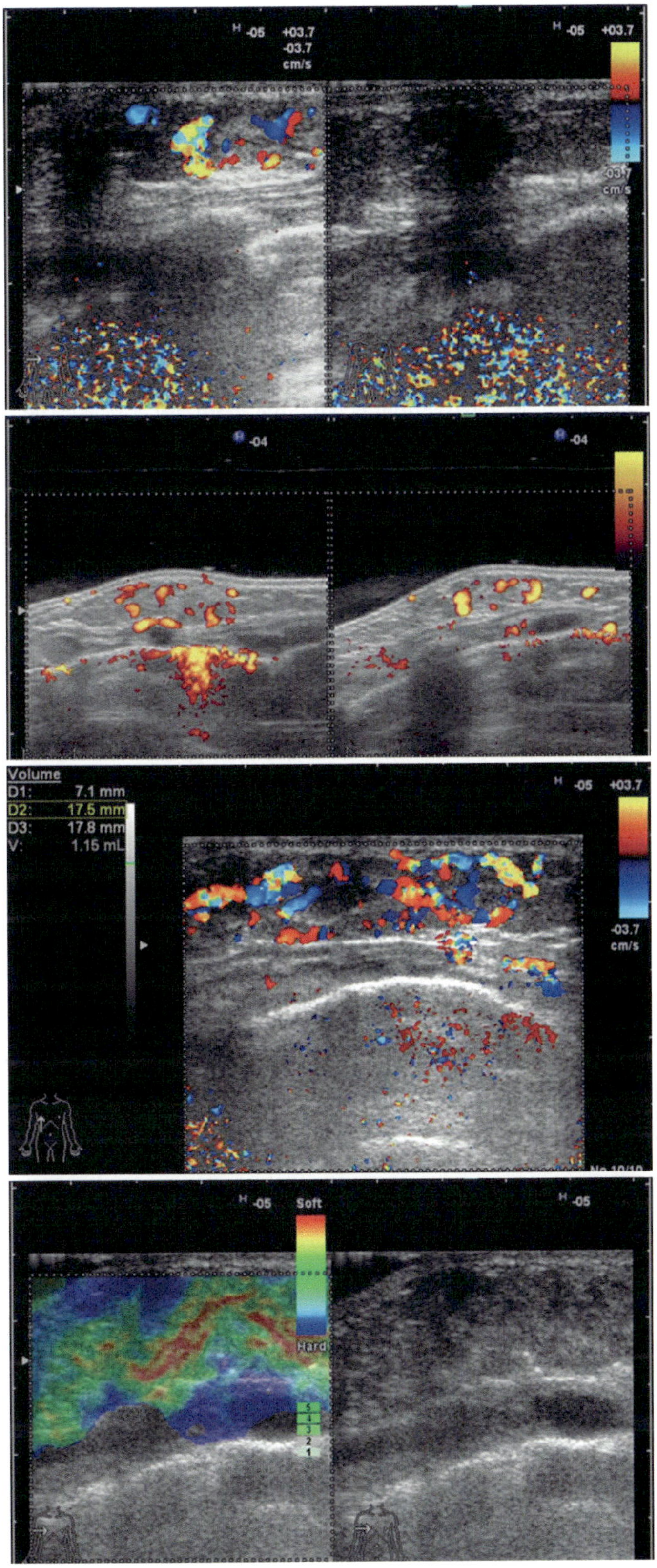

Fig. 9.6 Hemangiolipoma in a 2-month-old boy encompassing the inner-lower quadrant of the right mammary bud; comparative breasts (*upper image*), Doppler assessment of the tumor with aliasing and connection with the intercostal vessels (*middle images*), and SE with soft tumor surrounding the mammary bud (*lower image*)

pathology. Especially in the gynecomastia, the glandular architecture organized in true mammary lobes similar to the female breast was not recognized.

The volume rendering of the whole breast as 3D or 4D images with possibilities of various digital subtraction for better illustration of the breast anatomy is yet insufficient developed in US; there are not yet available linear transducers for 4D acquisitions, neither Doppler 3D reconstructions for the small parts, but some researches were done with the 3D SE. A global 3D breast reconstruction is suitable both for ultrasonographers, for better understanding of the breast anatomy and to locate the radial and antiradial scanning, and for therapists, either surgeons or radiotherapists. The lobar anatomy in gynecomastia is real and could be demonstrated with 3D reconstructions of multidetector computed tomography (MDCT) acquisitions (Figs. 9.7 and 9.8).

The lobar anatomy of the gynecomastia appears in the FBU scanning with three anatomical components in various proportions according to the patient age, to the etiology, and to the stage of the dishormonal condition [18]. No other method of radiological imaging diagnosis in use has illustrated and correlated the anatomical and physiological-pathological changes of the male breast before the publication of the ductal echography of Teboul, in 1995 [14] and 2003 [15], which was further developed under the concept of FBU, few years after the SE was largely presented in the ECR Vienna, in 2004 [19]. These three anatomical elements of the gynecomastia are mandatory in the positive diagnosis:

1. *The breast parenchyma*, represented by the retroareolar mammary bud, with initial increasing size according to the development of the breast, appearing as a triangular or discoid hypoechoic mass, with the larger diameter toward the pectoral fascia; the development is usually asymmetrical for the both breasts, but rarely there is a unilateral change; as the development progresses, the peripheral borders of the mammary bud become irregular, with branching ducts usually more elongated toward the upper-outer quadrant, which is the largest as in woman breast; the ducts have distinct hypo-/isoechoic thin walls usually delimited by a hyperechoic central line representing the wall interfaces, named the *central line sign* that is pathognomonic for the virtual ductal lumen, and thus certify the anatomical nature (Fig. 9.9).

The usual thickness of the galactophorous ducts in gynecomastia that could be detected by ultrasound ranges between 0.4 and 1 mm, being dependent on the frequency of the transducers; usually the ducts are thinner in young and in adulthood male breast, but some cases may present thickened ducts in the florid stage or in hyperplasia with usual diameter up to 2.0–2.5 mm. The radial technique of examination after Teboul allows the demonstration of the connection between the ducts misinterpreted as *dendritic features*, *fingerlike projections*, or *spider legs* with the retroareolar core of the glandular bud described classically as *hypoechoic lesion* or *nodule*. The branching ductal range is small in infants and pubertal cases mimicking a nodular tumor (Fig. 9.10), but in the radial ultrasonography, we can follow up to three or four divisions in adulthood. In rare cases of gynecomastia, there are identified ductal ending small lobules, of <2–3 mm size, especially in endogenous tumoral hyperestrogenism [18]; they appear oval shaped, iso-/hypoechoic, without salient vasculature, and with benign-type strain, scored 1 and 2 Ueno (Fig. 9.11).

In some pathological gynecomastia, the hyperestrogenism is expressed by ductal hyperplasia, with diffuse increasing of their thickness, or ductal ectasia secondary to hyperprolactinemia, with milky secretion, similar to woman galactorrhea (Figs. 9.12, 9.13, and 9.14).

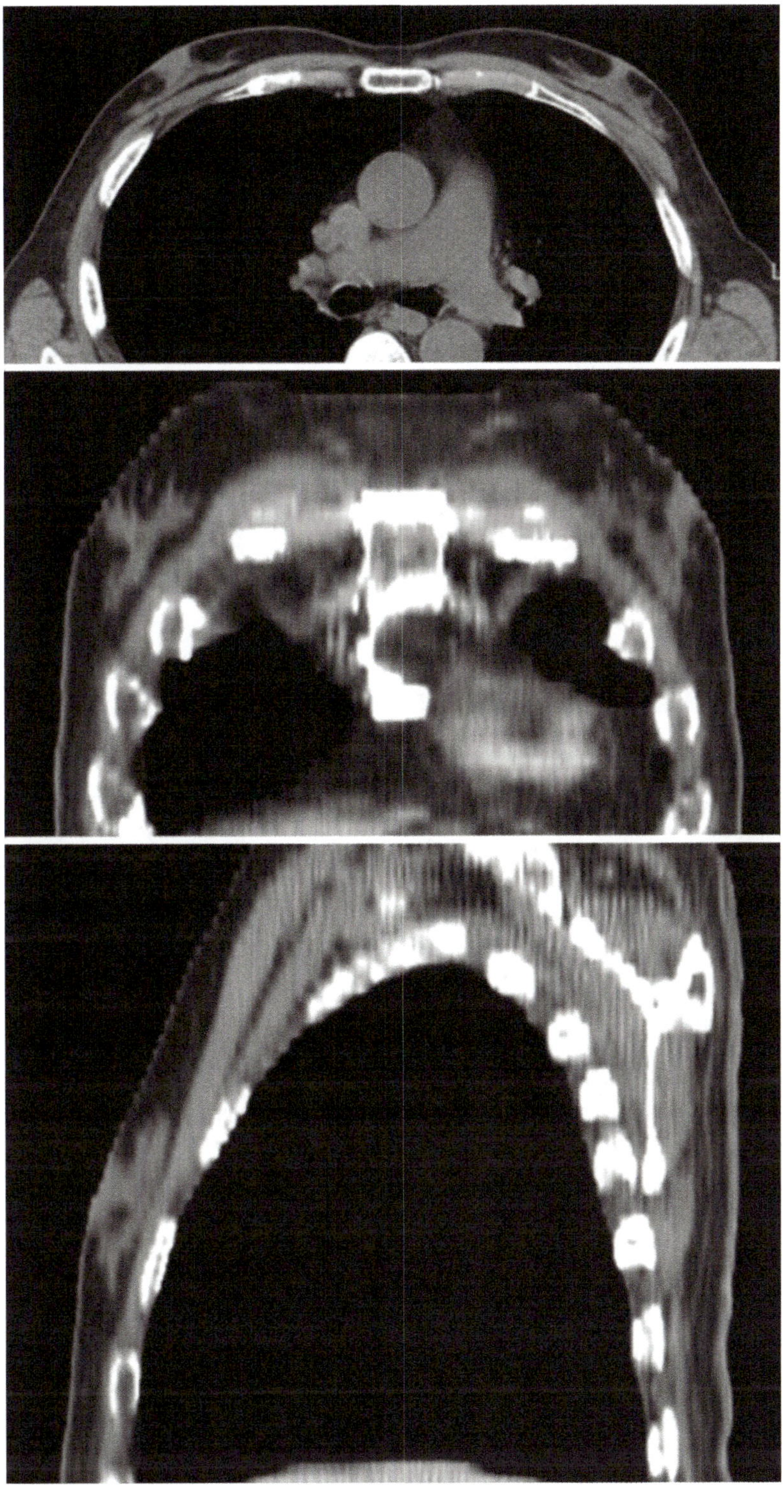

Fig. 9.7 MDCT in a 69-year-old patient with florid gynecomastia: the axial, coronal, and sagittal reconstructions demonstrate the branching ducts at the periphery of the mammary bud, but without global understanding of the mammillae

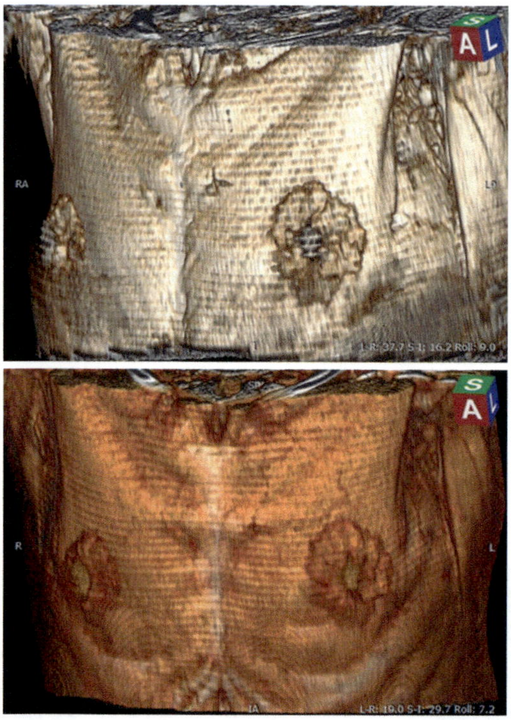

Fig. 9.8 The same case: MDCT with volume rendering illustrates the lobar architecture comparable with the anatomical preparations of woman breast by Sir A. P. Cooper in 1840

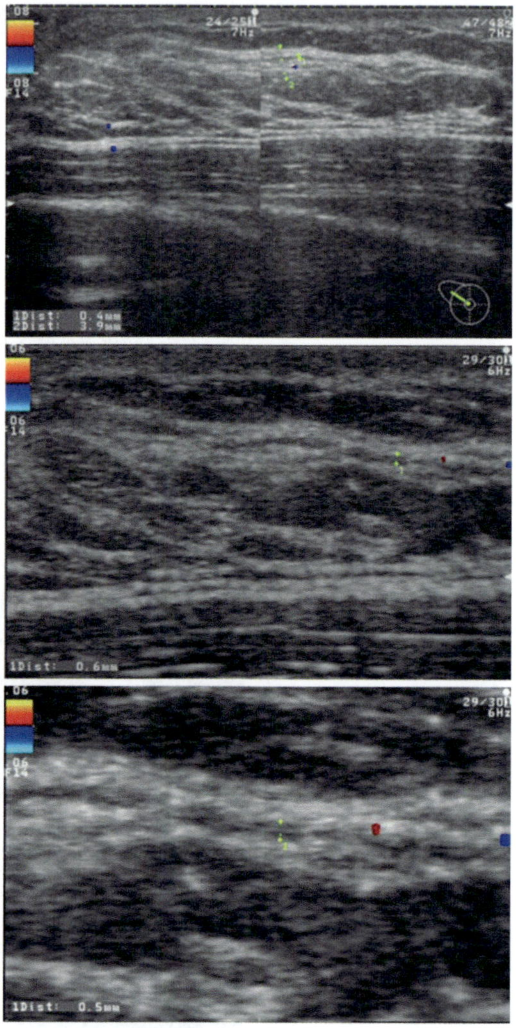

Fig. 9.9 Chronic gynecomastia in a 16-year-old patient with renal failure: the ductal echography demonstrates the lobar radial architecture with tinny ducts of 0.5 mm diameter; high-frequency transducer illustrates *the ductal central line sign* that is pathognomonic

2. *The glandular stromal tissue*, with hyperechoic aspect, named in the classical US *diffuse hyperechoic fibrous breast tissue* or simply neglected, represents the second breast glandular element. The specific stroma is an essential element of the breast architecture, both in woman and man, with complex histology, not only a fibrous network but a real tissue with stromal cells, it is essential in the development of the glandular parenchyma, both in normal, "benign" breast and in the development of malignancy. In gynecomastia, the amount of the hyperechoic layer is proportional with the development of the mammary bud and of the branching ducts, stroma being illustrated by the radial US as a layer in the periphery of the breast and as strips between the mammary ducts (Figs. 9.15, 9.16, 9.17, and 9.18). The hyperechoic stroma is not developed in pseudo-gynecomastia and represents the main element in the differential diagnosis; the fibrous network of the stroma develops thin Cooper ligaments that are neglected or even denied by the classical

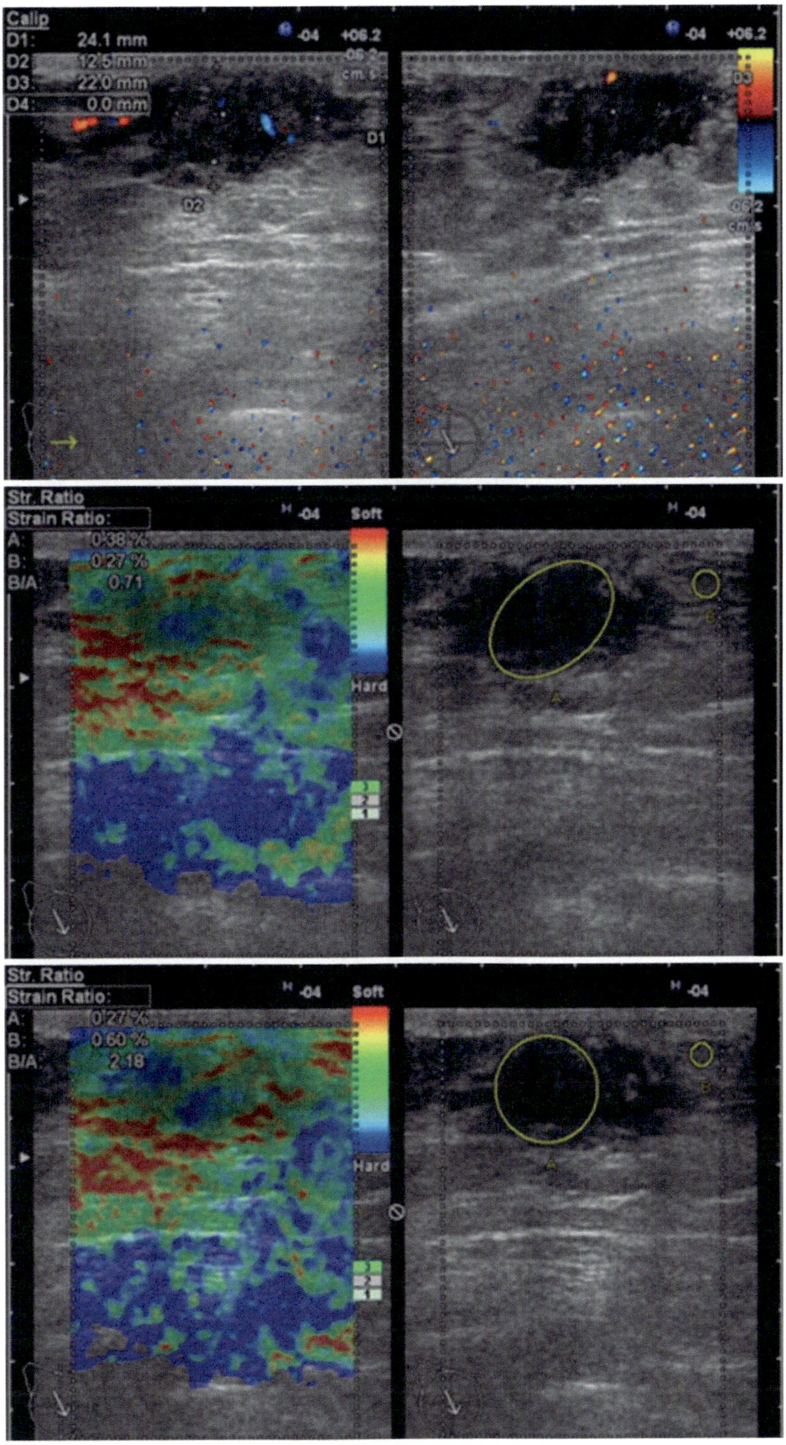

Fig. 9.10 Pseudonodular type of gynecomastia in a 9-year-old boy with enlarged mammary bud and short primary ducts with specular aspect; the stroma is discrete, the new formation vasculature is salient, and the SE shows a heterogeneous strain-type score 3 Ueno

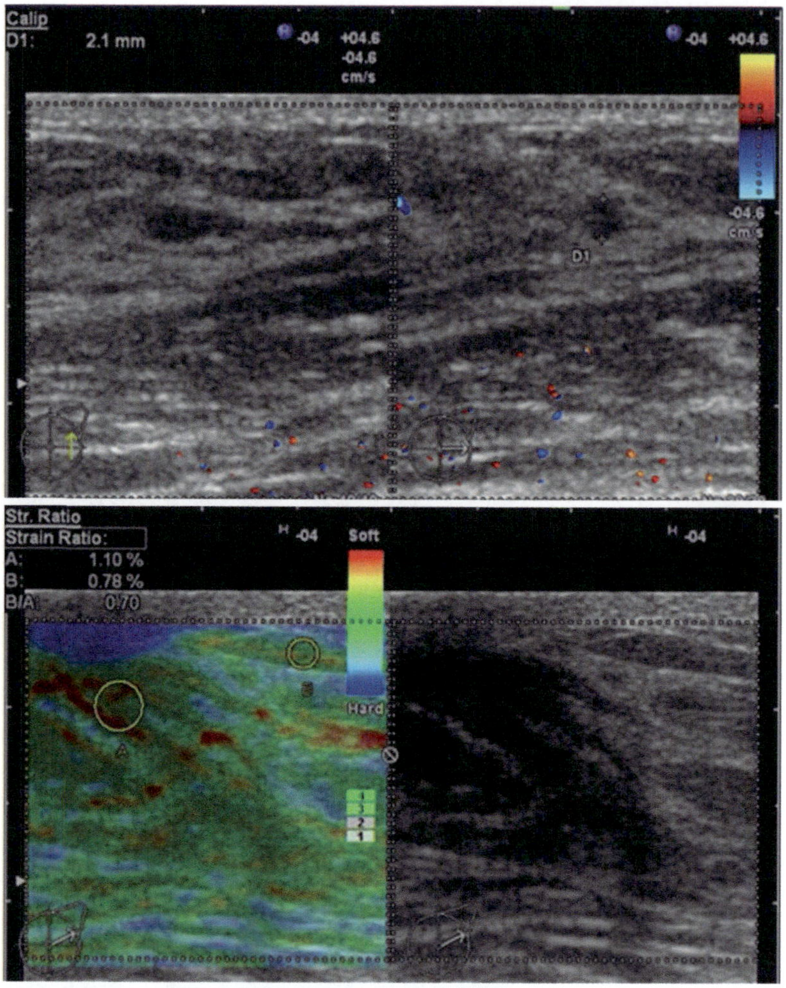

Fig. 9.11 Lobule of 2.1 mm diameter with ductal connection (L 3:00, antiradial and radial scans) and central thickening of the ducts in a 19-year-old patient with gynecomastia; normal SE with a score 1 Ueno for the breast parenchyma (epithelium), except the nipple with clear borders of score 4 Ueno

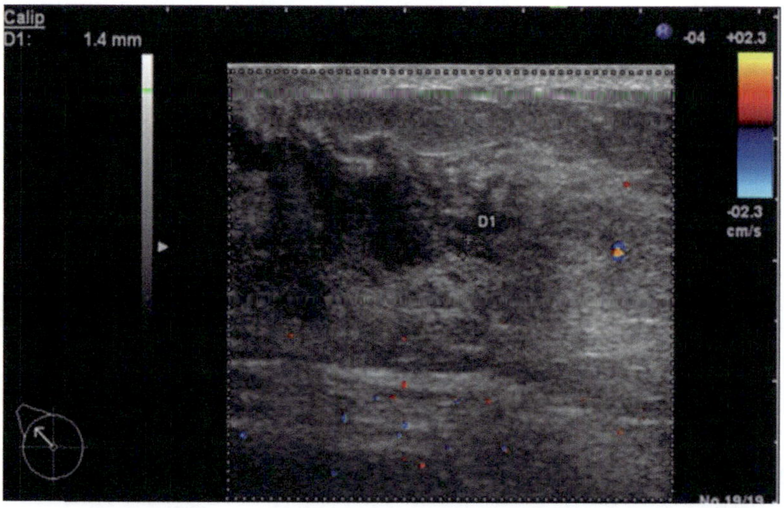

Fig. 9.12 Ductal hyperplasia in a 70-year-old man with pathological gynecomastia: ducts of 1.4 mm diameter with preservation of the "central line sign"

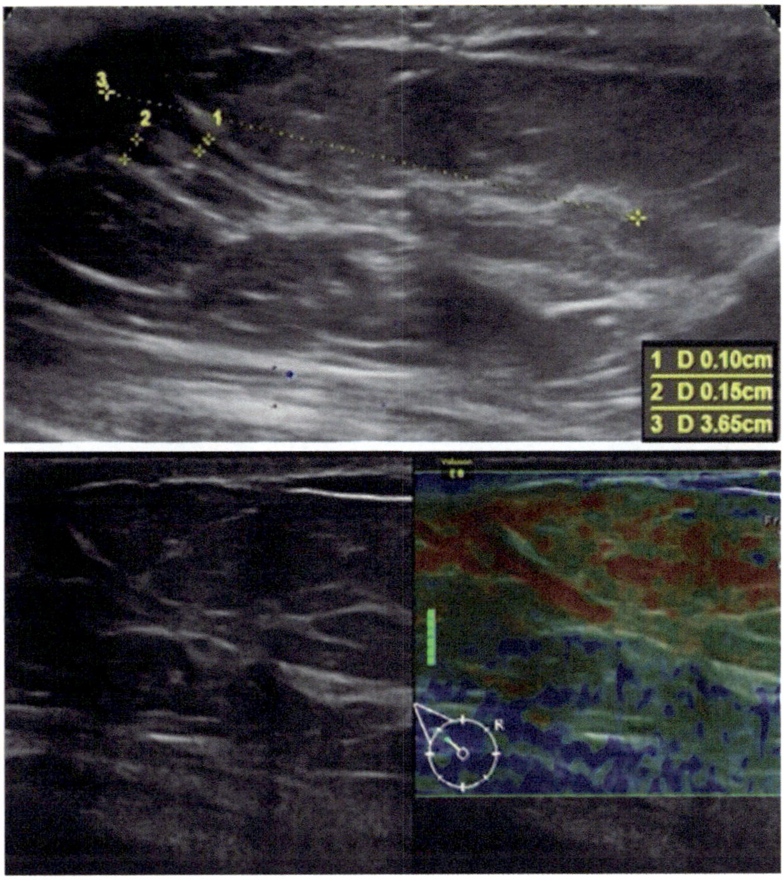

Fig. 9.13 FBU in gynecomastia with thin ductal ectasia with transonic fluid and a score 1 Ueno

breast male imaging (Figs. 9.19, 9.20, and 9.21). Moreover, the malignant tumors may present a stromal reaction similar to the woman breast cancer, identified in mammography as peritumoral spicules, in 2D US as a halo and in SE determining the score 5 Ueno.

3. *The new formation breast vasculature* is the third element of gynecomastia, with various intensities (mapping, vessel diameters, and velocities), and represents the argument of the breast development active process; the normal mammary bud has no salient vasculature in Doppler examination with the actual equipment in use, and the pseudo-gynecomastia rarely demonstrates few thin vessels with no relation with the retroareolar area. The gynecomastia illustrates increasing periareolar vasculature, proportional with the size of the breast parenchyma and stroma and with the active growing stage, associated with tenderness or pain; in the chronic stage of gynecomastia, with clinical no complaints, the new formation vasculature is reduced, and the vessels become thinner or less salient (Fig. 9.22). The periareolar site is determined by the normal mapping of the breast vasculature similar in man and woman, with afferent vessels from the axillary, intercostal, and internal mammary arteries converging to the periareolar vascular ring, better demonstrated by the 3D MRI reconstructions.

These anatomical elements are easy to demonstrate with the actual high-frequency transducers, and the interpreting of the scans becomes feasible to everyone by using the radial scan,

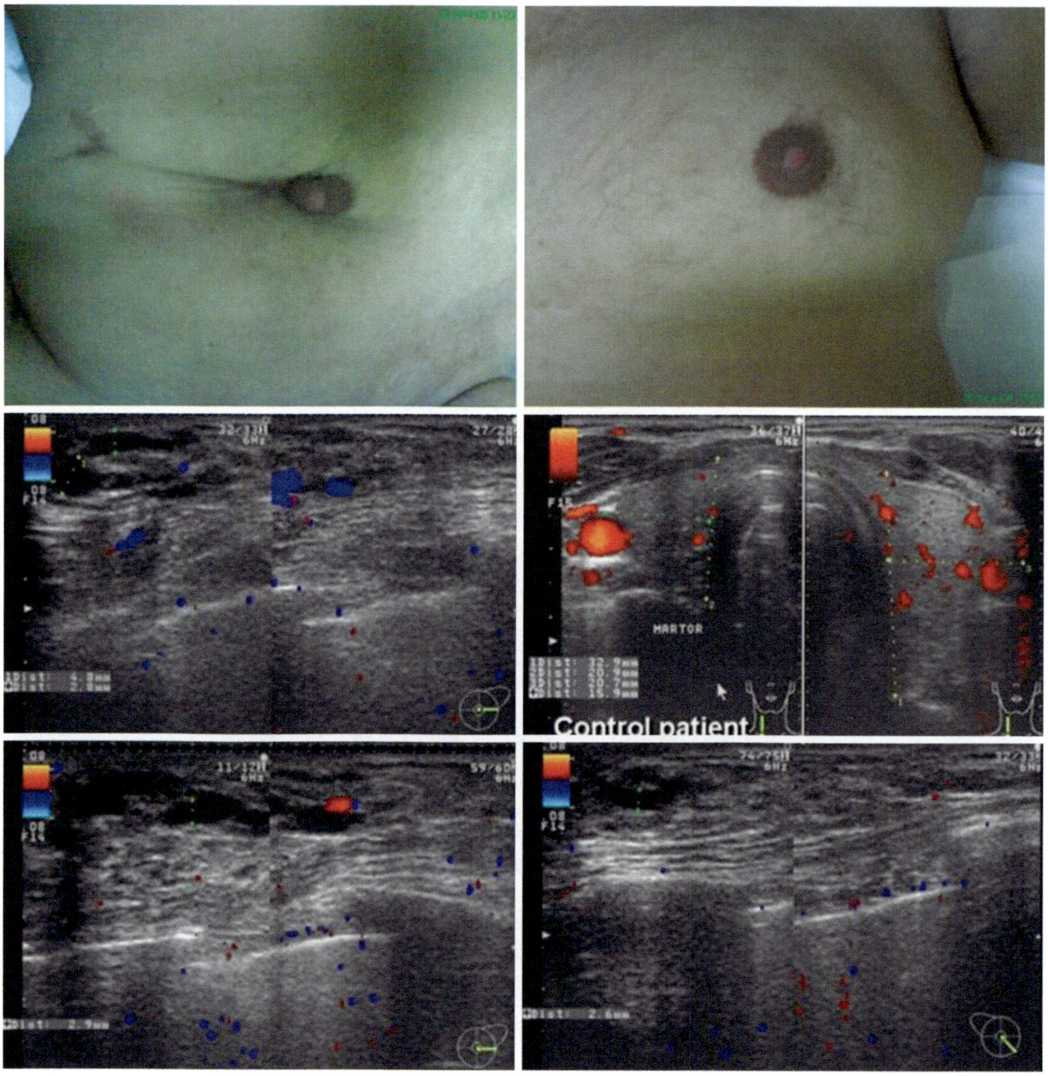

Fig. 9.14 Galactorrhea in man: 54-year-old male patient after right gynecomastia, misdiagnosed, and partially removed (segmentectomy), with local evolution and finally contralateral development equally. The patient presented exophthalmia, and Doppler US demonstrated diffuse goiter with moderate increasing of the power Doppler signal compared to a control patient [Atlas of Full Breast Ultrasonography, Chapter 10 - Physiological and Pathological Aspects of Full Breast US in Men and Children, 2016, p. 343, Aristida Colan-Georges, "With permission of Springer"]

with the nipple conventionally sited in the left-upper corner of the screen. In dense, large mammary bud, with significant acoustic shadow, the differential diagnosis with a malignancy can be quickly acquired adding the Doppler and SE that demonstrates a score 1 Ueno for the mammary bud and ducts and an overall score 2 Ueno for the global mammary glandular structures (including stroma). The small duct ectasia usually appears with a score 1 Ueno for the small size, the ductal walls in green on both sides, and the central fluid in red, while the largest ducts may appear in BGR (blue-green-red) sonoelastogram, similar to the cystic lesions (Figs. 9.13 and 9.14).

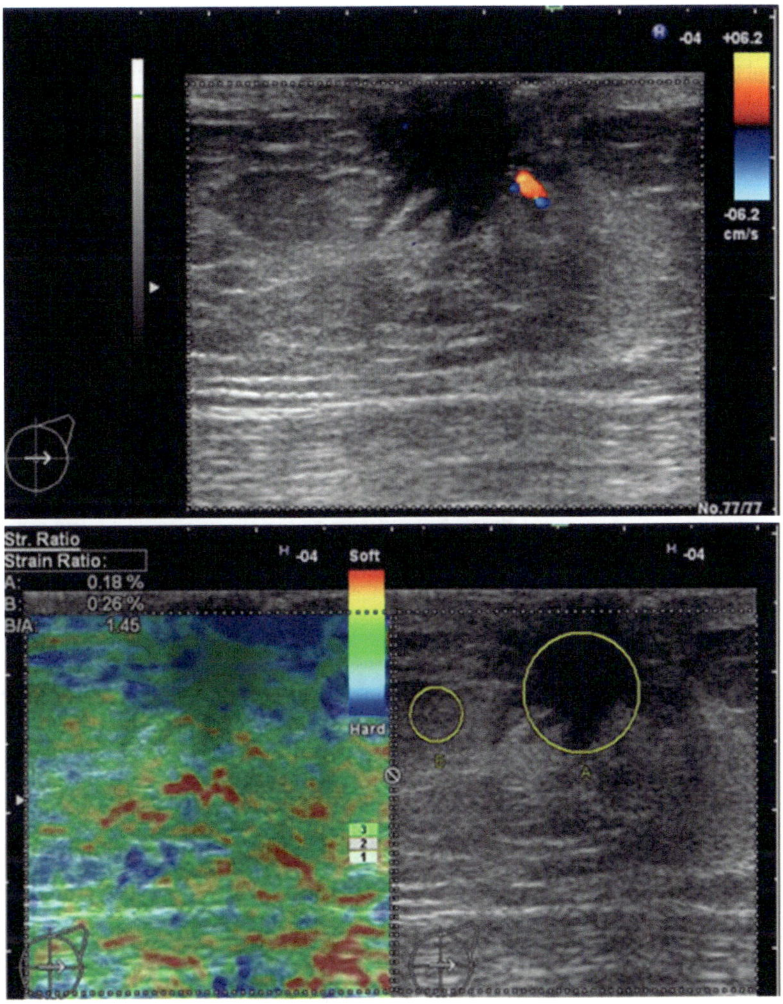

Fig. 9.15 FBU in a 13-year-old boy with physiological gynecomastia: hypoechoic mammary bud with dendritic incipient duct formation, new formation vasculature, hyperechoic stroma, and normal glandular reduced stiffness behind the harder nipple-areolar complex

9.2 Gynecomastia with Parenchymal Secondary Lesions

According to Olsson and col. [20], there are some pathological conditions found in a male breast with gynecomastia, similar to those found in woman breast; when examined by FBU, they illustrate some specific findings:

Ductal hyperplasia: Some galactophorous/lactiferous ducts emerging from the mammary bud can be thicker, over 1.5 mm, and more hypoechoic than the ordinary ducts, sometimes with *the central hyperechoic line sign* preserved, and there are no salient focal periductal vasculatures; the SE demonstrates a score 1 Ueno for the ducts; lobular hyperplasia is not described in male breast, but lobules may be present of small size, <2 mm, associated with ductal hyperplasia (Fig. 9.23).

Ductal ectasia (galactorrhea): The lactiferous ducts are thickened by luminal milky content, with *a doubled central hyperechoic line sign* present in small ectasia and a tubular shape being visualized in larger ducts; the fluid contents are variable, from transonic to isoechoic, according to the protein amount; no salient periductal focal vasculature is detected by Doppler. A typical

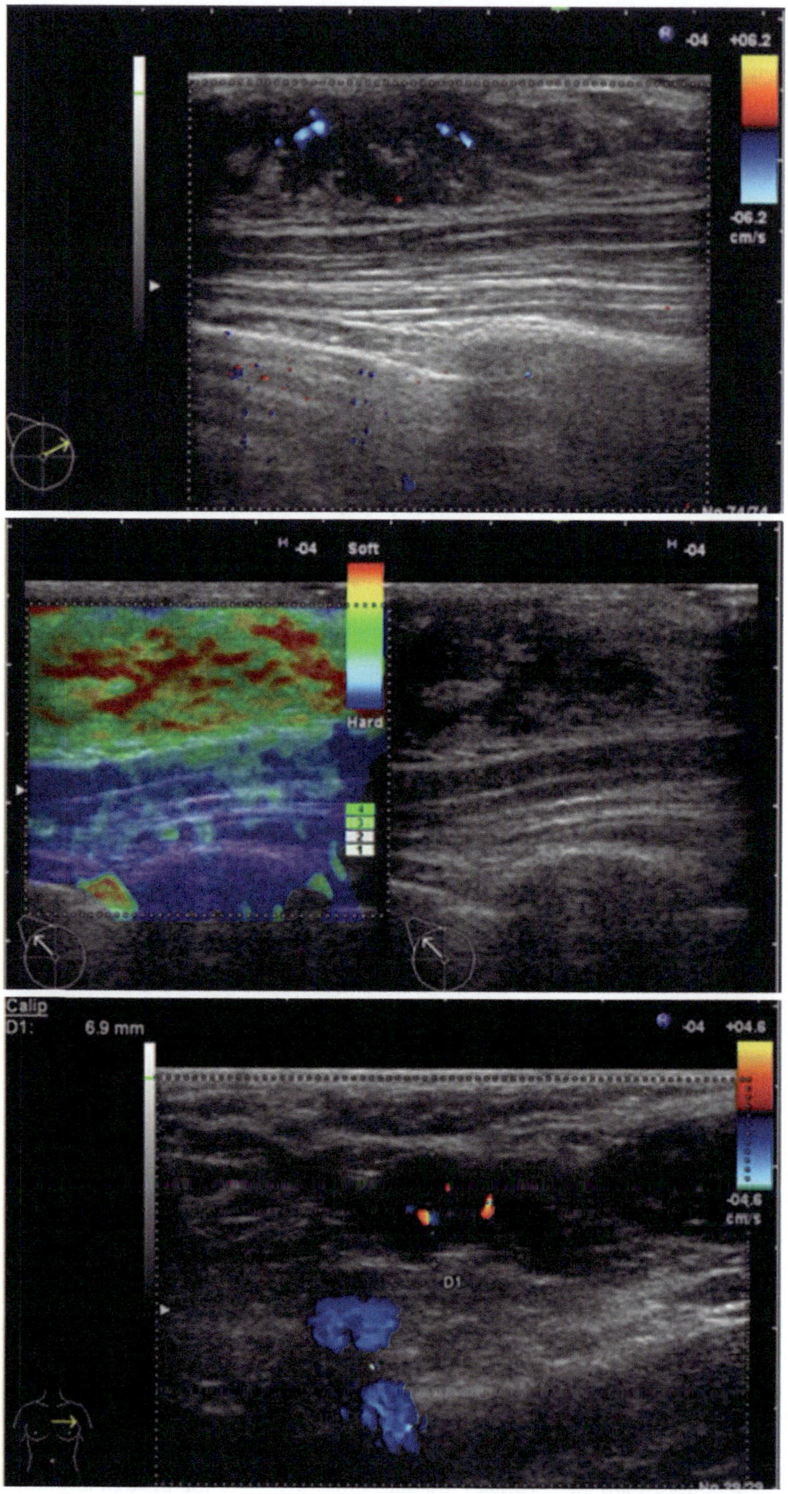

Fig. 9.16 Comparative FBU aspect of a florid pubertal gynecomastia in a different 13-year-old teenager: thick hypoechoic mammary bud and ducts of score 1 Ueno, peripheral glandular stroma, and salient new formation vasculature; note the reactive axillary satellite lymph node with thickened cortex and centrifugal vasculature

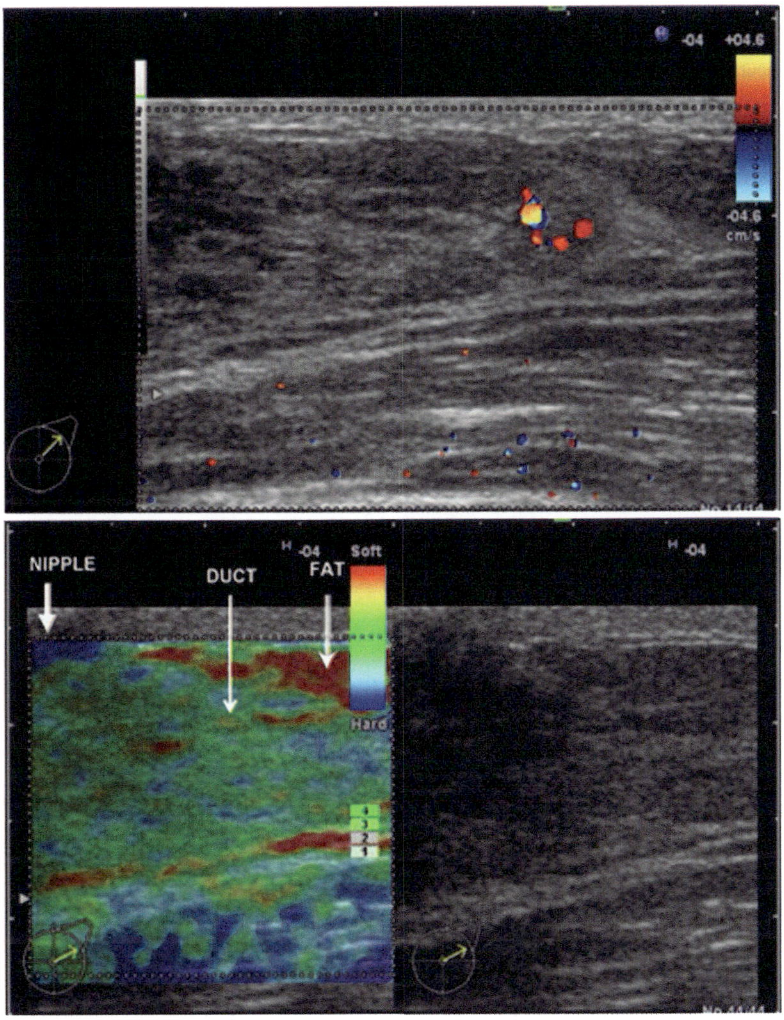

Fig. 9.17 FBU in an acute postpubertal gynecomastia in a 17-year-old boy: branching hypoechoic ductal tree with high elasticity, glandular hyperechoic stroma in light blue at SE, and new formation vasculature in the periphery of the lobe where some lobular formations are ending the ducts

aspect *in sandwich* may be described in SE for the small ectasias, with the score 1 Ueno for the ducts, which illustrates a central reddish fluid delineated by the yellow-green peripheral ductal walls (Fig. 9.13); the largest ectasias, very rare in man, may determine a BGR scoring upon the Ueno classification.

Papillomas are extremely rare in man and represent focal thickening of the ductal walls, rarely a pedunculated mass, with a vascular axe in the largest lesions not always salient in Doppler; because the nipple is small, with the pores usually not completely developed, the bloody nipple surge associated to the papilloma is unusual finding in man. The aspect of a large papilloma has a mosaic mapping in SE with a score 2 or 3 Ueno; the differential diagnosis is made with the segmental ductal hyperplasia that has no salient vasculature and illustrates a score 1 Ueno and with the DCIS, which is an uncommon disease, accounting for approximately 7% of all male breast carcinomas, most cases being papillary and intracystic papillary types [21]. The central papilloma is more common in male breast than the peripheral type; the association with atypical ductal hyperplasia or with DCIS is very rare but when occurs may do the differential diagnosis more difficult. The smallest papilloma may be not visualized or may appear as irregular thickening of the ductal walls associated with duct ectasia. Despite the proliferative character, ductal papilloma is not a real premalignant

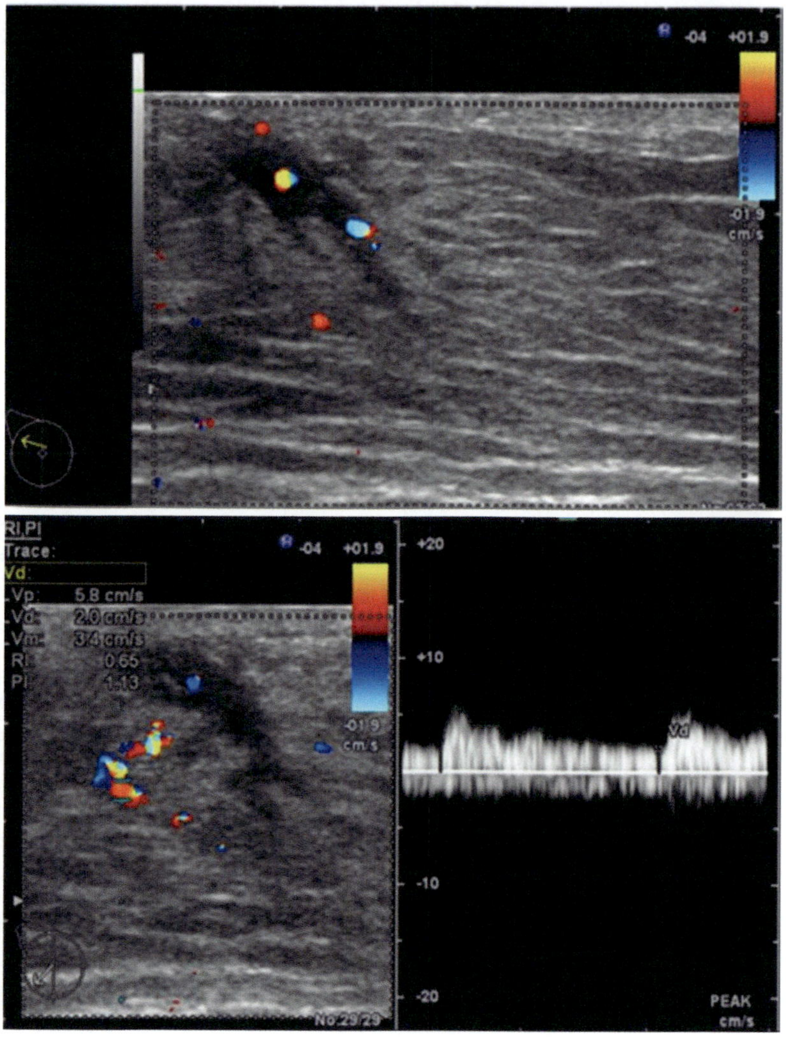

Fig. 9.18 Doppler ductal echography in an acute/florid postpubertal gynecomastia in a 19-year-old teenager: branching ducts surrounded by hyperechoic stroma with new formation periductal vasculature of reduced indices of velocimetry

lesion; it is usually central and may be associated with secretory pathology and overinfection, while breast cancer is usually located eccentrically to the nipple and has malignant characters from the first millimeter size of the beginning proliferation.

Adenoma is a benign-type mass that respects the Stavros criteria with benign posterior acoustic findings upon Kobayashi [22]; it may determine clinical complaints, but the aspect in the FBU has no suspect findings, and the biopsy is not necessary: the mass is connected to the ducts and has benign-type vasculature with peripheral few polar vessels with an arcuate course and a sonoelastogram with a score 1-2-3 Ueno according to the tumoral size. In the male breast, adenoma is usually a unique lesion, and the surgical treatment is suitable.

Fibrocystic changes may be rarely visualized in gynecomastia with galactorrhea, sometimes secondary to previous invasive maneuvers (biopsies, surgical scars); the size and number of the cysts are rarely very important, except for the cystic mastitis. FBU demonstrates the ductal connection of the lesions with the mammary bud; the fluid content may be more or less hypoechoic, and the elasticity may determine a score 2 Ueno for the smallest lesions or a typical BGR score if more than 4–5 mm size; in the absence of SE, the tissue harmonic imaging

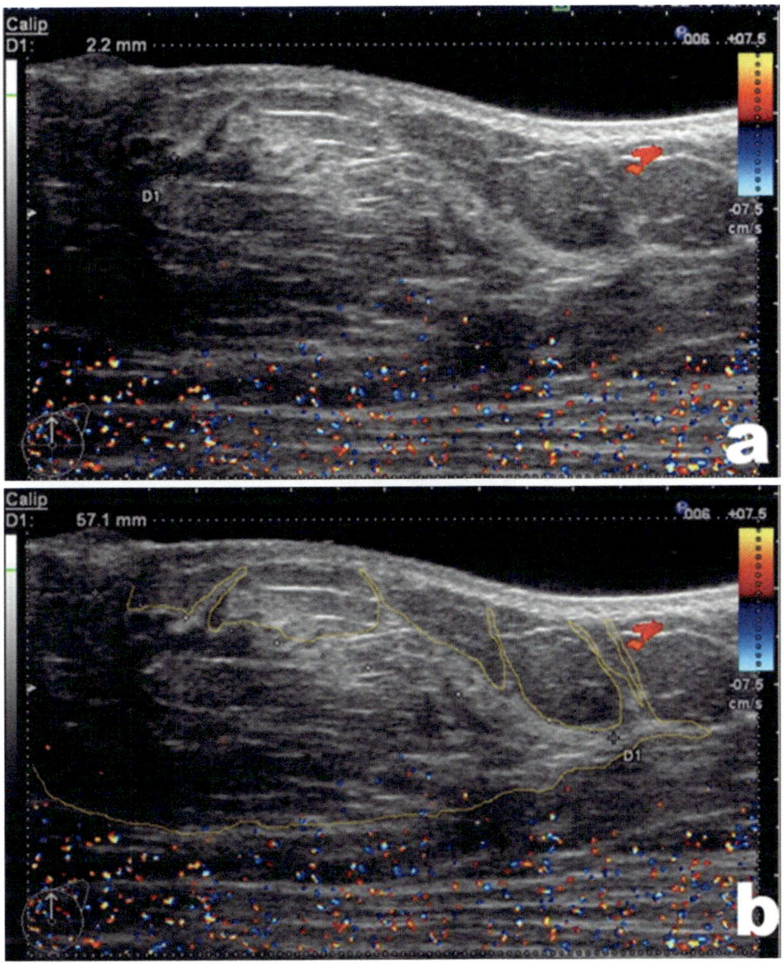

Fig. 9.19 Chronic painful gynecomastia in a 56-year-old male patient with hypercortisolism with full development of the breast and periareolar ductal hyperplasia of 2.2 mm diameter (**a**); (**b**) the delineation of the mammary lobe and the glandular extension along the Cooper ligaments

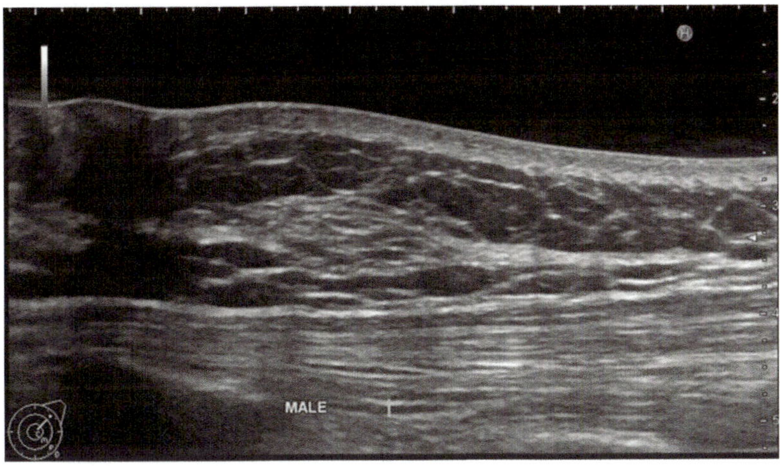

Fig. 9.20 Adult-type gynecomastia in the radial scan presenting thin ducts surrounded by significant amount of stroma; note the Cooper ligaments in the pre-mammary and in the retromammary fatty layers, and the superficial fascia corpora dividing the pre-mammary fat (courtesy of Dr. D. Amy)

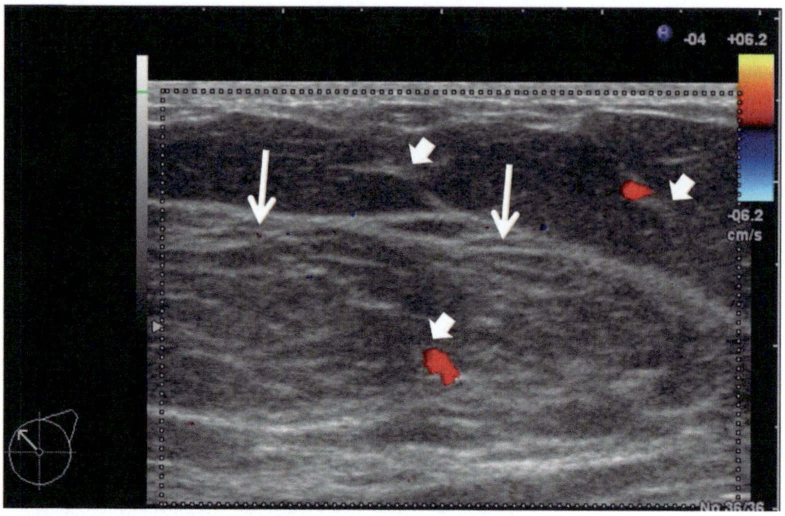

Fig. 9.21 Ductal echography: a radial scan in a 43-year-old man with gynecomastia demonstrates thin ducts surrounded by hyperechoic stroma (*arrows*) and Cooper ligaments with salient new formation vasculature (*thick arrows*)

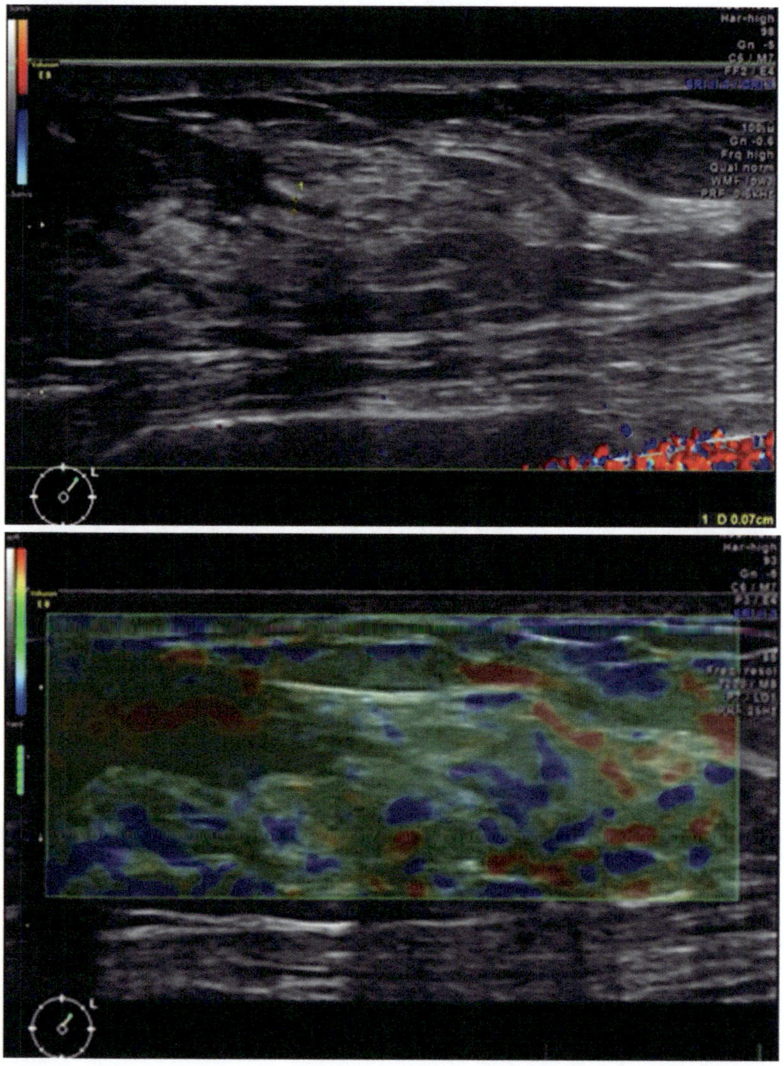

Fig. 9.22 FBU in a chronic, pathological gynecomastia in a 77-year-old patient with kidney failure: large breast without suspect findings; the absent signal in Doppler signifies good prognosis

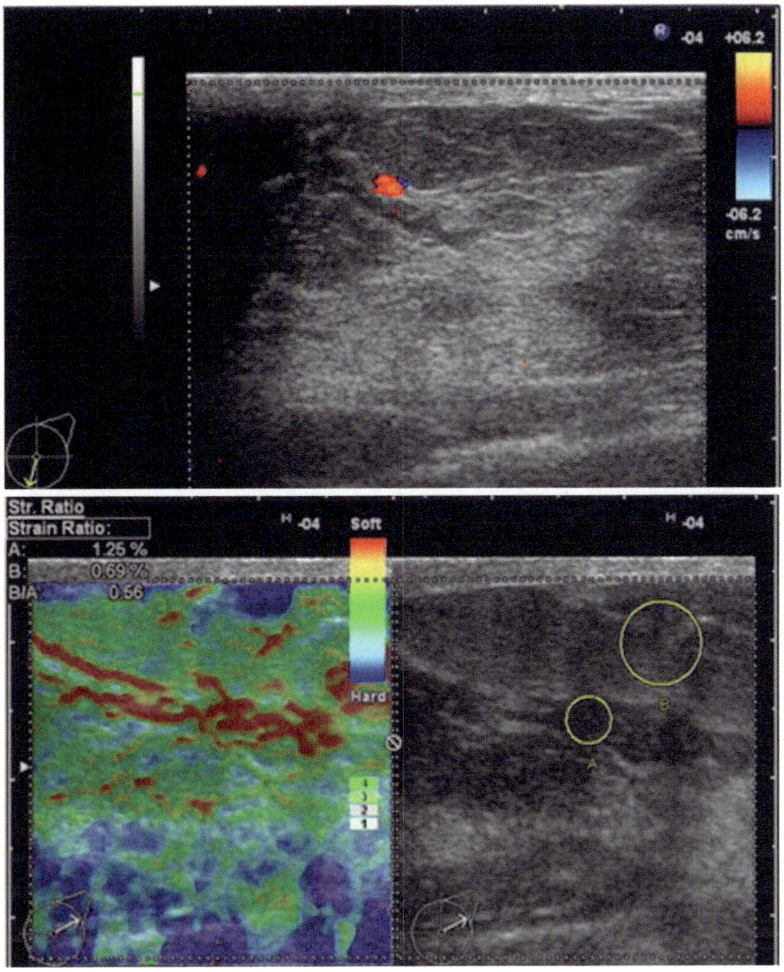

Fig. 9.23 FBU in a 38-year-old man with ductal hyperplasia with pseudo-tumoral aspect in 2D Doppler US, but with score 1 and 2 Ueno; there was a hyperestrogenism associated to adrenal hypercortisolism

(THI) may be useful for increasing the contrast in the gray scale (Fig. 9.24).

Diabetic mastopathy is not rare, but it is neglected in man; when significant development, the clinical and mammographic pseudo-malignant aspect may determine the indication for biopsy. Sometimes it appears as a hypoechoic mass, with irregular shape, heterogeneous structure, and increased strain, and it may be suspect in ultrasound, but the absence of the malignant-type vasculature is the main differential criterion in the FBU.

Paget's disease (more frequent in man than in woman) may develop a nipple-areolar clinical complex various lesions such as ulceration, eczema, nipple discharge, bleeding, and crust formation; the 5-year survival is worse in males than in females' Paget's disease, because of late presentation, 50 % of the male patients having nipple-areolar changes associated with palpable breast mass, positive lymph nodes, or both [23]. Pathologically breast Paget's disease is characterized by the invasion of nipple epidermis by Paget's cells via the ductal way; they are malignant glandular epithelial cells with enlarged pleomorphic and hyperchromatic nuclei presenting discernible but not prominent nucleoli, and with abundant pale, clear cytoplasm, which often contains mucin and sometimes melanin pigment [24]. The pathological reports in the literature detected almost always an underlying intraductal carcinoma (DCIS) [25] or in advanced stages DCIS combined with invasive ductal carcinoma (IDC). Because of the rarest incidence of cases, there are few descriptions of the classical US in male Paget's disease: the findings are nonspe-

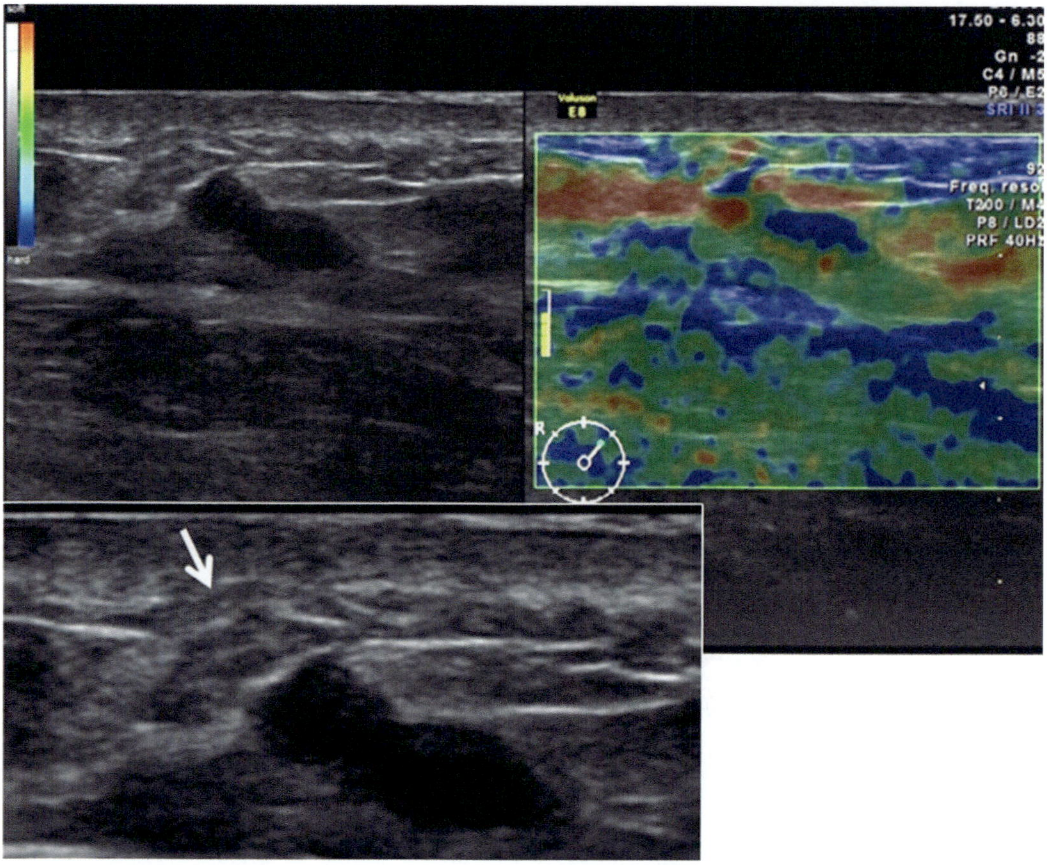

Fig. 9.24 FBU in male illustrates clustered cysts with complex BGR score; some tinny superficial ducts with *the central line sign* demonstrate the gynecomastia

cific and mimic breast infection: parenchymal heterogeneousness, hypoechoic areas, small mass, skin thickening, or dilated ducts [26]. However, the mammary bud is enlarged and hypoechoic in all gynecomastia, the dilated ducts are always present in benign ductal ectasia, and the skin changes are better evaluated by the clinical examination.

Mammography and the breast MRI do not add specific findings to assess malignancy and to suspect Paget's disease.

In FBU examination, the anatomical technique allows the proving of the ductal way of spreading of the disease, the nipple being connected by thickened ducts with the peripheral mass with malignant features upon Stavros; the malignancy is characterized by the new formation vasculature in Doppler, and the SE demonstrates the increased strain of the assembly nipple-areolar complex, connective ducts, and underlying/peripheral breast tumor.

Breast cancer is by far the most important pathology of the male breast, and it will be detailed in the following section.

9.3 Male Breast Cancer: Positive and Differential Diagnosis by the Anatomical Full-Breast US

Usually the male breast cancer is eccentrically located under the nipple-areolar complex and appears as a palpable mass that is unilateral, firm, fixed, peripheral to the nipple, and sometimes associated with nipple discharge or skin changes (usually skin bulge, rarely skin retraction); satellite lymphadenopathy is frequent, because of the late presentation of the patients in the absence of the painful breast.

Breast cancer in men was considered a rare disease, accounting for ≈1% of all breast cancer cases [27], but the modern society seems to increase the risk, due to the changes in food hormonal contaminants, to the treatments for optional sex changes, and other factors such as genetic and environmental factors.

Some general assumptions largely accepted in the literature are useful in the clinical imaging diagnosis:

- Breast cancer occurs in older men, as a unifocal lesion in one breast.
- Most cases of gynecomastia have no cancer associated; however, a sudden increase of a single breast in a man over 50 years old is suspect.
- Breast cancer in man presents clinical signs similar to woman breast cancer: a mass hard to touch, in a single breast, usually without pain or nipple discharge, but sometimes may be detected due to the esthetical complaint (Fig. 9.25).
- The only way to confirm the malignancy is by performing a biopsy.

However, the new noninvasive imaging techniques are more feasible than the biopsies, which

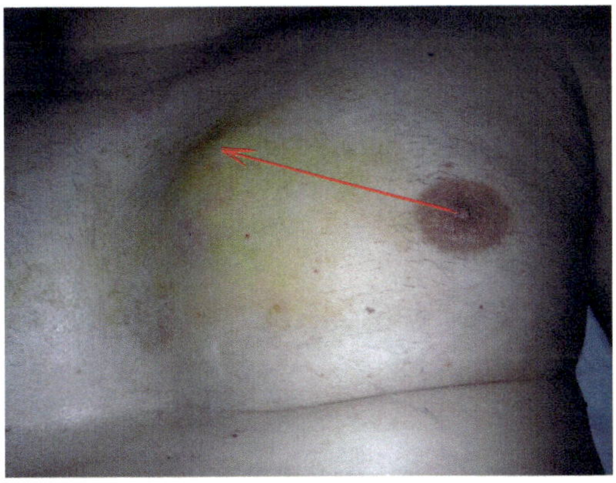

Fig. 9.25 Male breast cancer, clinical aspect after FNA: UIQ tumor, distant from the nipple, with large size and increased stiffness with bulging of the skin

have up to 25% risk of false-positive or false-negative results [28] and a high risk of secondary hematoma [29], due to the new formation vasculature more large, tortuous, and abundant than the rest of the breast vessels, as are revealed by the Doppler examination [13]. This is the reason the biopsy should be preserved to precise the histological type of the malignancy in the cases with large masses, with radiological imaging malignant features, eventually with satellite malignant-type lymph nodes, which should be temporized for the surgical treatment, and initial chemotherapy and/or radiotherapy would be useful to reconvert the staging of the breast cancer.

The challenge in the classical assumptions may be represented by the FBU examination; the aspect of the breast cancer in men is similar to the cancer descriptors in woman, but the examination is easier to perform, because the breast size is smaller and the variability in the breast architecture is less important than in female breasts where the hormonal age-related changes are complex. This technique is useful especially for demonstrating the connection between the abnormal mass/lesion with the mammary bud or the ductal tree for certifying the breast parenchymal etiology, and the radial scanning is mandatory to precise the anatomical elements and the location upon the clockwise notation.

The tumoral descriptors based on the Stavros criteria [30, 31] and the ACR BI-RADS assessment edition 2003 and 2013 [32, 33] are well known, and they are unchanged in the radial scanning upon Teboul used in the FBU technique. In addition, FBU develops the role of the new formation vasculature detected by Doppler (color or power) and the correlation of the vascular pattern with the strain of the tumor and of the surrounding tissues demonstrated by SE (Figs. 9.26, 9.27, 9.28, and 9.29).

The aspect of the vasculature of the pathological mass must be carefully analyzed to avoid overdiagnosis: the malignant vessels are larger, more tortuous, with high velocities, and sometimes with aliasing artifact at the same parameters of acquisition that are used to demonstrate normal velocities in the other breast vessels. The number of vascular poles is according with the

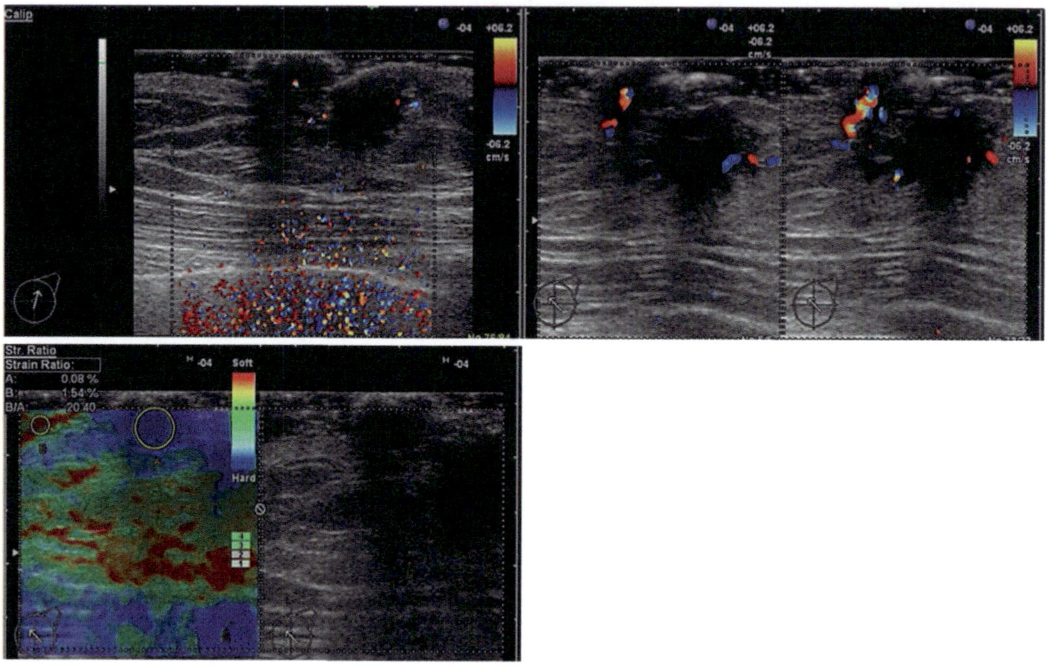

Fig. 9.26 L 5:00 central breast cancer in a 69-year-old male: FBU demonstrates the malignant features based on Stavros, the connection to the nipple, the new formation vasculature, the whole assembly tumor-connecting nipple ducts [Atlas of Full Breast Ultrasonography, Chapter 10 - Physiological and Pathological Aspects of Full Breast US in Men and Children, 2016, p.351, Aristida Colan-Georges, "With permission of Springer"]

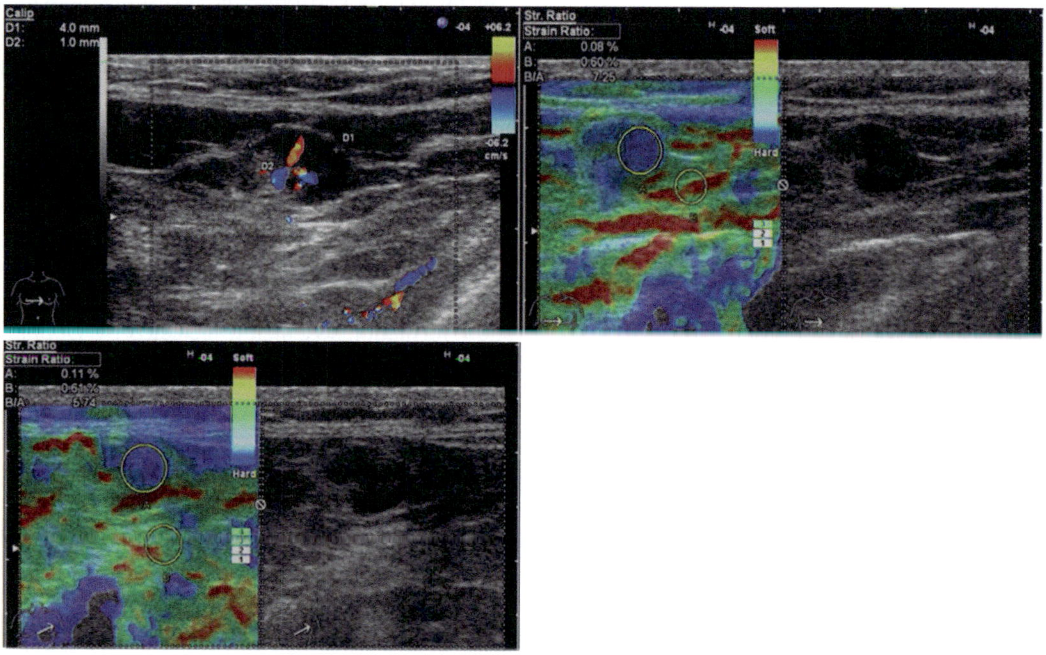

Fig. 9.27 L 5:0 The same case: suspected findings of intramammary lymph node in the lower-inner quadrant (upper right and left images) and left axillary lymph node (bottom image) [Atlas of Full Breast Ultrasonography, Chapter 10 - Physiological and Pathological Aspects of Full Breast US in Men and Children, 2016, p.351, Aristida Colan-Georges, "With permission of Springer"]

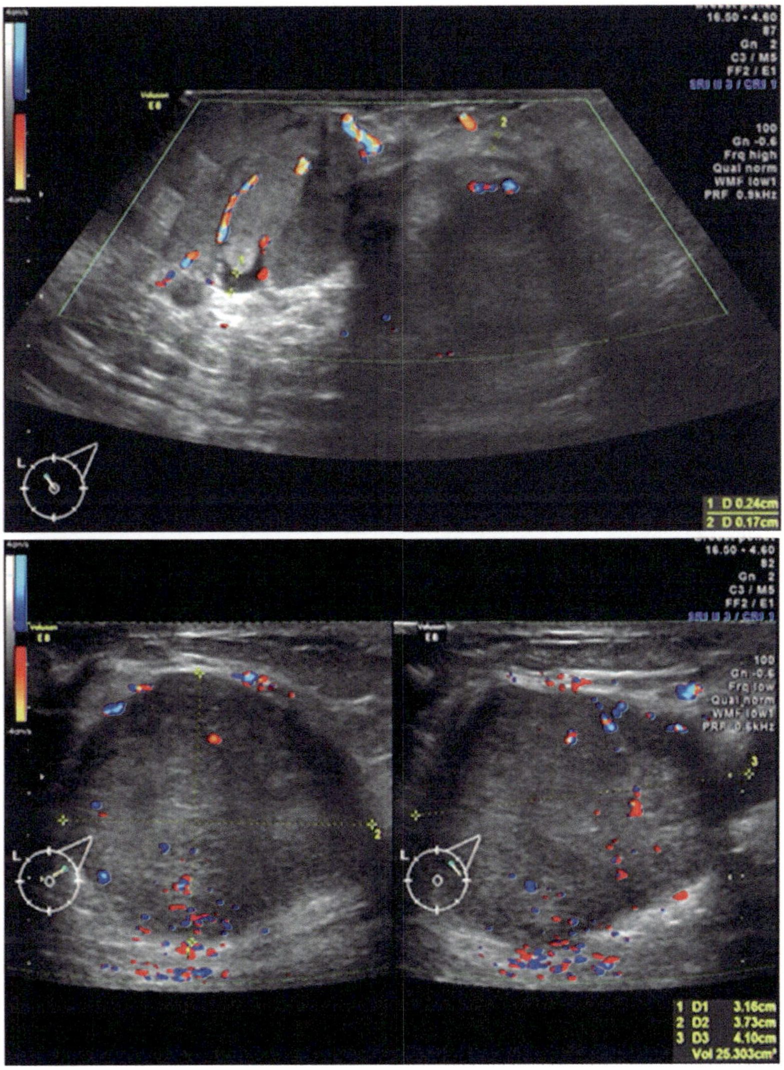

Fig. 9.28 FBU in a 47-year-old man with bifocal large IDC (G3) in the left UEQ that can be better visualized with a long linear probe using the radial scanning that allows the depiction of the ductal connection (upper image); the increase of the probe frequency allows a better illustration of the peripheral multipolar new formation vasculature with internal distribution for the second centrifugal mass, apparently without internal vessels (below image). Note the suspect multi-lobulated contour but the benign posterior findings upon Stavros [31]

tumor size, but more specific is the plunging arterial angle that is incident in malignant tumors, while in the benign ones, it is acute, tangential to the tumoral surface [34]. 3D/4D Doppler reconstructions are spectacular and useful for the therapeutic approach (Fig. 9.30), but less specific than the incident angle of the plunging artery, which was equally proved useful in the diagnosis of the woman breast cancer and in other small part malignancies.

The SE is recommended in the differential diagnosis of suspect masses, but its role was either overvalued, or minimized, because it was used as a unique technique of examination, with inconsistent results when compared with the classical US or other techniques. However, when using SE as an application integrated in the US and Doppler assessment, the results are more accurate, the sensibility and specificity of this full examination exceeding 95% and 99%, respectively [35]. This concept is logical, because each other technique of examination, mammography, tomosynthesis, or MRI, is using all disposable applications for concluding the diagnosis. The unstandardized variants of the SE offered by different providers conducted to various reporting scores for the same lesion, but the most used by different manufacturers and the best correlated with the US BI-RADS assessment is the Ueno (Tsukuba) scoring, exemplified in this chapter.

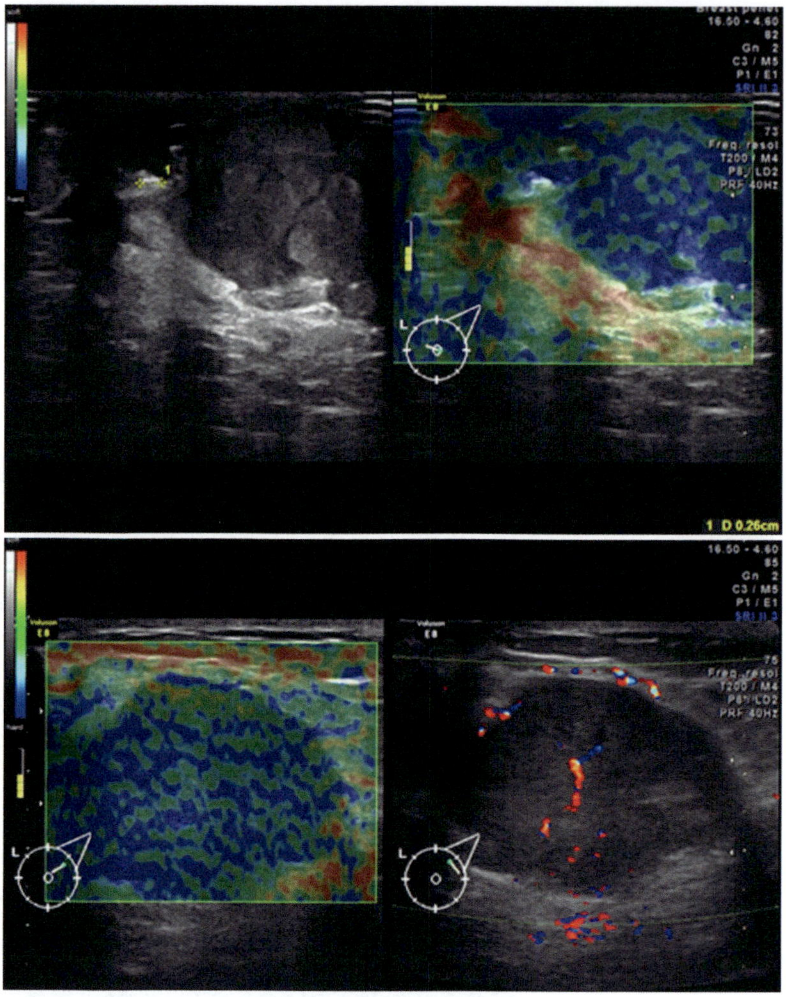
Fig. 9.29 FBU in a 47-year-old man, the same case: SE illustrates a score 4 Ueno for both masses, suggesting malignancy; the centripetal tumor is connected to an ampullary ectasia

The illustration of the ductal connection with the suspect masses is essential in the diagnosis of male breast cancer, because similar to women, most cases are invasive ductal carcinomas (IDC) [36, 37], while lobular carcinomas are rarer in men because of less previous anatomical lobular development [38].

In our experience, by using the FBU, it is easier to detect breast cancer in men than in women, because of the small breast volume; indeed, it is easier to completely scan the male breast with the actually linear high-frequency transducers in use, without missing errors. Moreover, there are few glandular structures surrounding the tumor, easily to compare with the abnormal findings; thus the sensibility of the method is ≈100% [13]. The stages of cancer development at the presentation for an US should be earlier due to psychological and economic factors, US being no painful and more available. In a 10-year follow-up of cases with gynecomastia usually with tenderness or pain, we did not find occurrence of male breast cancer of interval, but we found breast cancer occurrence in previous asymptomatic patients; we did not find multicentric breast cancer in men, concordant with the literature reports, but in advanced stage, a bifocal cancer was found associated with multiple axillary lymphadenopathy. 4D US should be performed if available, even with conventional convex probe, for better illustrating of the voluminous breast masses and for proving the connection between lesions and the anatomical structures (Fig. 9.30).

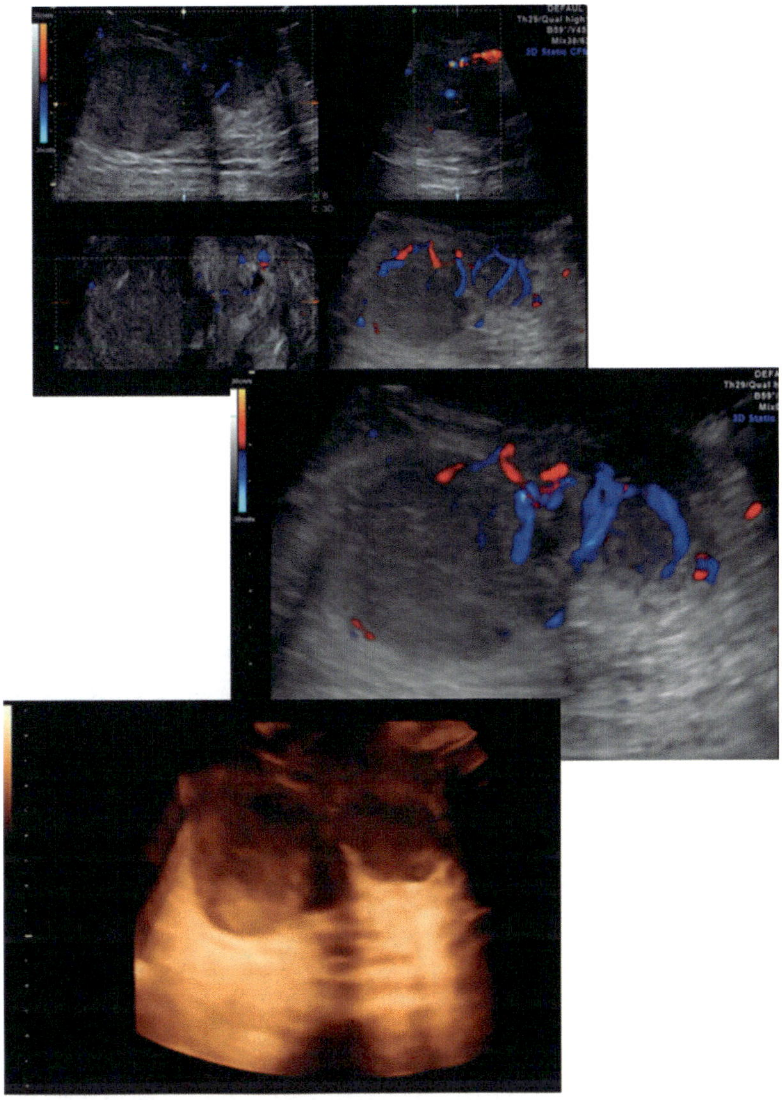

Fig. 9.30 The same case: Doppler 3D and US 4D are useful in illustrating simultaneously both masses with their vascular mapping; the local extension of the disease is important for the therapeutic decision

The differential diagnosis of any suspect male breast mass should include lesions that are not associated with the hormonal breast changes type gynecomastia, according to Olsson and col. [20]:

Non-Gynecomastia lesions:

- Pseudo-gynecomastia
- Lipoma
- Myofibroblastoma
- Granular cell tumor (neural origin)
- Epidermal inclusion cyst
- Cystic lymphangioma
- Varix
- Leiomyoma
- Pleomorphic hyalinizing angiectatic tumor of soft tissues

This pathological group of lesions is heterogeneous, and their importance is different according to their occurrence; the most frequent differential diagnosis of the suspect male breast masses is lipoma and pseudo-gynecomastia, easily to precise by FBU; for the non-mammary tumors (lymphoma, metastases) it is demonstrated the missing of any connection with the mammary ductal tree. Some specific female breast lesions are not encountered in male breast, or are exceptionally found, such as fibroadenomas, phyllodes tumor, or lobular carcinoma.

The diagnosis of the breast cancer using the FBU must include the satellite lymph node description:

- The site: axillary, supra- and subclavicular, thoracic lateral, and internal mammary.
- The number of abnormal nodes visualized: the prognosis is changed if many abnormal nodes are detected, but it is assumed the real number is underestimated by all techniques of imaging diagnosis.
- The transverse diameter: it is the most significant parameter for the size changing in lymphadenopathy, due to the developing metastasis by cortical involvement, via the afferent cortical lymphatic vessels (already invisible in all radiological imaging diagnostic techniques); the size of the abnormal/suspect lymph node should be compared with the ipsilateral or contralateral lymph nodes without detectable anomalies, rather than with statistical cutoff values, because of the large variability between individuals (Fig. 9.31).
- The anatomical lymph node architecture:
  - The cortex: normal, thin, or thickened.
  - Medullary: presence, size, and echogenicity (normal large and hyperechoic, or large with reduced echogenicity in chronic reactive/inflammatory nodes (Fig. 9.29), and reduced size or absent in malignancies).
  - Hilum vascular Doppler signal: normal artery and veins undetectable/reduced;

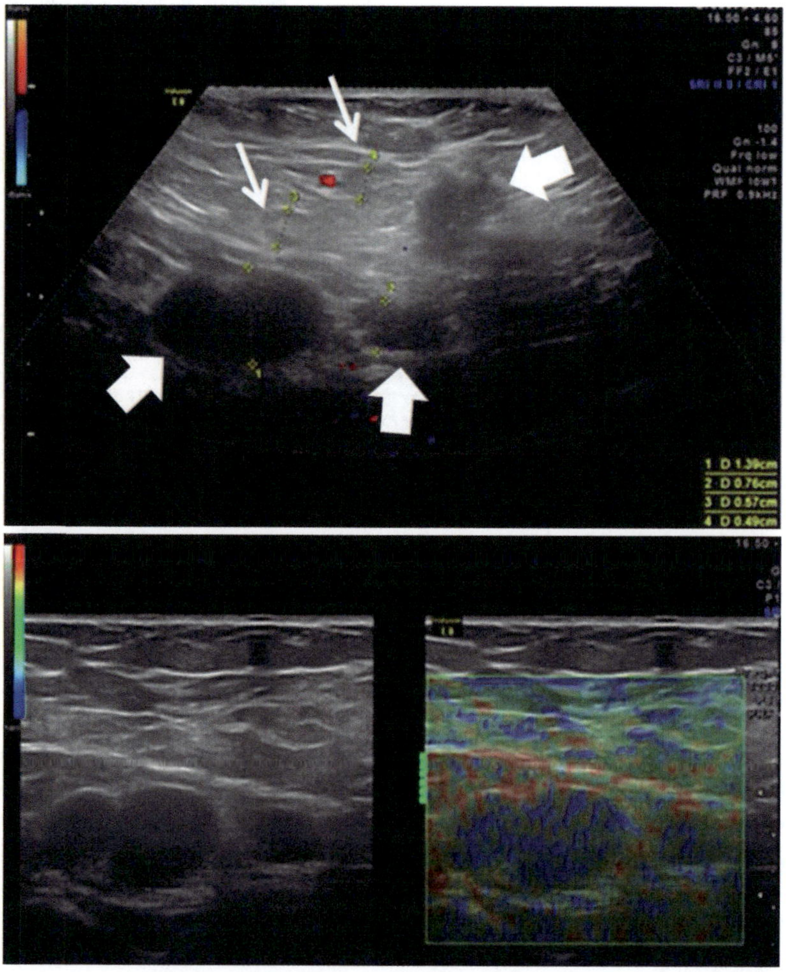

Fig. 9.31 The same case. FBU of the satellite axillary lymph nodes demonstrates some small normal nodes with thin cortex and the transverse diameter <6 mm (*arrows*), together with multiple lymphadenopathies with thickened hypoechoic cortex, the transverse diameter increased up to 14 mm (*thick arrows*), and the strain increased with a score 4 Ueno

  increased vasculature with centrifugal orientation toward the cortex in benign node-type lymphadenitis.
  - Suspect vasculature: peripheral pericapsular and cortical new vessel formation, concordant with the cortical thickening in node metastasis.
  - The afferent pericapsular lymphatic vessels and the efferent hilar lymphatic vessel are undetectable by all radiological and imaging techniques of diagnosis except the contrast lymphangiography.
- SE scoring: usually the normal or the benign lymph nodes illustrate the score 2 Ueno (Fig. 9.32), sometimes with focal BGR score for edematous changes, rarely the score 3 or 4 Ueno in cases with benign node calcification-type tuberculosis; the malignant nodes may illustrate the score 3 Ueno for the focal cortical vascularized thickening (partial involvement) and the score 4 Ueno for the whole node involvement; the score 5 Ueno is not commonly found, but if the strain ratio is available, it has high values according to the diagnosis, but usually of inferior value compared with the strain ratio of the primary breast tumor.

In conclusion, the role of the US in the diagnosis of the male breast must increase according to the technical development of the ultrasound devices: long probes with possibilities to study the anatomical views in large radial and antiradial scans without "blind" spaces and increased sensibility, high-frequency probes with better

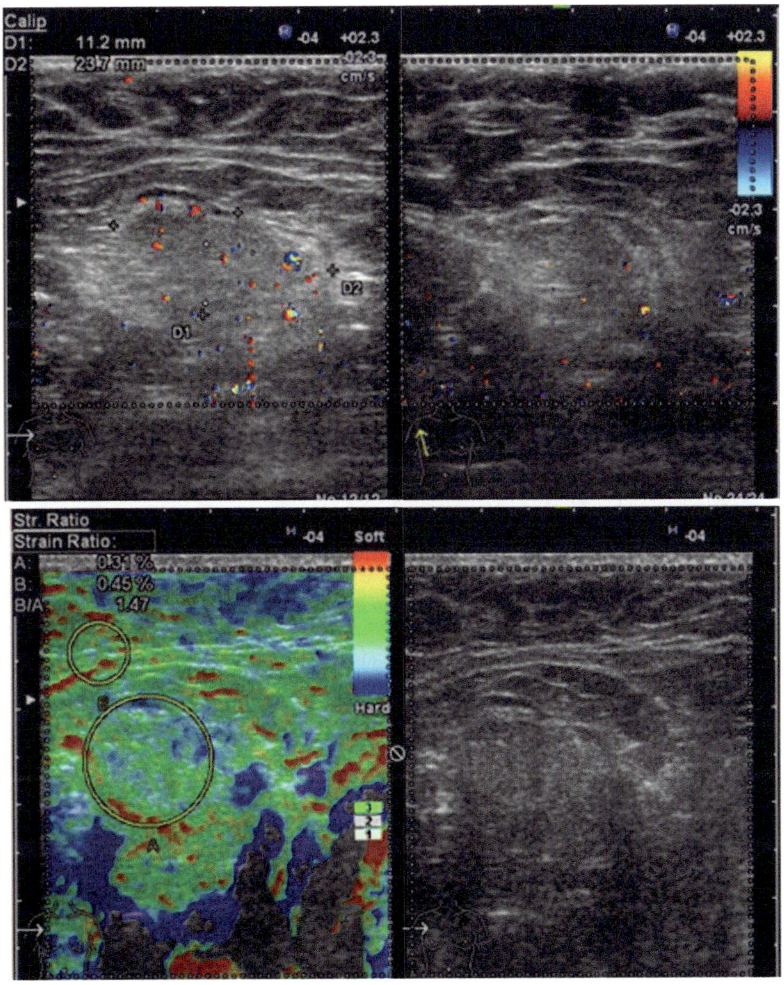

Fig. 9.32 Lymph node differential diagnosis: Doppler US aspect of some enlarged benign axillary lymph nodes in a 70-year-old patient with gynecomastia, of 11 × 23 mm size, but presenting a thin cortex, enlarged medullary area with reduced hyper echogenicity and minimal central vasculature, suggesting a benign lymphadenomegaly (term more specific than benign lymphadenopathy)-type reactive histiocytosis; the SE is concordant with a score 2 Ueno and low FLR up to 1.50

resolution allowing a detailed study of the breast epithelium of <1 mm size, better sensibility of Doppler with possibilities of 3D mapping, and development of the SE with increased specificity of the overall US examination, which becomes complete, designed as "FBU."

The engineering development of the US is more advanced nowadays than the medical modality of examination and interpreting upon the classical approach; the devices should be fully exploited and improved by evolving possibilities of 3D and 4D examinations with high-resolution probes and better differentiation of the anatomical structures with better subtraction-type threshold applications, etc. The final aim is to realize an anatomical breast US examination and interpreting more accurate, reproducible, and useful as first intention method available for all patients, including children and men, without risk of irradiation and avoiding unnecessary biopsies.

References

1. Braunstein GD. Gynecomastia. N Engl J Med. 2007;357(12):1229–37.
2. Georgescu A, Enachescu V. The diagnosis of gynecomastia by Doppler ductal US: etiopathogenic, endocrine and imaging correlations. Vienna: ECR; 2010. http://dx.doi.org/10.1594/ecr2010/C-0420.
3. Johnson ER, Murad M. Gynecomastia: pathophysiology, evaluation, and management. Mayo Clin Proc. 2009;84(11):1010–5. http://www.mayoclinicproceedings.com.
4. Georgiadis E, Papandreou L, Evangelopoulou C, et al. Incidence of gynaecomastia in 954 young males and its relationship to somatometric parameters. Ann Hum Biol. 1994;21(6):579–87.
5. Niewoehner CB, Nuttal FQ. Gynecomastia in a hospitalized male population. Am J Med. 1984;77(4):633–8.
6. Nordt CA, DiVasta AD. Gynecomastia in adolescents. Curr Opin Pediatr. 2008;20(4):375–82.
7. McKiernan JF, Hull D. Breast development in the newborn. Arch Dis Child. 1981;56(7):525–9.
8. Hines SL, Tan WW, Yasrebi M, DePeri ER, Perez EA. The role of mammography in male patients with breast symptoms. Mayo Clin Proc. 2007;82(3):297–300.
9. Ganmaa D, Sato A. The possible role of female sex hormones in milk from pregnant cows in the development of breast, ovarian and corpus uteri cancers. Med Hypotheses. 2005;65(6):1028–37.
10. Murayama K, Oshima T, Ohyama K. Exposure to exogenous estrogen through intake of commercial milk produced from pregnant cows. Pediatr Int. 2010;52(1):33–8. https://doi.org/10.1111/j.1442-200x.2009.02890.x.
11. Marshall WA, Tanner JM. Variations in pattern of pubertal changes in girls. Arch Dis Child. 1969;44(235):291–303.
12. Evans GF, Anthony T, Turnage RH, et al. The diagnostic accuracy of mammography in the evaluation of male breast disease. Am J Surg. 2001;181:96–100.
13. Colan-Georges A. Atlas of full breast ultrasonography. New York, NY: Springer; 2016.
14. Teboul M, Halliwell M. Atlas of ultrasound and ductal echography of the breast. Oxford: Blackwell Science Inc; 1995.
15. Teboul M. Practical ductal echography: guide to intelligent and intelligible Ultrasound imaging of the breast. Madrid: Saned Editors; 2003.
16. Joyce JA, Pollard JW. Microenvironmental regulation of metastasis. Nat Rev Cancer. 2009;9(4):239–52.
17. Khamis ZI, Sahab ZJ, Sang Q-XA. Active roles of tumor stroma in breast cancer metastasis. Int J Breast Cancer. 2012;2012:574025. 10 pages. http://dx.doi.org/10.1155/2012/574025.
18. Georgescu A, Enachescu V. The diagnosis of gynecomastia by Doppler ductal US. Etiopathogenic, endocrine and imaging correlations – partial data. Med Ultrason. 2009;11(3):33–40.
19. Ueno E, Iboraki P. Clinical application of US elastography in the diagnosis of breast disease. ECR 5–9 March, Vienna, Austria. 2004.
20. Olsson H, Bladstrom A, Alm P. Male gynecomastia and risk for malignant tumours – a cohort study. BMC Cancer. 2002;2:26. https://doi.org/10.1186/1471-2407-2-26.
21. Camus MG, Joshi MG, Mackarem G, et al. Ductal carcinoma in situ of the male breast. Cancer. 1994;74(4):1289–93.
22. Kobayashi T. Clinical ultrasound of the breast. New York, NY: Springer; 1978.
23. Desai DC, Brennan EJ Jr, Carp NZ. Paget's disease of the male breast. Am Surg. 1996;62(12):1068–72.
24. Karakas C. Paget's disease of the breast. J Carcinog. 2011;10:31. https://doi.org/10.4103/1477-3163.90676.
25. Hayes R, Cummings B, Miller RA, Guha AK. Male Paget's disease of the breast. J Cutan Med Surg. 2000;4(4):208–12.
26. Gunhan-Bilgen I, Oktay A. Paget's disease of the breast: clinical, mammographic, sonographic and pathologic findings in 52 cases. Eur J Radiol. 2006;60:256–63.
27. Weiss RJ, Moysich BK, Swede H. Epidemiology of male breast cancer. Cancer Epidemiol Biomarkers Prev. 2005;14(1):20–6.
28. Jackman RJ, Nowels KW, Rodriguez-Soto J, et al. Stereo-tactic, automated, large core needle biopsy of nonpalpable breast lesions: false-negative and histo-

logic underestimation rates after long-term follow-up. Radiology. 1999;210:799–805.

29. Hertl K, Marolt-Musik M, Kocijancic I, et al. Haematomas after percutaneous vacuum-assisted breast biopsy. Ultraschall Med. 2007;30:33–6.
30. Stavros AT, Rapp LC, Parker HS. Breast ultrasound. Philadelphia, PA: Lippincott Williams & Wilkins; 2004.
31. Stavros AT, Thickman D, Rapp CL, Dennis MA, Parker SH, Sisney GA. Solid breast nodules: use of sonography to distinguish between benign and malignant lesions. Radiology. 1995;196:123–34.
32. American College of Radiology. Illustrated breast imaging reporting and data system (BI-RADS): ultrasound. Reston, VA: American Coll. of Radiology; 2003. http://www.acr.org/deparments/stand_accred/birads/us_assess.pdf.
33. D'Orsi CJ, Sickles EA, Mendelson EB, et al. ACR BI-RADS ® Atlas, breast imaging reporting and data system. Reston VA: American Coll. of Radiology; 2013.
34. Kujiraoka Y, Ueno E, Yohno E, et al. Incident angle of the plunging artery of breast tumors. In: Research and development in breast ultrasound. Tokyo: Springer; 2005. p. 72–5.
35. Georgescu A, Bondari S, Manda A, Andrei EM. The differential diagnosis between breast cancer and fibro-micro-cystic dysplasia by full breast US - a new approach. Vienna: ECR; 2012. https://doi.org/10.1594/ecr2012/C-0167. EPOS™.
36. Ruddy KJ, Winer EP. Male breast cancer: risk factors, biology, diagnosis, treatment, and survivorship. Ann Oncol. 2013;24:1434. https://doi.org/10.1093/annonc/mdt025.
37. Burga AM, Fadare O, Lininger RA, et al. Invasive carcinomas of the male breast: a morphologic study of the distribution of histologic subtypes and metastatic patterns in 778 cases. Virchows Arch. 2006;449(5):507–12.
38. Kornegoor R, Verschuur-Maes AH, Buerger H, et al. Molecular subtyping of male breast cancer by immunohistochemistry. Mod Pathol. 2012;25(3):398–404.

10 Lymph Node Staging with US (and FNA)

Dominique Fournier

Abbreviations

ALND	Axillary lymph node (surgical) dissection
AUS	Axillary ultrasound
FNA	Fine-Needle Aspiration
LN	Lymph node
SN	Sentinel node
NPV	Negative predictive value
PPV	Positive predictive value
SLNB	Sentinel lymph node (surgical) biopsy
US	Ultrasound
US-FNAB	US-guided fine-needle aspiration biopsy (with core biopsy needle)
US-FNAC	US-guided fine-needle aspiration cytology

10.1 Introduction

Take-Home Messages

- Ultrasound and US-guided fine-needle aspiration cytology (FNAC) is the most accurate and cost-effective method for the N staging of invasive breast cancer:
  - US *alone* is suggested for the preoperative staging of patients with early-stage breast cancer.
  - US-guided FNAC can identify 90% of *axillary and extra-axillary* lymph nodes (LNs) with metastatic deposit larger than 5 mm, avoiding sentinel lymph node biopsy.
  - US can *exclude heavy metastatic burden* when lymph nodes appear normal on US (≤3 mm cortical thickness).
- Looking systematically for *extra-axillary nodal basins* avoids the risk of overpassing N2/N3 nodal disease.
- Any *round* in shape LN, even <5 mm, should be considered as abnormal.
- Normal internal mammary LNs are not visible with US; therefore any mass effect adjacent to the internal mammary vessels or any bulge of the pleura is abnormal.
- A totally invaded *intramammary lymph node* might represent a source of error for multicentricity/multifocality.
- Doppler color flow imaging can demonstrate *micrometastasis* in a morphologically normal LN as an *avascular* cortical area.
- Fine-needle aspiration cytology (FNAC) is more frequently used worldwide than core biopsy.
- The liquid-based cytology (LBC) technique for fine needle aspirates significantly improved performance of FNAC.

Lymphatic dissemination can occur even during early stages of breast cancer. To determine if the cancer has spread to the lymph nodes (LNs)

D. Fournier, M.D.
Institut de radiologie, rue du Scex 2, CH-1950, Sion, Switzerland
e-mail: dominique.fournier@groupe3r.ch

D. Amy (ed.), *Lobar Approach to Breast Ultrasound*, https://doi.org/10.1007/978-3-319-61681-0_10

represents the most important prognostic factor for breast cancer recurrence and related death [1, 2]. The risk of metastases or death increases both with breast cancer size and number of axillary LN involved [3, 4]. Therefore, preoperative knowledge of regional LN status is essential before treatment planning because the detection of occult metastatic LNs changes the clinical stage and consequently the therapeutic options.

More than 30 years ago, patients with breast cancer had their 5-year survival rate decreasing from 87 to 75% when the clinical stage increased from I to II and to 46% when the clinical stage increased from II to IIIC [5]. For patients diagnosed with breast cancer during 2005–2009, the 5-year survival rate was up to 85% and higher [6]. More recently, a 96% 5-year survival rate was reported during 2006–2012, demonstrating improvements in all tumor and nodal stages compared to 1999–2005, and 100% for patients with tumors ≤1 cm. Comparing 1999–2005 and 2006–2012 patients, there was a little improvement in tumor size (≤T1 65% *vs.* 60%) and LN-negative tumors (N0 68% *vs.* 65%), but patients received increased chemotherapy, hormonal therapy, and targeted therapy (60% *vs.* 53%) [7]. This improvement can mainly be explained by early diagnosis of breast cancer with less nodal disease as well as better treatment options.

The answer to the question of nodal involvement and consequently the clinical stage of breast cancer depends on many factors, from the type of test method, size, and location of the metastasis to sampling techniques.

Ultrasound (US) is the primary imaging modality worldwide for evaluating axillary LN [8]. US-guided fine-needle aspiration cytology (US-FNAC) of axillary LN is a sensitive and very specific method to detect metastasis in breast cancer patients. When a preoperative US-FNAC result is positive, axillary LN dissection (ALND) can be planned safely instead of a sentinel LN dissection (SLNB) because of the excellent positive predictive value of US-FNAC.

The mean reported rate of SLNB avoidance is 20–30% [9–11] and could be more than 40% with additional experience [12].

10.1.1 The Importance of N3 Disease Demonstration

The seventh edition (2010) of the AJCC (American Joint Committee on Cancer) staging system for breast cancer defines a pathologically *positive axillary node* as containing a metastasis measuring at least 0.2 mm or containing >200 tumor cells.

Positive node status is further subdivided by four factors:

1. The size of the axillary metastasis: 0.2 mm (or >200 cells) up to 2 mm is a *micrometastasis* (pN1mic); >2 mm is a *macrometastasis*: pN1, pN2, and pN3, depending on total number of positive nodes.
2. The anatomic location of the node involved: positive *internal mammary nodes* affects pN depending on the status of other nodes (e.g., internal mammary *and* axillary is N3b); a positive *infraclavicular* (*axillary level III*) node is pN3a; a positive *supraclavicular* node is pN3c.
3. The total number of positive axillary nodes: total of 1–3 positive nodes is pN1, 4–9 positive nodes is pN2, and >9 positive nodes is pN3.
4. The method of detection (tissue biopsy versus FNAC or clinical detection).

Therefore demonstrating abnormal LN in another nodal basin draining the breast besides the axillary one (*extra-axillary nodes*) is of great importance because it changes the clinical stage:

- From stage I (no node involved or small groups of cancer cells not larger than 2 mm) to II for every N1 (metastasis >2 mm found in one to three axillary LNs but less than four lymph nodes *or* in the internal mammary LN if proved during a sentinel lymph node procedure and not otherwise clinically detected).
- From stage I to IIIC for every N3.

Complete axillary lymph node dissection (ALND) makes no sense in patients with N3 disease for whom a nonsurgical treatment is usually the first step. That is why screening for N3 disease is very important and should be done systematically in the preoperative staging.

10.1.2 What Is the Challenge for N Staging?

For an accurate N staging in breast cancer patients, the main challenge is to identify the N staging that changes the treatment options and affects the survival rate. Therefore the goal is to detect macrometastasis (>2 mm) because there is no significant difference for recurrence-free period and overall survival if the sentinel node (SN) is negative or if positive only with ≤2 mm micrometastatic or isolated tumor cells [13, 14]. Consequently the detection of micrometastasis is of less importance [15], and the prognostic significance of this low positivity in axillary LN is currently debated, as is its management [16].

But having identified suspicious LN macrometastatic deposits in the nodal basins draining the breast, cells are required from a suspicious LN for cyto- or histological analysis, which is still the gold standard to prove metastatic involvement in a LN. To do that with minimally invasive techniques and at low cost is a true challenge for society. This challenge can be overcome by wide use of US and US-guided fine-needle aspiration cytology (FNAC).

10.1.3 New Frontiers for Evaluation of Small Superficial Lymph Nodes with Ultrasound

To promote better understanding of modern US imaging for the analysis of early metastatic LN, it is important to underline new frontiers of ultrasound imaging:

- The very high spatial and contrast resolution boosted by *harmonic imaging* allows to demonstrate
  - Structures thinner than 1 mm such as the normal cortex of a small superficial lymph node (Fig. 10.1).
  - Small (<3–5 mm) metastatic deposits, such as the beginning of a cortical bulge corresponding to a macrometastasis (Fig. 10.2).
  - Tiny rounded superficial nodes as small as 3 mm (Fig. 10.3) allowing characterization of benign or malignant nodes

    In the skin: skip metastasis of a skin melanoma [17–20].

    In the neck: metastasis of a cervicofacial tumor [21, 22].
- The ultra-sensitive Doppler color flow imaging can demonstrate
  - Invisible blood vessels on B-mode, like arteries and veins in small anatomic structures such as in the cortex of a lymph node, less than 3 mm in short diameter (Fig. 10.1).
  - *Micrometastatic deposit* in a morphologically normal LN as an *avascular* area in the cortex (Fig. 10.4), something new in the field of imaging. The *avascularity* of small tumoral lesions is a well-known pathophysiological finding: most malignancies and metastases originate as an avascular mass and only induce the development of new vessels when beyond a few millimeters in size. The early metastases can grow up to a size of approximately 1–2 mm^3 before their metabolic demands are restricted due to diffusion limitation of oxygen and nutrients [23].

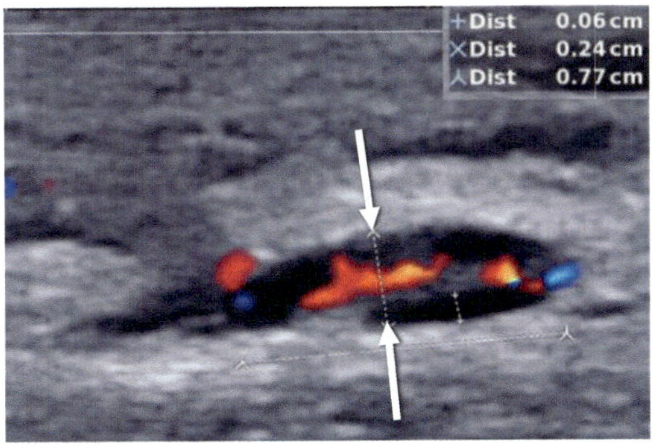

Fig. 10.1 Demonstration of high spatial resolution of ultrasound. A normal US-sentinel axillary lymph node (*longitudinal view*): 2.4 mm in short axis diameter (*long arrows*); 7.7 mm in long axis diameter; 0.6 mm thickness of the deep cortex; normal vascularization on color Doppler

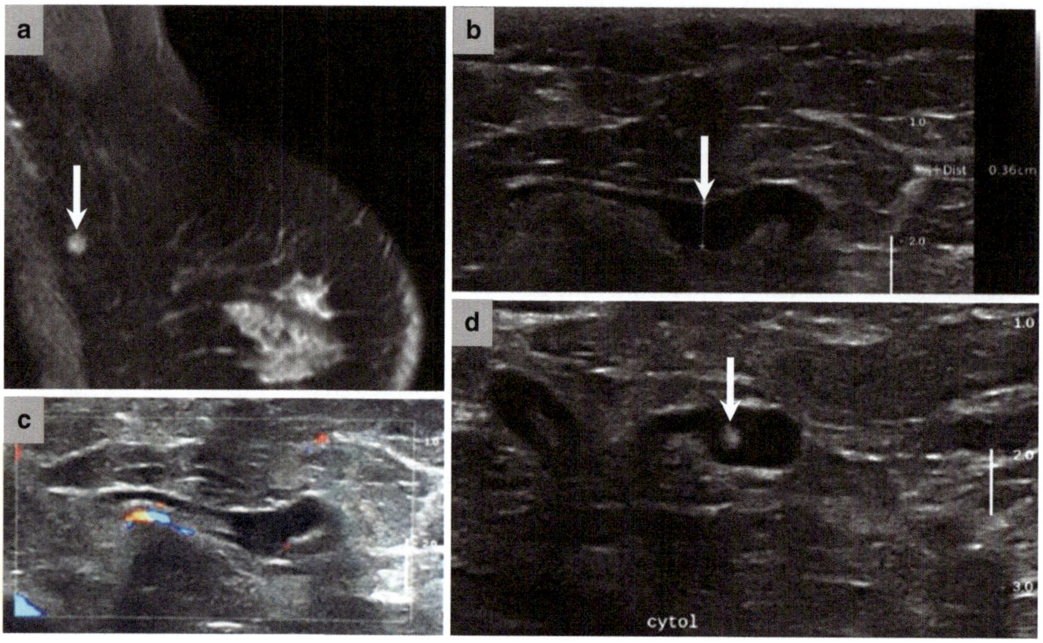

Fig. 10.2 Invasive ductal carcinoma of the left breast with an *early metastatic axillary LN*: MRI (saggital fat sat view): suspicious <1 cm axillary lymp node (**a**); US: suspicious focal 3.6 mm thickening of the cortex deforming the hilum (**b**);« avascular » on color Doppler (**c**), US-guided FNAC: *metastasis* (**d**)

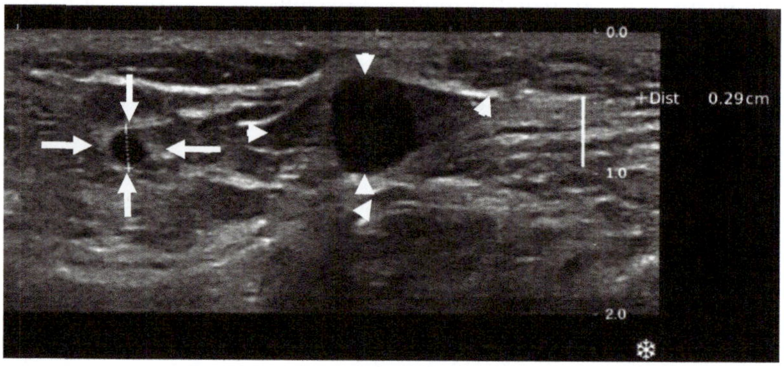

Fig. 10.3 High resolution (*harmonic imaging*) US image of two anechoic *metastases* in two axillary LN: a round metastasis, 2.9 mm in size within a 5 mm node (*arrows*); an ovoid metastasis, 7.7 mm within a 15 mm node (*arrowheads* marking the limits of the node)

- The high-resolution quantitative shear wave *elastography* allows:
  - Demonstration, when present, of higher stiffness at the periphery of the early (5–10 mm) intra-nodal growing metastasis (Fig. 10.5)
  - To challenge the common concept that the greater stiffness is in the cortex of metastatic LN [24–26]
  - Confirmation of the well-known pathophysiological principle that in the microenvironment of a growing tumor, the periphery is usually denser than the center [27], which may also be secondary to the compression of the surroundings by the growing metastasis (Fig. 10.6)

10.1.4 Differential Diagnosis of an Axillary Mass (See Table 10.1)

It is important to remember that lymphadenopathy in the nodal basins draining the breast may not be caused only by metastases of a breast cancer. General diseases and cancers other than

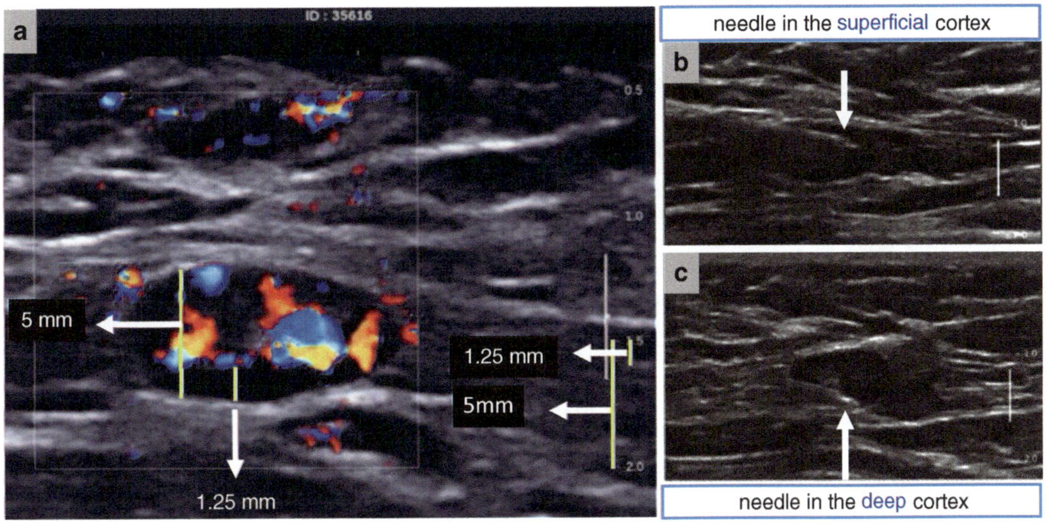

Fig. 10.4 *The smallest metastasis detected* with US and US-guided FNAC*: 1.25 mm thickness*. Analysis of the cortex of this «morphologically normal » oval 5 × 7 mm axillary US sentinel node (**a**): Deep cortex is more hypoechoïc than superficial cortex, no vessels on color-Doppler. Is that an early metastasis? US-guided FNA was performed on both side of the cortex (**b**, **c**); Cytologic results: *tumoral cells in the deep cortex*, normal lymphoïd cells in the superficial cortex

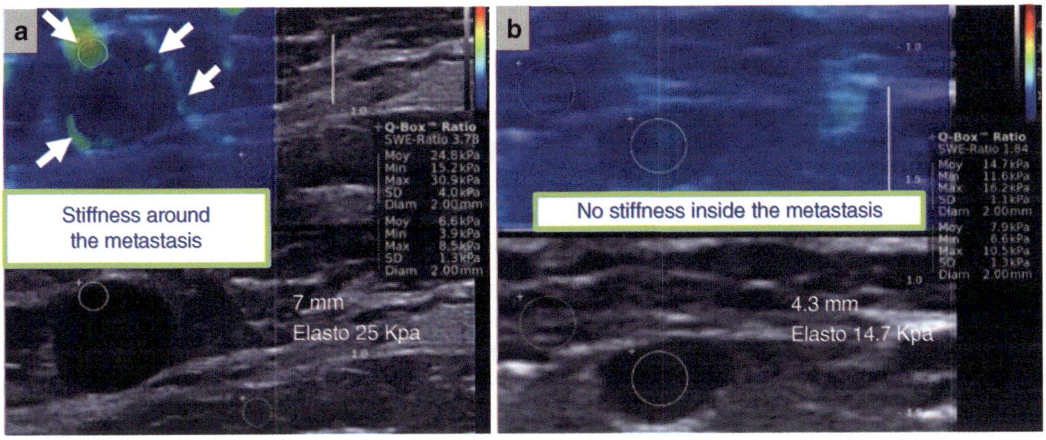

Fig. 10.5 Shear wave *elastography* US analysis of two different small *metastatic* LN: elastography showing the maximum (but low: 25 Kpa)) stiffness at the periphery (**a**) of a 8 mm metastasis within a 11 × 7 mm node: a completely replaced 4.3 mm metastatic node, with no stiffness inside or around (**b**)

breast cancer can produce *clinically* detectable lymphadenopathies anywhere in the body including the lymphatic basins draining the breast.

On imaging, occult axillary or internal mammary lymphadenopathies secondary to a general disease can be found in patients with or without breast cancer. In both situations, it is necessary to look at adjacent and contralateral nodal basins for the presence of similar nodes. When there are similar nodes in the symmetrical contralateral area, the probability of lymphadenopathies from a systemic disease is high and the probability of metastases of breast cancer is low. The clinical history of the patient may reveal a systemic disease. In the absence of a known systemic disease, one should look for such a disease.

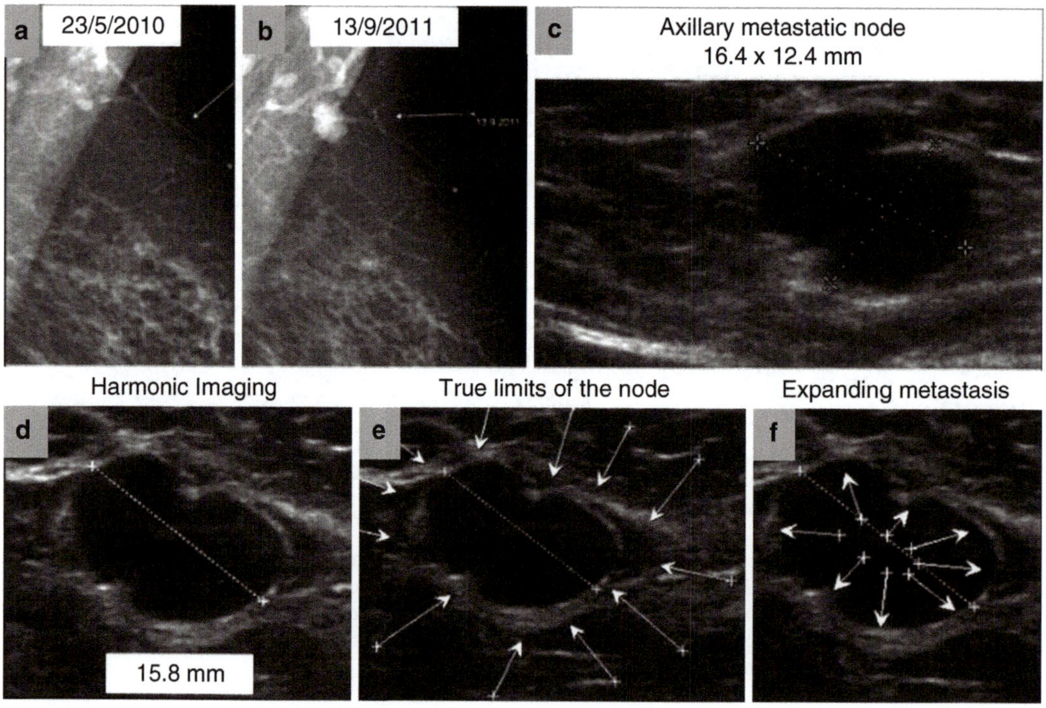

Fig. 10.6 Invasive ductal carcinoma of the left breast. Progression of an axillary lymph node over15 months on mammograms (**a**, **b**). Typical 16 mm macrometastatic LN on standard US (**c**). Harmonic imaging: better visibility of the contour of the metastasis (**d**), of the surounding compressed cortex of the LN (**e**), of the *growing metastasis* (**f**)

Table 10.1 Differential diagnosis of axillary lymphadenopathy

1. Benign
a. Reactive lymphadenopathy
i. Mastitis
ii. Loco-regional infection
iii. Cat scratch disease
iv. Loco-regional inflammation (subcutaneous cysts or abscesses)
v. Zona
vi. Silicone-induced adenitis
b. Systemic disease
i. Autoimmune diseases (rheumatoid arthritis, lupus…)
ii. Infectious mononucleosis
iii. HIV
c. Granulomatous disease
i. Sarcoidosis
ii. Tuberculosis
2. Malignant
a. Melanoma
b. Metastases (breast carcinoma,…)
c. Lymphoma/leukemia

10.2 The Nodal Basins Draining the Breast

Recent studies show that breast cancers induce remodeling of the local lymphatic vessels and the regional lymphatic network in the sentinel and distal LN. These changes include an increase in number and diameter of tumor-draining lymphatic vessels. Consequently, lymph flow away from the tumor is increased, which significantly increases tumor cell metastasis to draining LN and may contribute to systemic spread [28].

Within the node the lymph flows from the peripheral cortical sinuses into the medullary sinuses that converge at the hilum. The lymph leaves then the node via the efferent lymphatic vessels toward a more central LN. The common concept is that the first metastatic deposit is coming to the cortex and fixed there.

An important goal of imaging would be to detect the metastatic sentinel node (SN) at the stage of the early metastasis in the 2–3 mm thin cortex of the SN.

Lymphoscintigraphic studies for SLNB have demonstrated the lymph to drain in:

- Axillary nodes
- Extra-axillary nodes
  - Internal mammary (parasternal)
  - Intramammary
  - Intra- and interpectoral
  - Infraclavicular (axillary level III)
  - Supraclavicular
  - Mediastinal
  - Contralateral internal mammary
  - Contralateral axillary.

10.2.1 The Axillary Lymph Nodes

Most (75%) of the breast lymph goes to axillary LN, while the rest to internal mammary lymph nodes [29]:

- Inner and outer quadrants of the breast drain mainly in the axilla, while the second basin is the internal mammary nodes (IMN).
- The superficial system drains to the axilla, usually to a LN posterior to the pectoralis minor muscle.
- The deep system drains to the axilla and also anastomoses with the perforating system, which drains to the IMN [30, 31].

However, *extra-axillary* nodal basins, such as internal mammary chains and infra-/supraclavicular regions, can be involved in up to 56% of breast cancer [32–34].

Advanced nodal involvement was reported as an important cause of false-negative SLNB, because of lymphatic drainage being possibly deviated by macrometastatic axillary LN occluding the natural lymphatic draining routes [35]. Other causes of axillary false-negative staging can be related to variations of lymphatic breast drainage, either from anatomic variants or surgically acquired as for patients with previous aesthetic or oncologic breast surgery or any thoracotomy affecting their lymphatic routes.

10.2.2 The Extra-axillary Lymph Nodes

LNs are considered *extra-axillary* when localized out of the two first levels of the axilla. Among patients with non-axillary SN, 7–10% had no SN in the axilla at all [31]. Patients with inner-quadrant (IQ) breast cancer demonstrated a sixfold greater frequency of isolated extra-axillary metastasis, and such findings were associated with triple the risk for disease progression [36].

Krause et al. [37] reported that in 6 (40%) of 15 patients with a central or medial localized tumor, the SN was observed in the infraclavicular (n = 3), parasternal (n = 2), or contralateral axilla (n = 1); for the latter, the SN of the contralateral axilla showed metastases, whereas the simultaneous SNs, and all removed lymph nodes from the ipsilateral axilla, were uninvolved.

In the study of Altinyollar et al. [38], 20% of patients had suspicious infraclavicular LN on US (N3b). The specificity of US in the identification of metastatic LN in the infraclavicular region was 98%, with a sensitivity of 47%, a positive predictive value of 95%, a negative predictive value of 74%, and an overall accuracy of 78%.

Unusually situated SN can be present in 12% of the patients (outside the axilla and internal mammary chain), as found in the study of van Rijk et al. [39]: of which

- 47% in the breast
- 29% in the infraclavicular fossa
- 17% between the pectoral muscles
- 6% within the supraclavicular bed.

Metastasis was positive for 17% of LN and the treatment adjusted accordingly.

Key point: in the staging of breast cancer patients, one should systematically look for extra-axillary nodal basins to avoid the risk of overpassing N2–3 nodal disease, thus understaging the cancer in these patients with higher risk of undertreatment and disease progression.

10.3 Preoperative Detection of Lymph Node Involvement

Various preoperative examination methods are used to evaluate the nodal status but, while none can detect the nodal disease with 100% accuracy, on the other hand, exclusion of early metastatic nodal disease is impossible with any imaging technique because up to 25% of nodal metastases are ≤5 mm in size, below the reliable limit for detection [40].

Currently, in developed countries with breast screening programs, patients with breast cancer rarely have an obvious clinically metastatic axillary LN involvement (cN2-cN3) but usually present with normal or discrete asymmetric axillary LN (on palpation or imaging), associated with early stage of breast cancer. Only 20% [41] to 30% suffer from axillary disease and 60–70% of patients have negative LN [42].

In order to differentiate the expression "clinical detection" from the "detection by physical examination," it is important to remember that the TNM classification defines as clinically detected: *detected by imaging studies (excluding lymphoscintigraphy) or by clinical examination and having characteristics highly suspicious for malignancy or a presumed pathologic macrometastasis, based on fine-needle aspiration biopsy with cytological examination.*

10.3.1 Physical Examination

Physical examination is the oldest method to evaluate the nodal status in breast cancer patients but has a low sensitivity of about 30% and is limited by adiposity, small size of early metastatic LN, and metastatic LN in inaccessible (internal mammary, infraclavicular) locations [43, 44].

Positive physical examination: a metastatic nodal involvement can be suspected by physical examination in the axilla and more rarely in the infra- and supraclavicular regions. These situations of advanced breast cancer are rare nowadays.

A positive physical axillary examination is inaccurate in evaluating the nodal status, because only 49% of patients presenting with clinically palpable LN have metastases at FNAC [45]. The large proportion of false positives (50%) in patients with moderately suspicious LN decreases (23%) in patients with highly suspicious LN [46].

Negative physical examination: a negative physical axillary examination is more frequent as the majority of breast cancer patients present with an early-stage cancer and clinically negative LN [41, 42]. Imaging can however demonstrate metastatic LNs in the axillary region or, more importantly in extra-axillary regions, (internal mammary, infraclavicular basins) inaccessible to palpation.

Therefore, with or without suspicious physical examination, imaging techniques are needed for better evaluation of the LN status than physical axillary examination.

10.3.2 Imaging Techniques for the N Staging in Patients with Breast Cancer

Imaging techniques are more sensitive than physical examination for the characterization of a suspicious axillar lymphadenopathy: morphological imaging as mammography, US, MRI, and CT helps analyze size, shape, and contours of the LN, while functional imaging (diffusion and MR spectroscopy, lymphoscintigraphy, and FDG PET/CT) will reflect angiogenesis and tumoral metabolism [47, 48].

10.3.2.1 Mammography

Mammography is the oldest imaging technique for the breast and was for a long time the sole method to evaluate the axillary region. The sensitivity is low (14–39%) for LN staging because only the lower part of the axilla is visible [44, 49].

As shown in Table 10.1, there are many causes of axillary abnormalities other than metastatic nodes from breast cancer. Among axillary abnormalities seen mammographically, the most common are abnormal LNs:

- 80% lymphadenopathy
  - 29% nonspecific benign
  - 26% metastatic breast cancer
  - 17% LLC or well-differentiated lymphocytic lymphoma
  - 29% collagen vascular disease and lymphomas other than well-differentiated lymphocytic lymphoma, metastatic disease from nonbreast primary site, and metastatic disease from unknown primary site, sarcoidosis
- 20% other than lymphadenopathy, epidermal most prevalent (30%)

When a length greater than 33 mm is used as predictor for malignancy, the specificity and sensitivity are 97% and 31%, respectively. There can be association between malignancy and nonfatty LN with ill-defined or spiculated margins, but in most cases, benign and malignant LN cannot be distinguished from each other mammographically [50].

Non-screening Mammography

Enlarged LNs on otherwise normal mammograms are usually benign (Fig. 10.7). The clinical history is essential and can reveal possible causes of nodal enlargement. Among patients with malignant LN, all had a known history of non-breast malignancy in the study from Lee et al. [51].

However, for patients with breast cancer, if suspicious LNs are identified on mammography (Fig. 10.6), they are highly likely (99.5% specificity) to be malignant [52].

The sonographic assessment of suspicious abnormal LN for patients with breast cancer has a 100% sensitivity and 100% NPV, and when an isolated abnormal axillary LN is identified on mammography, only 30% are malignant, but the majority are metastatic lymph nodes from a breast cancer [53].

Screening Mammography

The incidence of axillary "lymphadenopathy" detected on screening mammography (based on two or more of the following criteria: size >2 cm, replacement of fatty hilum, rounded shape, and

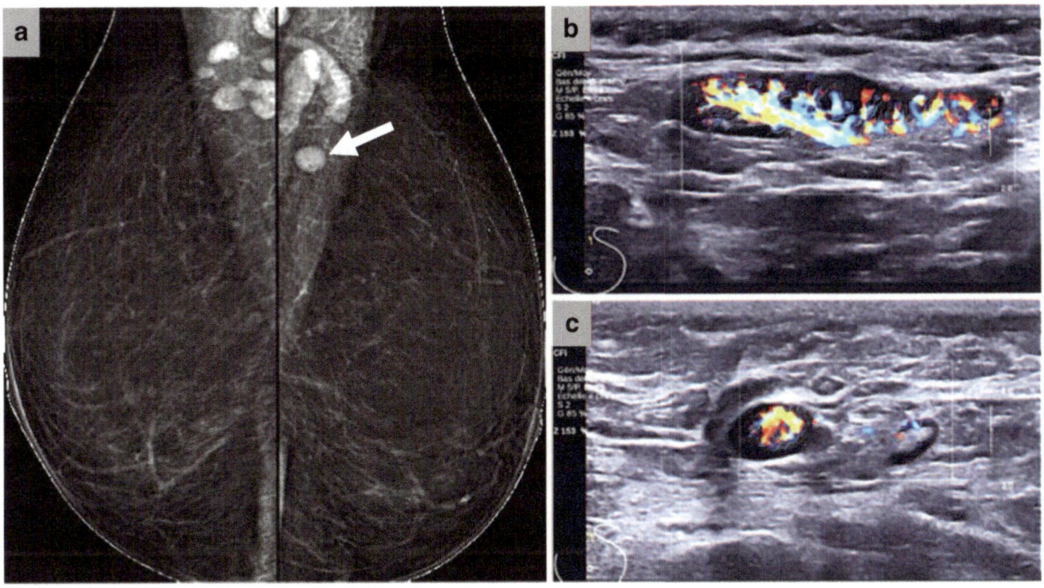

Fig. 10.7 Mammo-sonographic correlation of *normal axillary LN* from the same patient: symetric oblique mammographic view of breasts (**a**): multiple oval axillary LN with a rounded asymetric one (*arrow*) in the lower part of the left axilla (see DD Table 10.1); US sagittal (**b**) and transverse (**c**) view with color-Doppler of the left axilla: 12.8 × 6.6 mm normal LN with a < 3 mm cortex, normal branching vasculature

generalized increased density) is very low, only 0.04%. But if lymphadenopathy is present, the incidence of malignant LN involvement is high (62%), and 50% of such patients had underlying malignancy other than breast cancer [54].

10.3.2.2 CT

CT is superior to physical examination but not usually used for the regional staging of breast cancer. LN size alone is a poor predictor of the presence of metastasis. In the 1990s, considering LN greater than or equal to 1 cm as abnormal, irregular, and spiculated margins with surrounding fatty infiltration, as signs for extracapsular LN extension, the PPV for axillary metastases was of 89% with 50% sensitivity, 75% specificity, and 20% negative predictive value [55].

Measurement of the short axis diameter by itself in a manner similar to that used for CT evaluation of mediastinal or retroperitoneal nodes is not useful. However, a long axis to short axis ratio of less than 2 (rounded node) has 97% specificity for malignancy, and LN with an irregular-appearing or eccentrically thickened cortex should be considered suspicious. Nodes with concentric cortical thickening—defined as >2 mm—and nodes with absent fatty hilum are indeterminate [56].

The performances of CT have improved with technological developments and currently achieve 93% sensitivity, 58% specificity, 72% accuracy, 59% positive predictive value, and 93% negative predictive value for the regional staging of breast cancer [49].

10.3.2.3 PET/CT

FDG PET/CT is mainly used in patients with advanced breast cancer for staging locoregional as well distant metastases and for monitoring response to therapy [57].

Limited observations suggest that FDG PET/CT has advantages over conventional modalities in detecting occult extra-axillary LN, especially internal mammary LN, upstaging the disease and impacting on the adjuvant management. But the performance of the technique currently remains below what is required to replace assessment of axillary LN status by surgical biopsy and histological assessment [40, 58] because of its limitations:

- Sensitivity for LN staging ranges from 20 to 100% and specificity from 65 to 100%.
- Low spatial resolution precludes the detection of small LN metastases [32].
- Only as sensitive as US for detecting axillary LN metastases [59].
- Not sufficient to predict lymphatic spread (false-negative rate of 52%) or micrometastasis because FDG avidity is mainly influenced by the size of the metastasis [60].

The dependence on radioisotopes limits the use of the procedure to only about 60% of eligible patients in developed countries and is negligible elsewhere [61].

10.3.2.4 Sentinel Lymph Node Biopsy (SLNB): Lymphoscintigraphy

Since the introduction of the method into clinical practice in 1994 [62], the sentinel lymph node surgical biopsy procedure is the common standard for axillary LN staging in breast cancer patients with a normal axilla on physical examination and imaging. The technique of SLNB is performed with a radioisotope or blue dye. Lymphoscintigraphy is used to identify the lymphatic drainage basins of the tumor, determine the number of SN, locate the SN in an unexpected location, and mark the SN over the skin for surgical biopsy.

SLNB is equivalent to axillary dissection in the detection of metastasis in regional LNs, with up to 75% less morbidity, in patients with early-stage disease [63] and represents a relevant advance in the treatment of patients with clinically negative axilla, obtaining less than 1% of axillary recurrence in patients with negative SLNB [64–66]. Axillary LN dissection can be safely omitted in clinically node-negative patients with negative sentinel LN, as well as in a selected group of patients with limited (micrometastasis) SN involvement [67] decreasing the incidence of surgical arm and shoulder morbidity [68]. On the contrary, for positive axillary

SLNB patients, a classical complete axillary lymph node surgical dissection (ALND) is still the rule, sometimes in a second surgical procedure when immediate frozen sections are false negative.

The drawbacks of SLNB are:

- False negatives up to 10% in localization of sentinel node
- Expensive technique
- Irradiation
- Time-consuming
- Not available outside developed countries.

Therefore the current challenge is to reduce the rate of SLNB. New developments on US and MRI [69] and cost-effective strategies in the workup of patients with early breast cancer, who are a majority of the cases in the developed countries, will decrease under 50% the proportion of patients undergoing SLNB [70].

10.3.2.5 Magnetic Resonance Imaging (MRI)

MRI has several advantages over other imaging modalities, such as the lack of ionizing radiation (compared to PET/CT) or less intra- and interobserver variation (common in ultrasound examinations). Despite its limitations (claustrophobia, accessibility, cost), MRI is increasingly used for the pre-therapeutic evaluation of breast cancer. MRI has a broad sensitivity range reported as 36–78% and 93–100% specificity for detecting axillary metastasis [49, 71–73] and allows an accurate evaluation of axillary LN, levels I–III, as well as the internal mammary nodes.

There is a large variation in the criteria for distinguishing positive from negative LN: size, short/long axis ratio, LN >4 mm, short axis diameter >5 or >10 mm, shape, irregular margins, lobulated margins, presence of fatty hilum, cortical thickening, cortical thickness >3 mm, asymmetric cortex, unclear margins, perinodular edema, anatomic location of the LN, signal intensity time curves, heterogeneous uptake of USPIO, lack of USPIO uptake, T2* values, high signal intensity on DWI, early-stage enhancement, apparent diffusion coefficient (ADC) values, visual inspection of DWI and ADC, and detectability on DWI [69]. We would point out other interesting criteria reported in recent years:

- When using a signal intensity increase in the LN of >100% during the first post-contrast images as a threshold for malignancy, sensitivity is 83%, specificity 90%, and accuracy 88%; these results are not improved when LN size and morphology are used as additional criteria [72].
- Asymmetry and irregular margin are also significant predictors for present metastasis (90% sensitivity, 90% specificity 90%, PPV 100%), whereas the absence of asymmetry and homogeneous internal structure of LN are highly predictive of absent metastasis (NPV 94.3%) [74].
- Diffusion-weighted (DW) MRI gives better results than ultrasound to predict axillary LN metastases. The mean ADC value of the metastases was significantly lower than that of the benign axillary LN [75].
- A washout ratio of >49% shows the greatest diagnostic accuracy [76].
- The comet tail sign has a specificity of 95% and the loss of fatty hilum a PPV of 100%.
- MRI is superior to other imaging modalities when evaluating the axilla, having highest sensitivity of 85% [77].

The diagnostic performance of some MRI protocols for excluding axillary LN metastases approaches the NPV needed to replace SLNB, with 85% sensitivity and 95% negative predictive value (NPV) [69]. Before to decide if MRI evaluation of axillary LN can replace SLNB, differentiation between minimal and more advanced nodal disease (high nodal disease burden being defined as >3 metastatic nodes in the majority of studies) must be clear.

As other authors, we perform an extended MR mammography (MRM) protocol, including axillae, supraclavicular nodes, and cervical nodes, to combine local staging (T staging)

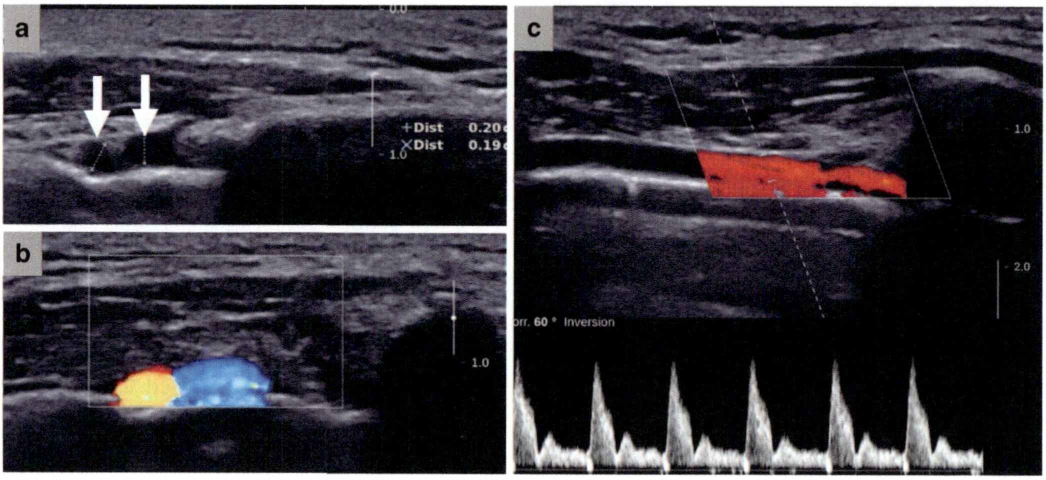

Fig. 10.8 High spatial resolution. Sonographic demonstration of the small right internal thoracic vessels on parasternal position: transverse view of the *1.9 mm in diameter* internal thoracic artery and the (2.0 mm vein (**a**); color-Doppler imaging (**b**); *saggital view* of the internal thoracic artery on color-Doppler imaging with a >80 cm/s systolic peak (**c**)

and locoregional staging (N staging) of breast cancer within one single examination [35].

Key point: after identification of a suspicious LN on MRI, the demonstration of the metastatic involvement is usually confirmed with US-guided FNAC (Fig. 10.8).

10.3.2.6 US

The first role of US is as a triage tool for breast cancer staging. The second role of US is as guidance for percutaneous needle sampling. These issues are dealt with under Section 6 below.

10.4 The Problem of the Internal Mammary Nodes (IMNs)

The internal mammary lymph nodes (IMNs) represent the second regional basin of lymph drainage of the breast. The IMN are located along the internal thoracic artery. The drainage to the IMN occurs in 32% of tumors from the upper inner quadrant, 52% from the lower inner quadrant, 29% from the lower outer quadrant, 10% from the upper outer quadrant, and 24% from the center of the breast. Moreover, non-palpable lesions tended to drain toward the IMN more frequently than palpable tumors [78]. Metastases to the IMN have been described as occurring in 4–65% in patients with clinical N2 or N3 locally advanced breast cancer, increasing in frequency with medial tumor location and greater axillary LN involvement [79–83].

IMN metastasis has similar prognostic importance as axillary nodal involvement and is also considered a major prognostic factor in breast cancer [80, 84, 85] associated with higher rates of distant metastasis and lower overall survival rates [32, 86]. Most IMN metastases have concomitant axillary metastases, but 8–10% of patients with breast cancer may present with IMN metastases only [81].

Although routine IMN evaluation might be indicated, it has not been routinely performed, perhaps because IMN drainage with lymphoscintigraphy is more difficult to demonstrate than axillary drainage. Pleural lesion and internal mammary artery bleeding after surgical biopsy during the SLNB for IMN were found in 7.2 and 5.2% of patients, respectively [87]. According to TNM staging, ipsilateral IMLN metastases are considered as stage N3b, which is accepted as inoperable. The presence of IMLN involvement also affects the area that should undergo irradiation.

Key point: in our experience, normal internal mammary LNs are not visible on US, but sometimes on MRI. Consequently, when doing US evaluation of IMN, we consider as an abnormal LN any mass adjacent to the internal thoracic artery or any bulge to the pleura. We must however keep in mind that internal mammary lymphadenopathy may be associated with diseases other than breast carcinoma (see Table 10.1).

10.4.1 Imaging Methods for Detection of Metastatic IMN

Scatarige et al. published in 1990 [88] the first report illustrating the criteria for diagnosing internal mammary lymphadenopathy on imaging.

10.4.1.1 Lymphoscintigraphy: SLNB

In the axilla, SLNB lymphoscintigraphy is still the current procedure to identify the (normal or metastatic) SN in the internal mammary chain. However, a surgical sampling of the internal mammary SN is not routinely performed [89, 90] because the current contribution from IMN treatment is unclear [30]. Approximately only 20% of internal mammary SN are metastatic. This can change staging (13%) of patients with non-axillary sentinel LN and their treatment strategy 17% [31, 91]. QIU et al. [87] reported a change in LN staging in 8.1% of patients, and systemic treatment changed in only 0.7%. Internal mammary chain radiotherapy was guided by this result.

10.4.1.2 CT FDG PET/CT

FDG PET/CT is most helpful in staging recurrent or metastatic breast cancer and in evaluating the response to treatment of locally advanced and metastatic breast cancer.

In patients with advanced breast cancer (N3), Zhang et al. [92] reported an overall incidence of IMN involvement of 14%, detected on ultrasound (most used technique), thoracic CT, breast MRI, and/or positron emission tomography/CT. The median size of the enlarged IMN was 1.3 cm (range 0.5–3.0 cm). This study revealed two complementary points of interest:

1. Intercostal spaces involved:
   (a) First: 55%
   (b) Second: 58%
   (c) Third: 22%
   (d) Fourth: 1%
2. Associated involved basins:
   (a) IMN nodal involvement only (N2b) in 9%
   (b) IMN and axillary or infraclavicular nodal disease (N3b) in 59%
   (c) Supraclavicular and IMN involvement, with or without axillary or infraclavicular nodal involvement (N3c) in 32%

Surgical biopsy of the IMN was not routine as most patients (81%) had simultaneous confirmed metastases in the axillary or the supraclavicular LNs that were sampled by US-guided fine-needle aspiration. Although less than 10% of breast cancer patients have positive IMN on PET/CT performed for initial staging or restaging, a positive IMN indicates a very high likelihood of malignant involvement (80%) on US-guided FNAC [93].

10.4.1.3 MRI

Malignant and benign IMN may be seen on breast MRI. Few studies have been published on the utility of MRI for detection of abnormal IMN despite the numerous MRI breast examinations done for breast cancer patients.

Kinoshita et al. [94] reported a 91% accuracy, 93% sensitivity, and 89% specificity, considering a size of more than 5 mm as a positive finding (ranged from 7 to 22 mm) on MRI. In a more recent study, before neoadjuvant chemotherapy for patients with clinical stage IIA to IIIA disease, the prevalence of IMN adenopathy was 16% on MRI and 14% on PET/CT [86]. In 7 of these 14 patients (50%), more than one IMN was detected. In patients with operable breast cancer, Cheon et al. [95] reported to increase to have IMN adenopathy at initial staging with PET/CT and MRI. Inner tumor location and especially a positive axillary LN status were associated with IMN adenopathy.

10.4.1.4 Ultrasound

US evaluation of internal mammary nodes in patients with breast cancer is quick to perform and should be done for any patient. The high spatial resolution of US allows good visualization of the internal thoracic artery and vein, with a diameter of about 2 mm (Fig. 10.8). Fortuitously, IMNs are situated in front of the intercostal spaces, which give perfect acoustic windows to look for lymphadenopathy. An obvious abnormal internal mammary node greater than 5–10 mm is usually seen at first glance as a rounded hypoechoic nodule nearby the internal thoracic vessels (Figs. 10.9 and 10.10a). The location of metastatic IMN is mainly in the first and second intercostal spaces. If multiple IMNs are visible, one should think of an underlying systemic disease (Fig. 10.10d) and look for lymphadenopathy in other regions (see Table 10.1).

10.4.2 And What to Do with IMN?

Among 10% of patients with positive internal mammary (IM) US findings, only 1.3% had isolated IM involvement according to Dogan et al. [96], and ultrasound resulted in N status change for 8% of patients as well as the clinical stage for 6.4% patients.

The finding of a tumor-positive SN in the internal mammary chain would indicate the need for radiation therapy to these nodes. However, IMN irradiation can cause increased cardiac morbidity and is not recommended unless pathologically proven IMNs have been produced in early breast cancer [91, 97].

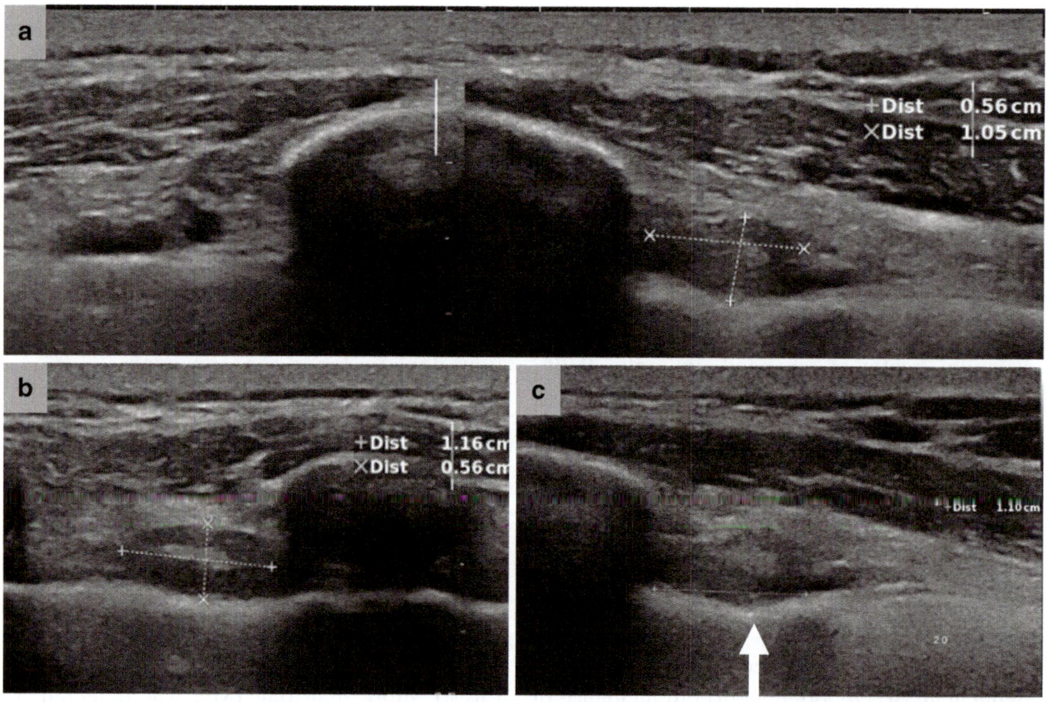

Fig. 10.9 Internal mammary lymphadenopathy secondary to chronic capsulitis of the left breast prothesis; (**a**) transverse symetric view of internal mammary chains on both side of the sternum, with asymetry: normal artery and veins on the *right* and a 5.6 × 10.5 mm internal mammary lymphadenopathy on the *left* (**c**), blurring the mammary vessels, displacing the pleural line (*arrow*), (**b**) sagittal view demonstrating better the central fatty hilum and the regular thickness of the <3 mm cortex

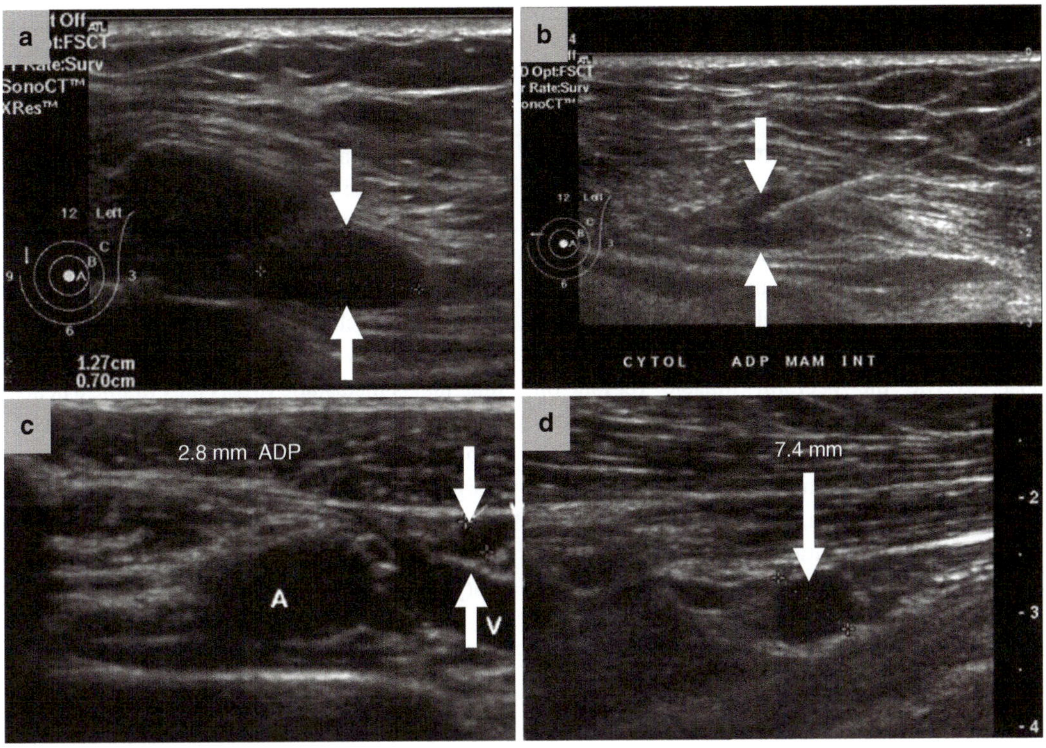

Fig. 10.10 Abnormal *extra-axillary LN* well demonstrated in year 2004. (**a**) 12.7 × 7 mm *internal mammary* node, below the cartilage of a rib. US-guided FNAC (**b**): *metastasis* (N3c); (**c**) Another patient with a round *2.8 mm infraclavicular metastasic LN* on FNAC (N3a); (**d**) Another patient with *a 7.4 mm pseudo metastatic infraclavicular node*. US-guided FNAC: lymphoid reactive cells (chronic inflammatory disease: *lupus*)

Currently, the question of the consequences of the presence of macrometastasis in internal mammary chains is under debate.

10.5 The Lymph Nodes in the Breast

It is important to know that LNs surrounding the breast are not only located in the axillary region but also in the breast region; most often a low axillary LN (level I) is seen at the periphery of the outer upper quadrant. Less frequently, some LNs are situated outside of "the normal axillary area":

- An *intramammary lymph node* (*IMLN*), surrounded by breast tissue, may be present in every breast quadrant.
- An *axillary ectopic inferior node* can be found below the equatorial plane of the breast, at the periphery of the fibroglandular tissue.
- An *axillary ectopic posteroinferior node* can be found in low and posterior location, under the latissimus dorsi muscle.
- A *node of the inframmamary fold.*

The latter location is underestimated but was reported by Gui et al. [98] who analyzed 50 inframammary fold specimens from 42 patients who underwent mastectomy: three specimens (6%) containing fibro-fatty tissue without breast parenchyma had IMN within the inframammary fold and one patient (2%) who had a mastectomy for invasive ductal carcinoma had inframmamary fold tissue containing a lymph node with breast cancer metastasis. A normal

LN of the inframmamary fold is rarely reported but can be visible on MRI (Personal data).

10.5.1 The Intramammary Lymph Nodes (IMLNs)

By definition, intramammary lymph nodes should be completely surrounded by breast parenchyma, a criteria which helps in distinguishing them from inferior axillary LN which also overlie the pectoral muscle region on mammography. Intramammary lymph nodes are involved in a variety of clinical situations including benign situations, tumor metastasis, breast lymphoma, and breast cancer [99]. Benign breast conditions are responsible for 51% of IMLN and 49% are found in association with primary breast carcinoma [100]. Metastatic disease to IMLN may be the first clinical and/or radiological sign of breast cancer. The presence of IMLN metastases is an independent predictor of poor outcome in patients with breast carcinoma [101].

The incidence of IMLN ranges between 0.7% (on imaging) and 48% (on mastectomy specimen) [102]. Their role in lymphatic drainage of breast regions is important although it is not known if they represent true SN or if lymphatic drainage to them comes from independently developed pathways.

In patients with breast cancer, the involvement of the IMLN is rare (0.1%) and the nodes are usually larger than 1 cm in size [103].

Shen et al. [104] analyzed 196 IMLN specimens collected for 20 years and demonstrated that 18% of patients had IMLN that were identified preoperatively by either mammographic or US methods. In 82% of other cases, IMLN were detected only on pathologic examination of surgical breast specimens. Metastases in IMLN were found in 28% of all cases ($n = 36$). Most patients who had IMLN metastases (81%) also had axillary metastases, and isolated IMLN metastases were documented in six (5%) patients.

On mammograms, normal IMLNs are circumscribed oval or reniform masses with a central or peripheral lucency that represents fat within the hilum, and the majority (72%) are situated within the upper-outer quadrant [105]. Intramammary nodes represent 0.5% of palpable or mammographically detected masses [106] and have been reported in approximately 5% of patients undergoing mammography [107].

On US, the typical normal IMLN appears as a solid hypoechoic reniform mass with a fatty hilum typically showing flow on color Doppler imaging. A metastatic IMLN may mimic a benign mass: absence of fatty hilum and completely hypoechoic, round-shaped, and well-delineated margins. If a synchronous benign-appearing nodule is present in a breast with cancer this should raise the possibility of a metastatic intramammary lymph node, especially if the nodule is close to an artery and in the upper outer quadrant [102, 105, 108, 109].

On preoperative SLNB lymphoscintigraphy, Nogareda et al. [110] reported the presence of IMLN in 2.2% (38/1725) of patients. No lymphatic tissue was found at pathology for 3/38 (8%), and one was not found during surgery; of the remaining 34, 10 (26%) were metastatic and 24 (63%) were metastasis-free.

The literature is scarce on MRI studies dealing with IMLN: two case reports [111, 112] and a study on 93 cases of breast cancer of Vijan et al. [113] confirming that 75% of them are found incidentally (intraoperatively by the surgeon or on pathologic review) and 25% preoperatively (evident on mammography, US, MRI, or lymphogram) and are histologically negative.

If a breast cancer metastasis is identified in an IMLN, additional axillary LN disease is common, regardless of the method of detection of the IMLN [113].

Mastectomy specimens showed IMLN in 48% of patients; 10% of these patients were upstaged (lymph node stage), and 1/76 patient received additional systemic treatment, as a result of the upstaging [102].

A rare condition in the breast region such as herpes zoster infection may also be a cause of painful intramammary lymphadenopathy [114].

If appearing before the cutaneous eruption as a prodromal lymphadenopathy, this may clinically simulate an inflammatory lesion of the upper outer quadrant of the breast; ultrasound with color Doppler analysis depicts a simple benign reactive lymphadenopathy (personal data).

10.5.2 IMLN Totally Replaced: A Cause of Multicentricity/Multifocality?

The knowledge of the existence of IMLN is of some importance in the following clinical situation: when a woman with a breast tumor presents with a second well-circumscribed malignant lesion in the same breast, this should raise the differential diagnosis of a true second breast cancer or of a totally replaced metastatic IMLN. This possibility seems rarely mentioned in radiological reports and in the literature but can occur in 8% of breast cancer [110]. On imaging, some features in favor of that hypothesis are:

- A second well-circumscribed tumoral lesion
- Localization in the upper outer quadrant
- Along the lateral thoracic artery (external mammary artery)
- Complete disappearance after the first round of chemotherapy, an indirect evidence, as for the internal metastatic mammary nodes [86].

In that case, the workup should be as for one single breast tumor with N+ staging, in order to avoid unnecessary upstaging to multicentricity/multifocality that would lead to a more aggressive treatment, as mastectomy, which is no longer the only option since breast conservation therapy has become a safe option for selected patients with multifocal tumors [115, 116]. Avoiding the axillary lymphadenectomy (ALND) when a metastatic IMLN is present without axillary involvement seems reasonable [110].

10.6 US and US-Guided FNAC for the Diagnosis of Lymph Node Metastasis

Modern imaging with CT, MR, and PET/CT for N staging of breast cancer patients can demonstrate obvious/suspicious metastatic LN involvement. But currently no imaging technique per se is sufficiently accurate to allow choosing the most adequate therapeutic option because of:

- Low specificity due to other causes of axillary lymphadenopathy (see Table 10.1)
- Inaccurate sensitivity to detect early metastatic axillary and extra-axillary LN
- Low rate (20%) of positive SLNB for IMN
- For micrometastasis in the SN, 0% sensitivity.

Accordingly, whatever the result of the test and the location of the target, the unavoidable best practice step is to sample cells from suspicious LN for cytological/histological analysis.

This is no doubt optimally performed with preoperative US and US-guided fine-needle aspiration cytology (FNAC) of suspicious *axillary and extra-axillary* LN in terms of precision, speed, simplicity, and cost-effectiveness.

The criticism that US cannot detect metastasis less than 5 mm is unfounded because other morphologic and functional imaging modalities are not any better. Furthermore, metastasis less than 3 mm in size can be identified and sampled with US (Figs. 10.2 and 10.4).

10.6.1 Ultrasound as a Triage Tool

The first role of US is as a triage tool for breast cancer staging. US was already used in the 1980s for further characterization of isolated abnormal axillary lymph nodes identified on mammography or palpable lymphadenopathy [44, 117]. The cut-off was very simple: normal nodes were not visible [118]. Thereafter many authors have underlined the role of ultrasound as the standard noninvasive imaging modality for the evaluation of axillary lymph nodes and

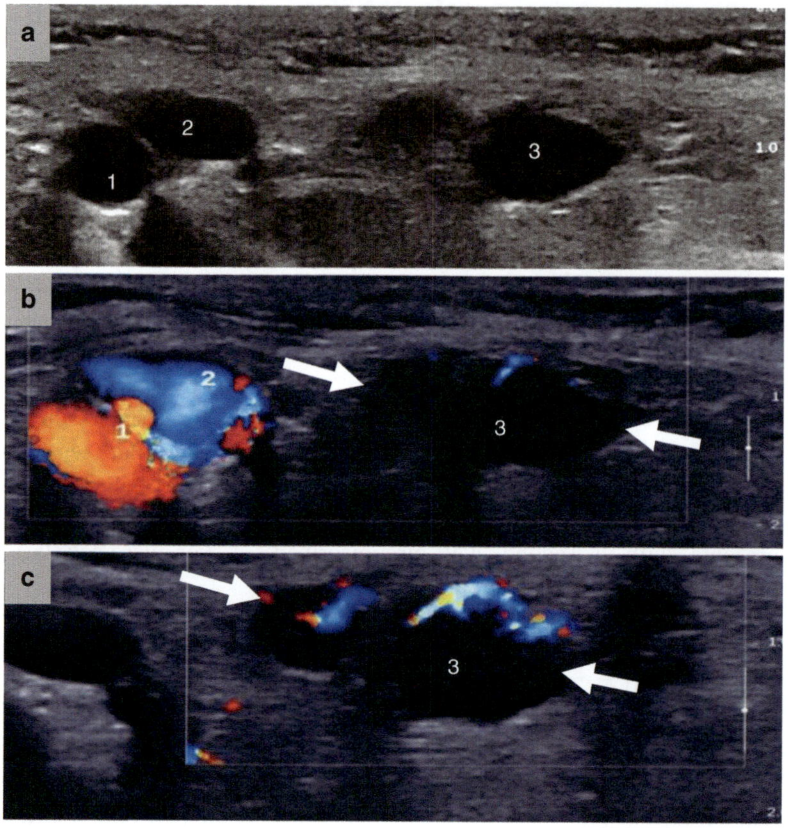

Fig. 10.11 False positive axillary LN. US of the left axilla in a 59 year old woman during her yearly dense breast screening with US: B mode (**a**), color-Doppler (**b**, **c**) of the same region showing three well circumscribed structures: 1 = axillary artery; 2 = axillary vein; 3 = *lymphadenopathy*:(i) asymetric (not shown) (ii) 13 × 7 mm (iii) lobulated (iv) no fatty hilum (v) abnormal vasculature. US-guided FNAC: *reactive lymphadenopathy*. Clinical history: surgery for skin melanoma of the shoulder with axillary dissection 20 years ago

described the criteria and the scanning technique [47, 48, 119]. US and US-guided FNAC can detect all cases of axillary involvement with three or more lymph nodes, and 93% of those with metastatic deposit measuring more than 5 mm are detected [120].

Key point: triage US can demonstrate suspicious metastatic axillary lymphadenopathy at first glance when there is more than the two normal nodular hypoechoic anatomic structures—the axillary artery and vein—on the sagittal view of the axilla (Fig. 10.11). But one shall not forget the rare false positives (Table 10.1, Figs. 10.11 and 10.17).

10.6.2 Ultrasound Guidance for Percutaneous Needle Sampling

The second role of US is as guidance tool for percutaneous needle sampling. US-guided sampling has well-known advantages and can be performed during the same session as diagnostic US. Like numerous authors, we used, over 20 years of experience, US combined with FNAC as the most suitable method for preoperative evaluation of axillary LN in women with breast cancer because it can both evaluate more nodal basins (e.g., the supraclavicular fossa) than MRI and guide needle sampling with fine-needle aspiration to confirm the status of any indeterminate node (including internal mammary nodes) within minutes [43, 48, 121–127].

10.6.3 Sonographic Criteria for Malignant Lymph Nodes

Various criteria have been proposed to differentiate metastatic LN from benign [47, 128, 129]. The morphological characteristics are the most useful: the absence of a hilum and cortical thickness (<4 mm) are most strongly associated with malignancy [130] (Fig. 10.12).

When a cut-off point of a cortical thickness of 2.5 mm was used, sonographic classification showed 85% (35/41) sensitivity and 78% (117/150) specificity [131].

In the daily practice, one should consider three categories based on US appearance [129]:

1. *Mass-like appearance*
2. *Focal nodular cortical thickening* (fatty hilum preservation and thickening > than 2 mm)
3. *Diffuse cortical thickening* (fatty hilum preservation and thickening >2 mm).

Mass-like appearance is observed in 45% of metastatic lymph nodes (Figs. 10.3 and 10.12) followed by diffuse cortical thickening in 35% (Fig. 10.13a) and focal nodular cortical thickening in 20%.

The focal cortical bulge or thickening is considered to be the earliest detectable morphologic change in the presence of metastasis, but this criterion is difficult to apply and has a low positive predictive value because it is nonspecific. This finding is therefore considered indeterminate. A true abnormal cortical bulge is seen as focal thickening of the cortex that does not follow the margin of the echogenic hilum and should be distinctly hypoechoic (Fig. 10.2). This sign is more accurate if associated with another finding such as the presence of cortical, in addition to hilar, blood flow on color Doppler [47].

Key point: in our experience, as for every superficial LN, when a round node is visible (>2 mm), it should be considered abnormal and FNAC will return positive for a metastasis. Such round nodes are most often located in axillary level III, infra- and supraclavicular regions (Figs. 10.10c and 10.13c).

Bedi et al. [128] classified the benign and malignant LN into six types:

- Type 1, without visible cortex (Fig. 10.14)
- Type 2, cortex ≤3 mm (Fig. 10.15)
- Type 3, cortex >3 mm (Fig. 10.16a, b)
- Type 4, generalized cortical lobulation (Fig. 10.16c)
- Type 5, with focal hypoechoic cortical lobulation (Fig. 10.2 and 10.13b)
- Type 6, hypoechoic node with absent hilum (Figs. 10.3, 10.5, 10.6, 10.10, 10.11, 10.17c, d)

Types 1–3 are considered benign. Types 5 and 6 are considered metastatic with indication for FNAC. Reactional changes are frequently observed in type 3. Type 4 is considered as probably benign, since this type comprised some false-negative results (9%). False positives are not rare, even for type 6, and pseudotumoral lymphadenopathy can be related to lupus (Fig.10.10d), silicone (Fig. 10.17), and previous surgery (Figs. 10.11 and 10.18); see Table 10.1.

- Morphological criteria of a metastatic node:
  - focal asymetric thickening +++
  - compression of hilum by a cortical nodule
  - partial/total hypoechoïc transformation
  - rounded form = long/short axis > 1.5-2
  - > 10 mm thickness
  - mass like with no hilum visible
- Color-Doppler: disorganized vasculature

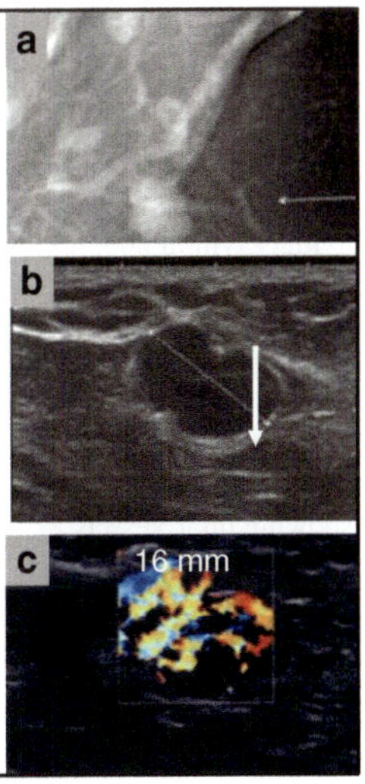

Fig. 10.12 US *criteria of metastatic lymph nodes*. Mammographic (**a**) and sonographic correlation (**b**) of a typical left axillary metastatic *mass-like* lymph node, 16 mm in long diameter, with disorganized vasculature (**c**)

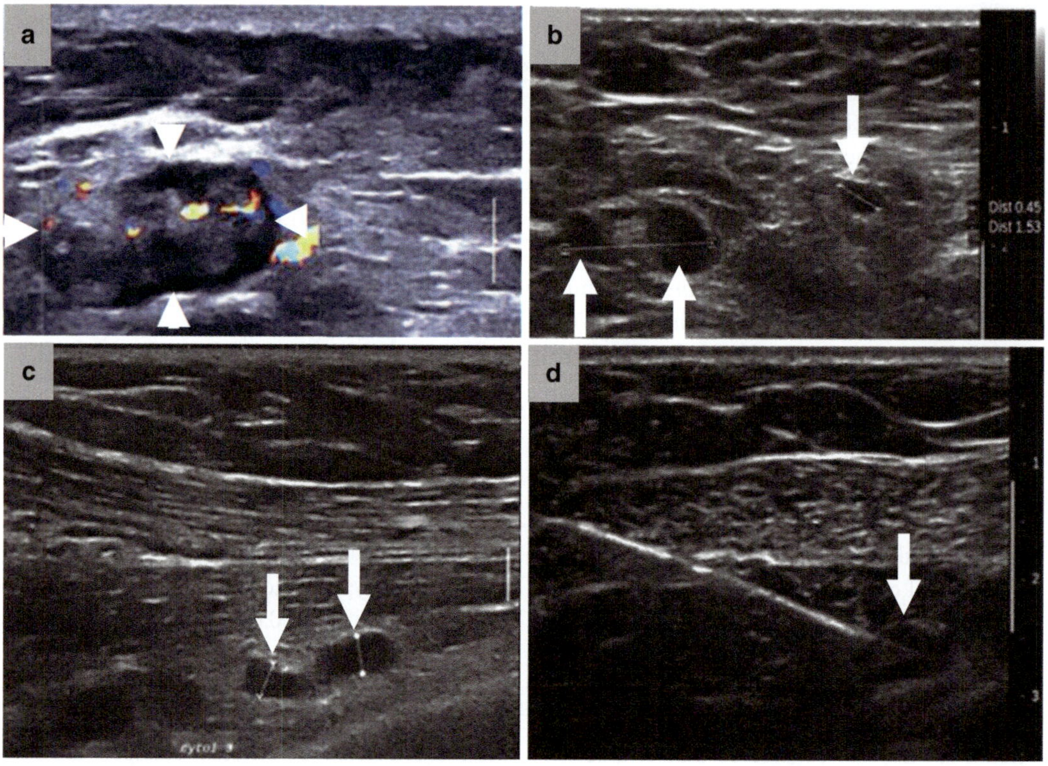

Fig. 10.13 71-year-old woman with a right breast cancer. US changes the N-staging. *Multiple suspicious LN*: 12 mm oval *axillary* LN with heterogenous hilum, irregular cortex, abnormal vasculature (**a**); a round hypoechoïc 4.5 mm *axillary* LN; another 15.3 × 7 mm LN, with polar nodules (**b**); two round hypoechoïc 3.4–3.6 mm *infra-clavicular nodes* (**c**); FNAC of a 4 mm *infra-clavicular LN* more distally located: *metastasis* = *N3a* (**d**)

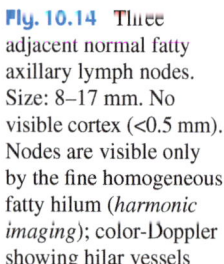

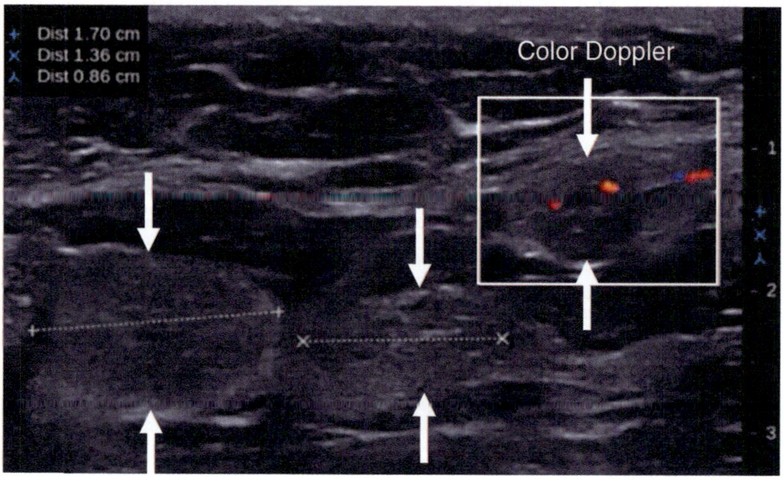

Fig. 10.14 Three adjacent normal fatty axillary lymph nodes. Size: 8–17 mm. No visible cortex (<0.5 mm). Nodes are visible only by the fine homogeneous fatty hilum (*harmonic imaging*); color-Doppler showing hilar vessels

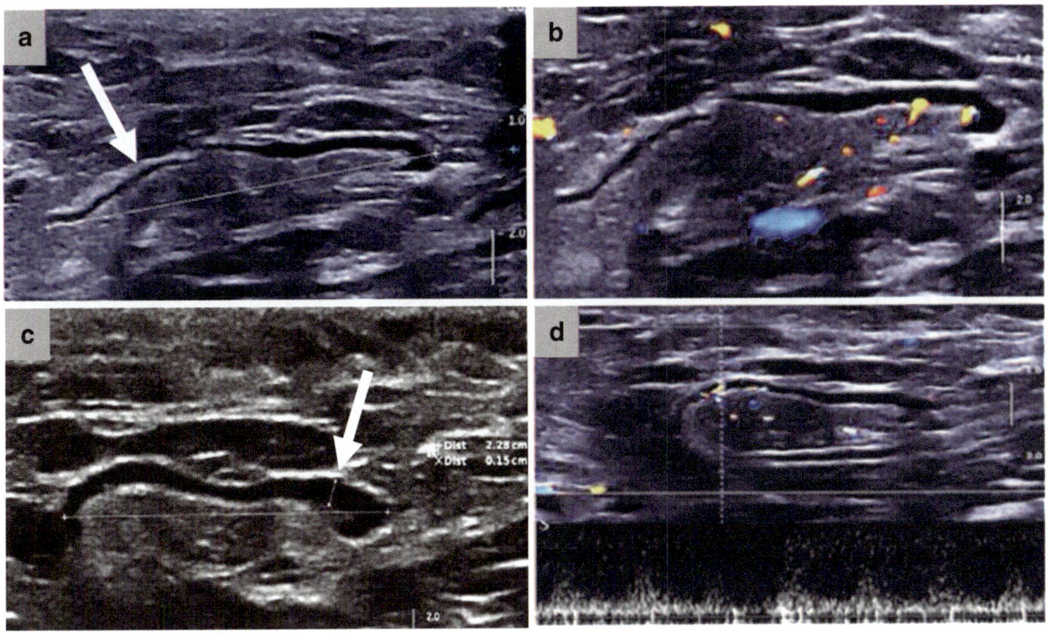

Fig. 10.15 High resolution (*harmonic imaging*) US of two normal axillary LN: 40 mm and 23 mm in long axis diameter; less than 1.5 mm thickness of the cortex (**a**, **c**); Color-Doppler (**b**, **d**): small arteries within the fatty hilum and at the basis of the cortex

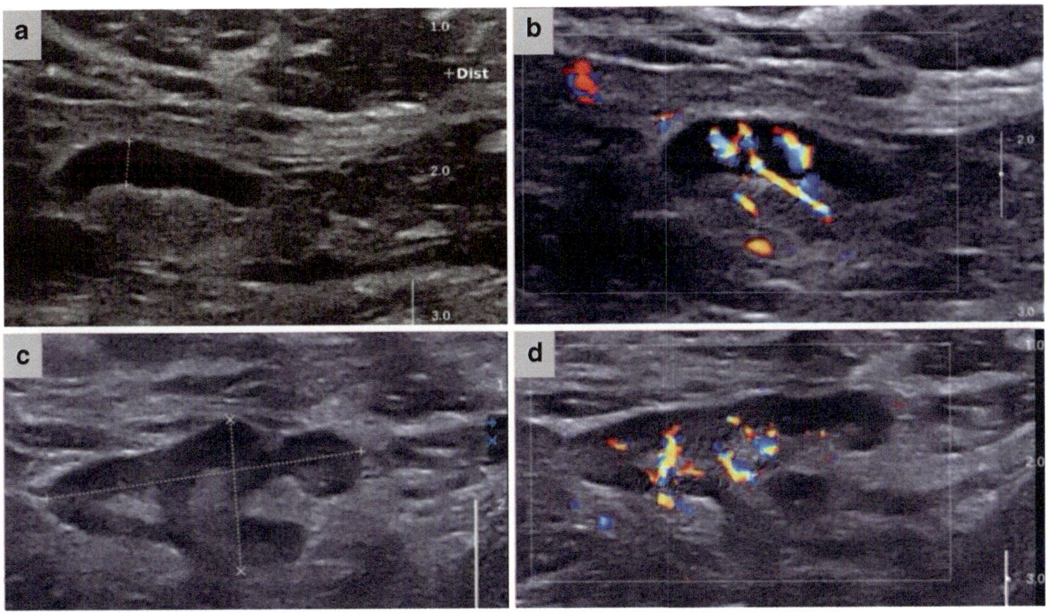

Fig. 10.16 Axillary *inflammatory lymphadenopathies* (two different patients): (**a**, **c**) 3 mm diffuse thickened cortex secondary to a breast abcess; (**b**, **d**) lobulated thickened cortex secondary to a breast mastitis; normal vasculature on Colo-Doppler

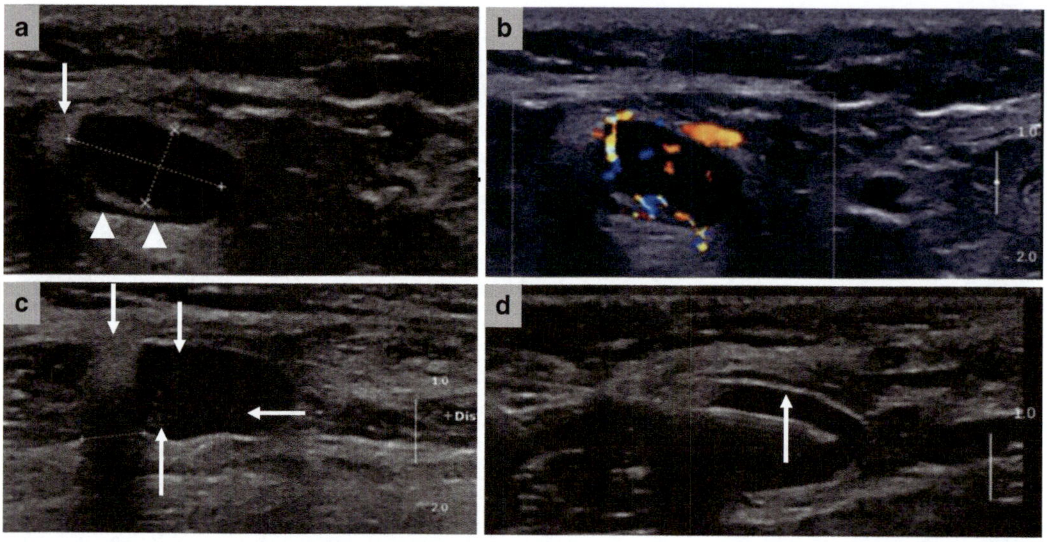

Fig. 10.17 *False positive* "metastatic "axillary lymph node. Clinical history: extracapsular breast *implant rupture* 10 years ago. A 11.6 × 5.8 mm LN on B-mode US (**a**, **c**), with silicone deposits mainly at the periphery of the node (*arrows*). The deep cortex is normal, non reactive (*arrowheads*); on color-Doppler vascularization is desorganized (**b**). US-guided FNAC (**d**): *reactive lymphadenopathy*

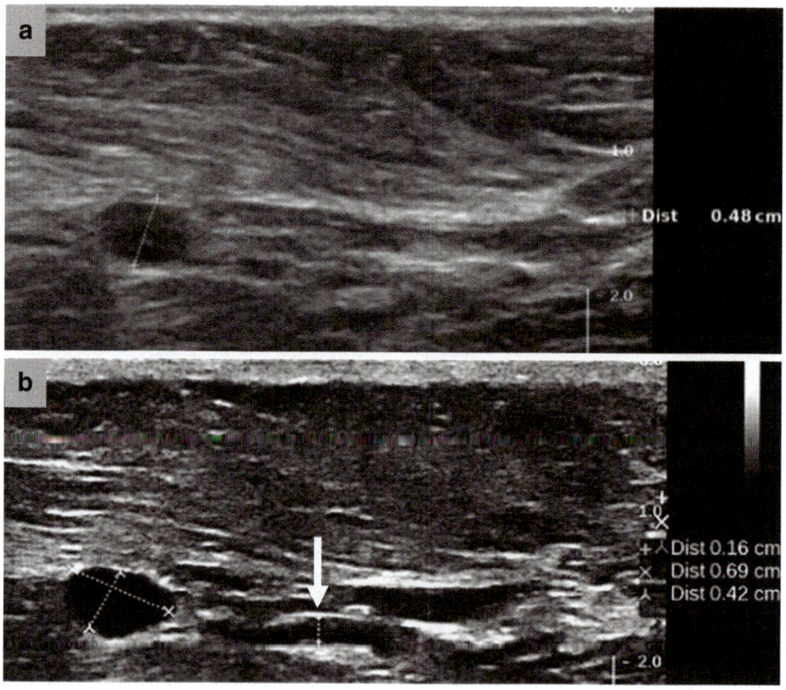

Fig. 10.18 Comparison of image quality (spatial and contrast resolution) between usual B-mode US (**a**) and *Harmonic imaging* (**b**) of the same nodule. Patient coming for her annual US follow-up 8 years after lumpectomy in the right breast: round shape 7 × 4.2 mm hypoechoic nodule in the lower axilla (without vessels inside on color Doppler, not shown): *metastatic node with necrosis*? US-guided FNAC result: normal lymphoid cells. No change at 6-months follow-up. Normal adjacent node, with 1.6 mm thickness cortex (*arrow*)

Ultrasound is also a multiparameter imaging technique with option to use simultaneously B-mode, color Doppler, or elastography to demonstrate the vascularization and stiffness of LN for better characterization.

10.7 Factors Affecting the Accuracy of Ultrasound and US-Guided FNAC

To demonstrate small early metastatic LN, basic prerequisite requirements are dependent on

- Sonographer: expertise in US imaging of small parts and slow displacement of the probe on the region of interest using image magnification
- Ultrasound device: >12 MHz linear-array transducer, tissue harmonic imaging, and color Doppler
- Patient: obese or not, heavy or low axillary tumor burden.

10.7.1 Harmonic Imaging

Harmonic and real-time compounding imaging improves image resolution and lesion characterization by reducing reverberation and near-field artifacts [132–134]. These features make it easier to identify the normal LN: the cortex, even with a thickness of <1 mm, is visible and more hypoechogenic compared to the surrounding fatty tissue and fatty hilum (Fig. 10.15). More importantly, this facilitates the identification of the earliest metastatic changes in a LN: the focal thickening (Figs. 10.2, 10.3, 10.4, 10.6).

10.7.2 Color Doppler

The use of color Doppler imaging allows

- Improved characterization of a normal LN by demonstrating vessels in the fatty hilum of a normal LN with unapparent cortex (Fig. 10.14)
- Better demonstration of abnormal vascularization criteria in metastatic LN (Fig. 10.12c, 10.13a, 10.17b)
- Better demonstration of normal vasculature in reactive lymphadenopathy (Fig. 10.16)
- Confirmation of "avascularity" of a benign lesion which can simulate an abnormal LN such as complex cyst/lymphocele or fat necrosis.

Contrast-enhanced color Doppler can be used for preoperative localization and evaluation of sentinel nodes [135].

10.7.3 Elastography

Imaging tissue elastography can provide important additional information on tissues and lesions as for breast cancers [136]. In the diagnosis of breast cancer, a sensitivity of 82% has been reported for elastography, versus 94% for conventional gray-scale US [137–139].

We have for 10 years used the Aixplorer ultrasound system developed by SuperSonic Imagine (France) that offers revolutionary technology with ShearWave elastography in breast imaging. In our experience, this complementary tool is of relative additional value to the B-mode and color Doppler analysis in characterization of LN, in concordance with reports by other authors [124]. For small (<5 mm) focally or completely invaded LN, there is no significant stiffness difference between theses nodes (or LN) and the surroundings. For larger (>8 mm) metastasis, moderate stiffness can be mainly observed at the periphery of growing metastasis, probably due to a compression effect on surroundings (Fig. 10.5).

10.7.4 The Impact of Obesity

Obesity does impact accuracy of preoperative AUS. Searching for small metastatic LN in obese patients may be more difficult than in a thin one, but Dighe et al. [123] recently reported that the performance of US was significantly improved in these, with a 2.5-fold increase in sensitivity and 100% specificity compared to those with a BMI < 30 kg/m2 assumedly because abnormal hypoechoic LN with thickened cortex are readily differentiated from the hyperechoic surrounding fat [140].

However, in our experience, US-guided FNAC for sampling small (5 mm) LN at depths of more than 3 cm can be less precise and give false-negative results. For suspicious LN greater than 10 mm, obesity is not a limiting factor to reach the target.

10.7.5 The Impact of Heavy or Low Axillary Tumor Burden

The accuracy of preoperative US in early-stage breast cancer patients depends mainly on the size and number of axillary LN metastases, primary tumor size [141], and tumor grade [119]. Gross (significant/macroscopic) extracapsular extension (ECE) [142] or >3 positive SLNs is considered as a *heavy tumor burden* while pT1–2, cN0 with <3 positive SLNs as a *low tumor burden* [143, 144]. The presence of four or more involved axillary LNs is associated with lymphovascular space invasion (LVSI), increased number of involved SN, increased size of SN metastasis, and *lobular* histology [145, 146].

With screening, patients have currently a low axillary tumor burden. In their cohort study, Stachs et al. [40] reported a low axillary tumor burden with 45.2% of pN + (sn) patients having a maximum size of lymph node metastases ≤ 5 mm and 43.3% having only one metastatic LN after completion of ALND. Only 11.6% of patients had three or more positive LNs.

In patient with heavy axillary tumor burden, preoperative US-guided FNAC from radiologically suspicious LN is highly efficient in detecting metastases and is easy to perform [147]. Tahir et al. [148] reported sensitivity to be 47.1%, specificity 100%, PPV 100%, NPV 70%, and overall accuracy 76.3%. When two or more LNs were involved, the sensitivity raised to 80% and negative predictability to 93.3%. Kramer et al. [149] confirmed 90% accuracy of US-FNAC to detect three or more positive LNs. But most importantly, preoperative axillary US excluded 96% of N2 and N3 invasive ductal metastases [150].

In patients with low axillary tumor burden, having clinically negative LN, the sensitivity of US-guided FNAC was about 50% a few years ago [151]. With a low nodal macrometastatic burden, the performance of US-guided FNA decreases with a substantial number of false negatives [40, 123, 152]. Rocha et al. [153] reported the sensitivity was 69.6%, 83.7%, and 100% in the assessment of invasive breast tumors in stages T1, T2, and T3. Micrometastases are not frequently detected with US-FNAC: according to the study of Britton et al. [130], core biopsy had 26.7% sensitivity, whereas FNAC could not identify micrometastatic deposits.

10.7.6 Size of the Sentinel Node Metastasis

About 25% of nodal metastases are ≤5 mm in size and are therefore below the reliable limit for detection by imaging techniques [40]. Some studies however report nodal metastatic infiltration less than 5 mm in size that can be detected with US [124, 129] (Figs. 10.3, 10.4, 10.5). With the high resolution of current US devices, we can expect now to see early detectable morphologic change as a focal cortical bulge or thickening, which is considered the earliest detectable morphologic change in the presence of metastasis [47] (Fig. 10.2b).

Metastatic involvement is more specific when presenting as mass-like nodes. As stated earlier, in our experience, every round lymph node is malignant, whatever the size (Figs. 10.3, 10.5, 10.10c, 10.13b, c), until proven otherwise with FNAC to exclude the rare false positives (Figs. 10.11, 10.17, 10.18).

As AUS accurately excludes—sensitivity of 76% and NPV of 89%—clinically significant (>2.0mm) axillary LN disease in patients with clinical T1–T2, N0 breast cancer, AUS may be an alternative to SLNB for these patients, where axillary surgery is no longer considered therapeutic [154].

10.7.7 Invasive Lobular Cancer (ILC)

Invasive lobular cancers (10% of breast cancers) may have uncommon metastatic spread, different from invasive ductal cancers (IDC). Invasive lobular cancers and invasive ductal cancers are biologically distinct entities with different LN involvement patterns, ILC having a tendency to metastasize to more nodes than IDC with a diffuse metastatic morphological pattern compared to the sinusoidal pattern of IDC. This difference was not associated with a significant impact on patient outcome in the study of Fernández et al. [155]. Brouckaert et al. [156] did however report different results: in LN-negative patients, ILC carries a better prognosis regarding distant metastasis-free interval, with a trend toward improved breast cancer-specific survival. In LN-positive patients, both are significantly worse for ILC, especially after longer follow-up (>4–5 years).

The false-negative rate for N2 and N3 invasive lobular cancer is significantly higher (17%) than that for invasive ductal cancer (4.1%), which suggests that axillary US cannot be used to exclude N2 and N3 metastases in these patients [150]. Cases of invasive lobular carcinoma are more common in the false-negative smears [157]. In our experience, invasive lobular cancers have more false-negative LNs on US-FNAC. Dellaportas reported one case of a metastasis from an invasive lobular cancer on 3/50 false-negative US-FNAC, with the other two being micrometastasis [135]. This type of cancer usually has a low cellular component of non-cohesive cells in the tumor; it may also be similar in the metastatic LN.

10.8 Percutaneous US-Guided Sampling of Suspicious Lymph Node

US-guided FNAC is the best technique to sample cells from superficial tissues and LNs. Percutaneous needle sampling of palpable suspicious LN is more accurate under US guidance for its intrinsic advantages and because positive physical examination has low accuracy of 70% and low PPV of 80% in confirming metastatic involvement [43]. Core biopsy can be used if the node is greater than 5–10 mm and readily accessible. FNA is a good alternative when a smaller needle is desired due to the small size and the location of the LN as for other patient-related factors (e.g., anticoagulation) [158].

10.8.1 Fine-Needle Aspiration Cytology (FNAC) Is More Frequently Used than Core Biopsy

Literature repeatedly reports that core biopsy has gained increased popularity in the presurgical diagnosis of axillary metastatic involvement compared to fine-needle aspiration. But the reality is the opposite: only 5% of US-guided percutaneous samplings are performed with a core biopsy needle and 95% with a fine needle (21–32 G) [159]. In a review on 31 studies, Diepstraten et al. [160] reported 21 teams using FNA for all, 3 using FNA more than 90% of the time, only 5 using core biopsy alone, and 2 both techniques.

FNA has gained popularity due to its fast and easy approach, inexpensiveness, and lesser frequency of complications [161]. The rate of inadequate aspiration is influenced by the nature of the lesion, the available technology, and both experience and personal choices from the operator. The nature of the lesion is the most common cause (68%) of inadequacy of FNAC, followed (32%) by the operator experience [162]. In our own experience, the high cellularity of a metastatic node always results in a representative aspiration material, as long as the tip of the needle has positively reached the target. False negatives are rare: some early metastatic nodes from lobular cancers, sampling in the necrotic area of a large metastatic LN or in metastatic LN, healed after neoadjuvant chemotherapy.

Core biopsy has some drawbacks and is less precise for suspicious LN smaller than 10 mm. Core biopsy will usually require more than one sample. That may generate air or bleeding after the first pass, obscuring the small target for next sample. Some anatomic limitations while sampling with core biopsy are the vicinity of the suspicious node with the subclavian and axillary arteries but also of the pleura. The reasons for false negatives are failure to sample the LN (45%) or failure to sample the metastatic disease in the LN (55%) [163]. The positive predictive value reaches 97% and negative predictive value 80% [129].

Considering combined advantages and drawbacks of both techniques, we continued performing sampling of suspicious LN with FNA under US guidance for more than 20 years. We use a 23 gauge needle with a 40 cm extension tube, itself connected at the other end to a 20 ml disposable plastic syringe mounted on a syringe holder (Fig. 10.19). This makes FNAC easier and very accurate even for small lesions.

Key point: in order to maximize the performance of FNAC for small (<5 mm) target, it is of the utmost importance that the operator minimizes weight in his hand to optimize targeting accuracy. This is achieved by maintaining the needle between the thumb and index finger in the dominant hand. Holding directly the syringe in one's hand is suboptimal. This method requires the aid of a third person to take care of the syringe.

10.8.2 Liquid-Based Cytology (LBC) for Cell Preservation

LBC technique was developed to screen women for cervical cancer and was fast becoming a useful method in evaluating both gynecological and non-gynecological preparations, including FNAC. The slides are easier and less

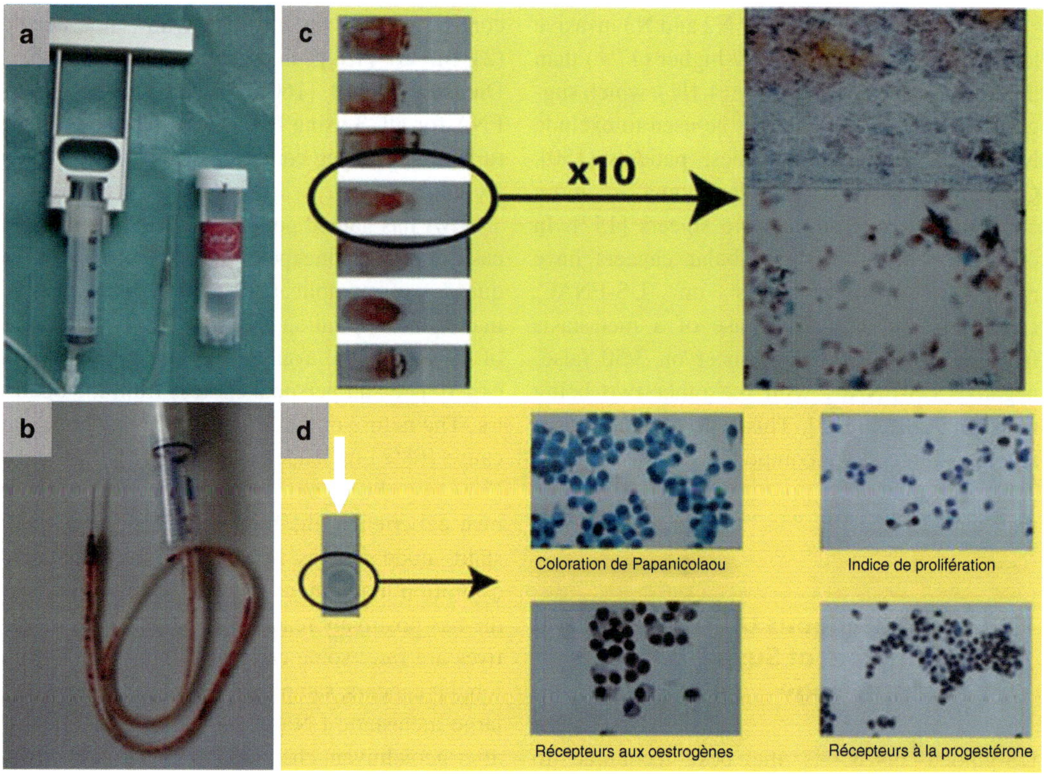

Fig. 10.19 Material for FNA and liquid based cytology (**a**). Blood contamination in needle and tube during FNA (**b**): Magnification of standard smears slides with blood contamination (**c**): many slides with poor visibility. On single slide (*arrow*) after LBC preparation (**d**): magnification of slides stained for different tests, containing a monolayer of well-stained and preserved cells (even when FNA had blood contamination)

time-consuming to screen and interpret, because the cells are limited to a defined area (20 mm in diameter) on the slide, with a clear background and excellent cellular presentation [164–167].

For almost 20 years, we use the LBC technique for our fine-needle aspirates (Fig. 10.19). This has dramatically improved our performance for FNAC, increasing representative specimens from 69 to 92% and decreasing poorly representative aspirates from 18% to 6% and insufficient aspirates from 12 to 1% [125, 168, 169]. Our technique of FNAC sampling with LCB was detailed at ECR 2012 [125]. As with other authors, we advocate the use of this procedure also for cytological analysis of suspicious LN in breast cancer patients [93, 151, 170].

Key point: one of the main advantages of using LBC is that, even with obvious blood contamination, we can continue sampling because there is blood cells and clot destruction during the process of the specimen preparation.

10.8.3 Which Targeted Lymph Node to Sample?

The most suspicious LN, usually the sentinel one, should be the first node to sample. But even when there are evident axillary metastatic LNs on imaging, it remains necessary to look for suspicious LN in other nodal basins because of potential clinical stage changes if an *extra-axillary* LN is metastatic on US-guided FNAC.

Key point: for the most accurate N staging, if suspicious *extra-axillary* LN are identified, one should sample the node in the worst location (supraclavicular, infraclavicular, internal mammary).

US-FNAC (cytology) or FNAB (core biopsy) of a *normal appearing* LN on US (cortex <3 mm) is rarely reported [127, 129]. In our study on US-guided FNAC in clinically node-negative patients, we identified 7% more metastatic LN by sampling *normal appearing* SN, usually at the pole nearest to the tumor (Fig. 10.4) [125]. Some additional precisions are important to optimize accuracy of FNAC depending on the size of the metastatic deposit. The target should be:

- The cortical metastatic nodule or the thickened/lobulated cortex of a small (<10 mm) LN
- The periphery of a larger (>10 mm) metastatic LN to avoid false-negative results related to sampling in a necrotic central area
- The same location (second attempt) or in another suspicious one in order to improve accuracy if the first aspirate is not representative.

Key point: one pass is sufficient for an accurately performed FNAC with good technique and using the LBC procedure for cell preservation and cell preparation.

10.8.4 Detecting Sentinel Node (SN) with Ultrasound: Contrast?

The location of the SN is possible with US. In a study of the relative position of 36 nodes identified as sentinel to other nodes, 81% represented the lowest node identified in the axilla, 11% were the second lowest, and 8% were the third lowest node [171].

In patients with early breast cancer without evident axillary abnormal LN, contrast-enhanced US may be helpful to identify SN. Contrast-enhanced ultrasound (CEUS) shows potential to improve the accuracy of US for the differential diagnosis of benign and malignant LN [172–174]. A malignant node enhances more than a benign one after contrast material administration and displays a heterogeneous pattern of enhancement of the cortex, whereas a benign node is homogeneously dyed and has centrifugal enhancement [175]. In addition, there is higher peripheral vessel distribution in malignant node, which is emphasized after contrast material administration, and the enhancement lasts longer compared to benign node [176]. In a study on 50 patients, contrast-enhanced US had 90% negative predictive value and 75% positive predictive value for detecting SN involvement [135].

Few teams are using CEUS for the SN identification and characterization because native US alone can detect the SN easily when abnormal. Moreover, if no abnormal LN is detected on high-resolution US, it is not important to know which LN is the SN because when US is normal, the probability of having more than three macrometastatic lymph nodes is too low to impact on patients' workup.

10.9 Cost Savings

The detection of metastatic LN with US-FNAC, *avoiding the SLNB*, has the following positive consequences:

- Reduction of time and costs related to
  - Anesthesia
  - Operative identification of SN
  - Intra-/postoperative SN analysis
- Diminishing potential associated complications of SLNB
- No radioactive isotope and blue dye injection
- Reduction of total time
  - To definitive pathological diagnosis
  - Before starting the adjuvant treatment
- Reduction of total costs for the patients, hospitals, and insurances.

By avoiding SLNB with positive preoperative FNAC, the cost savings to the health care system are mainly related to the one-step axillary surgery. The cost balanced is by a 12% reduction of SLNBs and a marked reduction of unnecessary axillary lymph node dissections (ALND) resulting from false-positive clinical staging [177].

In our study on 86 patients with early-stage breast cancer (cN = 0) and candidates for primary breast surgery, US-guided FNAC had 100% specificity, 100% PPV, 73% sensitivity, and 71% NPV. Many patients (37/86) with positive FNAC had one stage axillary surgery thus avoiding an unnecessary SLNB for the 43% positive cases. The costs were reduced by 37 × 3000 euros, avoiding the sole lymphoscintigraphy procedure [12]. The reduction rate of SLNB may be further improved with the operator expertise. If a 40% rate of SLNB avoided, as in our study, is applied to the current rate (70%) of SLNB in developed countries, this would represent significant health costs economy [178].

ALND decreased from 78 to 21% ($p < 0.001$) after publication of ACOSOG Z0011 recommendations. The mean overall cost of SLNB was $41,059 per patient, while SLNB with completion ALND was $50,999 ($p < 0.001$). Intraoperative frozen section decreased from 95% to 66% ($p = 0.015$). Omitting the frozen section decreased mean costs from $4319 to $2036. ACOSOG Z0011 trial significantly impacted axillary management resulting in a 20% reduction in the mean overall cost per patient by omitting ALND [179] and resulted in a 64% reduction in inpatient hospital days as an 18% reduction of early perioperative costs [180].

For SLNB specifically, by injecting the radioactive colloid without obtaining a preoperative lymphoscintigram, McMasters et al. [181] reported that patient charges were reduced by $545 and concluded that considering the extra time and cost required, the use of routine lymphoscintigraphy for identification of axillary SLNs was not justified.

10.10 The Recent Evolution in the Management of Axilla

Since the first study of Giuliano et al. [62], SLNB has been established as the common standard of care for axillary staging in most patients with invasive breast carcinoma. Twenty years later, methods of axillary evaluation in invasive breast cancer continue to evolve and converge to the diminution of SLNB.

Before the American College of Surgeons Oncology Group Z0011 trial (ACOSOG Z0011), we worked to identify axillary metastases preoperatively mainly with AUS-guided FNAC, allowing appropriate patients to directly undergo ALND and without the need for SLNB.

10.10.1 Avoiding unnecessary complete axillary lymph node dissection

Based on the first results of Z0011 and other similar recommendations (the 2011 St. Gallen Consensus Conference [182], EORTC AMAROS trial [144]) new evidence emerged regarding daily practice: *complete axillary lymph node dissection (ALND) is unnecessary in patients with early breast cancer, especially when the SN is minimally (micrometastases in a single SN) involved or when there are one to two positive sentinel lymph nodes (SLNs)*. There would be no benefit in terms of survival and local recurrence for these patients, but also because the criteria used for ALND (≥3 SNs, extracapsular extension) reliably identifies patients at high risk for residual axillary disease [183].

This was also confirmed recently with a 6.2% rate for 10-year cumulative locoregional recurrence of ALND and 5.3% with SLNB alone ($p = 0.36$). Despite the potential for residual axillary disease after SLNB, SLNB without ALND offers excellent regional control for selected patients with early metastatic breast cancer treated with breast-conserving therapy and adjuvant systemic therapy [184]. Taking into account this recommendation, there were a significantly lower number of axillary clearances performed in SLNB-positive patients in the post-Z0011 period (71.4%) compared to the pre-Z011 period (93.7%) [185].

Parallel to this, a new trial was designed comparing SLNB vs. observation when axillary ultrasound is negative for patients with small breast cancer candidates to breast-conserving surgery [186, 187].

10.10.2 A New Role for the Radiologists?

In view of all this, radiologists might need to redefine their role regarding preoperative assessment of the axilla and raise questions on how aggressively we should pursue percutaneous sampling of axillary nodes [188]. Using the current performance of US and US-FNAC for N staging in patient with breast cancer, the key point for preoperative imaging remains to detect macrometastasis (>2 mm) in LN because *micrometastasis and ≤ 2 positive axillary nodes do not affect recurrence-free period and overall survival.* With its current performance, US can reach this goal.

US can confirm heavy metastatic axillary burden avoiding a large proportion of SLNB:

- There is 91% sensitivity for three or more positive *axillary and extra-axillary* LNs; therefore US-identified metastasis should be treated as clinically node-positive disease and is appropriate even in patients planning breast-conserving surgery [149, 189].
- US-guided FNA can identify 93% of LN with metastatic deposit measuring more than 5 mm [120, 129].

US can exclude heavy metastatic axillary burden:

- Patients with *a normal gray-scale US* (LN with ≤3 mm cortical thickness) are unlikely to have extensive axillary disease and may be ideally suited for axillary conservation because [190]
  - Only 2.2% false negative for pT1–2 breast cancers [40, 191].
  - Recurrence-free survival equivalent to patients with pathologic N0 disease [154].
  - Ninety-six percent exclusion of N2 and N3 invasive ductal metastases but less accurate for lobular metastasis [150].

10.11 What Does the Future Hold?

Based on the review of the current literature and our experience, the pragmatic "best patient management" could be to use only ultrasound for the N staging of invasive breast cancer.

But this requires greater education to reach sufficient expertise in order to have a PPV and NPV as good as SLNB. Specialized training in both US and US-guided FNA (adequate sampling) is required to reduce false diagnosis.

New trends will come from ongoing studies for the N staging in patients with breast cancer:

- US *alone* is suggested for the preoperative staging of patients with early-stage breast cancer [42].
- When US is negative in early-stage breast cancer patient candidates to breast-conserving surgery, observation alone could be an alternative to SLNB [186].
- Not to perform axillary surgery as staging procedure in clinically and sonographically negative axilla [40].

Thus, in the near future, the recommended triage method for N staging would be US with two options:

1. *No* axillary/extra-axillary *abnormal node* = no heavy macrometastatic burden = no axillary surgery.
2. *Abnormal nodes*: either a single round node, of any size without a fatty hilum, or >3 abnormal nodes in any nodal basin draining the breast = macrometastasis = different treatment options according to patient and tumor features.

Promoting this protocol, based on us only, for workup of patients with breast cancer, compared to other imaging techniques and surgical procedures, would be beneficial to patients in terms of irradiation and time to diagnosis and treatment.

Moreover in terms of cost-effectiveness, US-guided FNAC for N staging of patients with breast cancer is cost-effective, both in developing countries, having restricted access to high-level technologies as MRI, PET/CT, and SLNB and in First World countries which are faced with a permanent increase in health expenditure.

References

1. Nemoto T, Natarajan N, Bedwani R, Vana J, Murphy GP. Breast cancer in the medial half. Results of 1978 National Survey of the American College of Surgeons. Cancer. 1983;51(8):1333–8.
2. Saez RA, McGuire WL, Clark GM. Prognostic factors in breast cancer. Semin Surg Oncol. 1989;5(2):102–10. Review
3. Colzani E, Liljegren A, Johansson AL, Adolfsson J, Hellborg H, Hall PF, Czene K. Prognosis of patients with breast cancer: causes of death and effects of time since diagnosis, age, and tumor characteristics. J Clin Oncol. 2011;29:4014–21.
4. de Boer M, van Dijck JA, Bult P, Borm GF, Tjan-Heijnen VC. Breast cancer prognosis and occult lymph node metastases, isolated tumor cells, and micrometastases. J Natl Cancer Inst. 2010;102:410–25.
5. Fisher B, Bauer M, Wickerham DL, Redmond CK, Fisher ER, Cruz AB, Foster R, Gardner B, Lerner H, Margolese R, et al. Relation of number of positive axillary nodes to the prognosis of patients with primary breast cancer. An NSABP update. Cancer. 1983;52(9):1551–7.
6. Allemani C, Weir HK, Carreira H, Harewood R, Spika D, Wang XS et al.; CONCORD Working Group. Global surveillance of cancer survival 1995–2009: analysis of individual data for 25,676,887 patients from 279 population-based registries in 67 countries (CONCORD-2). Lancet. 2015;385(9972):977–1010.
7. Saadatmand S, Bretveld R, Siesling S. Tilanus-Linthorst. Influence of tumour stage at breast cancer detection on survival in modern times: population based study in 173,797 patients. BMJ. 2015;351:h4901.
8. Ojeda-Fournier H, Nguyen JQ. Ultrasound evaluation of regional breast lymph node. Semin Roentgenol. 2011;46(1):51–9.
9. Baruah BP, Goyal A, Young P, Douglas-Jones AG, Mansel RE. Axillary node staging by ultrasonography and fine-needle aspiration cytology in patients with breast cancer. Br J Surg. 2010;97(5):680–3.
10. Deurloo EE, Tanis PJ, Gilhuijs KG, Muller SH, Kröger R, Peterse JL, Rutgers EJ, Valdés Olmos R, Schultze Kool LJ. Reduction in the number of sentinel lymph node procedures by preoperative ultrasonography of the axilla in breast cancer. Eur J Cancer. 2003;39:1068–73.
11. Diaz-Ruiz MJ, Arnau A, Montesinos J, Miguel A, Culell P, Solernou L, Tortajada L, Vergara C, Yanguas C, Salvador-Tarrasón R. Diagnostic accuracy and impact on management of ultrasonography-guided fine-needle aspiration to detect axillary metastasis in breast cancer patients: a prospective study. Breast Care (Basel). 2016;11(1):34–9.
12. Huber D, Duc C, Schneider N, Fournier D. Ultrasound-guided fine needle aspiration cytology in staging clinically node-negative invasive breast cancer. Gynecol Surg. 2012;9:185.
13. Francissen CMTP, Dings PJM, van Dalen T, Strobbe LJA, van Laarhoven HWM, de Wilt JHW. Axillary recurrence after a tumor-positive sentinel lymph node biopsy without axillary treatment: a review of the literature. Ann Surg Oncol. 2012;19(13):4140–9.
14. Giuliano AE, Hunt KK, Ballman KV, Beitsch PD, Whitworth PW, Blumencranz PW, Leitch AM, Saha S, McCall LM, Morrow M. Axillary dissection vs. no axillary dissection in women with invasive breast cancer and sentinel node metastasis: a randomized clinical trial. JAMA. 2011;305:569–75.
15. Maaskant-Braat AJ, van de Poll-Franse LV, Voogd AC, Coebergh JW, Roumen RM, Nolthenius-Puylaert MC, Nieuwenhuijzen GA. Sentinel node micrometastases in breast cancer do not affect prognosis: a population-based study. Breast Cancer Res Treat. 2011;127(1):195–203.
16. Tallet A, Lambaudie E, Cohen M, Minsat M, Bannier M, Resbeut M, Houvenaeghel G. Locoregional treatment of early breast cancer with isolated tumor cells or micrometastases on sentinel lymph node biopsy. World J Clin Oncol. 2016;7(2):243–52.

17. Blum A, Schlagenhauff B, Stroebel W, Breuninger H, Rassner G, Garbe C. Ultrasound examination of regional lymph nodes significantly improves early detection of locoregional metastases during the follow-up of patients with cutaneous disease: result of a prospective study of 1288 patients. Cancer. 2000;88(11):2534–9.
18. Tregnaghi A, De Candia A, Calderone M, Cellini L, Rossi CR, Talenti E, Blandamura S, Borsato S, Muzzio PC, Rubaltelli L. Ultrasonographic evaluation of superficial lymph node metastases in melanoma. Eur J Radiol. 1996;24(3):216–21.
19. Voit C, Mayer T, Kron M, Schoengen A, Sterry W, Weber L, Proebstle TM. Efficacy of ultrasound B-scan compared with physical examination in follow-up of melanoma patients. Cancer. 2001;91(12):2409–16.
20. Mandava A, Ravuri PR, Konathan R. High-resolution ultrasound imaging of cutaneous lesions. Indian J Radiol Imaging. 2013;23(3):269–77.
21. Dudea SM, Lenghel M, Botar-Jid C, Vasilescu D, Duma M. Ultrasonography of superficial lymph nodes: benign vs. malignant. Med Ultrason. 2012;14(4):294–306.
22. Kristo B, Krišto B, Buljan M. The lymph node roundness index in the evaluation of lymph nodes of the neck. Coll Antropol. 2015;39(1):165–9.
23. Hillen F, Griffioen AW. Tumour vascularization: sprouting angiogenesis and beyond. Cancer Metastasis Rev. 2007;26(3–4):489–502. Review
24. Chiorean L, Barr RG, Braden B, Jenssen C, Cui XW, Hocke M, Schuler A, Dietrich CF. Transcutaneous ultrasound: elastographic lymph node evaluation. current clinical applications and literature review. Ultrasound Med Biol. 2016;42(1):16–30.
25. Kilic F, Velidedeoglu M, Ozturk T, Kandemirli SG, Dikici AS, Er ME, Aydogan F, Kantarci F, Yilmaz MH. Ex vivo assessment of sentinel lymph nodes in breast cancer using shear wave elastography. J Ultrasound Med. 2016;35(2):271–7.
26. Wojcinski S, Dupont J, Schmidt W, Cassel M, Hillemanns P. Real-time ultrasound elastography in 180 axillary lymph nodes: elasticity distribution in healthy lymph nodes and prediction of breast cancer metastases. BMC Med Imaging. 2012;12:35.
27. Gkretsi V, Stylianou A, Papageorgis P, Polydorou C. Stylianopoulos T. Remodeling components of the tumor microenvironment to enhance cancer therapy. Front Oncol. 2015;5:214.
28. Ran S, Volk L, Hall K, Flister MJ. Lymphangiogenesis and lymphatic metastasis in breast cancer. Pathophysiology. 2010;17(4):229–51.
29. Suami H, Pan WR, Mann GB, Taylor GI. The lymphatic anatomy of the breast and its implications for sentinel lymph node biopsy: a human cadaver study. Ann Surg Oncol. 2008;15(3):863–71.
30. Manca G, Volterrani D, Mazzarri S, Duce V, Svirydenka A, Giuliano A, Mariani G. Sentinel lymph node mapping in breast cancer: a critical reappraisal of the internal mammary chain issue. Q J Nucl Med Mol Imaging. 2014;58(2):114–26.
31. Tanis PJ, Nieweg OE, Valdés Olmos RA, Peterse JL, Rutgers EJ, Hoefnagel CA, Kroon BB. Impact of non-axillary sentinel node biopsy on staging and treatment of breast cancer patients. Br J Cancer. 2002;87(7):705–10.
32. Liu Y. Role of FDG PET-CT in evaluation of locoregional nodal disease for initial staging of breast cancer. World J Clin Oncol. 2014;5(5):982–9.
33. Robertson IJ, Hand F, Kell MR. FDG-PET/CT in the staging of local/regional metastases in breast cancer. Breast. 2011;20(6):491–4.
34. Hong J, Choy E, Soni N, Carmalt H, Gillett D, Spillane AJ. Extra-axillary sentinel node biopsy in the management of early breast cancer. Eur J Surg Oncol. 2005;31(9):942–8.
35. Baltzer PA, Dietzel M, Burmeister HP, Zoubi R, Gajda M, Camara O, Kaiser WA. Application of MR mammography beyond local staging: is there a potential to accurately assess axillary lymph nodes? Evaluation of an extended protocol in an initial prospective study. AJR Am J Roentgenol. 2011;196(5):W641–7.
36. Tran A, Pio BS, Khatibi B, Czernin J, Phelps ME, Silverman DH. 18F-FDG PET for staging breast cancer in patients with inner-quadrant versus outer-quadrant tumors: comparison with long-term clinical outcome. J Nucl Med. 2005;46(9):1455–9.
37. Krause A, Dunkelmann S, Makovitzky J, Küchenmeister I, Schümichen C, Reimer T, Friese K, Gerber B. Detection of atypical site of "sentinel lymph nodes" by lymph drainage scintigraphy in patients with breast carcinoma. Zentralbl Gynakol. 2000;122(10):514–8.
38. Altinyollar H, Dingil G, Berberoglu U. Detection of infraclavicular lymph node metastases using ultrasonography in breast cancer. J Surg Oncol. 2005;92(4):299–303.
39. van Rijk MC, Tanis PJ, Nieweg OE, Olmos RA, Rutgers EJ, Hoefnagel CA, Kroon BB. Clinical implications of sentinel nodes outside the axilla and internal mammary chain in patients with breast cancer. J Surg Oncol. 2006;94(4):281–6.
40. Stachs A, Göde K, Hartmann S, Stengel B, Nierling U, Dieterich M, Reimer T, Gerber B. Accuracy of axillary ultrasound in preoperative nodal staging of breast cancer—size of metastases as limiting factor. Spring. 2013;2:350.
41. Khout H, Richardson C, Toghyan H, Fasih T. The role of combined assessment in preoperative axillary staging. Ochsner J. 2013;13(4):489–94.
42. Gipponi M, Fregatti P, Garlaschi A, Murelli F, Margarino C, Depaoli F, Baccini P, Gallo M, Friedman D. Axillary ultrasound and fine-needle aspiration cytology in the preoperative staging of axillary node metastasis in breast cancer patients. Breast. 2016;30:146–50.
43. Feng Y, Huang R, He Y, Lu A, Fan Z, Fan T, Qi M, Wang X, Cao W, Wang X, Xie Y, Wang T, Li J, Ouyang T. Efficacy of physical examination, ultrasound, and ultrasound combined with fine-needle

aspiration for axilla staging of primary breast cancer. Breast Cancer Res Treat. 2015;149(3):761–5.
44. Pamilo M, Soiva M, Lavast EM. Real-time ultrasound, axillary mammography, and clinical examination in the detection of axillary lymph node metastases in breast cancer patients. J Ultrasound Med. 1989;8(3):115–20.
45. Usmani S, Ahmed N, Al Saleh N, abu Huda F, Amanguno HG, Amir T, al Kandari F. The clinical utility of combining pre-operative axillary ultrasonography and fine needle aspiration cytology with radionuclide guided sentinel lymph node biopsy in breast cancer patients with palpable axillary lymph nodes. Eur J Radiol. 2015;84(12):2515–20.
46. Specht MC, Fey JV, Borgen PI, Cody HS 3rd. Is the clinically positive axilla in breast cancer really a contraindication to sentinel lymph node biopsy? J Am Coll Surg. 2005;200(1):10–4.
47. Dialani V, James DF, Slanetz PJ. A practical approach to imaging the axilla. Insights Imaging. 2015;6(2):217–29.
48. Ecanow JS, Abe H, Newstead GM, Ecanow DB, Jeske JM. Axillary staging of breast cancer: what the radiologist should know. Radiographics. 2013;33(6):1589–612.
49. Wu PQ, Liu CL, Liu ZY, Ye WT, Liang CH. Value of mamography, CT and DCE-MRI in detecting axillary lymph node metastasis of breast cancer. Nan Fang Yi Ke Da Xue Xue Bao. 2016;36(4):493–9.
50. Walsh R, Kornguth PJ, Soo MS, Bentley R, DeLong DM. Axillary lymph nodes: mammographic, pathologic, and clinical correlation. AJR Am J Roentgenol. 1997;168(1):33–8.
51. Lee CH, Giurescu ME, Philpotts LE, Horvath LJ, Tocino I. Clinical importance of unilaterally enlarging lymph nodes on otherwise normal mammograms. Radiology. 1997;203(2):329–34.
52. Valente SA, Levine GM, Silverstein MJ, Rayhanabad JA, Weng-Grumley JG, Ji L, Holmes DR, Sposto R, Sener SF. Accuracy of predicting axillary lymph node positivity by physical examination, mammography, ultrasonography, and magnetic resonance imaging. Ann Surg Oncol. 2012;19(6):1825–30.
53. Shetty MK, Carpenter WS. Sonographic evaluation of isolated abnormal axillary lymph nodes identified on mammograms. J Ultrasound Med. 2004;23:63–71.
54. Murray ME, Given-Wilson RM. The clinical importance of axillary lymphadenopathy detected on screening mammography. Clin Radiol. 1997;52(6):458–61.
55. March DE, Wechsler RJ, Kurtz AB, Rosenberg AL, Needleman L. CT-pathologic correlation of axillary lymph nodes in breast carcinoma. J Comput Assist Tomogr. 1991;15:440–4.
56. Uematsu T, Sano M, Homma K. In vitro high-resolution helical CT of small axillary lymph nodes in patients with breast cancer: correlation of CT and histology. AJR Am J Roentgenol. 2001;176(4):1069–74.
57. Chudgar A, Clark A, Mankoff D. Applications of PET/CT in breast cancer, NCCN guidelines and beyond. J Nucl Med. 2016;57:1304.
58. Peare R, Staff RT, Heys SD. The use of FDG-PET in assessing axillary lymph node status in breast cancer: a systematic review and meta-analysis of the literature. Breast Cancer Res Treat. 2010;123:281–90.
59. Riegger C, Koeninger A, Hartung V, Otterbach F, Kimmig R, Forsting M, Bockisch A, Antoch G, Heusner TA. Comparison of the diagnostic value of FDG-PET/CT and axillary ultrasound for the detection of lymph node metastases in breast cancer patients. Acta Radiol. 2012;53(10):1092–8.
60. Fujii T, Yajima R, Tatsuki H, Oosone K, Kuwano H. Implication of ^{18}F-fluorodeoxyglucose uptake of affected axillary lymph nodes in cases with breast cancer. Anticancer Res. 2016;36(1):393–7.
61. Ahmed M, Purushotham AD, Douek M. Novel techniques for sentinel lymph node biopsy in breast cancer: a systematic review. Lancet Oncol. 2014;15(8):e351–62.
62. Giuliano AE, Kirgan DM, Guenther JM, Morton DL. Lymphatic mapping and sentinel lymphadenectomy for breast cancer. Ann Surg. 1994;220:391–8.
63. Kell MR, Burke JP, Barry M, Morrow M. Outcome of axillary staging in early breast cancer: a meta-analysis. Breast Cancer Res Treat. 2010;120:441–7.
64. Straver ME, Meijnen P, van Tienhoven G, van de Velde CJ, Mansel RE, Bogaerts J, Demonty G, Duez N, Cataliotti L, Klinkenbijl J, Westenberg HA, van der Mijle H, Hurkmans C, Rutgers EJ. Role of axillary clearance after a tumor-positive sentinel node in the administration of adjuvant therapy in early breast cancer. J Clin Oncol. 2010;28(5):731–7.
65. Veronesi U, Viale G, Paganelli G, Zurrida S, Luini A, Galimberti V, Veronesi P, Intra M, Maisonneuve P, Zucca F, Gatti G, Mazzarol G, De Cicco C, Vezzoli D. Sentinel lymph node biopsy in breast cancer: ten-year results of a randomized controlled study. Ann Surg. 2010;251:595–600.
66. Zavagno G, De Salvo G L, Scalco G. et al.; GIVOM Trialists. A randomized clinical trial on sentinel lymph node biopsy versus axillary lymph node dissection in breast cancer: results of the SENTINELLA/GIVOM trial. Ann Surg. 2008;247:207–13.
67. Maguire A, Brogi E. Sentinel lymph nodes for breast carcinoma: a paradigm shift. Arch Pathol Lab Med. 2016;140(8):791–8.
68. Husted Madsen A, Haugaard K, Soerensen J, Bokmand S, Friis E, Holtveg H, Peter Garne J, Horby J, Christiansen P. Arm morbidity following sentinel lymph node biopsy or axillary lymph node dissection: a study from the Danish Breast Cancer Cooperative Group. Breast. 2008;17(2):138–47. Epub 2007 Oct 24
69. Kuijs VJL, Moossdorff M, Schipper RJ, Beets-Tan RGH, Heuts EM, Keymeulen KBMI, Smidt ML, Lobbes MBI. The role of MRI in axillary lymph node imaging in breast cancer patients: a systematic review. Insights Imaging. 2015;6:203–15.

70. Rahman RL, Crawford SL, Siwawa P. Management of axilla in breast cancer: the saga continues. Breast. 2015;24(4):343–53.
71. Yoshimura G, Sakurai T, Oura S, Suzuma T, Tamaki T, Umemura T, Kokawa Y, Yang Q. Evaluation of axillary lymph node status in breast cancer with MRI. Breast Cancer. 1999;6:249–58.
72. Kvistad KA, Rydland J, Smethurst HB, Lundgren S, Fjosne HE, Haraldseth O. Axillary lymph node metastases in breast cancer: preoperative detection with dynamic contrast-enhanced MRI. Eur Radiol. 2000;10:1464–71.
73. García Fernández A, Fraile M, Giménez N, Reñe A, Torras M, Canales L, Torres J, Barco I, González S, Veloso E, González C, Cirera L, Pessarrodona A. Use of axillary ultrasound, ultrasound-fine needle aspiration biopsy and magnetic resonance imaging in the preoperative triage of breast cancer patients considered for sentinel node biopsy. Ultrasound Med Biol. 2011;37:16–22.
74. Harnan SE, Cooper KL, Meng Y, Ward SE, Fitzgerald P, Papaioannou D, Ingram C, Lorenz E, Wilkinson ID, Wyld L. Magnetic resonance for assessment of axillary lymph node status in early breast cancer: a systematic review and meta-analysis. Eur J Surg Oncol. 2011;37(11):928–36.
75. Chung J, Youk JH, Kim JA, Gweon HM, Kim EK, Ryu YH, Son EJ. Role of diffusion-weighted MRI: predicting axillary lymph node metastases in breast cancer. Acta Radiol. 2014;55(8):909–16.
76. Yun SJ, Sohn YM, Seo M. Differentiation of benign and metastatic axillary lymph nodes in breast cancer: additive value of MRI computer-aided evaluation. Clin Radiol. 2016;71(4):403.e1–7.
77. Arslan G, Altintoprak KM, Yirgin IK, Atasoy MM, Celik L. Diagnostic accuracy of metastatic axillary lymph nodes in breast MRI. Spring. 2016;5(1):735.
78. Estourgie SH, Nieweg OE, Olmos RA, Rutgers EJ, Kroon BB. Lymphatic drainage patterns from the breast. Ann Surg. 2004;239(2):232–7.
79. Freedman GM, Fowble BL, Nicolaou N, Sigurdson ER, Torosian MH, Boraas MC, Hoffman JP. Should internal mammary lymph nodes in breast cancer be a target for the radiation oncologist? Int J Radiat Oncol Biol Phys. 2000;46(4):805–14. Review.
80. Veronesi U, Cascinelli N, Bufalino R, Morabito A, Greco M, Galluzzo D, Delle Donne V, De Lellis R, Piotti P, Sacchini V, et al. Risk of internal mammary lymph node metastases and its relevance on prognosis of breast cancer patients. Ann Surg. 1983;198:681–4.
81. Huang O, Wang L, Shen K, Lin H, Hu Z, Liu G, Wu J, Lu J, Shao Z, Han Q, Shen Z. Breast cancer subpopulation with high risk of internal mammary lymph nodes metastasis: analysis of 2,269 Chinese breast cancer patients treated with extended radical mastectomy. Breast Cancer Res Treat. 2008;107:379–87.
82. Ragaz J, Olivotto IA, Spinelli JJ, Phillips N, Jackson SM, Wilson KS, Knowling MA, Coppin CM, Weir L, Gelmon K, Le N, Durand R, Coldman AJ, Manji M. Locoregional radiation therapy in patients with high-risk breast cancer receiving adjuvant chemotherapy: 20-year results of the British Columbia randomized trial. J Natl Cancer Inst. 2005;97:116–26.
83. Colleoni M, Zahrieh D, Gelber RD, Holmberg SB, Mattsson JE, Rudenstam CM, Lindtner J, Erzen D, Snyder R, Collins J, Fey MF, Thürlimann B, Crivellari D, Murray E, Mendiola C, Pagani O, Castiglione-Gertsch M, Coates AS, Price K, Goldhirsch A. Site of primary tumor has a prognostic role in operable breast cancer: the international breast cancer study group experience. J Clin Oncol. 2005;23:1390–400.
84. Cody HS, Urban JA. Internal mammary node status: a major prognosticator in axillary node-negative breast cancer. Ann Surg Oncol. 1995;2:32–7.
85. Noguchi M, Koyasaki N, Ohta N, Kitagawa H, Earashi M, Thomas M, Miyazaki I, Mizukami Y. Internal mammary nodal status is a more reliable prognostic factor than DNA ploidy and c-erb B-2 expression in patients with breast cancer. Arch Surg. 1993;128:242–6.
86. Jochelson MS, Lebron L, Jacobs SS, Zheng J, Moskowitz CS, Powell SN, Sacchini V, Ulaner GA, Morris EA, Dershaw DD. Detection of internal mammary adenopathy in patients with breast cancer by PET/CT and MRI. AJR Am J Roentgenol. 2015;205(4):899–904.
87. Qiu PF, Liu YB, Wang YS. Internal mammary sentinel lymph node biopsy: abandon or persist? Onco Targets Ther. 2016;9:3879–82.
88. Scatarige JC, Boxen I, Smathers RL. Internal mammary lymphadenopathy: imaging of a vital lymphatic pathway in breast cancer. Radiographics. 1990;10(5):857–70. Review
89. Glass EC, Essner R, Giuliano AE. Sentinel node localization in breast cancer. Semin Nucl Med. 1999;29:57–68.
90. van der Ent FW, Kengen RA, Pol HA, Povel JA, Stroeken HJ, Hoofwijk AG. Halsted Revisited: Internal Mammary Sentinel Lymph Node Biopsy in Breast. Ann Surg. 2001 Jul;234(1):79–84.
91. Chen RC, Lin NU, Golshan M, Harris JR, Bellon JR. Internal mammary nodes in breast cancer: diagnosis and implications for patient management—a systematic review. J Clin Oncol. 2008;26(30):4981–9.
92. Zhang YJ, Oh JL, Whitman GJ, Iyengar P, Yu TK, Tereffe W, Woodward WA, Perkins G, Buchholz TA, Strom EA. Clinically apparent internal mammary nodal metastasis in patients with advanced breast cancer: incidence and local control. Int J Radiat Oncol Biol Phys. 2010;77:1113–9.
93. Wang CL, Eissa MJ, Rogers JV, Aravkin AY, Porter BA, Beatty JD. (18)F-FDG PET/CT-positive internal mammary lymph nodes: pathologic correlation by ultrasound-guided fine-needle aspiration and assessment of associated risk factors. AJR Am J Roentgenol. 2013;200(5):1138–44.
94. Kinoshita T, Odagiri K, Andoh K, Doiuchi T, Sugimura K, Shiotani S, Asaga T. Evaluation of

small internal mammary lymph node metastases in breast cancer by MRI. Radiat Med. 1999;17:189–93.
95. Cheon H, Kim HJ, Lee SW, Kim DH, Lee CH, Cho SH, Shin KM, Lee SM, Kim GC, Kim WH. Internal mammary node adenopathy on breast MRI and PET/CT for initial staging in patients with operable breast cancer: prevalence and associated factors. Breast Cancer Res Treat. 2016;160(3):523–30.
96. Dogan BE, Dryden MJ, Wei W, Fornage BD, Buchholz TA, Smith B, Hunt K, Krishnamurthy S, Yang WT. Sonography and sonographically guided needle biopsy of internal mammary nodes in staging of patients with breast cancer. AJR Am J Roentgenol. 2015;205(4):905–11.
97. Farrús B, Vidal-Sicart S, Velasco M, Zanón G, Fernández PL, Muñoz M, Santamaría G, Albanell J, Biete A. Incidence of internal mammary node metastases after a sentinel lymph node technique in breast cancer and its implication in the radiotherapy plan. Int J Radiat Oncol Biol Phys. 2004;60(3):715–21.
98. Gui GP, Behranwala KA, Abdullah N, Seet J, Osin P, Nerurkar A, Lakhani SR. The inframammary fold: contents, clinical significance and implications for immediate breast reconstruction. Br J Plast Surg. 2004;57(2):146–9.
99. Troupis T, Michalinos A, Skandalakis P. Intramammary lymph nodes: a question seeking for an answer or an answer seeking for a question? Breast. 2012;21(5): 615–20.
100. Nassar A, Cohen C, Cotsonis G, Carlson G. Significance of intramammary lymph nodes in the staging of breast cancer: correlation with tumor characteristics and outcome. Breast J. 2008;14(2):147–52.
101. Abdullgaffar B, Gopal P, Abdulrahim M, Ghazi E, Mohamed E. The significance of intramammary lymph nodes in breast cancer: a systematic review and meta-analysis. Int J Surg Pathol. 2012;20(6):555–63.
102. Rampaul RS, Dale OT, Mitchell M, Blamey RW, Macmillan RD, Robertson JF, Ellis IO. Incidence of intramammary nodes in completion mastectomy specimens after axillary node sampling: implications for breast conserving surgery. Breast. 2008;17(2):195–8.
103. Gunhan-Bilgen I, Memiş A, Ustun EE. Metastatic intramammary lymph nodes: mammographic and ultrasonographic features. Eur J Radiol. 2001;40(1):24–9.
104. Shen J, Hunt KK, Mirza NQ, Krishnamurthy S, Singletary SE, Kuerer HM, Meric-Bernstam F, Feig B, Ross MI, Ames FC, Babiera GV. Intramammary lymph node metastases are an independent predictor of poor outcome in patients with breast carcinoma. Cancer. 2004;101(6):1330–7.
105. Svane G, Franzén S. Radiologic appearance of nonpalpable intramammary lymph nodes. Acta Radiol. 1993;34:577–80.
106. Gordon PB, Gilks B. Sonographic appearance of normal intramammary lymph nodes. J Ultrasound Med. 1988;7(10):545–8.
107. Stomper PC, Leibowich S, Meyer JE. The prevalence and distribution of well circumscribed nodules on screening mammography: analysis of 1500 mammograms. Breast Dis. 1991;4:197–203.
108. Kim SJ, Ko EY, Shin JH, Kang SS, Mun SH, Han BK, Cho EY. Application of sonographic BI-RADS to synchronous breast nodules detected in patients with breast cancer. AJR Am J Roentgenol. 2008;191(3):653–8.
109. Edeiken-Monroe BS, Monroe DP, Monroe BJ, Arnljot K, Giaccomazza M, Sneige N, Fornage BD. Metastases to intramammary lymph nodes in patients with breast cancer: sonographic findings. J Clin Ultrasound. 2008;36:279–85.
110. Nogareda Z, Álvarez A, Perlaza P, Caparrós FX, Alonso I, Paredes P, Vidal-Sicart S. Presence of intramammary lymph nodes in the preoperative lymphoscintigraphy to locate the sentinel lymph node. Clinical significance. Rev Esp Med Nucl Imagen Mol. 2015;34(2):83–8.
111. Mahajan A, et al. Diagnosis of a malignant intramammary node retrospectively aided by mastectomy specimen MRI-Is the search worth it? A case report and review of current literature. Korean J Radiol. 2013;14(4):576–80.
112. Kembhavi SA, Choudhary H, Deodhar K, Thakur MH. Reactive intramammary lymph node mimicking recurrence on MRI study in a patient with prior breast conservation therapy. J Cancer Res Ther. 2013;9(1):111–3.
113. Vijan SS, Hamilton S, Chen B, Reynolds C, Boughey JC, Degnim AC. Intramammary lymph nodes: patterns of discovery and clinical significance. Surgery. 2009;145:495–9.
114. Aksoy Ozcan U, Tezcanli E, Yildirim Y, Garipagaoglu M. The great mimicker: zona zoster at the mastectomy site causing contralateral intramammary lymph node enlargement. Case Rep Oncol Med. 2012;2012:468576.
115. Houvenaeghel G, Tallet A, Jalaguier-Coudray A, Cohen M, Bannier M, Jauffret-Fara C, Lambaudie E. Is breast conservative surgery a reasonable option in multifocal or multicentric tumors? World J Clin Oncol. 2016;7(2):234–42.
116. Lynch SP, Lei X, Hsu L, Meric-Bernstam F, Buchholz TA, Zhang H, Hortobágyi GN, Gonzalez-Angulo AM, Valero V. Breast cancer multifocality and multicentricity and locoregional recurrence. Oncologist. 2013;18(11):1167–73.
117. Bruneton JN, Caramella E, Héry M, Aubanel D, Manzino JJ, Picard JL. Axillary lymph node metastases in breast cancer: preoperative detection with US. Radiology. 1986;158(2):325–6.
118. Mustonen P, Farin P, Kosunen O. Ultrasonographic detection of metastatic axillary lymph nodes in breast cancer. Ann Chir Gynaecol. 1990;79(1):15–8.
119. Ciatto S, Brancato B, Risso G, Ambrogetti D, Bulgaresi P, Maddau C, Turco P, Houssami N. Accuracy of fine needle aspiration cytology (FNAC) of axillary lymph nodes as a triage test

in breast cancer staging. Breast Cancer Res Treat. 2007;103(1):85–91.
120. Krishnamurthy S, Sneige N, Bedi DG, Edieken BS, Fornage BD, Kuerer HM, Singletary SE, Hunt KK. Role of ultrasound-guided fine-needle aspiration of indeterminate and suspicious axillary lymph nodes in the initial staging of breast carcinoma. Cancer. 2002;95(5):982–8.
121. Alvarez S, Añorbe E, Alcorta P, et al. Role of sonography in the diagnosis of axillary lymph node metastases in breast cancer: a systematic review. AJR Am J Roentgenol. 2006;186:1342–8.
122. Choi YJ, Ko EY, Han BK, Shin JH, Kang SS, Hahn SY. High-resolution ultrasonographic features of axillary lymph node metastasis in patients with breast cancer. Breast. 2009;18(2):119–22.
123. Dihge L, Grabau DA, Rasmussen RW, Bendahl PO, Rydén L. The accuracy of preoperative axillary nodal staging in primary breast cancer by ultrasound is modified by nodal metastatic load and tumor biology. Acta Oncol. 2016;55(8):976–82.
124. Fornage BD. Local and regional staging of invasive breast cancer with sonography: 25 years of practice at MD Anderson Cancer Center. Oncologist. 2014;19(1):5–15.
125. Fournier D, Huber D, Duc C, Laswad T, Moreau J, Villemain AM, Schneider N. The role of ultrasonography guided-fine-needle-aspiration in axillary lymph node staging of breast cancer. Case series of 108 patients. ECR 2012/C-2585. Vienna. March 1–5 2012.
126. Houssami N, Ciatto S, Turner RM, Cody HS 3rd, Macaskill P. Preoperative ultrasound-guided needle biopsy of axillary nodes in invasive breast cancer: meta-analysis of its accuracy and utility in staging the axilla. Ann Surg. 2011;254(2):243–51.
127. Mainiero MB, Cinelli CM, Koelliker SL, Graves TA, Chung MA. Axillary ultrasound and fine-needle aspiration in the preoperative evaluation of the breast cancer patient: an algorithm based on tumor size and lymph node appearance. AJR Am J Roentgenol. 2010;195(5):1261–7.
128. Bedi DG, Krishnamurthy R, Krishnamurthy S, Edeiken BS, Le-Petross H, Fornage BD, Bassett RL Jr, Hunt KK. Cortical morphologic features of axillary lymph nodes as a predictor of metastasis in breast cancer: in vitro sonographic study. AJR Am J Roentgenol. 2008;191(3):646–52.
129. Duchesne N, Jaffey J, Florack P, Duchesne S. Redefining ultrasound appearance criteria of positive axillary lymph nodes. Can Assoc Radiol J. 2005;56(5):289–96.
130. Britton PD, Goud A, Godward S, Barter S, Freeman A, Gaskarth M, Rajan P, Sinnatamby R, Slattery J, Provenzano E, O'Donovan M, Pinder S, Benson JR, Forouhi P, Wishart GC. Use of ultrasound-guided axillary node core biopsy in staging of early breast cancer. Eur Radiol. 2009;19(3):561–9.
131. Cho N, Moon WK, Han W, Park IA, Cho J, Noh DY. Preoperative sonographic classification of axillary lymph nodes in patients with breast cancer: node-to-node correlation with surgical histology and sentinel node biopsy results. AJR Am J Roentgenol. 2009;193(6):1731–7.
132. Fournier D. Ultrasound assessment of sentinel lymph node on breast cancer. Contribution of Aixplorer and its harmonic imaging. Swiss Congress of Radiology. Luzern. 30. Mai – 1. Juni 2013.
133. Kubota K, Ogawa Y, Nishigawa T, Yoshida S. Tissue harmonic imaging ultrasound of the axillary lymph nodes: evaluation of response to neoadjuvant chemotherapy in breast cancer patients. Oncol Rep. 2003;10(6):1911–4.
134. Shapiro RS, Wagreich J, Parsons RB, Stancato-Pasik A, Yeh HC, Lao R. Tissue harmonic imaging sonography: evaluation of image quality compared with conventional sonography. AJR Am J Roentgenol. 1998;171(5):1203–6.
135. Dellaportas D, Koureas A, Contis J, Lykoudis PM, Vraka I, Psychogios D, Kondi-Pafiti A, Voros DK. Contrast-enhanced color Doppler ultrasonography for preoperative evaluation of sentinel lymph node in breast cancer patients. Breast Care (Basel). 2015;10(5):331–5.
136. Sarvazyan A, Hall TJ, Urban MW, Fatemi M, Aglyamov SR, Garra BS. An overview of elastography—an emerging branch of medical imaging. Curr Med Imaging Rev. 2011;7(4):255–82.
137. Cosgrove DO, Berg WA, Doré CJ, Skyba DM, Henry JP, Gay J, Cohen-Bacrie C, BE1 Study Group. Shear wave elastography for breast masses is highly reproducible. Eur Radiol. 2012;22(5):1023–32.
138. Liu B, Zheng Y, Huang G, Lin M, Shan Q, Lu Y, Tian W, Xie X. Breast lesions: quantitative diagnosis using ultrasound shear wave elastography—a systematic review and meta-analysis. Ultrasound Med Biol. 2016;42(4):835–47.
139. Thomas A, Kümmel S, Fritzsche F, Warm M, Ebert B, Hamm B, Fischer T. Real-time sonoelastography performed in addition to B-mode ultrasound and mammography: improved differentiation of breast lesions? Acad Radiol. 2006;13(12):1496–504.
140. Shah AR, Glazebrook KN, Boughey JC, Hoskin TL, Shah SS, Bergquist JR, Dupont SC, Hieken TJ. Does BMI affect the accuracy of preoperative axillary ultrasound in breast cancer patients? Ann Surg Oncol. 2014;21(10):3278–83.
141. Koelliker SL, Chung MA, Mainiero MB, Steinhoff MM, Cady B. Axillary lymph nodes: US-guided fine-needle aspiration for initial staging of breast cancer—correlation with primary tumor size. Radiology. 2008;246(1):81–9.
142. Gooch J, King TA, Eaton A, Dengel L, Stempel M, Corben AD, Morrow M. The extent of extracapsular extension may influence the need for axillary lymph node dissection in patients with T1-T2 breast cancer. Ann Surg Oncol. 2014;21(9):2897–903.
143. Giuliano AE, McCall L, Beitsch P, et al. Locoregional recurrence after sentinel lymph node dissection with or without axillary dissection in patients with sentinel lymph node metastases: the American College of

Surgeons Oncology Group Z0011 randomized trial. Ann Surg. 2010;252:426–32. discussion 32–3

144. Rutgers EJ, Donker M, Straver ME, et al. Radiotherapy or surgery of the axilla after a positive sentinel node in breast cancer patients: final analysis of the EORTC AMAROS trial (10981/ 22023). J Clin Oncol. 2013;31(Suppl; abstract):LBA1001.
145. Katz A, Niemierko A, Gage I, Evans S, Shaffer M, Smith FP, Taghian A, Magnant C. Factors associated with involvement of four or more axillary nodes for sentinel lymph node-positive patients. Int J Radiat Oncol Biol Phys. 2006;65(1):40–4.
146. Beriwal S, Soran A, Kocer B, Wilson JW, Ahrendt GM, Johnson R. Factors that predict the burden of axillary disease in breast cancer patients with a positive sentinel node. Am J Clin Oncol. 2008;31(1):34–8.
147. Sauer T, Kåresen R. The value of preoperative ultrasound guided fine-needle aspiration cytology of radiologically suspicious axillary lymph nodes in breast cancer. Cytojournal. 2014;11:26.
148. Tahir M, Osman KA, Shabbir J, Rogers C, Suarez R, Reynolds T, Bucknall T. Preoperative axillary staging in breast cancer-saving time and resource. Breast J. 2008;14(4):369–71.
149. Kramer GM, Leenders MW, Schijf LJ, Go HL, van der Ploeg T, van den Tol MP, Schreurs WH. Is ultrasound-guided fine-needle aspiration cytology of adequate value in detecting breast cancer patients with three or more positive axillary lymph nodes? Breast Cancer Res Treat. 2016;156(2):271.
150. Neal CH, Daly CP, Nees AV, Helvie MA. Can preoperative axillary US help exclude N2 and N3 metastatic breast cancer? Radiology. 2010;257(2):335–41.
151. Schiettecatte A, Bourgain C, Breucq C, Buls N, De Wilde V, de Mey J. Initial axillary staging of breast cancer using ultrasound-guided fine needle aspiration: a liquid-based cytology study. Cytopathology. 2011;22(1):30–5.
152. van Wely BJ, de Wilt JH, Schout PJ, et al. Ultrasound-guided fine-needle aspiration of suspicious nodes in breast cancer patients; selecting patients with extensive nodal involvement. Breast Cancer Res Treat. 2013;140:113–8.
153. Rocha RD, Girardi AR, Pinto RR, de Freitas VA. Axillary ultrasound and fine-needle aspiration in preoperative staging of axillary lymph nodes in patients with invasive breast cancer. Radiol Bras. 2015;48(6):345–52.
154. Tucker NS, Cyr AE, Ademuyiwa FO, Tabchy A, George K, Sharma PK, Jin LX, Sanati S, Aft R, Gao F, Margenthaler JA, Gillanders WE. Axillary ultrasound accurately excludes clinically significant lymph node disease in patients with early stage breast cancer. Ann Surg. 2016;264(6):1098–102.
155. Fernández B, Paish EC, Green AR, Lee AH, Macmillan RD, Ellis IO, Rakha EA. Lymph-node metastases in invasive lobular carcinoma are different from those in ductal carcinoma of the breast. J Clin Pathol. 2011;64(11):995–1000.
156. Brouckaert O, Laenen A, Smeets A, Christiaens MR, Vergote I, Wildiers H, Moerman P, Floris G, Neven P; MBC Leuven. Prognostic implications of lobular breast cancer histology: new insights from a single hospital cross-sectional study and SEER data. Breast. 2014;23(4):371–7.
157. Boerner S, Sneige N. Specimen adequacy and false-negative diagnosis rate in fine-needle aspirates of palpable breast masses. Cancer. 1998;84(6):344–8.
158. Ganott MA, Zuley ML, Abrams GS, Lu AH, Kelly AE, Sumkin JH, Chivukula M, Carter G, Austin RM, Bandos AI. Ultrasound guided core biopsy versus fine needle aspiration for evaluation of axillary lymphadenopathy in patients with breast cancer. ISRN Oncol. 2014;2014:703160.
159. Holwitt DM, Swatske ME, Gillanders WE, Monsees BS, Gao F, Aft RL, Eberlein TJ, Margenthaler JA. Scientific Presentation Award: the combination of axillary ultrasound and ultrasound-guided biopsy is an accurate predictor of axillary stage in clinically node-negative breast cancer patients. Am J Surg. 2008;196(4):477–82.
160. Diepstraten SC, Sever AR, Buckens CF, Veldhuis WB, van Dalen T, van den Bosch MA, Mali WP, Verkooijen HM. Value of preoperative ultrasound-guided axillary lymph node biopsy for preventing completion axillary lymph node dissection in breast cancer: a systematic review and meta-analysis. Ann Surg Oncol. 2014;21(1):51–9.
161. Mendoza P, Lacambra M, Tan PH, Tse GM. Fine needle aspiration cytology of the breast: the nonmalignant categories. Patholog Res Int. 2011;2011:547580.
162. Scopa CD, Koukouras D, Androulakis J, Bonikos D. Sources of diagnostic discrepancies in fine-needle aspiration of the breast. Diagn Cytopathol. 1991;7(5):546–8.
163. Britton PD, Provenzano E, Barter S, Gaskarth M, Goud A, Moyle P, Sinnatamby R, Wallis M, Benson JR, Forouhi P, Wishart GC. Ultrasound guided percutaneous axillary lymph node core biopsy: how often is the sentinel lymph node being biopsied? Breast. 2009;18(1):13–6.
164. Karnon J, Peters J, Platt J, Chilcott J, McGoogan E, Brewer N. Liquid-based cytology in cervical screening: an updated rapid and systematic review and economic analysis. Health Technol Assess 2004;8(20).
165. Mayor S. NHS cervical screening programme to introduce liquid based cytology. BMJ. 2003;327(7421):948.
166. Saqi A. The state of cell blocks and ancillary testing: past, present, and future. Arch Pathol Lab Med. 2016;140(12):1318–22.
167. Tripathy K, Misra A, Ghosh JK. Efficacy of liquid-based cytology versus conventional smears in FNA samples. J Cytol. 2015;32(1):17–20. https://doi.org/10.4103/0970-9371.155225.
168. Fournier D, Joris F, Pauzé JL, Gaudin G, Vogel J. Avantages pratiques du transport en milieu liquide lors de ponction à l'aiguille fine des lésions du sein : à propos de750 ponctions dont 210 cancers. 21es journées Nationales de la Société Française de Sénologie et de Pathologie Mammaire, 20–22 oct 1999.

169. Joris F, Pauzé JL, Fournier D, Gaudin G, Vogel J. Cytologie des lésions du sein par ponction à l'aiguille : comparaison des potentialités du transport en milieu liquide et de l'analyse en couche mince par rapport à la méthode traditionnelle d'étalement sur lames. Erster Gemeinsamer Senologie Kongress der Deutschen-Österreichischen-Schweizer Gesellschaft für Senologie. Lugano. 5.-8 Juli 2000.
170. Jing X, Wey E, Michael CW. Diagnostic value of fine needle aspirates processed by ThinPrep® for the assessment of axillary lymph node status in patients with invasive carcinoma of the breast. Cytopathology. 2013;24:372–6.
171. Britton P, Moyle P, Benson JR, Goud A, Sinnatamby R, Barter S, Gaskarth M, Provenzano E, Wallis M. Ultrasound of the axilla: where to look for the sentinel lymph node. Clin Radiol. 2010;65(5):373–6.
172. Cox K, Sever A, Jones S, Weeks J, Mills P, Devalia H, Fish D, Jones P. Validation of a technique using microbubbles and contrast enhanced ultrasound (CEUS) to biopsy sentinel lymph nodes (SLN) in pre-operative breast cancer patients with a normal grey-scale axillary ultrasound. Eur J Surg Oncol. 2013;39(7):760–5.
173. Cui XW, Jenssen C, Saftoiu A, et al. New ultrasound techniques for lymph node evaluation. World J Gastroenterol. 2013;19:4850–60.
174. Sever AR, Mills P, Weeks J, Jones SE, Fish D, Jones PA, Mali W. Preoperative needle biopsy of sentinel lymph nodes using intradermal microbubbles and contrast-enhanced ultrasound in patients with breast cancer. AJR Am J Roentgenol. 2012;199(2):465–70.
175. Ouyang Q, Chen L, Zhao H, et al. Detecting metastasis of lymph nodes and predicting aggressiveness in patients with breast carcinomas. J Ultrasound Med. 2010;29:343–52.
176. Yang WT, Metreweli C, Lam PK, Chang J. Benign and malignant breast masses and axillary nodes: evaluation with echo-enhanced color power Doppler US. Radiology. 2001;220:795–802.
177. Genta F, Zanon E, Camanni M, Deltetto F, Drogo M, Gallo R, Gilardi C. Cost/accuracy ratio analysis in breast cancer patients undergoing ultrasound-guided fine-needle aspiration cytology, sentinel node biopsy, and frozen section of node. World J Surg. 2007;31(6):1155–63.
178. Glynn RW, Williams L, Dixon JM. A further survey of surgical management of the axilla in UK breast cancer patients. Ann R Coll Surg Engl. 2010;92(6):506–11.
179. Fillion MM, Glass KE, Hayek J, Wehr A, Phillips G, Terando A, Agnese DM. Healthcare costs reduced after incorporating the results of the American College of Surgeons Oncology Group Z0011 trial into clinical practice. Breast J. 2016;30.
180. Camp MS, Greenup RA, Taghian A, Coopey SB, Specht M, Gadd M, Hughes K, Smith BL. Application of ACOSOG Z0011 criteria reduces perioperative costs. Ann Surg Oncol. 2013;20(3):836–4.
181. McMasters KM, Wong SL, Tuttle TM, Carlson DJ, Brown CM, Dirk Noyes R, Glaser RL, Vennekotter DJ, Turk PS, Tate PS, Sardi A, Edwards MJ. Preoperative lymphoscintigraphy for breast cancer. Ann Surg. 2000;231(5):724–31.
182. Gnant M, Harbeck N, Thomssen C. St. Gallen 2011: summary of the consensus discussion. Breast Care (Basel). 2011;6(2):136–41.
183. Dengel LT, Van Zee KJ, King TA, Stempel M, Cody HS, El-Tamer M, Gemignani ML, Sclafani LM, Sacchini VS, Heerdt AS, Plitas G, Junqueira M, Capko D, Patil S, Morrow M. Axillary dissection can be avoided in the majority of clinically node-negative patients undergoing breast-conserving therapy. Ann Surg Oncol. 2014;21(1):22–7.
184. Giuliano AE, Ballman K, McCall L, Beitsch P, Whitworth PW, Blumencranz P, Leitch AM, Saha S, Morrow M, Hunt KK. Locoregional recurrence after sentinel lymph node dissection with or without axillary dissection in patients with sentinel lymph node metastases: long-term follow-up from the American College of Surgeons Oncology Group (Alliance) ACOSOG Z0011 randomized trial. Ann Surg. 2016;264(3):413–20.
185. Joyce DP, Lowery AJ, McGrath-Soo LB, Downey E, Kelly L, O'Donoghue GT, Barry M, Hill AD. Management of the axilla: has Z0011 had an impact? Ir J Med Sci. 2016;185(1):145–9.
186. Gentilini O, Veronesi U. Abandoning sentinel lymph node biopsy in early breast cancer? A new trial in progress at the European Institute of Oncology of Milan (SOUND: Sentinel node vs Observation after axillary UltraSouND). Breast. 2012;21(5):678–81.
187. Reimer T, Hartmann S, Stachs A, et al. Local treatment of the axilla in early breast cancer: concepts from the National Surgical Adjuvant Breast and Bowel Project B-04 to the planned Intergroup Sentinel Mamma trial. Breast Care (Basel). 2014;9:87–95.
188. Humphrey KL, Saksena MA, Freer PE, Smith BL, Rafferty EA. To do or not to do: axillary nodal evaluation after ACOSOG Z0011 trial. Radiographics. 2014;34(7):1807–16.
189. Reyna C, Kiluk JV, Frelick A, Khakpour N, Laronga C, Lee MC. Impact of axillary ultrasound (AUS) on axillary dissection in breast conserving surgery (BCS). J Surg Oncol. 2015;111(7):813–8.
190. Cox K, Weeks J, Mills P, Chalmers R, Devalia H, Fish D, Sever A. Contrast-enhanced ultrasound biopsy of sentinel lymph nodes in patients with breast cancer: implications for axillary metastases and conservation. Ann Surg Oncol. 2016;23(1):58–64.
191. Moorman AM, Bourez RL, Heijmans HJ, Kouwenhoven EA. Axillary ultrasonography in breast cancer patients helps in identifying patients preoperatively with limited disease of the axilla. Ann Surg Oncol. 2014;21(9):2904–10.

Lymphoscintigraphy and Sentinel Node Localization in Breast Cancer

11

Cornelis A. Hoefnagel

Take Home Messages

The sentinel lymph node biopsy (SLNB) is an important tool in breast cancer for nodal staging at the microscopic level.

Using the sentinel lymph node biopsy, radical lymphadenectomy can be avoided in the majority of breast cancer patients, leading to increased patient benefit and reduction of complications.

After intratumoral or closely peritumoral administration of the tracer, the lymphoscintigram will best represent the tumor's lymphatic drainage according to the lobar concept.

To ensure that the correct lymph node is identified and removed as "sentinel node," it is imperative that preoperative imaging is optimized by every possible means.

SPECT/CT is more sensitive and more accurate than planar lymphoscintigraphy, especially in locating non-axillary sentinel nodes, and this may influence the surgical approach.

The sentinel node lymph node biopsy is a safe procedure both for the patient and the hospital staff.

C.A. Hoefnagel
Nuclear Medicine Consultant, Fazantstraat 38, 1171 HS Badhoevedorp, The Netherlands
e-mail: keeshoefnagel@quicknet.nl

11.1 Introduction: Role of Nuclear Medicine in Breast Cancer

In view of the high incidence of breast cancer in women, this disease has always been an important indication for a variety of nuclear medicine procedures. In the era of planar scintigraphy, bone scintigraphy, tumor imaging, scintimammography, and lymphoscintigraphy, as well as the ejection fraction test monitoring potential cardiac side effects of chemotherapy were used.

Although bone scintigraphy remains important in the staging and follow-up of breast cancer, nowadays, the Sentinel Lymph Node Biopsy (SLNB) has become an important tool for staging of operable breast tumors at the nodal level, and hybrid imaging techniques are used, which, by combining functional parameters (provided by PET or SPECT), with anatomical reference (provided by CT or MRI), provide greater sensitivity, specificity, and accuracy.

SPECT/CT, performed in addition to planar bone scintigraphy, enables more accurate detection and localization of bone metastases. Moreover, it is helpful in differentiating metastases from hot spots due to a great variety of benign bone abnormalities.

Positron-emission tomography (PET) using ^{18}F-fluorodeoxyglucose (FDG) offers great sensitivity and accuracy for diagnosis, staging, restaging, and response monitoring [1]. Although MRI

D. Amy (ed.), *Lobar Approach to Breast Ultrasound*, https://doi.org/10.1007/978-3-319-61681-0_11

is the better technique for the T-staging of primary breast cancers, PET/CT is better than MRI in detecting nodal and distant metastases. Nevertheless, the SLNB remains the best technique for nodal staging at the microscopic level. For the detection of osteolytic and bone marrow metastases, FDG-PET/CT is better than bone scintigraphy, whereas the latter is better in osteosclerotic (osteoblastic) metastases. Breast carcinoma may have both types of skeletal metastases. PET/CT using ^{18}F as fluoride may be used for bone imaging and has a higher sensitivity than bone scintigraphy. ^{18}F-FDG-PET/CT is also useful in monitoring response to (preoperative) chemotherapy [2], as well as, during follow-up, in the detection of nodal recurrence and metastases.

Because not all tumors accumulate high amounts of FDG and this radiopharmaceutical is aspecific and it is difficult to access the breast for PET-guided biopsy, lately, a great number of more specific agents are being used and new technologies have been developed. The latter includes the use of dedicated breast PET techniques (PEM, Mammi PET) [3], allowing biopsy of the metabolically most active part of the tumor, and PET/MR, which combines the most sensitive (but little specific) technique for breast imaging (MR breast) with molecular imaging by PET, which increases the specificity and improves the detection and evaluation of lesions in (for MRI) more difficult areas [4].

This chapter will focus on lymphoscintigraphic techniques and sentinel lymph node mapping.

11.2 Lymphoscintigraphy in Breast Carcinoma

Since the early 1970s, a variety of lymphoscintigraphic applications, using a gamma camera after administration of technetium-99m-labeled microcolloids, have been used in breast cancer [5], including the study of lymphedema, the alterations of lymphatic drainage after surgery and the use of internal mammary lymphoscintigraphy in radiation therapy planning. From these early experiences lessons were learned, which are relevant to the more recent development, i.e., lymphatic mapping as an integral part of the sentinel lymph node biopsy procedure. A similar technique is used for radioguided occult lesion localization (ROLL).

A significant burden to patients may be the occurrence of lymphedema of the arm as a consequence of radical surgery and/or radiotherapy of regional lymph nodes. One of the very reasons to perform the sentinel node biopsy procedure is to avoid this mutilation by (in hindsight) unnecessary lymph node dissection and to carry out this surgery only when mandatory because of lymph node (micro)metastases.

If lymphedema occurs, the speed and pattern of lymphatic drainage of the extremity can be objectivated and assessed by lymphoscintigraphy in a semiquantitative way [6]. The results may help decide if lymphatic microsurgery is possible or conservative treatment is indicated and can determine the benefit of such treatments during follow-up [7].

Lymphoscintigraphy can also demonstrate the altered drainage pathways after breast surgery with lymph node dissection. In a study comparing preoperative and postoperative lymphoscintigraphy in patients with breast carcinoma undergoing mastectomy with radical axillary lymph node dissection, drainage to the homolateral axilla was visualized in 26/32 patients preoperatively; however, after surgery, drainage to the contralateral axilla was demonstrated in 8 patients (29%), which has consequences for follow-up and the management of a nodal recurrence in the contralateral axilla [8]. Where a contralateral lymph node metastasis was regarded more or less as a sign of distant metastases, in our current sentinel node concept, it would be regarded as the "new" sentinel node (neo sentinel node).

To facilitate radiation therapy to the internal mammary nodes in patients with breast cancer, the position of these nodes as well as alternative lymphatic pathways may be visualized by internal mammary lymphoscintigraphy. Indications for radiotherapy to these nodes are a medial or central localization of the primary tumor, axillary lymph node metastases, inoperable breast carcinoma, a tumor-positive subclavicular lymph node biopsy, and local tumor recurrence.

40–80 MBq (1–2 mCi) of ^{99m}Tc-nanocolloid in a small volume (0.1–0.2 ml) is injected intramuscularly into the abdominal anterior rectus muscle

Table 11.1 The prognostic significance of internal mammary lymphoscintigraphic (IML) findings

	Ege 1978 [10]	Bourgeois 1998 [13]
Nodal status	Relapse rates at 3 years	Relapse / progression rates
Axilla negative/IML negative	9%	4%
Axilla positive/IML negative	21%	28%
Axilla negative/IML positive	21%	13%
Axilla positive/IML positive	32%	45%
	5 -year survival	Relapse percentage
Normal IML	83%	21%
Pathological IML	50%	40%

on the side of the affected breast, in the direction of the homolateral axilla under a 45 degree angle and approximately after 2 h a static lymphoscintigram with ^{57}Co-markers indicating the sternal midline is made; subsequently, an injection is given into the contralateral rectus muscle and 2 h later scintigraphy is repeated with and without ^{57}Co-markers on the corners of the standard radiation field. This way it can be determined if all nodes are included in the standard radiation field (if not, this must be corrected) and what the minimal and maximal distances from the midline are (to see if the radiation field can be shrunk, to avoid irradiating too much lung tissue).

The lymphoscintigram is scored as normal, equivocal/suspected, or pathological, criteria for pathology being an incomplete chain of lymph nodes and obvious filling defects in nodes [5]. From histology, it is known that, in operable breast carcinoma, metastases to the internal mammary nodes are present in 9–24% of the patients [9], and the reported percentages of pathological lymphoscintigrams of 22–27% are in concordance with this [10, 11]. In addition, the scintigram may disclose the so-called crossing over phenomenon, i.e. contralateral nodes, which in most cases would be outside the standard radiation field.

Experience with this technique in many thousands of patients at the Netherlands Cancer Institute demonstrated an overall percentage of pathology of 27.9% and that this percentage increased with the stage of disease. Correction of the radiation field was required in 26.5% of the patients, and the crossing over phenomenon, nearly always requiring field correction, occurred in 14.0% of normal and 45.3% of abnormal lymphoscintigrams [11].

Of relevance to the sentinel node biopsy procedure is the observed great individual variability in lymphatic drainage and the fact that long-term follow-up studies by Ege [12] and Bourgeois [13] have demonstrated the prognostic significance of the internal mammary nodes, in analogy with the more accepted prognostic parameter of the axillary nodes: in patients with a normal lymphoscintigram, Ege found a 5-year survival rate of 83%, in contrast with 50% survival in patients with a pathological lymphoscintigram (Table 11.1).

11.3 Sentinel Lymph Node Biopsy: From Concept to Practice

In 1977, the urological surgeon Cabanas was the first to use the term "sentinel node," when he reported his (radiological) approach to the management of penile carcinoma [14]. But it was not till 1992, that the sentinel node biopsy procedure in surgical oncology was introduced in early stage melanoma by Morton [15]. The procedure is based upon the concept of an orderly progression of lymph node metastases: the tumor drains directly to one or few first lymph nodes, called sentinel node(s), from which further connections with so-called second echelon nodes exist [16].

First, the lymphatic drainage pathways from the tumor are mapped, and the sentinel node(s) is/are identified by lymphoscintigraphy and marked on the skin [17], so that, subsequently, these can be localized more easily during surgery, by combined use of an intraoperative probe and injection of patent blue dye and then selectively removed [18]. If, by pathology [19], these first tier node(s) is/are found to be free of tumor cells, more extensive nodal surgery, which may be associated with additional morbidity and complications, e.g., lymphedema, can be avoided.

This procedure represents a sensitive staging method. The detection rate of the combined approach in breast cancer ranges 93–100%, versus 66–82% for blue dye only, and 84–93% for using the probe without lymphoscintigraphic imaging [5]. The number of false-negative results is inversely related (Table 11.2).

The sentinel lymph node biopsy (SLNB) procedure is an important tool in surgical oncology for nodal staging of operable tumors. However, in order to base the entire treatment policy on the analysis of a single or few lymph node(s), it is imperative that the correct lymph node is identified as the sentinel node. To make this procedure as successful and reliable as possible, the lymphoscintigraphic studies must meet the highest-quality criteria, which can be achieved by using the right radiopharmaceutical (generally technetium-99m-labeled microcolloids with a diameter ranging 5–75 nm are preferred), meticulous tracer administration (depending on the indication) and by using a modern gamma camera, performing imaging at several time intervals both in the anterior and lateral projection (and for breast carcinoma in prone position), defining the body contour by means of transmission scanning using a ^{57}Co-flood source, and identifying and localizing the sentinel node(s) with the aid of a marker source or pen, marking its site on the skin with non-erasable ink in the position in which the patient will be operated [29].

After this technique was introduced for melanoma and breast carcinoma in the early 1990's, the number of clinical indications has expanded significantly, and the SLNB is now used in a great variety of tumor types, including penile carcinoma, vulvar carcinoma, testicular cancer, cervical carcinoma, prostatic cancer, bladder cancer, head and neck cancer, thyroid carcinoma, lung cancer, esophageal, gastric and colorectal cancers, anal carcinoma and Merkel cell tumor. For some indications, planar lymphoscintigraphy may suffice to locate the sentinel node. But for tumors or lymphatics located in anatomically more challenging regions (e.g. head and neck, abdominal and pelvic areas) more advanced technologies, e.g. SPECT/CT and use of an intraoperative mini gamma camera, are needed.

The major success determining factors for the sentinel node biopsy procedure are administered dose, colloid size, number of colloid particles (concentration), and route of administration, protocol, and quality of the lymphoscintigram. As there is a distinct learning curve for both nuclear medicine physicians, technologists, and surgeons, experience is an equally important factor, as is teamwork between nuclear medicine, surgery, and pathology departments [5].

Table 11.2 Sentinel node biopsy in breast cancer: techniques and results

Author	Number of patients	SN identified	False negative
Blue dye only			
Giuliano et al. [20]	174	0.66	0.11
Guenther et al. [21]	145	0.71	0.1
Flett et al. [22]	68	0.82	0.17
Probe only			
Crossin et al. [23]	50	0.84	0.13
Krag et al. [24]	443	0.93	0.11
Scan/dye/probe			
Doting et al. [25]	136	0.93	0.05
Cox et al. [26]	466	0.94	0.01
Chatterjee et al. [27]	60	0.97	0.05
V/d Ent et al. [28]	70	1	0.04

11.4 The Sentinel Node in Breast Carcinoma in View of the Lobar Concept

The axillary lymph node dissection (ALND) has always been regarded as an important staging procedure in breast cancer surgery. However, with the trend toward early diagnosis, the number of tumor-negative dissections is increasing, and the procedure is associated with a number of complications, e.g. pain, paresthesia, infection, lymphedema, and impaired shoulder function. After a learning phase and by adherence to criteria for high quality, also the sentinel lymph node biopsy (SNLB) procedure is an accurate staging method, which minimizes the number of unnecessary ALNDs, decreases the risk of avoidable morbidity, and may provide a better cosmetic result. The main indications for the sentinel node procedure are operable, palpable breast carcinoma without any clinical evidence of lymph node metastases and non-palpable tumors, for which the probe may be used both to detect the sentinel node and localize the non-palpable lesion.

Where the focus of interest for staging and prognostication was on the axilla, originally, lymphoscintigraphic studies have demonstrated that the drainage pathways from the breast are multiple and more complex and that the location of the sentinel node(s) shows great individual variability. Apart from drainage to the homolateral axilla, there may be drainage to the internal mammary nodes, to intramammary nodes, intra- and subpectoral nodes, subclavicular nodes, and contralateral axillary nodes. Therefore, lymphatic mapping of the sentinel node(s) requires high quality scintigraphic studies. The results of these studies may be influenced by many factors, and the procedure will be improved if these are taken into consideration.

Several routes of administration are being applied: subcutaneous, peritumoral, and intratumoral. Table 11.3 summarizes the characteristics of each of these approaches: four peritumoral injections closely around the tumor and a single intratumoral injection show comparable scintigraphic results, the more circumscript injection site being an advantage of the latter technique, enabling the visualization of intramammary lymphatic vessels and nodes, as well as axillary nodes close to the tumor (Fig. 11.1). Of the three techniques, lymphoscintigraphy after subcutaneous administration will reflect the tumor's drain-

Table 11.3 Sentinel node procedure in breast carcinoma: route of administration

	Subcutaneous	Peritumoral	Intratumoral
Injection	Single	Multiple	Single
Drainage (speed)	Fast	Slow	Fast/slow
Injection site on scintigram	Prominent	Very prominent	Circumscript
Internal mammary nodes	Rarely seen	++	++
Intramammary nodes	Never seen	+	++
Reflects tumor's drainage	+/–	+	++
Reflects lobar drainage	–	+	++

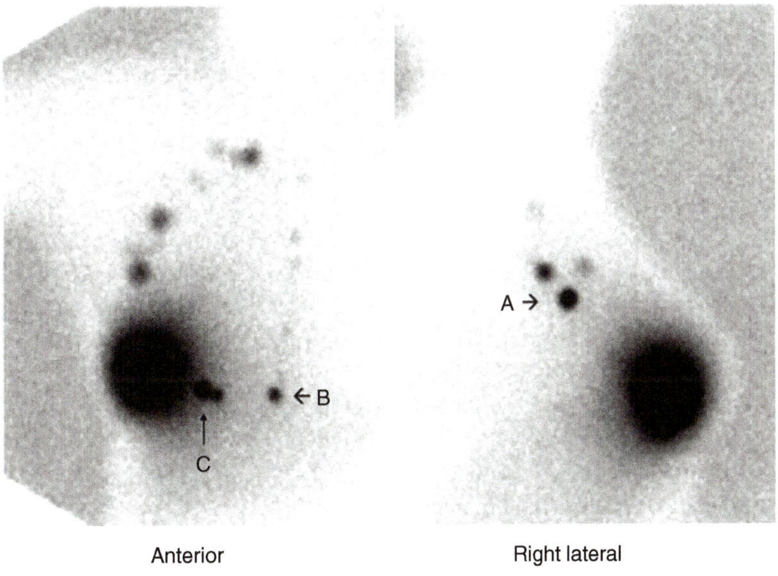

Fig. 11.1 Planar scintigrams of sentinel nodes in breast carcinoma after intratumoral injection, best matching the tumor's drainage in accordance with the lobar concept. Moreover, the circumscript injection site allows the detection of sentinel nodes in three lymphatic basins: in the axilla (**a**), the internal mammary chain (**b**), and intramammary (**c**)

age the least, as is apparent from the rare visualization of non-axillary lymph nodes. In a comparative study using both subdermal and peritumoral injections in 78 patients with carcinoma of the breast, Alazraki et al. [30] demonstrated that, although in 74/79 patients, the same axillary nodes were identified as sentinel nodes, the peritumoral technique showed internal mammary nodes, not visualized after subdermal injection, in 19 patients (21%).

In the context of the concept of the lobar approach, it should be emphasized that lobar lymphatic drainage is best demonstrated by lymphoscintigraphy after intratumoral administration, as it always reflects drainage of the tumor within its lobe, unlike lymphoscintigraphy after subcutaneous injection; (closely) peritumoral administration (four injections around the tumor) may also reflect lobar drainage but, in case of a tumor located near the edge of a lobe, may also represent drainage of the neighboring lob, if any of the injections have occurred into that lobe. In some centers, the subdermal route is favored for imaging of the axillary node, while for intraoperative localization of nonpalpable tumors, an intratumoral administration is done. However, both the tumor location and its lymphatic drainage can be demonstrated effectively and more reliable by a single procedure after intratumoral administration.

As in breast carcinoma patients, the lymphatic drainage is generally slower than is the case in melanoma after intracutaneous administration; it is important to make scintigrams at several time intervals in both anterior (supine) and lateral (prone) projection, as drainage may be fast or slow or a combination of both in patients with multiple sentinel nodes.

Of the first 549 breast carcinoma patients undergoing the SLNB procedure after intratumoral injection at The Netherlands Cancer Institute, 206 pathological sentinel nodes were found (37.5%), the majority of which in the homolateral axilla. Non-axillary sentinel nodes were detected in 149 patients (27%), 15 of whom without a sentinel node in the axilla [31]. They were either located in the internal mammary chain (104 patients; 19%), intramammary (38 patients), in the interpectoral nodes (9 patients), or in the infra- or supraclavicular nodes (12 patients). Overall, 128 (86%) of these nodes could be removed by the surgeon, 26 of which proved to be tumor positive (20%). As a consequence of this finding, the therapeutic management of these patients was altered. In analogy with a tumor-positive sentinel node in the axilla leading to surgical clearing of the affected axilla, the finding of a tumor-positive sentinel node in the internal mammary chain indicates the need for radiation therapy to these nodes.

Looking at the drainage patterns of ^{99m}Tc-nanocolloid in relation to the site of the primary breast tumor in 700 consecutive patients undergoing the sentinel node procedure with intratumoral administration, Estourgie et al. [32] found drainage to the internal mammary nodes to occur in 32.4% of tumors in the upper inner quadrant, 52.0% from the lower inner quadrant, 29.5% from the lower outer quadrant, 10.4% from the upper outer quadrant, and 23.7% from the center of the breast. Moreover, non-palpable lesions tended to drain toward the internal mammary nodes more frequently than palpable tumors.

The lymphoscintigraphic results can be further improved by optimalizing the administered dose and number of colloid particles: using a mean administered dose of 61.6 MBq ^{99m}Tc-nanocolloid in the first 100 patients at The Netherlands Cancer Institute, the scintigraphic sentinel node detection rate was 83%, and the overall identification rate (i.e. using scan, probe, and blue dye during surgery) was 90%. By increasing the dose in the subsequent 75 patients (mean dose 93.4 MBq), the detection rates rose to 93% and the identification rate to 97% [33]. By doubling the number of colloid particles at the same dose level in a third group (76 patients), the sentinel node was scintigraphically detected in 99% of the patients; moreover, lymphatic vessels, helpful in identifying the sentinel node, were more often shown, and the count rates of the sentinel node, facilitating the retrieval by the surgeon handling the probe, were higher, and, most importantly, more pathological nodes were found [34].

As breast cancer screening programs are progressively introduced in various countries, surgeons and diagnostic imaging departments are increasingly confronted with non-palpable breast lesions, which are not necessarily all malignant. If by mammography, ultrasonography and cytology the diagnosis breast carcinoma can be established; the sentinel node procedure is also applicable to this group of patients, which may have the greatest benefits of breast conserving surgery and sentinel lymph node biopsy. After intratumoral administration of the tracer, guided by ultrasonography or stereotaxis or an ^{125}I-seed, the sentinel lymph node biopsy, using the same imaging protocol, is performed with equally good results as in palpable tumors [35]. At the same time, the primary tumor can be located easily with the intraoperative probe for excision [36].

Radioguided occult lesion localization (ROLL) is a technique used for diagnostic excisional biopsy, instead of the traditional use of the hooked wire to guide the surgeon [37]. The radiopharmaceutical is injected intralesionally as described above, and, after scintigraphic confirmation, the surgeon excises the lesion. In case the lesion happens to be malignant, the sentinel lymph node biopsy occurs at a separate occasion.

11.5 The Role of Hybrid Imaging

In selected cases, single photon emission tomography combined with computerized tomography (SPECT/CT) may be added to planar scintigraphy for a great variety of indications, one of which is sentinel lymph node mapping [38]. Following planar scintigraphy, SPECT of the selected area is performed. Subsequently, an X-topogram of the area of interest is made, followed by a spiral CT-scan, either with low dose (which suffices in most cases) or with a higher ("diagnostic") dose and IV contrast. The reconstructed and attenuation corrected SPECT images are fused with the CT slices, resulting in a series of transaxial, coronal, and sagittal SPECT/CT fusion images.

SPECT/CT is of great value for the detection and proper localization of sentinel nodes of breast cancer, especially if it concerns the localization of non-axillary sentinel nodes, e.g., internal mammary, intramammary, interpectoral, and subpectoral nodes, and to exclude false-positive findings due to non-nodal tracer accumulation (e.g., intralymphatic or contamination). It provides the surgeon the anatomical detail needed to approach and resect sentinel nodes (Fig. 11.2). In case of non-visualization of a sentinel node by planar lymphoscintigraphy, the sentinel node can still be detected by SPECT/CT in half of the cases [39].

Sequential images of planar lymphoscintigraphy will remain important to identify lymph nodes appearing early as sentinel nodes. However, the anatomical localization of these sentinel nodes is better achieved by SPECT/CT

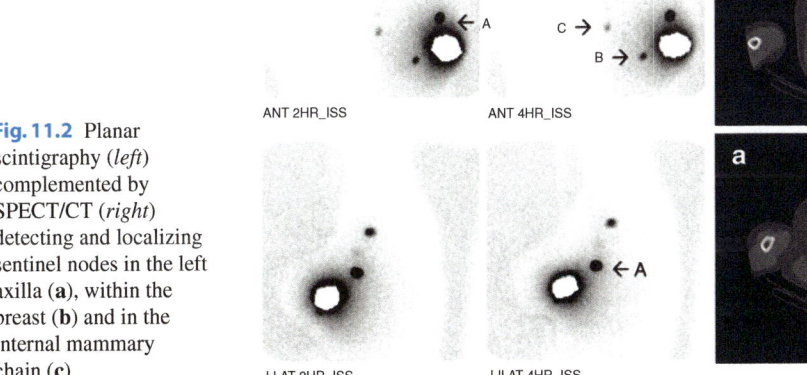

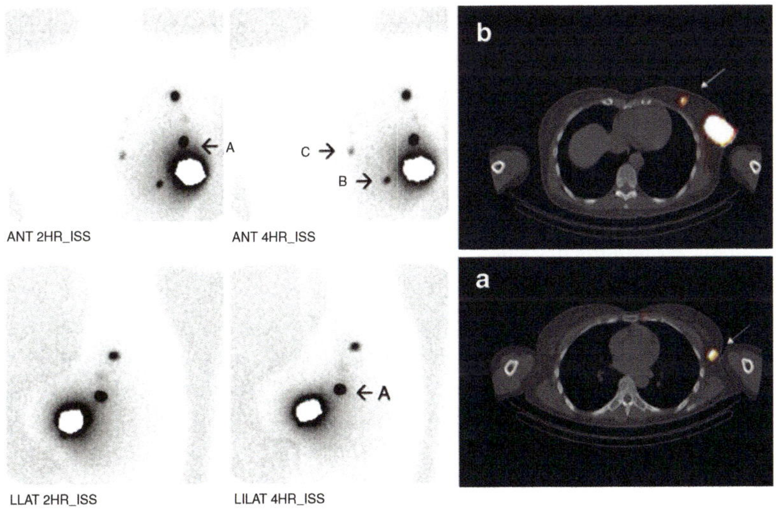

Fig. 11.2 Planar scintigraphy (*left*) complemented by SPECT/CT (*right*) detecting and localizing sentinel nodes in the left axilla (**a**), within the breast (**b**) and in the internal mammary chain (**c**)

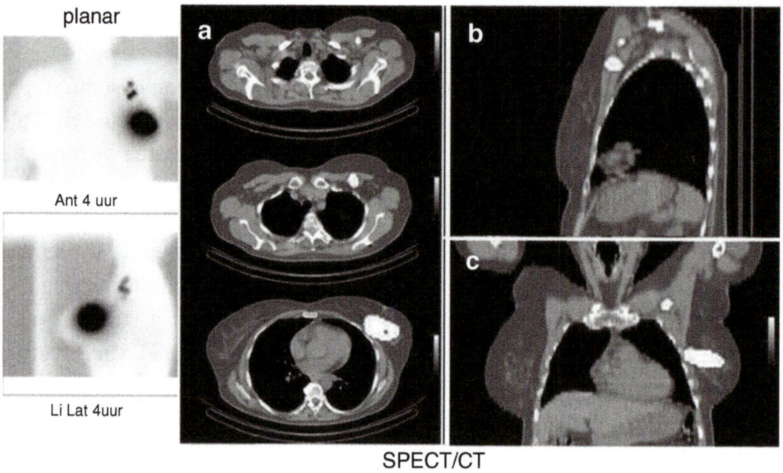

Fig. 11.3 Sentinel node mapping of a non-palpable breast carcinoma, centrally located in the upper outer quadrant of the *left* breast. Where the planar scintigram (*left*) might suggest drainage to the *left* axilla, SPECT/CT images in the transaxial (**a**), sagittal (**b**), and coronal (**c**) projection accurately localize the nodes between the two pectoral muscles, altering the surgical approach

(Fig. 11.3). Although PET/CT and PET/MR using ^{18}F-fluorodeoxyglucose (FDG) offer great sensitivity and accuracy for diagnosis, staging, restaging, and response monitoring in breast cancer, the sentinel node biopsy remains the best technique for nodal staging at the microscopic level.

Taking the SPECT/CT study one step further, it is possible to display the SPECT/CT fusion images in a two-dimensional way (transaxial, coronal, and/or sagittal sections) or in a three-dimensional way. For the latter, SPECT/CT fusion images are stacked and displayed in a volume-rendered way. The software allows to choose from a variety of parameters, by which the sentinel node(s) can be displayed within its surrounding environment, highlighting anatomical structures, such as the bone, muscle, and/or skin. Although the 3D volume-rendered images (either displayed in a static, rotational, or tilted mode) contain essentially the same information as the 2D-tomographic fusion images, the 3D volume-rendered display provides the surgeon with a three-dimensional road map, which is attractive and more easily interpretable (Fig. 11.4). Improved anatomical information to the surgeon may influence the surgical approach with the aim to preserve normal anatomical structures. New developments include the use of an intraoperative mini gamma camera during surgery and combination of gamma probe detection with fluorescence imaging during surgery after injecting a hybrid tracer (^{99m}Tc-nanocolloid + indocyan green).

11.6 Cost and Safety Issues

In many countries, the incidence of breast carcinoma is high. In the Netherlands, this disease accounts for 30.7% of all new cancer cases in women (0.1% in men), which means that 1 out of 10 women will encounter breast carcinoma during her lifetime.

A cost-benefit analysis of the sentinel lymph node biopsy versus radical lymphadenectomy in melanoma patients demonstrated significant savings together with a significantly lower number of complications [40]. In breast carcinoma, the financial benefit is less striking. Gemignani et al. [41] showed that overall hospital charges for the two procedures are similar, which is mostly due to the higher pathology charges and the use of frozen section analysis in the SLNB group. When the sentinel node is tumor negative, the hospital costs of the SLNB are lower than those of axillary lymph node dissection; however, when posi-

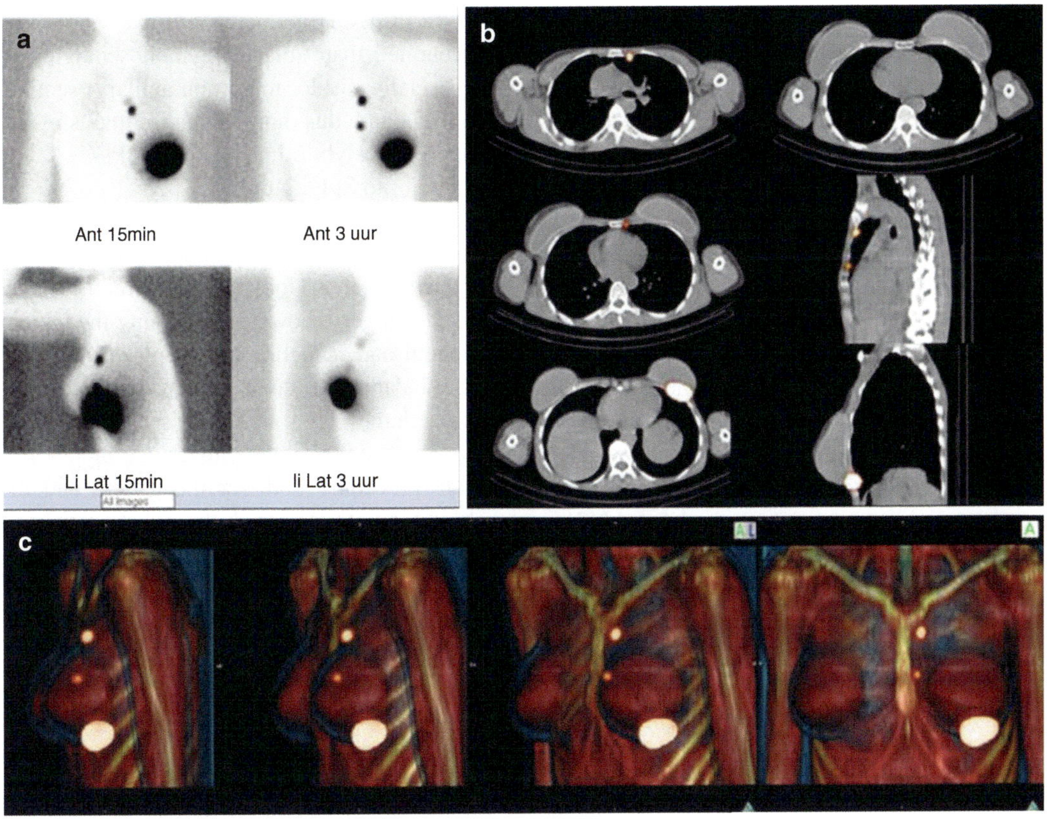

Fig. 11.4 Non-palpable breast carcinoma after bilateral breast implant with lymphatic drainage exclusively to the internal mammary nodes, as shown by planar scintigraphy (**a**), SPECT/CT (**b**) and 3D volume rendering (**c**)

tive, the costs are higher, especially when a correction of the pathology findings after immunohistochemistry leads to repeat admission for surgery. Nevertheless, the initial lack of financial gain must be balanced against the benefit of prevention of morbidity as a result of less extensive surgery, shorter anesthesia time, shorter hospital stay, fewer infections, fewer surgical complications, as well as the cosmetic effects and reduction in patient burden/suffering and social impact (e.g., the absence from work, inability to resume previous work, reeducation, acceptance). In a number of patients cost of radiotherapy to the internal mammary nodes and of conservative treatment or microsurgery of lymphedemic arms, which would be incurred later, are avoided.

The principal radiation safety issues to be considered are the absorbed radiation dose to the patient, the exposure and cumulative radiation burden to hospital staff and contamination of the environment. As lymphoscintigraphy is a routine nuclear medicine technique using a relatively low administered dose of technetium-99m, and the resected ^{99m}Tc-containing tissues are not readily disposed of, the environment is not at risk. The radiocolloid uptake in sentinel nodes is only a small fraction of the administered dose: at the Netherlands Cancer Institute the amount of activity in resected sentinel nodes has been measured in 51 patients with breast carcinoma, 24 h after administration of nominally 74 MBq ^{99m}Tc-nanocolloid. The mean uptake in the sentinel nodes was 6.5 kBq (range 0.03–102 kBq), which is 0.16% (range 0.001–2.5%) of the injected radiocolloid [42].

Due to the relatively low administered dose of technetium-99m, lymphoscintigraphy carries a low radiation burden to the patient; by far the greatest absorbed radiation dose is at the injection site, i.e., in case of intratumoral injection, the primary tumor, which will be resected. In comparison, the doses to the total body, bone marrow, ovaries, or testes are significantly lower (roughly ten times less than that of a routine bone scan).

As for the hospital staff, radiation protection measures for the SLNB must focus on reducing the exposure to external radiation (by limiting the duration of exposure, keeping distance where possible, shielding of radioactive materials, the timing of surgery, and monitoring personnel with thermoluminescence detectors and/or pocket dosemeters) and on avoiding internal contamination with radioactivity, i.e., by preventing inhalation (mask) and ingestion (gloves), avoiding accidental wounds, removing radioactive waste, and considering all used surgical instruments as contaminated [43].

The radiation burden to patient and personnel is low, and it can be extrapolated that a surgeon, operating 3–6 h after injection of 75 MBq ^{99m}Tc-microcolloid, can perform at least 2000 sentinel node biopsies per year before reaching the annual dose limit to the hands of the general public (50 mSv/yr) [44]. In practice this will not be reached.

Calculating the radiation exposure and dose to the hands and body for each of the staff members who are consecutively involved in the sentinel node procedure, it is shown that the highest dose will be to the hands of the nuclear medicine physician during the administration of the radiopharmaceutical. Subsequently, during the imaging phase, the nuclear medicine technologists receive a relatively low dose. With respect to the dose to the surgical staff, it should be noted that a surgeon can reduce the radiation dose to the hands and body by a factor 10 by operating 24 h instead of 4 h after the administration of the radiopharmaceutical. The radiation dose to the pathologist is negligible [5].

Conclusions

The sentinel lymph node biopsy is an important tool in breast cancer for nodal staging at the microscopic level.

To ensure that the correct lymph node is identified and removed as "sentinel node," it is imperative that preoperative imaging is optimized by every possible means.

SPECT/CT is more sensitive and more accurate than planar lymphoscintigraphy, especially in locating non-axillary sentinel nodes, and this may influence the surgical approach. Hybrid imaging with SPECT/CT is superior to SPECT only.

In breast carcinoma, the sentinel lymph node biopsy is not a particular cost-efficient procedure, if one looks at costs directly related to the surgery; however, weighing the patient benefit and reduction of complications bring the balance in favor of the sentinel node procedure.

The sentinel node lymph node biopsy is a safe procedure both for the patient and the hospital staff. Although the radiation risks to personnel are low, adequate radiation protection guidelines and timing of the procedure may further reduce the radiation dose to personnel.

References

1. Koolen BB, Vrancken Peeters MJTFD, Aukema TS, et al. 18F-FDG PET/CT as staging procedure in primary stage II and III breast cancer: comparison with conventional imaging techniques. Breast Cancer Res Treat. 2012;131:117–26.
2. Groheux D, Giacchetti S, Espie M, et al. Early monitoring of response to neoadjuvant chemotherapy in breast cancer with 18F-FDG PET/CT: defining a clinical aim. Eur J Nucl Med Mol Imaging. 2011;38:419–25.
3. Koolen BB, Vogel WV, Vrancken Peeters MJTFD, et al. Molecular imaging of breast cancer: from whole-body PET/CT to dedicated breast PET. J Oncol. 2012;2012:438647.
4. Pace L, Nicolai E, Luongo A, et al. Comparison of whole body PET/CT and PET/MRI in breast cancer patients: lesion detection and quatitation of 18F-deoxyglucose uptake in lesions and in normal organ tissues. Eur J Radiol. 2014;83:289–96.
5. Hoefnagel CA, Sivro-Prndelj F, Valdés Olmos RA. Lymphoscintigraphy and sentinel node procedures in breast carcinoma: role, techniques and safety aspects. World J Nucl Med. 2002;1:45–54.
6. McNeill G, Witte M, Witte C, et al. Whole-body lymphoscintigraphy: preferred method for initial assessment of the peripheral lymphatic system. Radiology. 1989;172:495–502.
7. Vaqueiro M, Gloviczki P, Fisher J, et al. Lymphoscintigraphy in lymphedema: aid to microsurgery. J Nucl Med. 1986;27:1125–30.

8. Perre CI, Hoefnagel CA, Kroon BBR, et al. Altered lymphatic drainage after lymphadenectomy or radiotherapy of the axilla in breast cancer patients: a lymphoscintigraphic study. Br J Surg. 1996;83:1258.
9. Haagensen CD. Metastasis of carcinoma of the breast to the periphery of the regional lymph node filter. Ann Surg. 1969;169:174–19.
10. Ege GN. Internal mammary lymphoscintigraphy: a rational adjunct to the staging and management of breast carcinoma. Clin Radiol. 1978;29:453–6.
11. Hoefnagel CA, Bartelink H, Heidendal Jeune M, Marcuse HR. Internal mammary lymphoscintigraphy for radiation therapy planning in breast carcinoma. J Eur Radiother. 1982;3:35–42.
12. Ege GN, Elhakim T. The relevance of internal mammary lymphoscintigraphy in the management of breast carcinoma. J Clin Oncol. 1984;7:774–81.
13. Bourgeois P, Frühling J. Lymphoscintigraphy in adult malignancy. In: Murray IPC, Ell PJ, editors. Nuclear medicine in clinical diagnosis and treatment. 2nd ed. Edinburgh: Churchill Livingstone; 1998. p. 783–90.
14. Cabanas RM. An approach to the treatment of penile carcinoma. Cancer. 1977;39:456–66.
15. Morton DL, Wen DR, Wong JH, et al. Technical details of intraoperative lymphatic mapping for early stage melanoma. Arch Surg. 1992;127:392–9.
16. Reintgen D, Cruse CW, Wells K, et al. The orderly progression of melanoma nodal metastases. Ann Surg. 1994;220:759–67.
17. Nieweg OE, Valdés Olmos RA, Jansen L, et al. Cutaneous lymphoscintigraphy. In: Nieweg E, Reintgen T, editors. Lymphatic mapping and probe applications in cancer. New York: Marcel Dekker; 2000. p. 43–70.
18. Rutgers EJT, Muller SH, Hoefnagel CA. The use of intraoperative probes in surgical oncology. In: Murray IPC, Ell PJ, editors. Nuclear medicine in clinical diagnosis and treatment. 2nd ed. London: Churchill Livingstone; 1998. p. 1025–36.
19. Van Diest PJ, Peterse HJ, Borgstein PJ, et al. Pathological investigation of sentinel lymph nodes. Eur J Nucl Med. 1999;26(suppl):S43–9.
20. Giuliano AE, Kirgan DM, Guenther JM, Morton DL. Lymphatic mapping and sentinel lymphadenectomy for breast cancer. Ann Surg. 1994;220:391–8.
21. Guenther JM, Krishnamoorthy M, Tan LR. Sentinel lymphadenectomy for breast cancer in a community managed care setting. Cancer J Sci Am. 1997;3:336–40.
22. Flett MM, Going JJ, Stanton PD, Cooke TG. Sentinel node localization in patients with breast cancer. Br J Surg. 1998;85:991–3.
23. Crossin JA, Johnson AC, Stewart PB, Turner WW Jr. Gamma-probe-guided resection of the sentinel node in breast cancer. Am Surg. 1998;64:666–8.
24. Krag D, Weaver D, Ashikaga T, et al. The sentinel node in breast cancer—a multicenter validation study. N Engl J Med. 1998;339:941–6.
25. Doting MH, Jansen L, Nieweg OE, et al. Lymphatic mapping with intralesional tracer administration in breast carcinoma patients. Cancer. 2000;88:2546–52.
26. Cox CE, Pendas S, Cox JM, et al. Guidelines for sentinel node biopsy and lymphatic mapping of patients with breast cancer. Ann Surg. 1998;227:645–51.
27. Chatterjee S, Menon M, Drew PJ, et al. Sentinel node biopsy in primary breast cancer: a prospective assessment of two complementary techniques. Eur J Surg Oncol. 1998;24:615–6.
28. Van de Ent FWC, Kengen RAM, Van der Poll HAG, Hoofwijk AGM. Sentinel node biopsy in 70 unselected patients with breast cancer: increased feasibility by using 10 mCi radiocolloid in combination with a blue dye tracer. Eur J Surg Oncol. 1999;25:24–9.
29. Uren RF, Hoefnagel CA. Lymphoscintigraphy. In: Thompson JF, Morton DL, Kroon BBR, editors. Melanoma. London: Martin Dunitz; 2004. p. 339–64.
30. Alazraki NP, Grant S, Styblo T, et al. Peritumoral (PT) vs subdermal (SD) injection methods for sentinel lymph node (SLN) imaging and intraoperative localization using 2 filtration sizes. J Nucl Med. 2000;41:71. (abstr)
31. Tanis PJ, Nieweg OE, Valdés Olmos RA, et al. Impact of non-axillary sentinel node biopsy on staging and treatment of breast cancer patients. Br J Cancer. 2002;87:705–10.
32. Estourgie SH, Valdés Olmos RA, Nieweg OE, et al. Lymphatic drainage patterns from the breast. Ann Surg. 2004;239:232–7.
33. Valdés Olmos RA, Jansen L, Hoefnagel CA, et al. Evaluation of mammary lymphoscintigraphy by single intratumoral injection for sentinel node identification. J Nucl Med. 2000;41:1500–6.
34. Valdés Olmos RA, Tanis PJ, Hoefnagel CA, et al. Improved sentinel node visualization in breast cancer by optimizing the colloid particle concentration and tracer dose. Nucl Med Commun. 2001;22:579–86.
35. Tanis PJ, Deurloo EE, Valdés Olmos RA, et al. Single intralesional tracer dose for radioguided excision of clinically occult breast cancer and sentinel node. Ann Surg Oncol. 2001;8:850–5.
36. Feggi L, Basaglia E, Corcione S, et al. An original approach in the diagnosis of early breast cancer: use of the same radiopharmaceutical for both non-palpable lesions and sentinel node localisation. Eur J Nucl Med. 2001;28:1589–96.
37. Luini A, Zurrida S, Paganelli G, et al. Comparison of radioguided excision with wire localization in occult breast lesion. Br J Surg. 1999;86:522–5.
38. Veit-Haibach P, Beyer T. State-of-the-art SPECT/CT: technology, methodology and applications. Eur J Nucl Med Mol Imaging. 2014;41(Suppl 1):S1–S149.
39. Van der Ploeg IMC, Valdes Olmos RA, Nieweg OE, et al. The additional value of SPECT/CT in lymphatic mapping in breast cancer and melanoma. J Nucl Med. 2007;48:1756–60.
40. Reintgen D, Albertini J, Milliotes G, et al. Investment in new technology research can save future health care dollars. J Fla Med Assoc. 1997;84:175–81.

41. Gemignani ML, Cody HS 3rd, Fey JV, et al. Impact of sentinel lymph node mapping on relative charges in patients with early-stage breast cancer. Ann Surg Oncol. 2000;7:575–80.
42. Jansen L, Muller SH, Nieweg OE, et al Uptake of radiocolloid in sentinel lymph nodes. In: Jansen L. Sentinel Node Biopsy, evolving from melanoma to breast cancer, Thesis, University of Amsterdam 1999. pp 151–168.
43. Miner TJ, Shriver CD, Flicek PR, et al. Guidelines for the safe use of radioactive materials during localization and resection of the sentinel lymph node. Ann Surg Oncol. 1999;6:75–82.
44. Persijn K, de Geest E. Sentinel node method: radiological protection. Tijdschr Nucl Geneesk. 2000;20:62. (abstract)

Non-mass Lesions on Breast Ultrasound Images

12

Ei Ueno

Breast lesions are classified into two categories: mass and non-mass abnormalities in ultrasound images [1, 2, 3]. A mass means a lump with components differing from the surrounding tissue; on the other hand, a non-mass abnormality means a lesion that is difficult to recognize as a mass on ultrasound images (Fig. 12.1).

To understand non-mass abnormality imaging, the genesis and progress of breast cancer must be understood.

12.1 Genesis and Progress of Breast Cancer

Multistep carcinogenesis is when breast cancer occurs progressively, and de novo type carcinogenesis is that which suddenly occurs.

Breast cancer occurs progressively with normal → ductal hyperplasia → atypical hyperplasia → DCIS and finally invasive ductal carcinoma in multistep carcinogenesis. The de novo type suddenly develops into invasive carcinoma with normal → (DCIS) → invasive ductal carcinoma [4, 5].

The multistep genesis type does not form a mass for a long time, and it is not rare that cancer is detected in this period by breast screening with mammography or ultrasound. Cancer cells mainly multiply in the duct and ductule of the terminal duct-lobular unit (TDLU) at the beginning. Ductules are extended while unfolding with the growth of cancer, and, as a result, lobules are expanded. Then, cancers spread along the mammary ducts, and lobules are observed to continue through mammary ducts on ultrasound images. Furthermore, cancers proliferate in mammary ducts and fuse with each other. Finally, mutation happens in a part of the DCIS and develops into invasive carcinoma (Fig. 12.2). On the other hand, the de novo type suddenly develops into an invasive cancer without passing through multisteps (Fig. 12.3). Non-mass lesions are detected in the middle of the multistep by sequence, and most are DCIS.

Non-mass abnormalities on breast ultrasounds are subdivided into four abnormalities:

1. Abnormalities of the ducts
2. Hypoechoic area in the mammary glands
3. Multiple small cysts
4. Architectural distortion

The assessment category is based on the features and distribution of these abnormalities, especially microcalcifications. I will interpret how to assess these lesions which were authorized by the Japan Association of Breast and Thyroid Sonology.

E. Ueno, M.D.
Tsukuba International Breast Clinic,
Tsukuba, Ibaraki, Japan
e-mail: ueno@tsukuba-breast.jp

D. Amy (ed.), *Lobar Approach to Breast Ultrasound*, https://doi.org/10.1007/978-3-319-61681-0_12

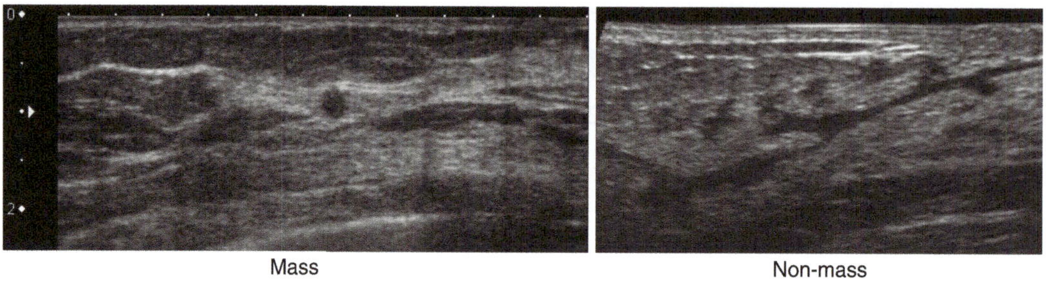

Fig. 12.1 Mass and Non-mass abnormalities: both are carcinomas

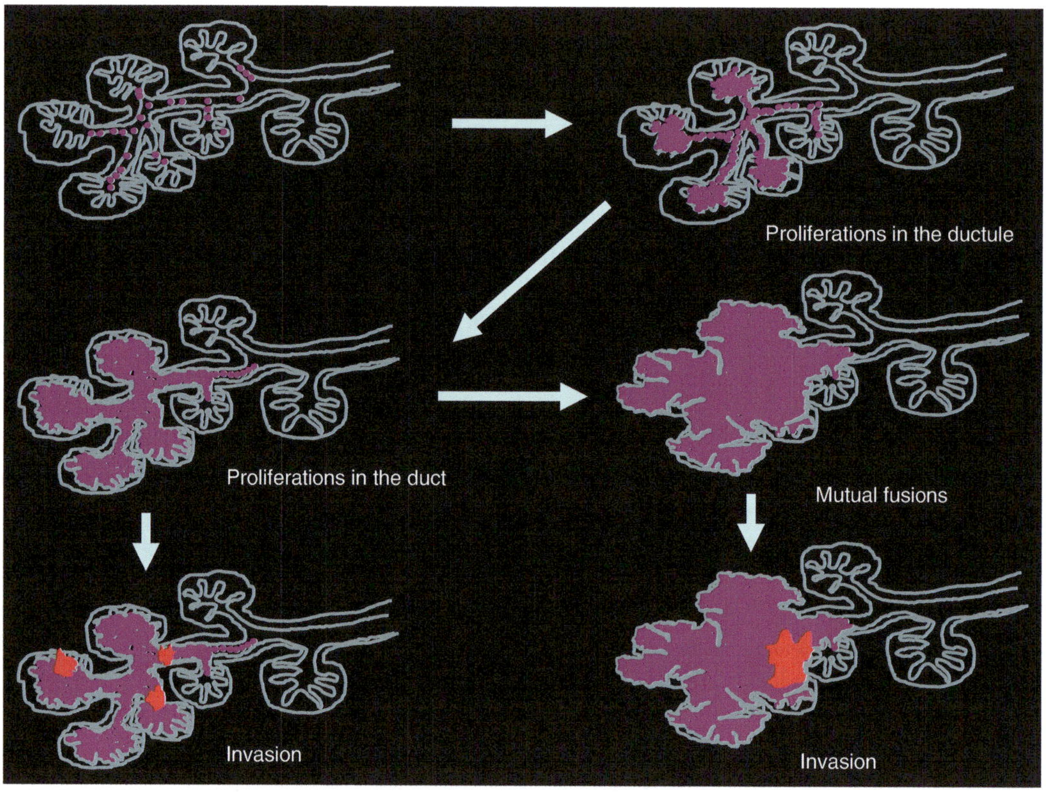

Fig. 12.2 Adenocarcinoma sequence

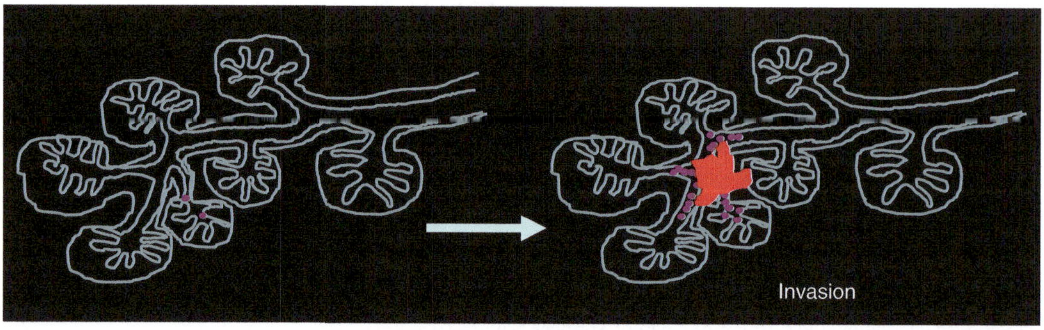

Fig. 12.3 Development of the De Novo type

12.2 Elasticity Score for Non-mass Lesions

The Tsukuba elasticity score is judged on the basis of color in the low echo area [6]. The hardness is displayed along a color spectrum: the soft tissues are displayed in red, and the hard tissues in blue. The lesions that have a low echo level and are shown in the red-green are classified in score 1, and the lesions in which blue is mixed with green are classified in score 2. The cases with much blue are classified in score 3, the cases which show as blue in the whole low echo area are classified in score 4, and the cases which appear blue over the low echo area are classified in score 5 (Fig. 12.4). It is extremely rare for the lesion to be malignant in the case of score 1. This elasticity score for non-mass lesion has not been authorized by JABTS.

12.2.1 Abnormalities of the Ducts

12.2.1.1 Definition

Abnormalities of the ducts are defined as lesions which are different from normal mammary ducts

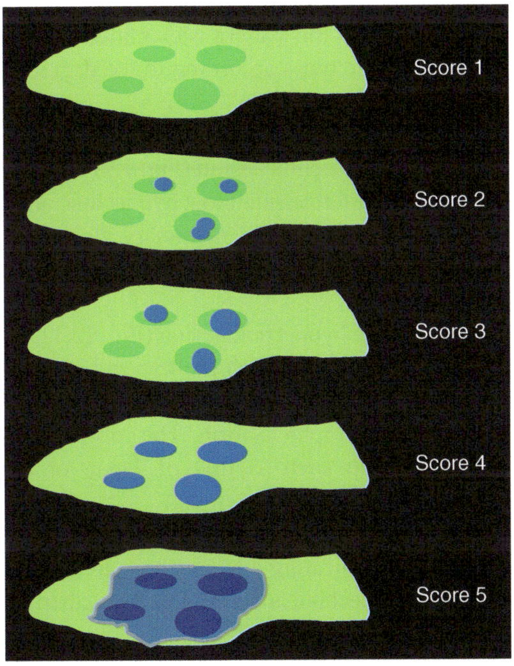

Fig. 12.4 Elasticity score for non-mass lesions

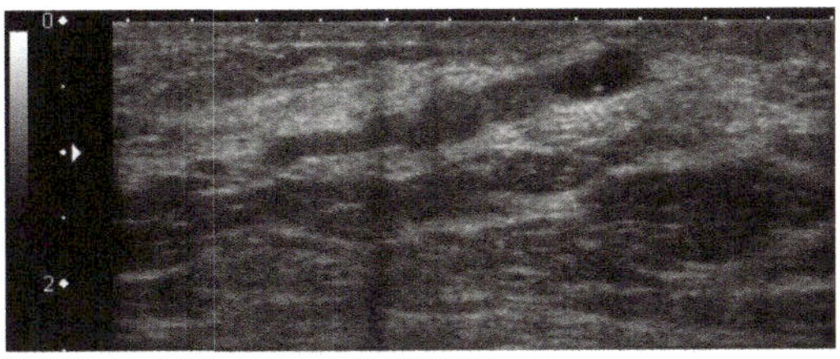

Fig. 12.5 Duct dilatation containing a solid part in a 49-year-old woman

in thickness of the duct, lumen, and wall. Such an abnormality is brought about by intraductal proliferation or the retention of the secretion accompanying the lesion (Fig. 12.5). Most lesions occur from TDLU but rarely occur from mammary ducts with the dilatation of the ducts.

Lesions occurring from TDLU include DCIS, ADH, and DH, and there are intraductal papilloma and intraductal papillomatosis of mammary duct origin. Abnormal findings include:

1. Duct dilatation
2. Duct with internal echoes which consist of:
   - Solid echoes
   - Floating echoes
   - Echogenic foci (Fig. 12.6)
   - Multiple small cysts
   - Linear high echoes
3. Thickening of the duct wall
4. A mammary stroma out of a duct is included as a wall by the ultrasound [4].
5. Irregularity of the duct caliber
6. Elasticity

12.2.1.2 Diagnosis

At first, duct dilatation is to be recognized as an abnormality of a mammary duct. The cascade of this judgment is shown in Fig. 12.7. When dilatation of a mammary duct extends over plural lobes, aberrations of normal development and involutions (ANDI) are considered, but, as for an abnormality limited to a segmental area or a local site, the existence of some kind of lesions must be considered [1, 7].

The properties of the intraductal echo are observed next. When a solid part is observed in a mammary duct, epithelium cell proliferation in the duct exists. There is a possibility of bleeding in the duct when the echoes have fluidity. When

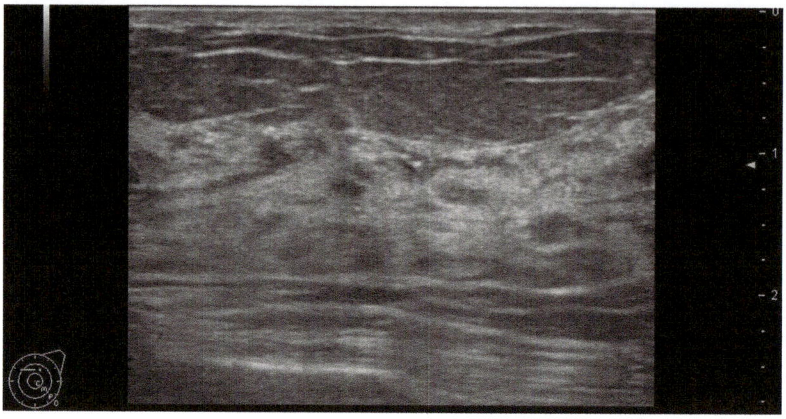

Fig. 12.6 Micro-calcifications are seen in the dilated duct. DCIS in a 65-year-old woman

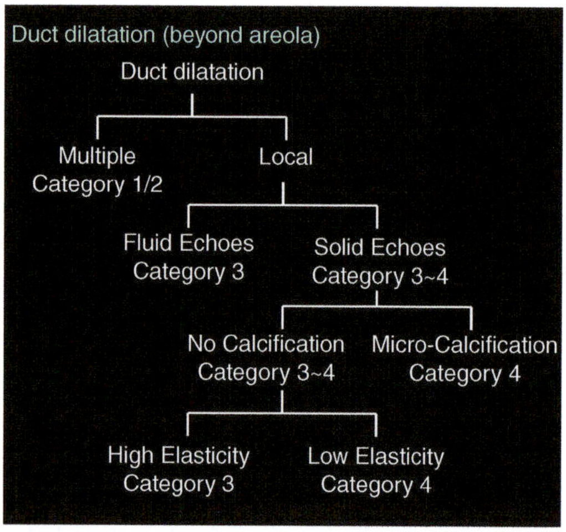

Fig. 12.7 Cascade of category for abnormalities of the ducts

microcalcification is confirmed in the solid part, it is more likely to be malignant. Because tissues are displayed in green by microcalcification in strain elastography, these findings are given priority over the elasticity score (Fig. 12.8). If the lesion does not have calcification and shows as blue, it is very likely that it is malignant. Double echo lines are sometimes seen in the inside of the tubular low echo (Fig. 12.9). As for this phenomenon, parenchyma around mammary ducts appears as a low echo in which the mammary duct wall is depicted as echo lines [8]. These are not calcifications.

12.2.2 Hypoechoic Lesions in the Mammary Glands

12.2.2.1 Definition

Echo levels are usually assessed on the basis of fat but here are based on an echo level of the mammary glands. When the level is lower than a mammary gland and higher than an echo level of the adipose tissue, the part is expressed with "hypoechoic."

Most breast diseases occur in the TDLU and show various forms by the quantity of cell proliferation. Ductal hyperplasia, atypical ductal hyperplasia, and ductal carcinoma in situ appear as this type, and this pattern is classified into the following three types according to the degree of the concrescence:

1. Mottled hypoechoic lesion (Fig. 12.10)
   It is a pattern that small low hypoechoic areas are interspersed in the mammary glands [1]. The lesion is in a condition to still remain in the TDLU.
2. Geographic hypoechoic lesion (Fig. 12.11)
   It is a pattern in which the hypoechoic area of the TDLU is concrescent and comes to have a geographical form. The form resembles a map such as that of Japan or the Philippines [3].
3. Indistinct hypoechoic lesion (Fig. 12.12) It is a pattern indicating a hypoechoic area where small hypoechoic areas are fused together.

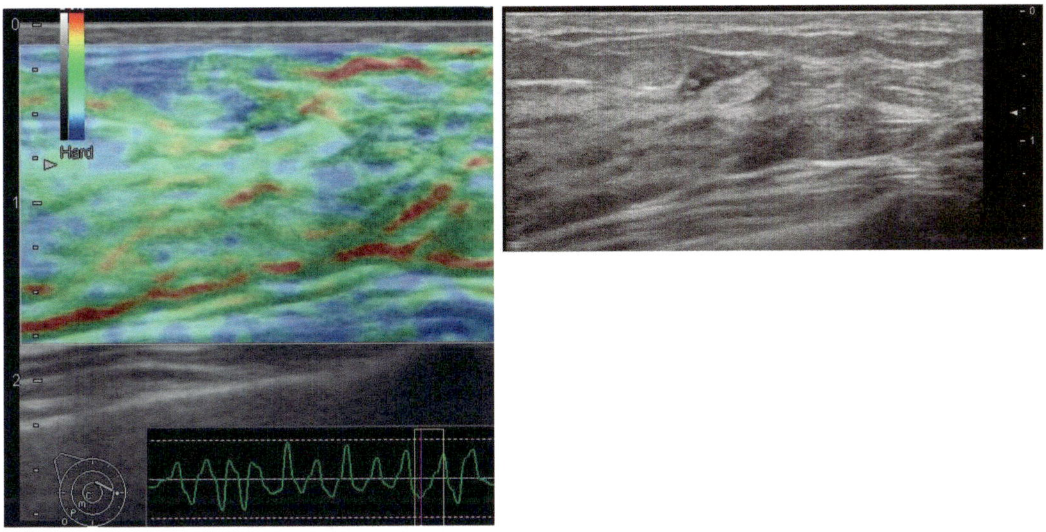

Fig. 12.8 Ductal carcinoma associated with microcalcification and micro-invasion

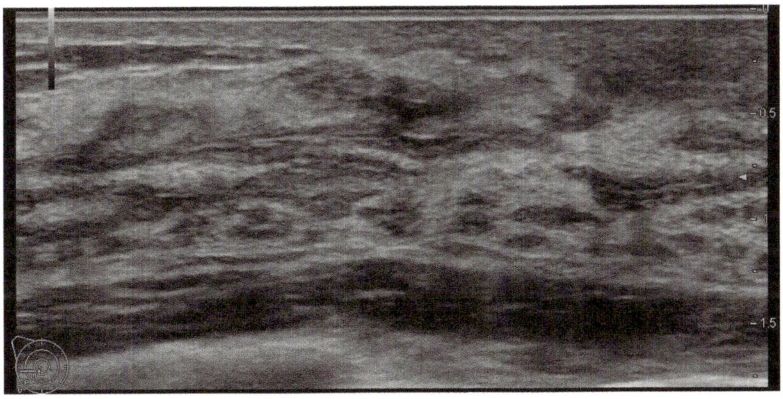

Fig. 12.9 Double lines in a 27-year-old woman

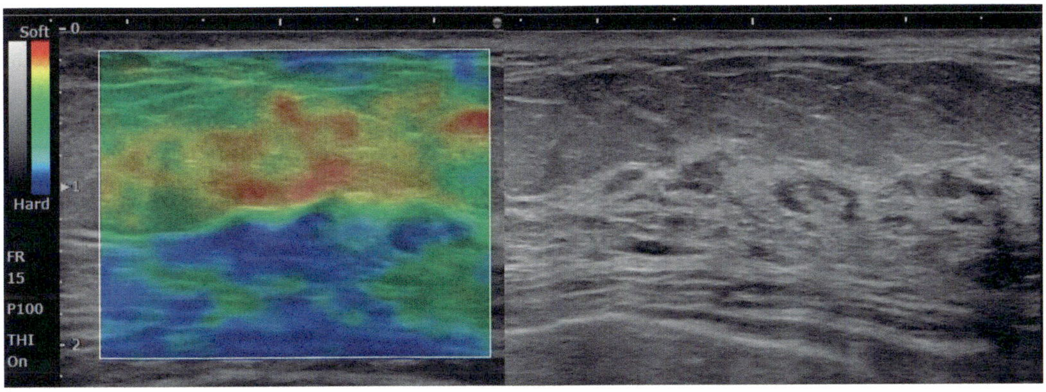

Fig. 12.10 Mottled pattern: DCIS

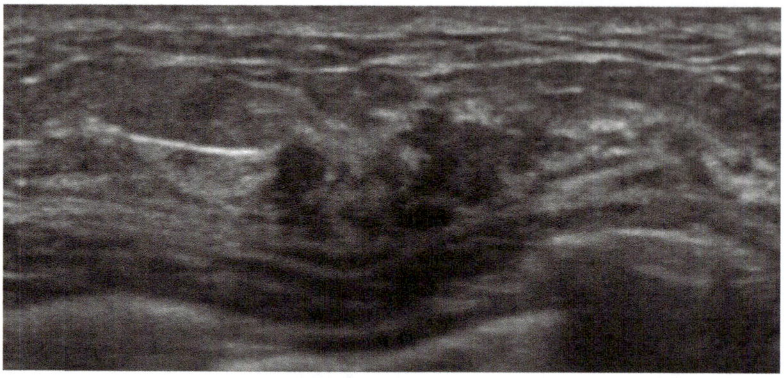

Fig. 12.11 Geographic pattern: DCIS

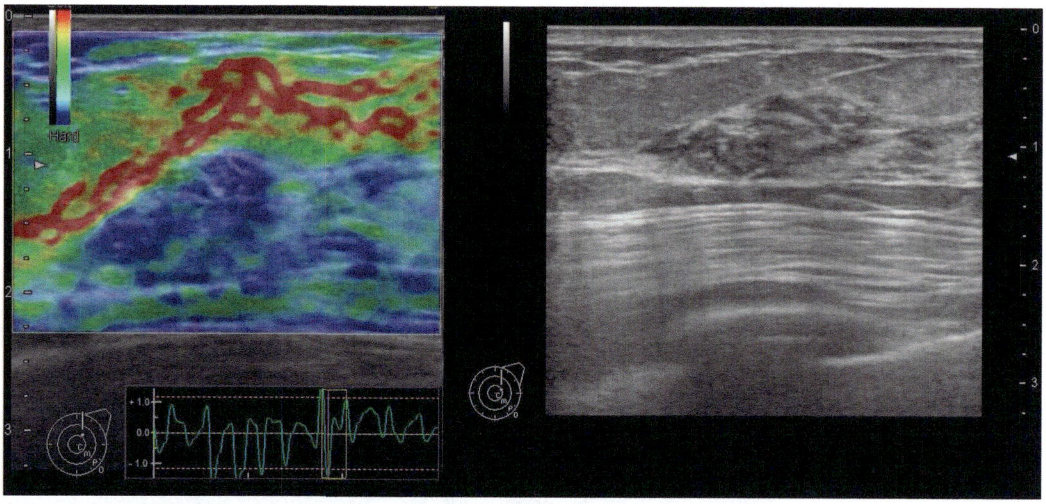

Fig. 12.12 Indistinct hypoechoic lesion: DCIS in a 68-year-old woman

12.2.2.2 Diagnosis

It is thought that the progression is in order of mottled, geographic, and indistinct hypoechoic lesions. Hyperplasia, atypical ductal hyperplasia, and ductal carcinoma in situ which occurred from plural terminal duct-lobular units (TDLU) multiply in the duct and form small polynesic and hypoechoic areas. DCIS gradually proliferates in the duct and expands the duct and forms a geographic pattern. Furthermore, when cancers multiply, lobules adhere to each other and come to appear as a hypoechoic large area. The tissue is dense in the same order. These lesions are diagnosed based on the abovementioned flow. Because there is much comedocarcinoma in the geographic pattern, calcification foci become an important point (Fig. 12.13). The procedure of the judgment is shown in Fig. 12.14.

12.2.3 Architectural Distortion

The collagenization of lesion tracts the circumference tissues and forms a distortion. Benign

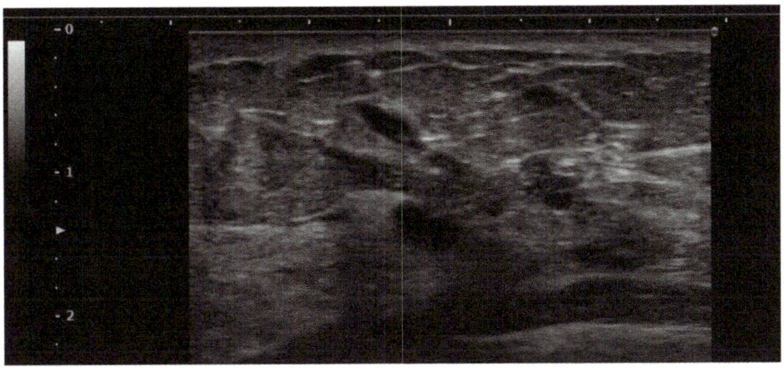

Fig. 12.13 Geographic pattern with micro-calcification: DCIS with microinvasion (Comedo type) in a 47-year-old woman

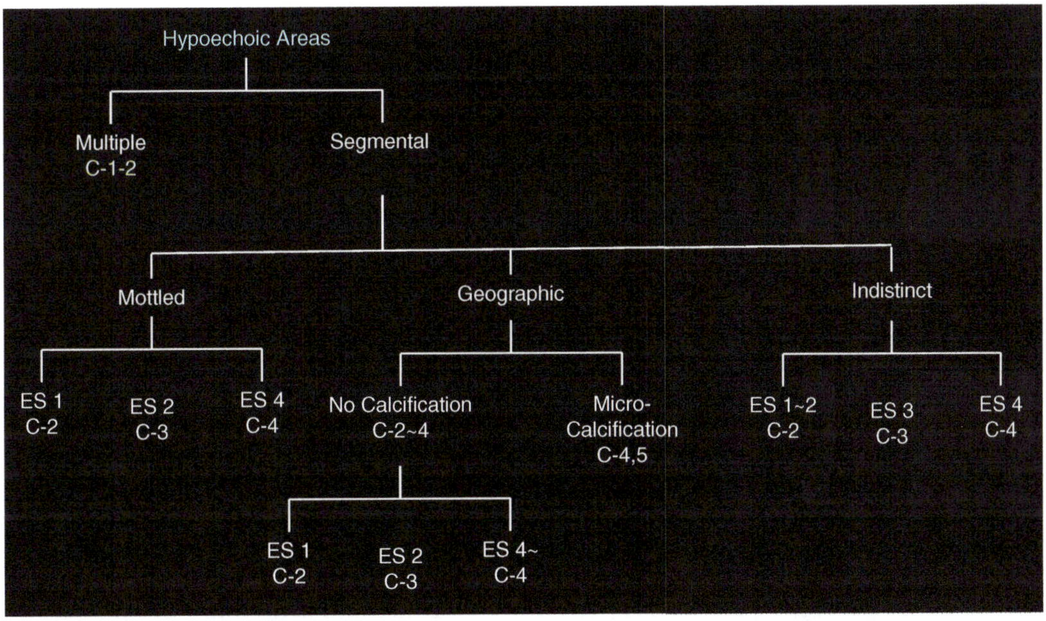

Fig. 12.14 Assessment category for hypoechoic area; Micoro-calcification is the most important finding in hypoechoic lesions

disorders indicating architectural distortion include sclerosing adenosis, radial scars, operation scars, etc. There are DCIS, lobular carcinoma, and scirrhous carcinoma with the malignancy. We must be careful not to excessively diagnose them because mammary glands show distortion in a woman in her late twenties in whom mammary gland atrophy starts. All diseases indicating architectural distortion have fewer Doppler signals than solid tumors in the color Doppler method. Because almost none of the hypoechoic area exists, it becomes either score 1 (Fig. 12.15) or 5 in elastography. Cancer indicates an elasticity of score 5 (Fig. 12.16). It is not accompanied by calcification. The cascade of this judgment is shown in Fig. 12.17.

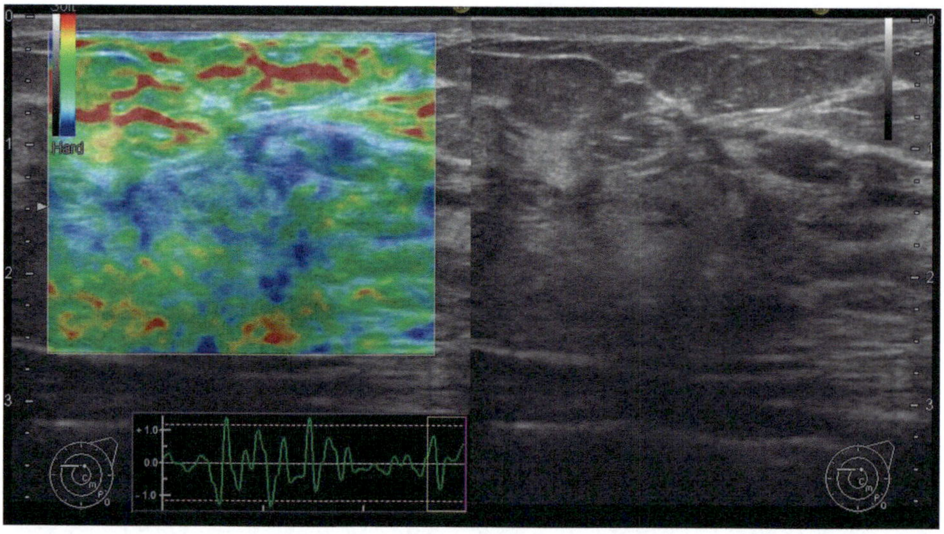

Fig. 12.15 Benign distortion in a 24-year-old woman

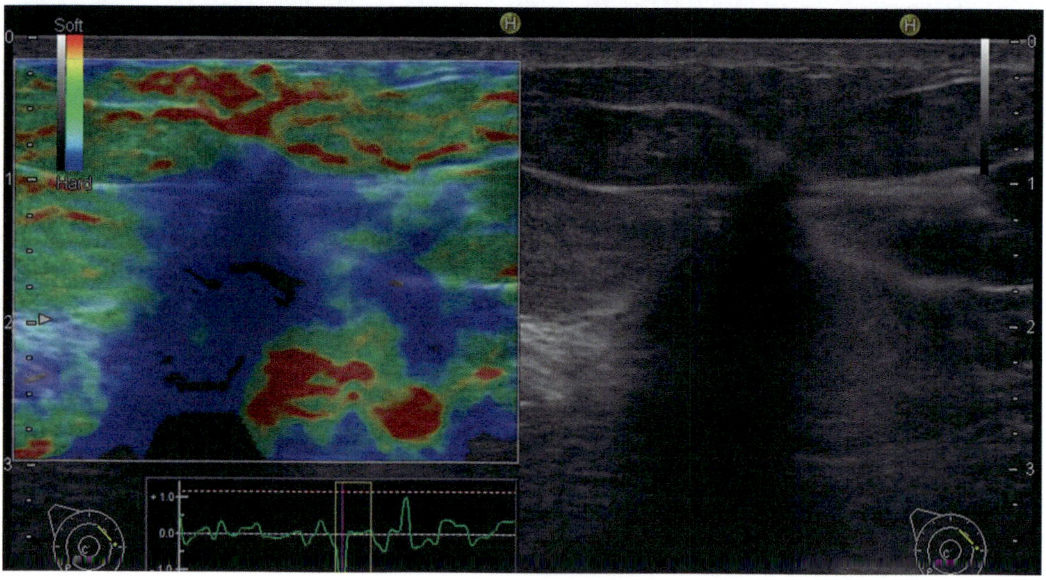

Fig. 12.16 Architectural distortion: Invasive ductal carcinoma in a 52-year-old woman

Fig. 12.17 Assessment category for architectural distortion

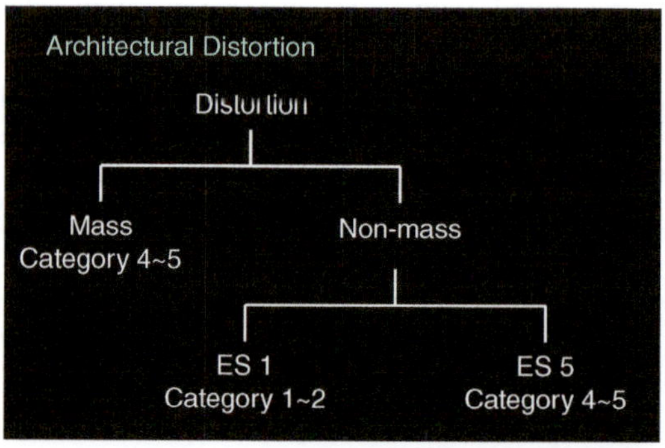

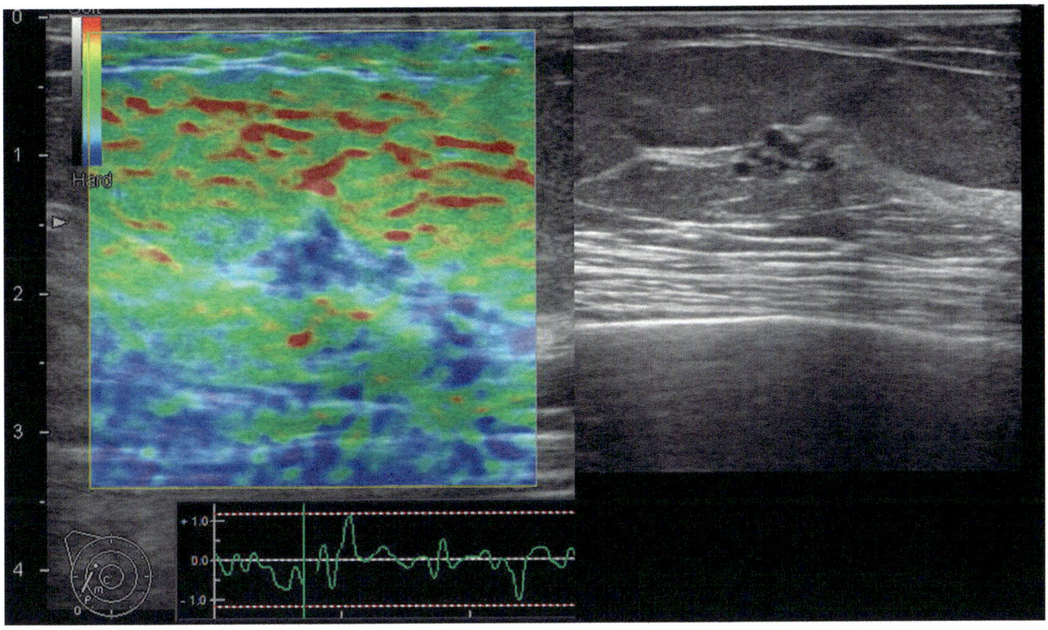

Fig. 12.18 Clustered microcyst: DCIS in a 65 year-old-woman

12.2.4 Clustered Microcysts

A pattern in which small cysts gather and look like a cluster of grapes. Most are benign disorders, but DCIS of low malignancies such as low papillary carcinoma is sometimes recognized. DCIS appears as score 5 in elastography (Fig. 12.18).

References

1. Ueno E. Real-time breast ultrasound. Tokyo: Nankodo; 1991. p. 60–3.
2. Endo T, Kubota M, Konishi Y, et al. Draft diagnostic guidelines for non-mass image-forming lesions by the Japan Association of Breast and Thyroid Sonology (JABTS) and the Japan Society of Ultrasonics in Medicine. Springer: Research and Development of Breast Ultrasound; 2005. p. 89–100.
3. Japan Association of Breast and Thyroid Sonology. Guideline for breast ultrasound/management and diagnosis. 3rd ed. Tokyo: Nankodo, Co., Ltd.; 2014.
4. Ueno E. Standpoint of the surgeon in diagnosis and treatment for breast—conserving therapy. Japanese Journal of Clinical Radiology. 1996;41:945–52.
5. Ueno E. Utility of breast ultrasound for breast conserving therapy—mainly intraductal components. Mamma. 1998;(30):1–4.
6. Itoh A, Ueno E, Tohno E, et al. Breast disease: clinical application of US elastography for diagnosis. Radiology. 2006;231:341–50.
7. Michel Teboul and Michael Halliwell: Atlas of ultrasound and ductal echography of the breast. Blackwell Science Ltd,1995
8. Izumori A, Horii R, Akiyama F, et al. Proposal of a novel method for observing the breast by high-resolution ultrasound imaging: understanding the normal breast structure and its application in an observational method for detecting deviations. Breast Cancer. 2013;20:83–91.

13 Mammographic Negative Cancer Detected by Ultrasound

Vedrana Buljević

13.1 Introduction

A few quotations from the book *Breast Cancer: A Lobar Disease* by Tibor Tot will be used as an introduction to this chapter, which will be followed by the presentation of several cases of early breast cancers invisible on mammography and detected by ultrasound. It is exactly through the presentation of the cases mentioned above that I will prove the theory stated in the sources claiming that breast cancer is a lobar disease, even at the earliest stages.

SOURCES:

CHAPTER 1: THE THEORY OF THE SICK LOBE—Tibor Tot (2007) [1].

1.3. The Hypotheses

1.3.2 The Theory of Biological Timing

"…Malignant transformation may appear in a single locus within the sick lobe, more than one locus at the same time or with considerable time difference. Or at a large number of loci…."

1.3.3 Similar Concepts

Ewing [2]

"DCIS grow in the distended ducts over considerable segments of the breast"

Gallagher and Martin [3]

V. Buljević, M.D.
Spinčićeva 2h, Split, Croatia
e-mail: dr.vedranab@gmail.com

"Human mammary carcinoma is not a focal process but a disease which affects breast epithelial diffusely"

Teboul and Halliwell [4]

"…Breast carcinoma as a malignant diffuse disease involving the whole epithelium of the affected lobe…."

1.4 Supporting Evidence

1.4.2 Genetic Evidence

Clarck et al. [5]

"…They found that a field of genetic instability can exist around a tumor in a morphologically normal tissue, and it may exist before the tumor develops. By mapping geographic zones of "normal" breast tissue adjacent to primary breast carcinoma by DNA methylation changes, a field of these changes extending as far as 4 cm from the primary lesion was demonstrated [6]. These findings are congruent with the average size of a sick lobe."

1.5 Breast Cancer at the Earliest Phase

1.5.1 Conditions for Perceiving Breast Carcinoma as a Lobar Disease

Tot [7]

Breast cancer is a lobar at its origin, but propagates to the nearby tissue beyond the borders of the sick lobe when advanced, large, and overtly invasive. We define early breast cancer as a purely in situ tumors and a tumors with invasive components of less than 15 mm. These tumors have a 10 year disease –specific survival of over 90%.

D. Amy (ed.), *Lobar Approach to Breast Ultrasound*, https://doi.org/10.1007/978-3-319-61681-0_13

1.5.3 Early Breast Cancer is Not Necessarily "Small"

Anderson et al. [8], Holland et al. [9], Faverly et al. [10], Foschini et al. [11]

"Breast cancer is not necessarily small at the earliest stages of its development; on the contrary, it is widespread and multifocal in the majority of cases." [8–11].

CHAPTER 8: LOBAR ULTRASOUND OF THE BREAST—Dominique Amy [12]

8.6 Multifocality, Multicentricity, and Diffuse Lesions

With introduction of ductal echography, a new definition of multiple lesions has become possible: multifocal cancers should now be defined as those developing within the same lobe along the ductal axis, while multicentric cancers develop in different lobes (they can also be solitary or multifocal). This definition is in agreement with histologic studies.

13.2 Diagnostic Procedures

Diagnostic procedures with all the patients consisted of the clinical examination (inspection and palpation), mammography, and ultrasound examination.

Lesions, detected by ultrasound, were cytologically verified under ultrasound control, and then an open biopsy was performed after a preoperative marcation under ultrasound control.

All the lesions were impalpable, invisible on mammography, and up to 10 mm long at the ultrasound examination.

Pathohistological analysis would confirm malignity of lesions detected by ultrasound but also the existence of additional malignant microscopic lesions around the primary process, which required reoperation—quadrantectomia.

Additional pathohistological detecting of microscopic foci in situ or microinvasive carcinoma in the tissue obtained by quadrantectomia (multifocality or diffusivity) would indicate subcutaneous mastectomy with primary reconstruction.

As an introduction to the ultrasound examination, it is important to begin with inspection and palpation and to carefully analyze mammographic images, in order to pay additional attention to irregularities during ultrasound examination.

This increases opportunities to detect breast carcinoma at the earliest stage. Early-stage carcinomas usually have very nonspecific morphological features that are more common with benign than with malignant lesions.

Breast inspection allows detection of changes on the breast skin, areola, and mamilla which can indicate malignity, even the one at its earliest stage such as Paget's disease that is not detectable by any of the screening methods.

Palpation is a further equally important part of the examination aimed at detecting asymmetrical tissue condensations which can lead to the diagnosis of well-differentiated carcinoma. These carcinomas are difficult to visualize by screening methods as they are morphologically very similar to the healthy breast tissue. Asymmetrical tissue condensations make us pay special attention to those places during ultrasound examination and possibly apply additional diagnostic procedures in case even the smallest change in the architecture is detected by ultrasound – this is particularly important for the early diagnosis of lobular and tubular carcinoma.

I advise my patients to undergo breast ultrasound examinations every 6 months. The reason for this is that even when the result of the examination is normal, in the breast tissue there can be a carcinoma at a subclinical undetectable stage. Within an interval of 6 months, such a carcinoma will be detectable at an early, still curable stage of disease, even then when it is about rapidly growing, poorly differentiated tumors.

13.2.1 Ultrasound Examination

A high-quality ultrasound examination requires a well-educated and trained expert, with a high-quality ultrasound device and a high-frequency probe—at least 10–14 MHz. Equally important is a good examination technique [12]

Personally, I perform ultrasound examination in three different sections: two of them being orientational (longitudinal, transversal), and after that I carefully apply the technique of ductal radial echography that follows the breast anatomy during scanning, which is not the case with the longitudinal and orthrogonal sections. In this way, each breast is scanned three times, which ensures a high degree of probability that not even the smallest part of the breast tissue will be omitted by the examination. The technique has been presented by Dr. Dominique Amy in many of her papers as well as by Dr. M. Tebule and Dr. M. Halliwell in the book entitled

Atlas of Ultrasound and Ductal Echography of the Breast [4, 12].

Cytological verification under ultrasound control is an important diagnostic method, especially for early carcinoma that is morphologically very often not clearly suspectable. Cytological puncture under ultrasound control is painless, simple, innocuous, cheap, and of high specificity (93–99%) as well as of high sensitivity (87–98%).

Examination results with early breast carcinoma are usually borderline. An insight into the necessity of a biopsy is obtained by integrating anamnestic data (family illness history, menarche, menopause, first-time birth, and data related to lactation), the results of the inspection, palpation, and mammographic and ultrasound examination, as well as the finding of the cytological analysis into a complete picture.

13.3 Case Reports

13.3.1 Case 1

G.S., aged 51

The patient comes to a regular breast ultrasound examination 6 months after the last examination.

The finding of the earlier inspection, palpation, and ultrasound examination was normal. (4).

The present finding of inspection and palpation is normal.

THE PRESENT ULTRASOUND EXAMINATION: in the left breast, in the lobe at 2 o' clock, two hypoechoic, not sharply outlined, irregular lesions, each 7 × 3 mm long, without attenuations which mutually confluate beside discretely changed architecture of the surrounding tissue (Figs. 13.1 and 13.2).

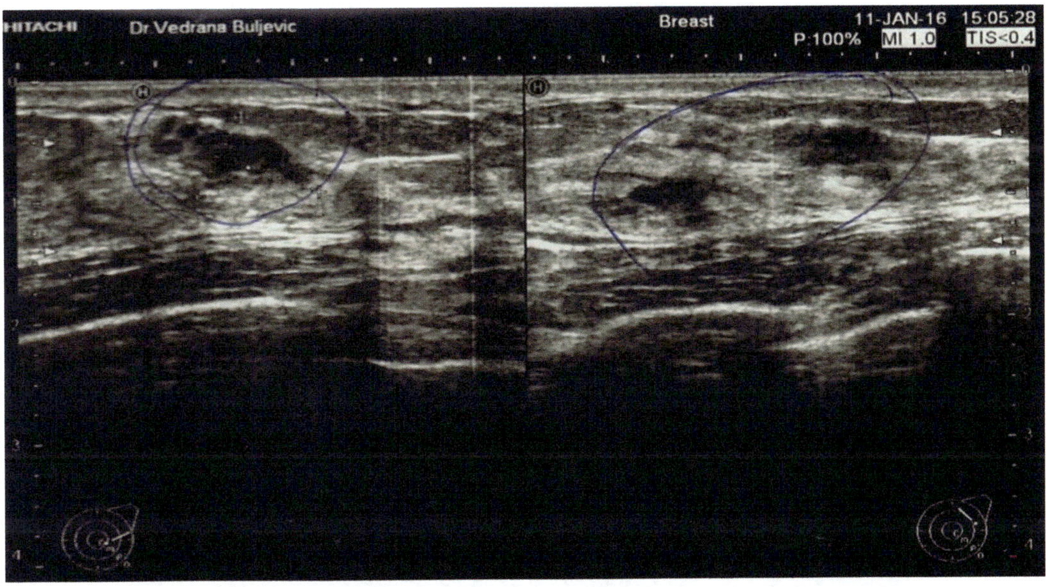

Fig. 13.1 ULTRASOUND: image of two small unspecific hypoechoic changes in upper outer quadrant of the left breast

MAMMOGRAPHY: does not differentiate suspected changes (Fig. 13.3).

THE RESULT OF CYTOLOGICAL ANALYSIS: ATYPICAL DUCTAL EPITHELIAL PROLIFERATION (**C4**) (Fig. 13.4).

Biopsy is indicated because it is about new changes that occurred within an interval of 6 months from the last examination, whereby atypical ductal epithelial proliferation is confirmed by a cytological analysis. The fact that the patient belongs to a risk group (aunt from mother side breast cancer) further confirms the decision to biopsy.

THE RESULT OF HISTOPATHOLOGICAL ANALYSIS OF BIOPSY: MALIGNANT.

After the malignity had been confirmed, a wider surgical procedure—quadrantectomia—was indicated.

RESULT OF HISTOPATHOLOGICAL ANALYSIS OF QUADRANTECTOMIA: CA DUCTALE IN SITU MAMMAE GR. II (Fig. 13.5).

In the FINAL PATHOHISTOLOGICAL FINDING of the tissue obtained by quadrantectomia, the size of DCIS could not be determined—because it cuts across a larger part of the sample, spreads up to the resection margins, is present in a several taken segments, and is focal at the margin—tumor is present in 10 out of 13 segments. It reaches the resection margins. It was

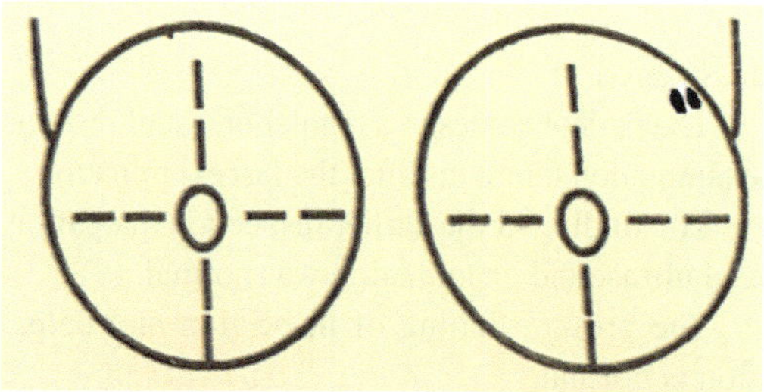

Fig. 13.2 SKETCH: ultrasound finding—two lesions in upper outer quadrant of the left breast. Example of multifocal lesion in the same lobe at 2 o' clock [8–12])

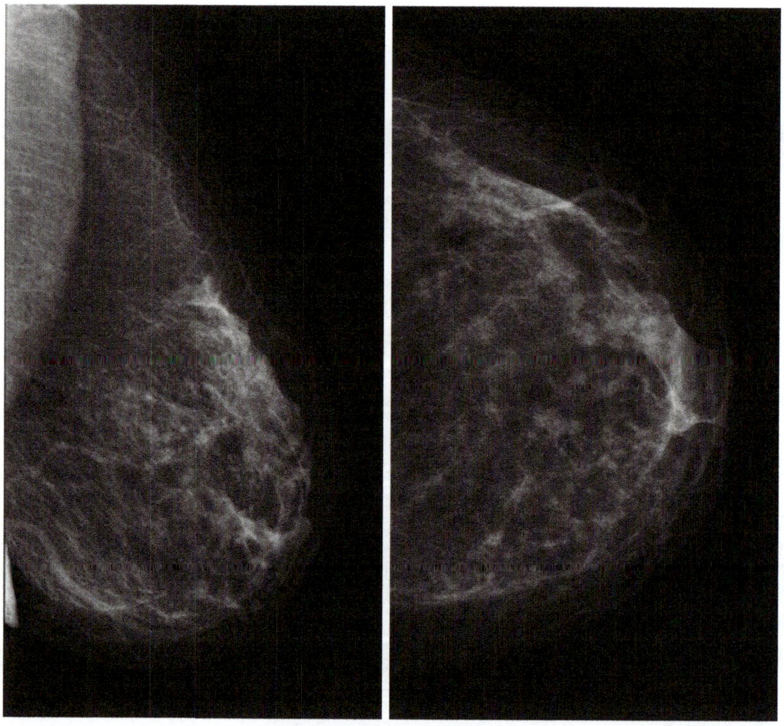

Fig. 13.3 MAMMOGRAPHY: MLO at CC projections of the left breast

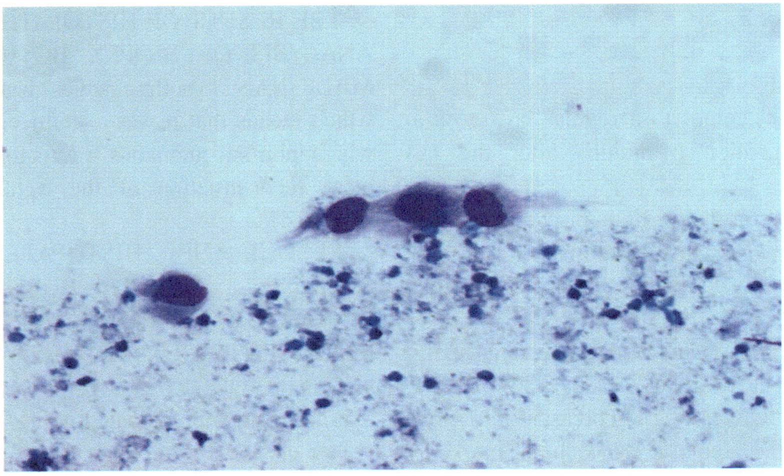

Fig. 13.4 CYTOLOGY: image of atypical ductal epithelium

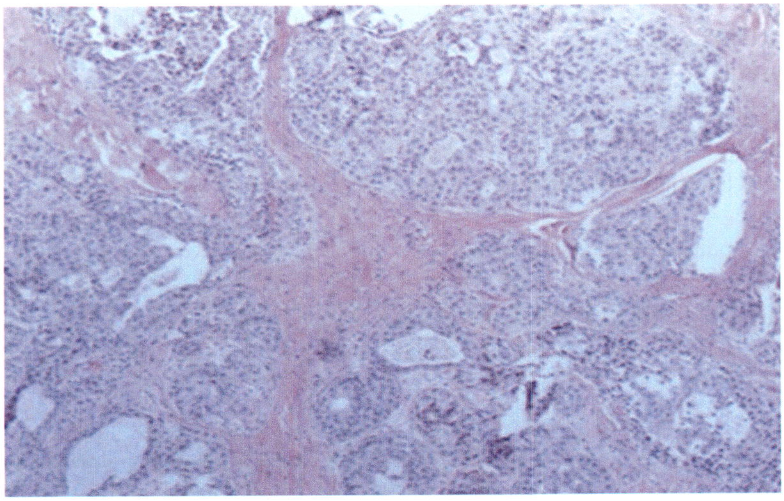

Fig. 13.5 PATHOHISTOLOGY: image of ductal carcinoma in situ gr. II

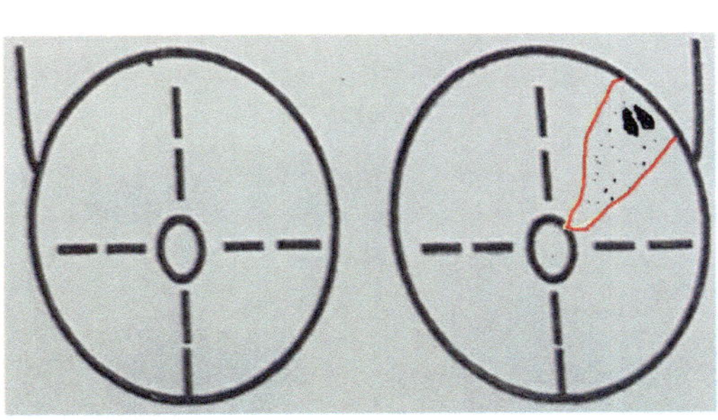

Fig. 13.6 SKETCH: two foci detected by ultrasound and wide area of carcinoma in situ on histopathology spaces tissue of quadrantectomia which corresponds to the average surface of lobe [4, 5, 7]

DCIS—clinging, cribriform, papillary with cancerization of lobules [5, 6, 12] (Fig. 13.6).

Due to the saturation of the whole tissue with in situ tumor and due to positive resection margins, subcutaneous mastectomy with primary reconstruction was indicated.

PHD of subcutaneous mastectomy: ONE FOCUS OF DCIS—a gr. III.

It can be clearly seen that in situ carcinoma has seized the whole lobe at 2 o'clock of the left breast, which is far wider than what had been visible at the preoperative procedure.

13.3.2 Case 2

M. J., aged 46

The patient comes to a regular breast ultrasound examination 6 months after the last examination.

The finding of the previous inspection, palpation, and ultrasound examination (4) was normal and so was the finding of the mammography 10 months ago.

Present palpation and inspection are normal.

THE PRESENT ULTRASOUND EXAMINATION: in the right breast at 11 o'clock 3 cm from the areola, a hypoechoic, markedly irregular change 6×6 mm in size. In the same breast, there is a similar change, also 6×6 mm in size, at the periphery of the lobe 8 o'clock (Figs. 13.7 and 13.8).

REPEATED MAMMOGRAPHY: DOES NOT DIFFERENTIATE SUSPECTED CHANGES (Fig. 13.9).

They are described on breast MRI as changes of suspected characteristics, 7×6 mm and 9×7 mm in size.

A cytological puncture under ultrasound control was indicated.

THE RESULT OF CYTOLOGICAL ANALYSIS OF BOTH LESIONS: ADENOCAR CINOMA (Fig. 13.10).

The patient was referred to a surgical biopsy with preoperative marcation under ultrasound control.

THE RESULT OF HISTOPATHOLOGICAL ANALYSIS OF BIOPSY BOTH LESIONS: MALIGNANT (both changes were malignant which means that it was a multicentric process, whereupon subcutaneous mastectomy with primary reconstruction of the right breast was indicated).

RESULT OF HISTOPATHOLOGICAL ANALYSIS OF SUBCUTANEOUS MASTECTOMY: CA MAMMAE INVASIVUM MULTICENTRICUM; CA MESTASTATICUM LYMPHONODORUM.

The histopathological finding reveals two malignant foci in the upper outer quadrant (one focus 9 mm in size is detected at the ultrasound examination as well as at the magnetic resonance). The largest microscopic focus is 2.5×1.5×2 cm in size, and in its surrounding, another focus 0.7 cm in size has been detected [12].

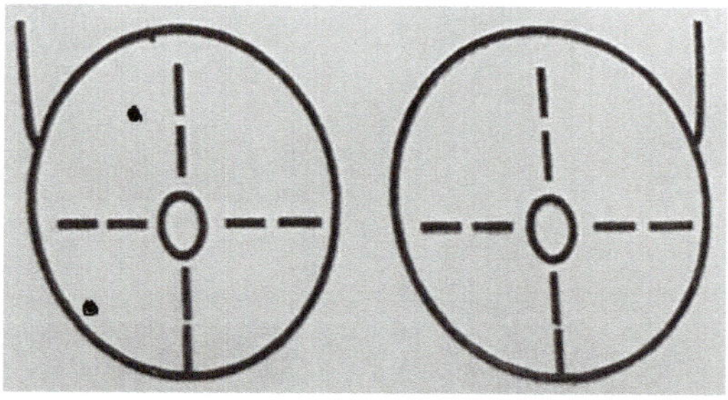

Fig. 13.8 SKETCH: two malignant foci in two different lobes of the right breast detected by ultrasound—multicentric carcinoma [1, 12]

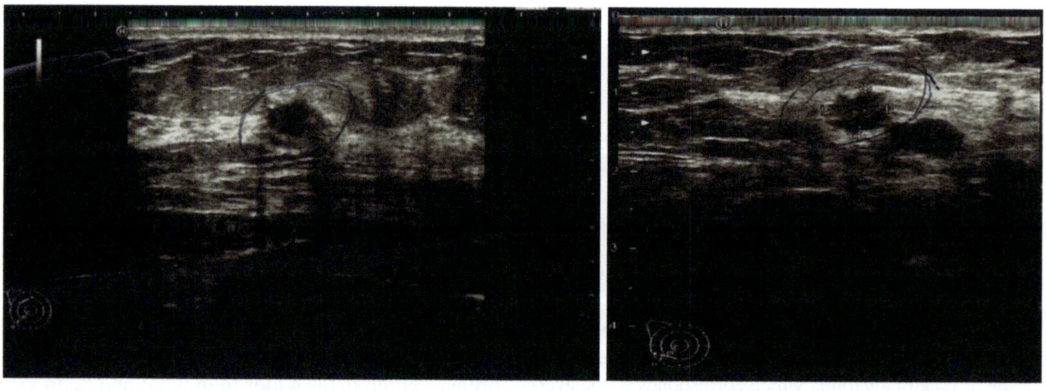

Fig. 13.7 ULTRASOUND: images of two small malignant foci within the two different lobes

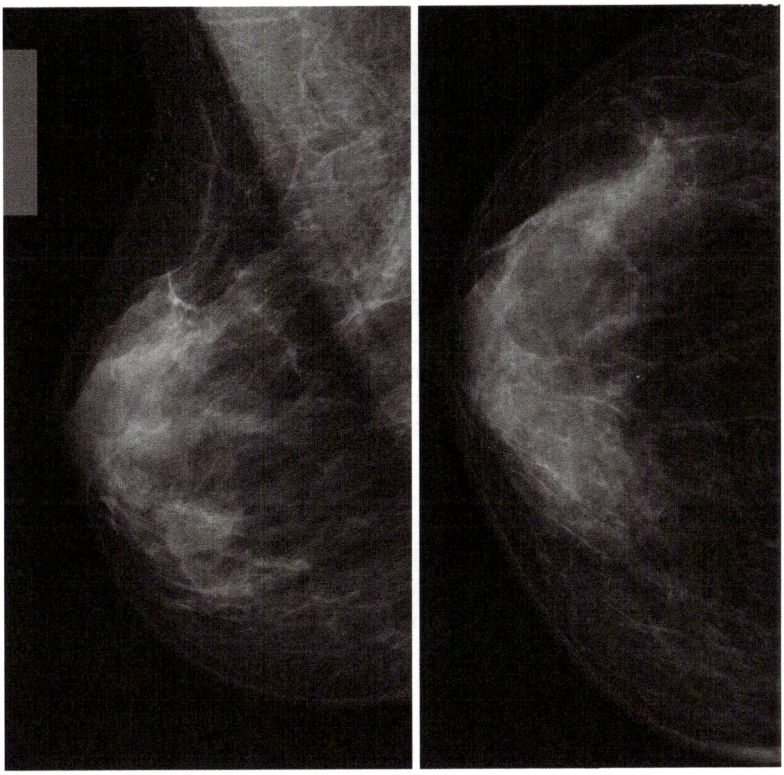

Fig. 13.9 MAMMOGRAPHY: right breast—MLO and CC projections

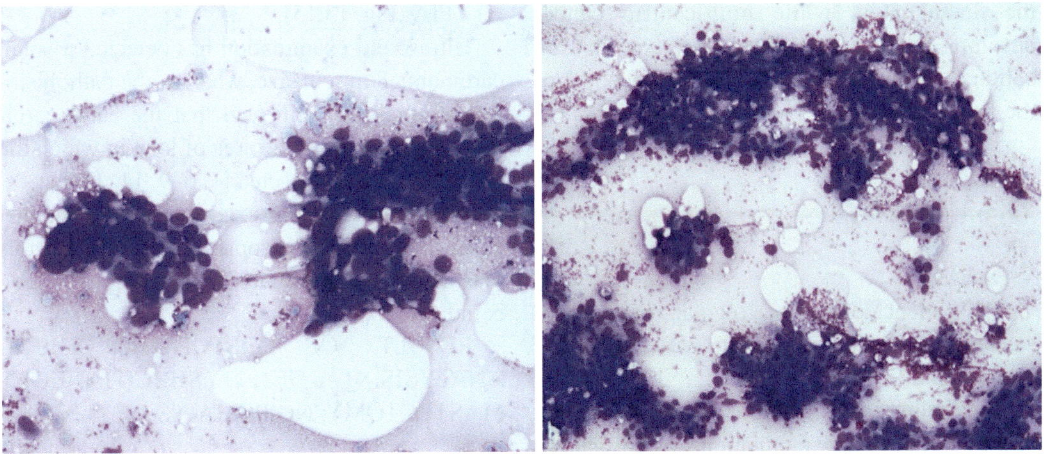

Fig. 13.10 CYTOLOGY: images of two malignant foci of the right breast—multicentric carcinoma

Microscopic carcinoma has spread to a large part of the tissue of the lobe at 11 o'clock and covers a far bigger surface than the one that can be detected by visual methods (1.2.3). It was a carcinoma of a medullary picture with cancerization of lobules, especially next to the mamilla base, and it spread also into the lower medial quadrant [1, 6–9, 11, 12].

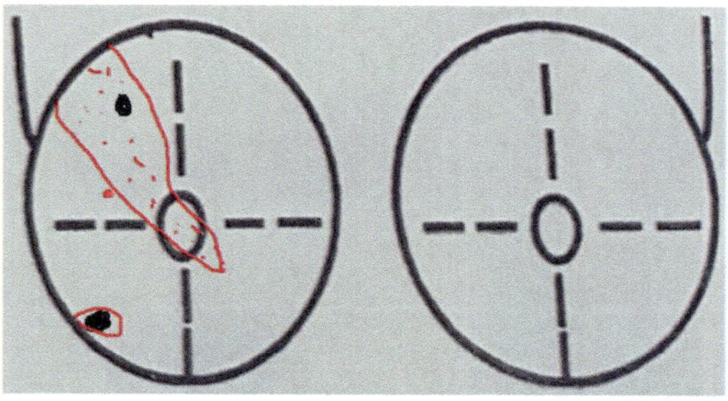

Fig. 13.11 SKETCH: two malignant foci detected by breast ultrasound and breast MRI and distribution of carcinoma in situ around foci in upper outer quadrant detected by histopathology of subcutaneous mastectomy which corresponds to the average surface of lobe [1, 6–9, 11, 12]

In the lower outer quadrant, the pathohistological analysis revealed a focus with a 0.7 mm diameter, which is in accordance with the findings of both ultrasound and magnetic resonances (Fig. 13.11).

This case is an illustration of the statements from the book mentioned in the introductory part, in which the author claims:

Multifocal cancers should now be defined as those developing within the same lobe along the ductal axis, while multicentric cancer develops in different lobes (they can also be solitary or multifocal). (Lobar Ultrasound of the Breast [12]).

13.3.3 Case 3

V. Đ., aged 46

The patient comes to a regular breast ultrasound examination 6 months after the last examination.

The finding of the previous inspection, palpation, and ultrasound examination was normal.

The present palpation and inspection examination is normal.

THE PRESENT ULTRASOUND EXAMINATION shows in the left breast, at the 2 o'clock in upper outer quadrant of left breast a hypoechoic change 8×5 mm in size, discretely irregular, lobuled with milder attenuations. It is a new change that was not described earlier (Fig. 13.12).

MAMMOGRAPHY: DOES NOT DIFFERENTIATE SUSPECTED CHANGES (Fig. 13.13).

A cytological puncture under ultrasound control is indicated.

THE RESULT OF CYTOLOGICAL ANALYSIS:

WELL-DIFFERENTIATED BREAST ADENOCARCINOMA (Fig. 13.14).

A biopsy is indicated.

THE RESULT OF HISTOPATHOLOGICAL ANALYSIS OF BIOPSY: MALIGNANT.

Whereupon a reoperation is indicated.

OP.: QUADRANTECTOMIA.

THE RESULT OF HISTOPATHOLOGICAL ANALYSIS OF QUADRANTECTOMIA: CA DUCTALE MICROINVASIVUM—EXTENSIVE CARCINOMA IN SITU OF CRIBRIFORM AND MICROPAPILLARY GROWTH WITH SEVERAL SOLID FOCI, OF MIDDLE, OCCASIONALLY HIGH-NUCLEAR GRADE, WITH COMEDONECROSIS, THE FOCUS OF MICROINVASION LESS THAN 1 mm, from the resection margin 2 mm, FLAT ATYPIA (Fig. 13.15).

Ultrasound examination has detected a small carcinoma 8 mm in size, whereas the pathohistological analysis confirmed that the early carcinoma cut across a wide area of lobe in which the process has been detected [1, 6–9, 11, 12].

With regard to the extensive malignant disease, detected microscopically, a subcutaneous mastectomy with primary implant reconstruction is indicated.

RESULT OF HISTOPATHOLOGICAL ANALYSIS OF SUBCUTANEOUS MASTECTOMY: NO REMAINS OF TUMOR.

13.3.4 Case 4

P. A., aged 39

The patient comes to a regular breast ultrasound examination 6 months after the last examination.

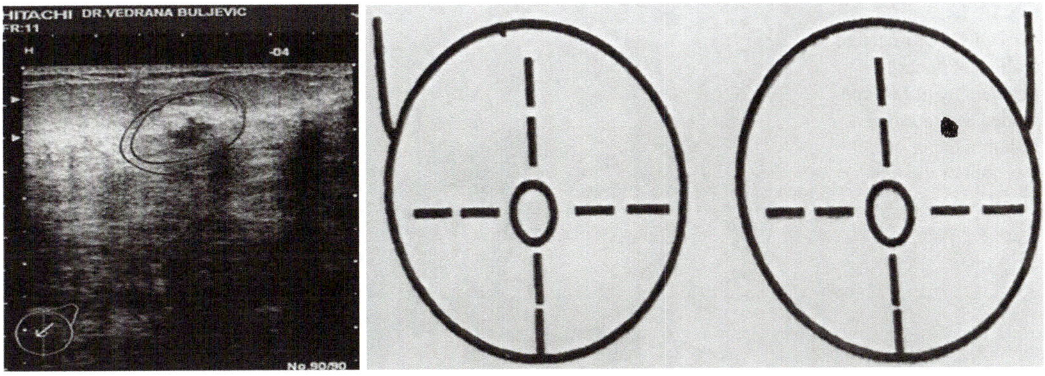

Fig. 13.12 ULTRASOUND: image of small malignant foci in the left breast and sketch of its position

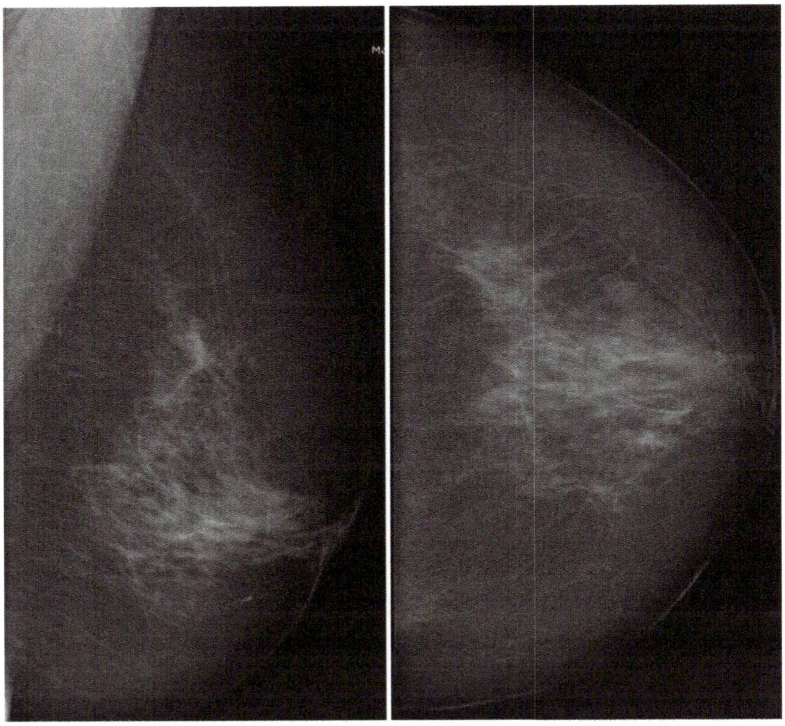

Fig. 13.13 MAMMOGRAPHY: left breast—MLO and CC projection

The finding of the palpation, inspection, and ultrasound examination 6 months ago was normal.

The present findings of palpation and inspection are normal.

THE PRESENT FINDING OF ULTRA SOUND EXAMINATION SHOWS in the left breast, in the upper outer quadrant at 2 o'clock, a hypoechoic benign change 11×7 mm in size (Fig. 13.16). MAMMOGRAPHY: DOES NOT DIFFERENTIATE SUSPECTED CHANGES (Fig. 13.17).

A cytological puncture of the new change is indicated.

THE RESULT OF CYTOLOGICAL ANALYSIS: DUCTAL EPITHELIAL PROLIFERATION.

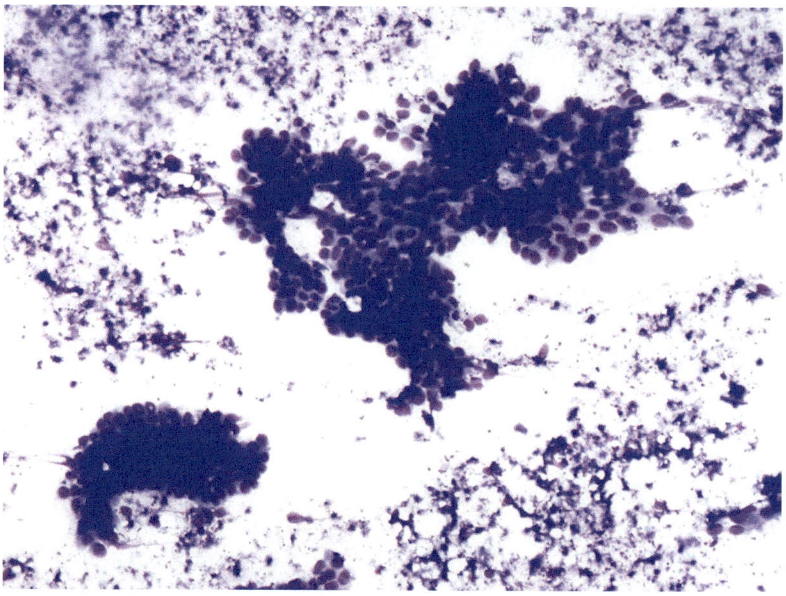

Fig. 13.14 CYTOLOGY: image of malignant material obtained by ultrasound-guided aspiration of lesion in upper outer quadrant of the left breast

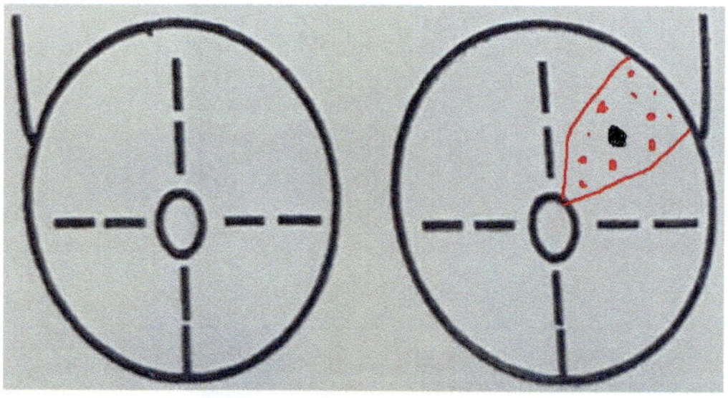

Fig. 13.15 SKETCH: small malignant foci in upper outer quadrant of the left breast and area of in situ carcinoma around it detected by histopathology of quadrantectomia which corresponds to the average surface of the lobe

Taking into consideration the facts: that there was a new change with the elements of proliferation in the cytological finding, that the change occurred within the interval of 6 months, that the patient belongs to a risk group (maternal grandmother and two aunts on her father's side had breast cancer) extirpation of the change in infirmary conditions with preoperative marcation under ultrasound control was indicated.

THE RESULT OF PATHOHISTOLOGICAL ANALYSIS OF BIOPSY: FIBROADENOMA, DCIS OF HIGH GRADE—CUTS ACROSS THE RESECTION MARGIN (in one resection margin, several small channels covered with irregular epithelium are detected) (Figs. 13.18 and 13.19).

By means of pathohistological analysis, the new change is confirmed as detected by ultrasound and cytologically verified as ductal epithelial proliferation—fibroadenoma. Beside the benign tumor, a focus of ductal in situ carcinoma of high grade has been detected, which spreads to the resection margin. Due to the positive resection margin, a reoperation—quadrantectomia—is indicated.

OP.: QUADRANTECTOMIA

THE RESULT OF PATHOHISTOLOGICAL ANALYSIS OF QUADRANTECTOMIA: DCIS (foci DCIS, which spread very close to the resection margin, are scattered around areal 4 cm) (Fig. 13.20).

Pathohistological analysis detects microscopic foci of DCIS on a wide area of 4 cm which corresponds to the average surface of the lobe. As it spreads again to the resection margin, a new operation is indicated—subcutaneous mastectomy.

RESULT OF PATHOHISTOLOGICAL ANALYSIS OF SUBCUTANEOUS MASTECTOMY: DCIS OF HIGH GRADE (in the middle part of the segment, approximately 1 cm under skin, there is a microscopic focus of DCIS of HIGH GRADE—it does not reach the resection margin).

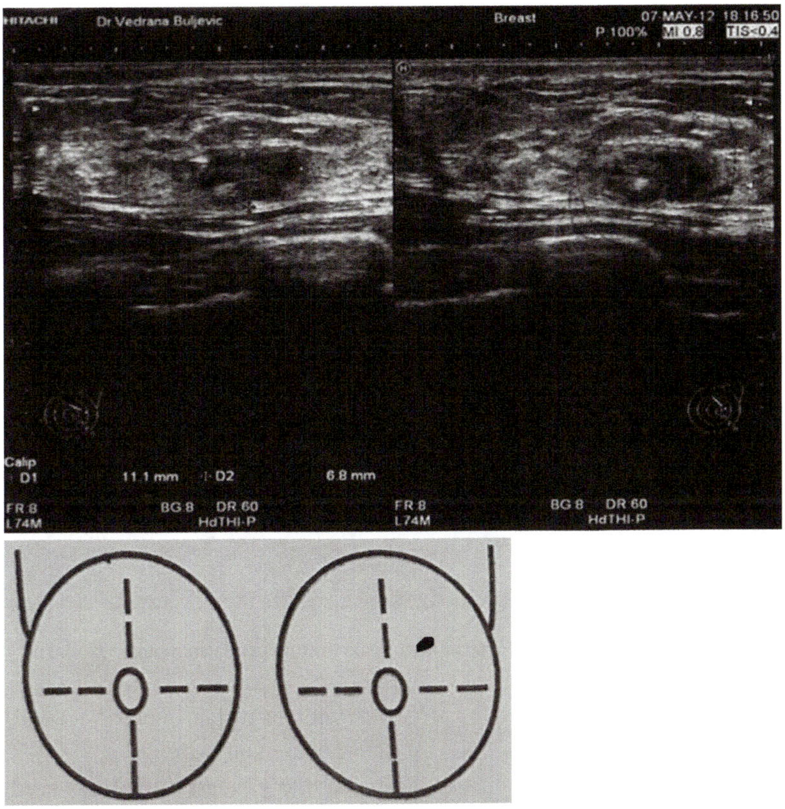

Fig. 13.16 ULTRASOUND: image and sketch of the small malignant foci in upper outer quadrant of the left breast

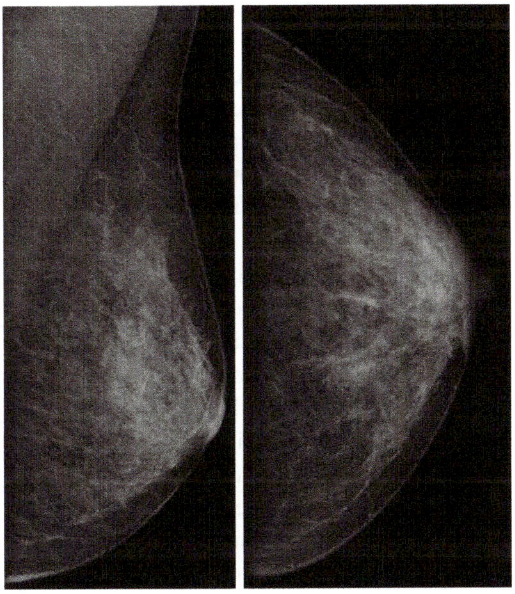

Fig. 13.17 MAMMOGRAPHY: MLO and CC projection of the left breast

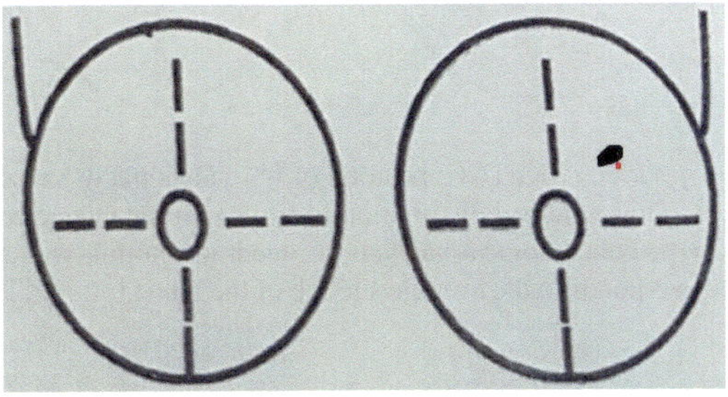

Fig. 13.18 SKETCH: position of microscopic foci in situ carcinoma beside the fibroadenoma (spot)

It can be concluded that the malignant disease in these cases was not detectable in its real proportions by visual methods, i.e., it is evident that the microscopic analysis detected malignant lesions on a wide area in the form of several individual microscopic malignant foci scattered around the area of one lobe either in the form of more in situ or in the form of more microscopically invasive

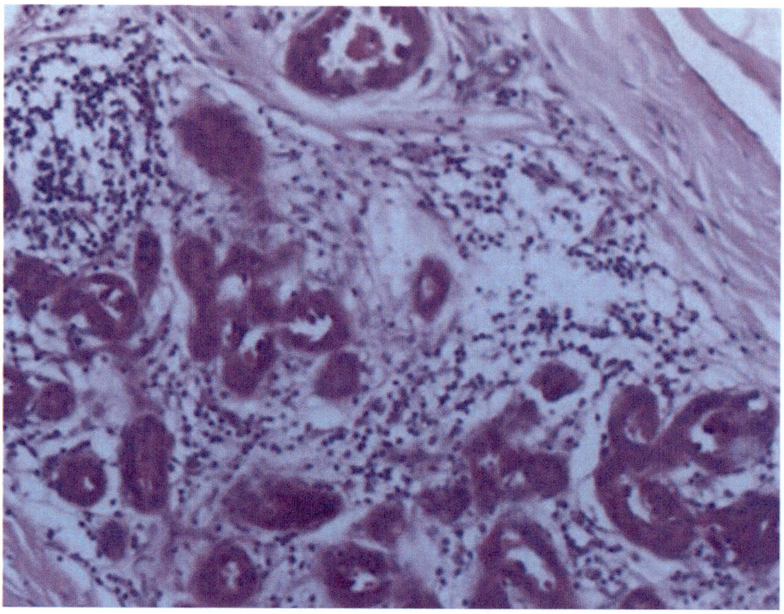

Fig. 13.19 PATHOHISTOLOGY: image of focus of high grade in situ ductal carcinoma

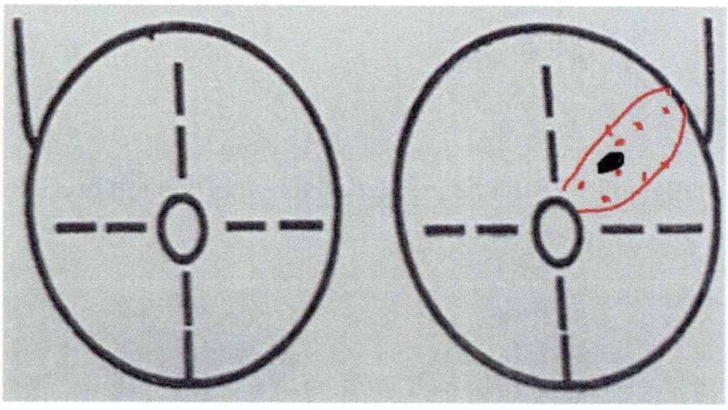

Fig. 13.20 SKETCH: position of fibroadenoma detected by ultrasound and distribution in situ carcinoma detected by pathohistological analysis of quadrantectomia which corresponds to the average surface of the lobe [1, 6–9, 11, 12]

individual foci or the malignant tissue spread all over the whole lobe [1, 6–9, 11, 12].

Conclusion

Early breast carcinoma diagnosis is the fundamental objective and purpose of the total breast disease diagnostics, particularly due to a very high percentage of healing (od 90–98%). The term of early breast carcinoma includes invasive carcinoma measuring up to 1 cm (without metastasis in the axilla and without distant metastasis) and in situ carcinoma of any size.

Early breast carcinomas need not be small, but can in the very beginning, at the microscopic level, affect a larger breast area—lobar disease. However, in spite of its diffusion to a large area of the glandular tissue, a high percentage of survival and healing is not reduced [8–11].

All the patients presented in this chapter have been regularly examined by palpation, inspection, mammography, and ultrasound. The results of the stated examinations have been compared with the findings of earlier examinations, which were crucial in detecting discrete new abnormalities – in this case, the abnormalities were detected during ultrasound examination (small lesions and discrete disarrangements of structures that had not been present before and the like).

All the breast carcinomas have their own subclinical phase during which they are not detectable by any of the examination methods.

In the next developmental phase, many of the carcinomas very often do not have developed morphological elements characteristic of malignity: ultrasound morphology is mostly nonspecific or has borderline features.

At an early stage, pathological neovascularization usually has not yet been developed, and it has not even come yet to the infiltration of the surrounding tissue. The results of the color Doppler analysis and elastography are often nonspecific and false negative.

Mammography is usually negative with very small carcinomas.

At an early stage, even the results obtained by magnetic resonance are not specific or it produces benign results.

However, if some of the discrete nonspecific, even benign abnormalities appear within the control interval, further treatment is indicated. In the cases described in this chapter, it was a cytological puncture under ultrasound control.

Knowledge of different pathomorphological features of individual types of breast carcinoma is extremely important as well as relating these features to the ultrasound and mammographic morphology.

I would like to place special emphasis on the importance of ultrasound diagnostics which was crucial in making an early diagnosis in the cases presented in this chapter [13].

A high-quality ultrasound device with high-frequency linear probe (10–18 MHz), along with a good examination technique (ductal echography) performed by well-educated experts, allows detecting very discrete changes that can hide carcinoma at an earliest possible detectable stage [4].

A decision regarding the need for biopsy can be reached upon incorporating the results of all the diagnostic procedures into a unified whole.

With initial breast carcinomas, due to their small dimensions, instead of core biopsy, an open biopsy is preferred after preoperative marcation under ultrasound control.

The examples stated above do not corroborate only the theory of breast carcinoma as a lobar disease but also the theory of synchronous occurring of early carcinoma in more different lobes in the form of tiny lesions, detectable by ultrasound, with microscopically detected spreading of initial malignant changes through a wide area of the adjacent lobe [4–7].

In order to avoid local recidives that make an early diagnosis futile, it is necessary to adapt the techniques of operative approach to the new ideas related to the lobar nature of early breast carcinoma [14].

We are called to a responsible attitude toward improving examination techniques and knowledges concerning early breast carcinoma diagnostics because each single early breast carcinoma diagnosis saves a life.

Whoever saves a life, it is considered as if he saved an entire world! Talmud.

References

1. Tot T. Breast cancer, a lobar disease. London: Springer; 2011.
2. Ewing J. Neoplastic diseases: a treatise of tumors. 4th ed. Philadelphia: Saunders WB; 1940. p. 568.
3. Gallagher HS, Martin JE. Early phases in the development of breast cancer. Cancer. 1969;24:1170–8.
4. Teboul M, Halliwell M. Atlas of ultrasound and ductal echography of the breast. Oxford: Blackwell Science; 1995.
5. Clarke MF, Dick JE, Dirks PB, Eaves CJ, Jammison CH, Jones DL, Visvader J, Weissman IL, Wahl GM. Cacer stem cells—prespectives on current status and future durectins. Cancer Res. 2006;66:9339–44.
6. Yan PS, Venkataramu C, Ibrahim A, Liu JC, Shen RZ, Diaz NM, Centeno B, Webel F, Lez UW, Shapiro CL, Eng C, Yeatman TJ, Huang TH. Mapping geographic zones of cancer risk with epigenetic biomarkers in normal breast tissue. Clin Cancer Res. 2006;12:6626–36.
7. Tot T. The theory of the sick breast lobe and the possible consequences. Int J Surg Pathol. 2007;1:68–71.
8. Anderson JA, Blichert-Toft M, Dyreborg U. In situ carcinomas of the breast. Types, growth pattern, diagnosis and treatment. Eur J Surg Oncol. 1987;13:105–11.
9. Holland R, Hendricks JH, Vebeek AL, Mravunac M, Schuurmans Stekhoven JH. Extent, distribution, and mammographic/histological correlation of breast ductal carcinoma in situ. Lancet. 1990;335:519–22.
10. Faverly DRG, Henricks JHCL, Holland R. Breast carcinoma of limited extent. Frequency, radiological-patologic characteristics, and surgical margin requirements. Cancer. 2001;91:647–59.

11. Foschini MP, Flamminio F, Miglio R, Calo DG, Cuccu MC, Masetti R, Eusebi V. The impact of large section on the study of in situ and invasive duct carcinoma of the breast. Hum Pathol. 2007;38:1736–43.
12. Amy D. Breast cancer a lobar disease. London: Springer; 2011. p. 153–62.
13. Amy D (2005) Millimetric breast carcinoma ultrasonic detection. In: Leading edge conference Pr. Goldberg B. USA.
14. Durante E. Multimodality imaging and interventional techniques. Ferarra, Italy: IBUS Course Abstracts; 2006.

14 Breast Implants

Jose Parada

Firstly, before talking about the ultrasound evaluation of breast implants, we must know there are different types of materials, shapes, content, etc.

For instance, there are prostheses filled with saline solution, more widely used in the USA, probably due to legal-medical issues, as silicone prevails in the rest of the world.

Many times, prior to the placement of prostheses, when dealing with a reconstruction after a mastectomy, expanders need to be used. There are several kinds of expanders, all of them equipped with valves that allow for progressive filling with saline solution to "create" the necessary space to place the final implant (Fig. 14.1).

Once the desired expansion is achieved, the plastic surgeon will decide which type of prosthesis is best suited to produce the best aesthetic result.

As we mentioned, there are saline solution-filled implants, prostheses with a smooth surface, and prostheses with a textured surface, each with their own special characteristics. For example, smooth implants, usually placed behind the pectorals, will be more likely to form a capsule, have less chances of creating a periprosthetic collection (known as seroma), and will be better tolerated post-op.

J. Parada, M.D.
Clinica por Imagenes Dres. Parada,
Montevideo, Uruguay
e-mail: jparada@clinicaparada.com.uy

Those with a textured surface will create seromas more frequently, and their location regarding the pectorals is indifferent.

An ultrasound is the first-line test to evaluate implants as it lets us know both their nature and their location regarding the pectoral; it is a perfectly tolerated and innocuous technique, which quickly at a considerably lower cost than an MRI provides us with detailed information about the health of the breast and the implants.

It is common to hear that an MRI is the ideal technique to study breast prothesis, and even though it is indeed very useful to study them, we usually choose to perform an MRI after a bad ultrasound by a technician with no knowledge of implants and with a report that is filled with doubts and inaccurate interpretations that force the clinician to perform an MRI.

We would like to remind you that when we perform a mammogram on breasts with implants, as long as the elasticity of the breast and the capsule allows it, we use Eklund technique, which pulls the implant back to obtain the cranial-caudal incidences almost free or free from the image of the prosthesis (Fig. 14.2).

In this way, we first evaluate the intra or extra-capsular ruptures.

As their name denotes, the confirmation of extracapsular ruptures will be easily interpreted by mammogram (Fig. 14.3).

However, the only differential diagnosis to consider if the implants were replaced is the presence

D. Amy (ed.), *Lobar Approach to Breast Ultrasound*, https://doi.org/10.1007/978-3-319-61681-0_14

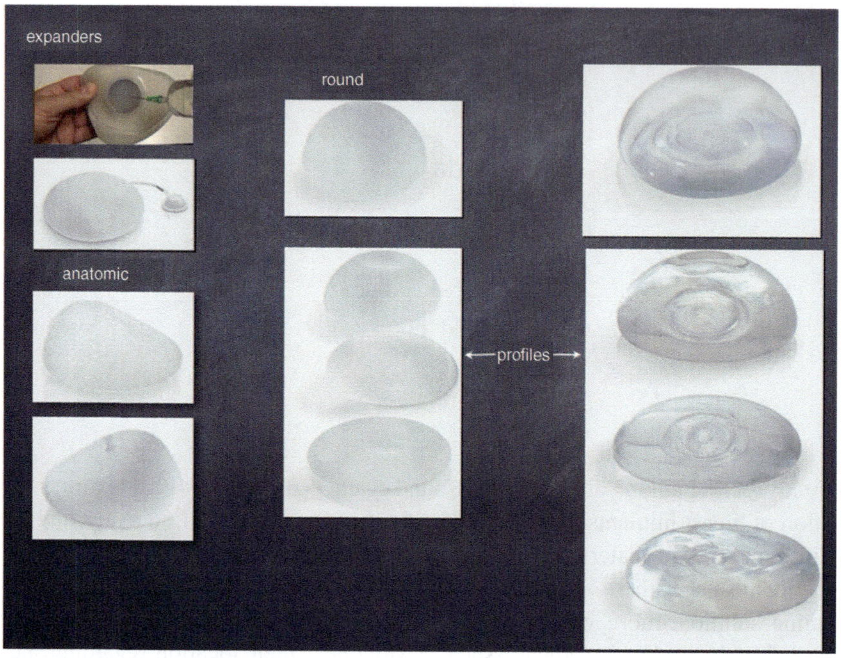

Fig. 14.1 Expanders and different kinds of implants

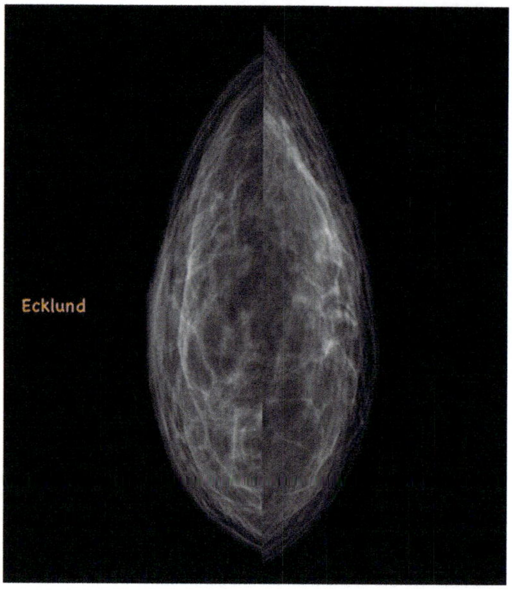

Fig. 14.2

of residue of pericapsular silicone from a previous rupture that can lead to confusion. Either way, if the internal echostructure of the implants is normal, i.e., virtually unechogenic, it is highly unlikely that the prosthesis is damaged (Fig. 14.4).

In the rupture of the intracapsular prosthesis, we basically make the diagnosis due to the alteration of the internal echostructure of the prosthesis. The regular homogeneity is lost, which can be checked by the presence of a heterogeneous, anarchic image (Fig. 14.5).

Another alteration we often see are the folds in the surface of the implants to which sometimes some meaning is attributed out of ignorance, especially when they are evident for the patient in sections in which the implant is subcutaneous or even in some reconstructions (Fig. 14.6).

Given how popular aesthetic implants are, it is our obligation to have a deep understanding of the ways in which these affect the study of mammary tissue in the first place and to understand the implants themselves which, as we can see, can have their own "pathology."

There are some limitations in the diagnosis for the radiologist given by the presence of implants, which is why we understand that every patient with implants sent for a yearly or biyearly control mammogram also has to undergo an ultrasound, always carried out with radial criteria, particularly in those cases in which the imaging semiology is somewhat distorted.

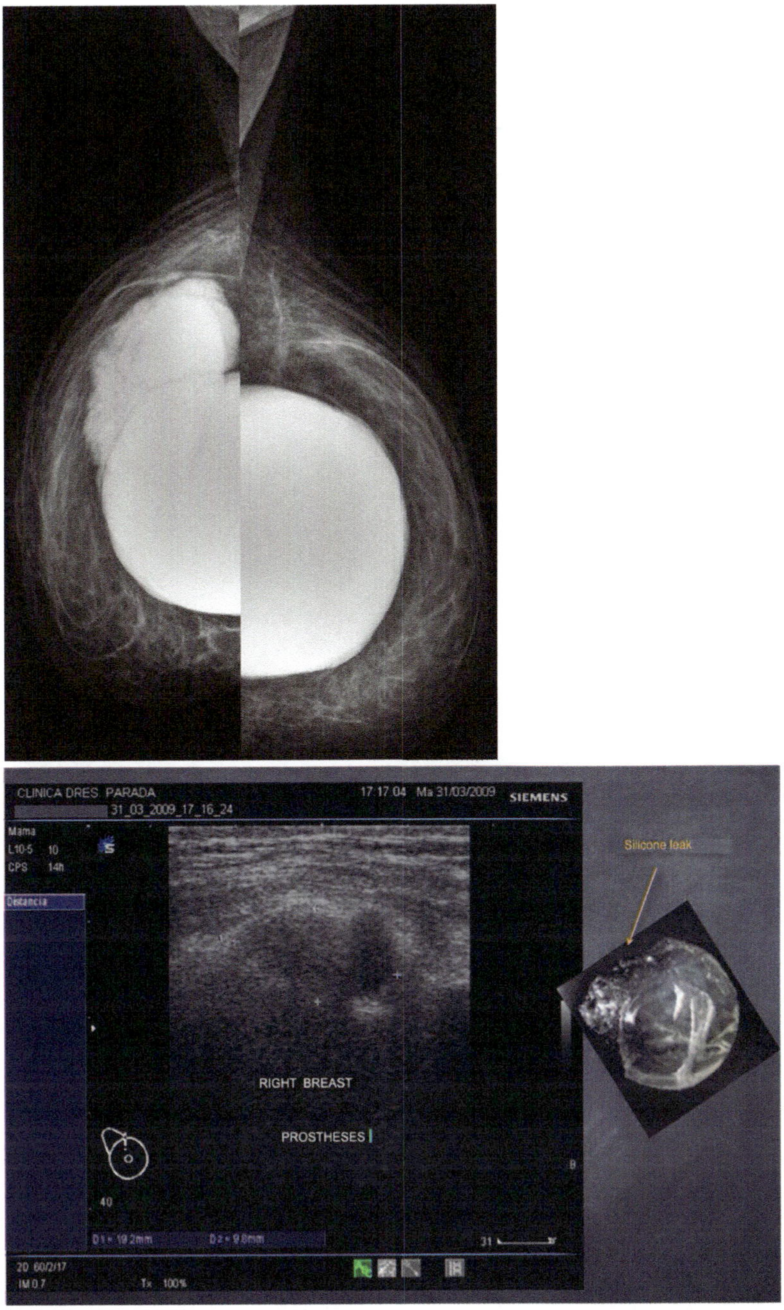

Fig. 14.3 Silicone material outside of the capsule

We quite often find periprosthetic fluid, which can show immediately after the operation or years later. This liquid often goes by unnoticed, and it must remain so as it is a thin layer that does not affect aesthetics or cause symptoms.

When this collection is greater, then the drainage of it is suggested, for which the ultrasound

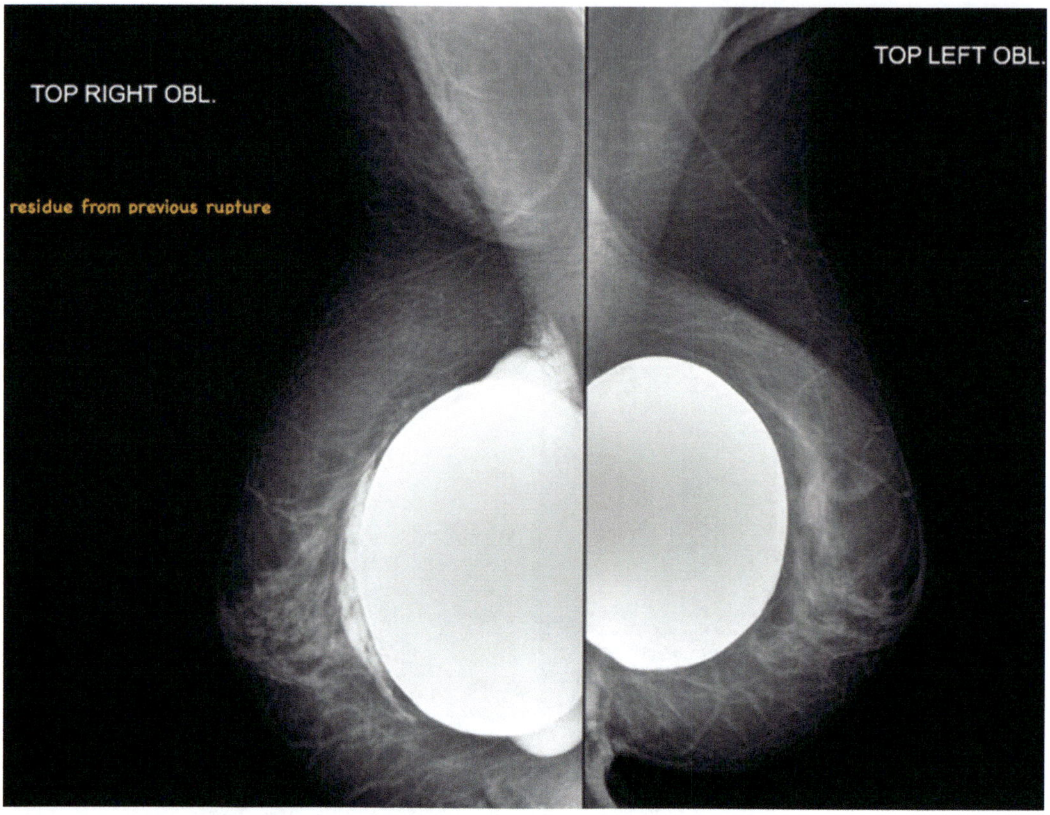

Fig. 14.4 Silicone remains from replacement

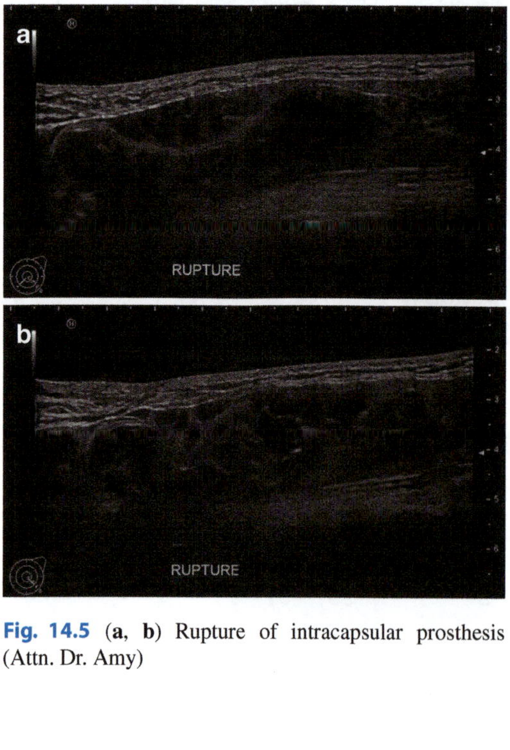

Fig. 14.5 (a, b) Rupture of intracapsular prosthesis (Attn. Dr. Amy)

guide is essential (Fig. 14.7) to preserve the indemnity of the implant and make sure it is completely drained. Furthermore, if when we remove the liquid it is transparent with no signs of contamination (turbidity), we inject corticosteroids in order to try to prevent its reoccurrence.

If we suspect contamination, a culture and antibiogram are performed.

A lot has been discussed about the cause of seromas without reaching any valid conclusions. However, there is an agreement on the fact that if we manage its reproduction after the draining puncture and the corticosteroid injection, we will have prevented a useless and expensive new intervention.

From a clinical point of view, a breast distended by a seroma is shocking (Fig. 14.8).

Of course the priority in the study of a breast with implants is to rule out simultaneous pathologies, which, as in every breast, can be benign or malignant.

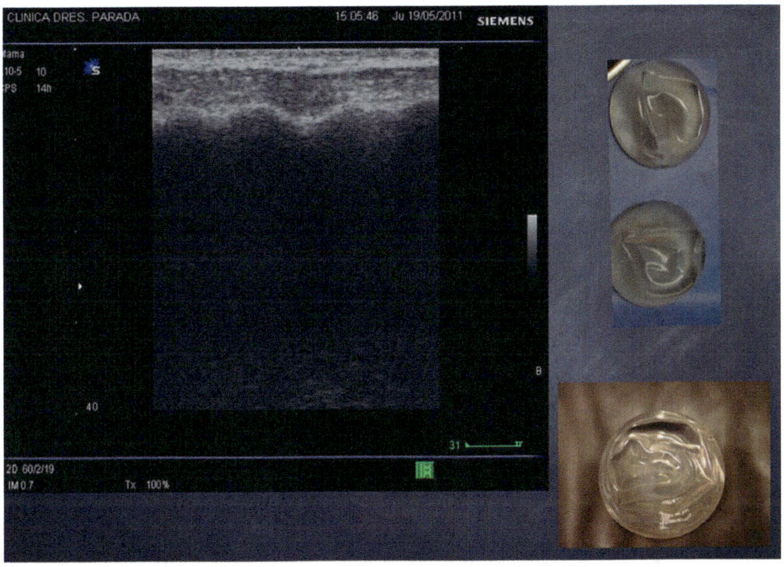

Fig. 14.6 Folds

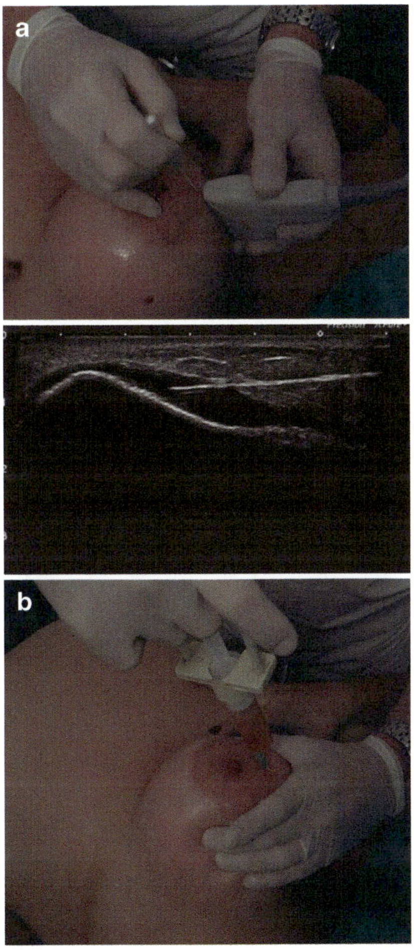

Fig. 14.7 (**a**, **b**) Ultrasound guide of the catheter. (**a**) periprosthetic seroma, 500 cc. (**b**) drainage

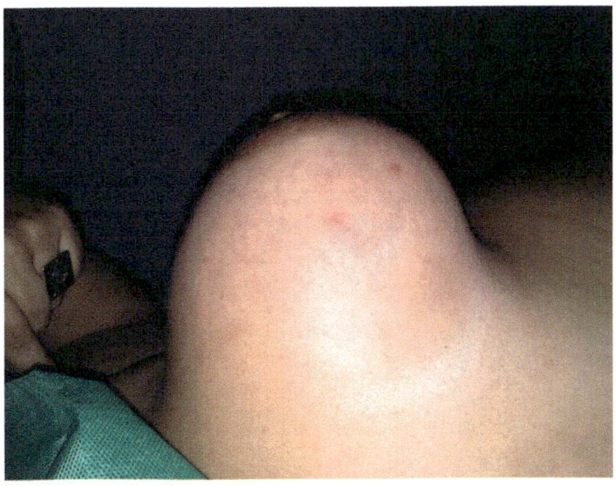

Fig. 14.8 Periprosthetic seroma

We must always keep in mind that the breast is studied with a ductal or radial technique if we intend to rule out multifocal lesions whether benign or malignant. The presence of implants sometimes prevents us from easily visualizing lesions that would otherwise be more easily seen. For this reason, and the multiple alterations we have mentioned that are characteristic of prostheses, we should always use ultrasound to evaluate breasts with prostheses.

Let's look at how, in this case, even though the Eklund technique was used, on the right, the opacity projected on the implant could have prevented diagnosis.

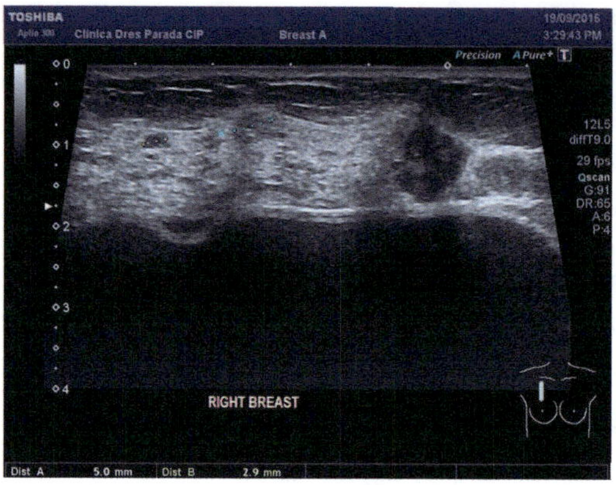

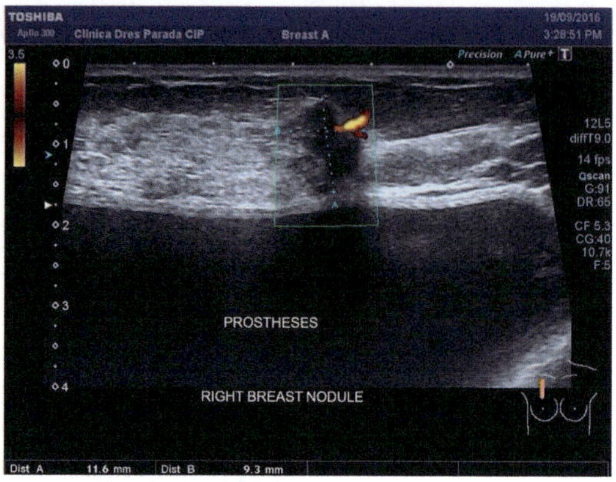

Of course, the ultrasound easily evidenced the presence of a solid vascularized nodule, with its main axis perpendicular to the skin. However, when we assess this with the ductal technique, we see there are two small images in the same lobule, close to the main nodule, that we puncture with a fine needle ruling out multifocality in this case.

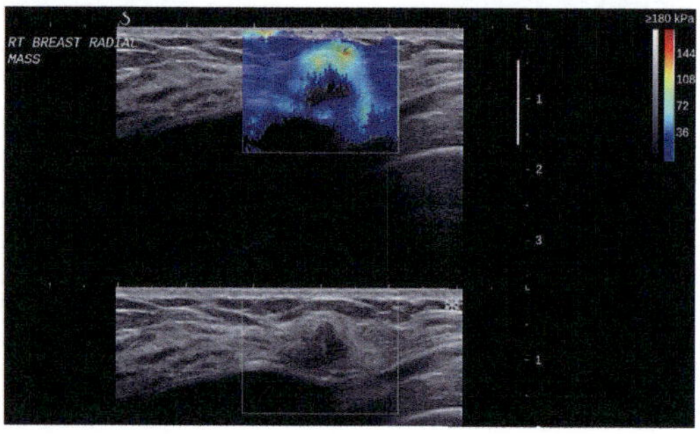

The main purpose of this chapter is to understand that an ultrasound is the first-line technique to evaluate breasts with implants due to its high sensitivity and specificity, as well as its higher accessibility due to cost and availability.

Our duty as radiologists, given the popularity of implants, is to know their characteristic pathologies, periprosthetic space, as well as their associated pathologies and to never forget that breasts should be studied with ductal ultrasound whether there are implants or not.

Bibliography

1. Kopans D. La mama en imágenes. Segunda edición, cap 5. España: Editorial Marban; 2003. p. 105.

Ultrasound-Guided Breast Interventional Procedure

15

Jose Parada

There are many varied instructions in the ultrasound guide for breast biopsies.

These include FNABs and cutting needle biopsies, as well as a core needle biopsy and a vacuum-assisted device, the placement of a metallic marker for a radiosurgical biopsy, and the need to leave a clip to locate the lesion after the neoadjuvant therapy.

Whatever the chosen method, the criteria used for the guide are exactly the same.

We always use freehand biopsy, that is to say, a biopsy where with one hand we hold the transducer and with the other we perform the puncture. Generally, the less skilled hand holds the transducer.

The movement we must make when puncturing the skin, as well as the internal advance of the needle, is sudden and fast. This is why proper training is essential.

This method reduces pain.

It is always best if we can use the long axis of the transducer to guide us.

The first thing we must do, once we've located the lesion and already have the device that is to be used, is to move the transducer over the lesion when we see the lesion on the screen so we can push it to the edge of the image, leaving a couple of centimeters between the lesion and the edge of the image in our screen, in order to visualize the initial trajectory before piercing the lesion. This first movement is the one we mentioned above. It has to be sudden and with little shifting, as the goal is to break through the skin in the least aggressive manner possible, after which we "gain momentum" again to break into the lesion.

When dealing with a fine needle and a solid mass, we will perform multiple forward and backward intralesional movements aspirating simultaneously and stopping once we consider we have enough material in the needle to spread it and for it to be representative of the lesion.

If we are aspirating a liquid mass, we aspirate until the edges of the capsule of the cyst or abscess collapse, and we take out the needle aspirating to achieve total drainage.

If we are dealing with thick abscesses, we can use larger gauge needles such as 18 and, if the pus is very thick, even 16. For this, we recommend using the same puncture point as when we used the smaller gauge needle (the smaller the gauge, the thicker the needle).

In general, if we perform the maneuver well, it is not necessary to apply prior local anesthesia, but this requires experience and skill that can be acquired only with practice.

When the lesions are close to the skin, the puncture is easier. We always puncture parallel to

J. Parada, M.D.
Clinica por Imagenes Dres. Parada, Montevideo, Uruguay
e-mail: jparada@clinicaparada.com.uy

D. Amy (ed.), *Lobar Approach to Breast Ultrasound*, https://doi.org/10.1007/978-3-319-61681-0_15

the length of the transducer, so we can follow the trajectory of the needle on the screen. The deeper the lesion, the farther we go from the transducer when we break through the skin, always trying to stay as parallel as possible to it.

We may need to angle the needle a little depending on the topography of the lesion. This is not inconvenient as it usually turns out to be quite practical to go in in parallel as usual, but as soon as we see the tip of the needle, we should angle it by raising the hand that is holding it. This may not be pleasant but it is a maneuver that can be used until we have the necessary skill and experience. Once we are more experienced, it is always better not to tilt the needle when we go in, in order not to cause discomfort.

In our personal experience, and since we work alongside an experienced cytologist, we currently reposition the fine needle aspiration puncture, always keeping in mind the multifocality of lesions and the need to analyze them before coming to a therapeutic decision.

We know we can gather more information from a tissue sample than from a handful of cells, but this cannot always be achieved; we are dealing with lesions that are often barely between 2 and 3 mm large.

We have a good understanding of the key concepts regarding ductal ultrasounds, as well as the concepts of multifocality or multicentricity, which have been introduced in other chapters. These allow us to understand why fine needle ultrasound-guided biopsies play, once again, a key role in the diagnosis of subclinical lesions prior to surgery.

We know that breast cancer cannot be prevented, as it is a multifactorial disease with an increasing incidence, especially in poorer countries. So far, our only weapon against it is early diagnosis, and the latest technological advancements have allowed us to do so in most cases to a subclinical level and to the millimeter. For this reason, together with the fact that it has been proven that this disease can affect the whole lobule, in more than 50% of cases with multicentric location, fine needle biopsies are a crucial technique.

This is why we need the assistance of an experimented cytologist to reliably tell us if the often scarce material we have obtained from the punctured "microcancers" is positive for atypical cells or not.

When the nodules are very small, we usually pierce them with the fine needle and, with it, carry the fat tissue and, many times, the scarce cells that represent the tumor. That is exactly why the intervention of a cytologist with experience and proper knowledge of this situation is crucial.

Of course, better information is obtained through a histologic puncture or a core biopsy, which is still a well-tolerated procedure when carried out under local anesthesia. But core biopsies are key procedures in nodules of 10 mm or more, which often require an immunohistochemical study to ensure a correct neoadjuvant therapy.

To carry out a **fine needle puncture,** we will use Fig. 15.1:

The length of the needle depends on the depth of the lesion that is to be punctured, but there is no need to use a needle with a greater gauge since that would cause a greater puncture hemorrhage and this finer needle is perfectly visible with modern echographs.

A fine needle is also less aggressive and painful for patients.

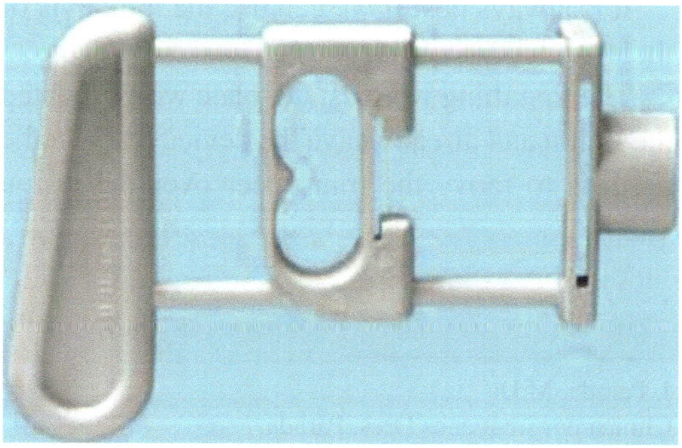

Fig. 15.1

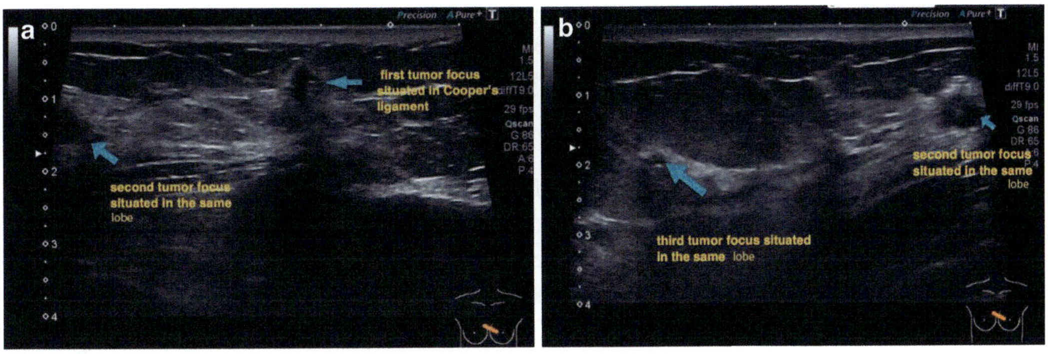

Fig. 15.2 (**a**, **b**) Multifocal cancer

When using a ductal echography technique, we can obtain multicentricity diagnoses. This is a good example of the above:

As shown by Fig. 15.2a, b, there are three tumor focus points. One of them is clearly invading Cooper's ligament, another is more internal, and the smallest one is closest to the areola, always in reference to the same duct, i.e., the same lobule.

It is important to remember that the start site for breast cancer is the terminal duct lobular unit and that the invasion of Cooper's ligament is common. The above case is a clear example of this.

The image has been magnified, but these are secondary lesions of no more than 4–5 mm in their maximum axis.

This patient was advised to undergo the puncture of a supposed sole nodule that was studied in a different health center. Before the usual puncture, we carried out a ductal echography to discard other smaller nodules, the presence of which was confirmed.

Since the biggest nodule was bigger than 1 cm and we proved that this was a multifocal process, on top of the fine needle puncture of the smaller nodules which demonstrated the multicentricity, we needed to complement this with a histologic puncture to understand the immunohistochemistry of the biggest tumor and to establish the appropriate neoadjuvant therapy for this case.

Clearly, if we have the training to guide a needle with ultrasound, we will be able to both place a metallic marker and perform a FNAB or carry out a core biopsy or, in the same way, place a metallic marker as a reference of the lesion's topography for future controls during adjuvant therapy.

It is important to recognize that, despite our best efforts, we can't always reach a precise conclusion, as the extracted material may be insufficient.

We can currently perform techniques such as contrast mammographies and/or magnetic resonances that allow us to confirm a multicentricity diagnosis and to establish the topography and determine the real dimensions of the lesions. Contrast mammography is advantageous since it allows for the exploration in the same workstation where we can visualize the mammography and the tomosynthesis. In this way, we can, for instance, overlap the topography of the microcalcifications with precision to see if there is an associated lesion (Fig. 15.3a, b).

To carry out a **contrast-enhanced spectral mammography** (CESM), an iodine nonionic contrast media is injected to a periphery vein in 1.5 cc per kilogram of body weight with an injection pump with a theoretical flow of 97 mL per minute. Two minutes after the injection is finished, the corresponding images are produced: a high-energy and a low-energy take per image.

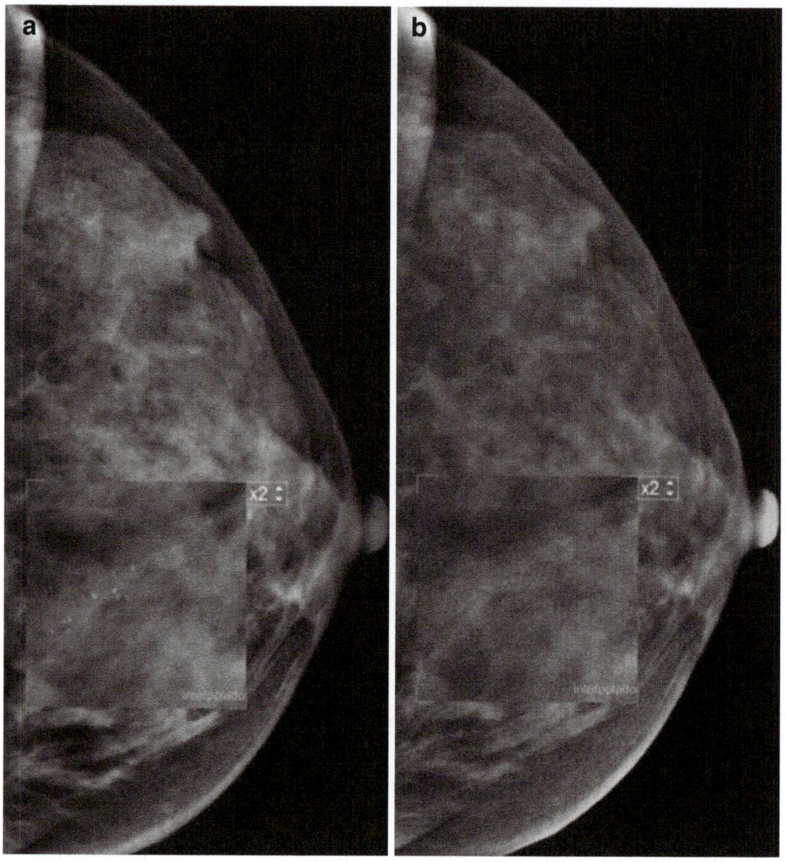

Fig. 15.3 (**a**, **b**) Microcalcifications with no associated lesions, low-grade CIS

The mammogram must have the necessary hardware and software.

One of the key features of this technique, as is the case with resonances, is the real measurement of the lesion (Fig. 15.4a, b) and the evaluation of multicentricity (Fig. 15.5a, b).

Patients must sign a consent form and undergo a study of their renal capacity as with any contrast radiography study.

Nowadays, we have practically all the possible imagenology tools to produce a correct and precise diagnosis before surgery so as to better plan the necessary neoadjuvant therapy, surgery, etc.

To carry out an **ultrasound-guided biopsy**, we need the following material:

- Alcohol gel
- Lidocaine + 20 cc syringe
- Puncturing system
- Scalpel blade
- Formaldehyde vials
- Gauzes
- Leukotape

The patient must not eat or drink for 4 h prior to the procedure and must provide recent coagulation studies which must have been performed no longer than 30 days before the puncture.

As a precaution, the patient must not take aspirin or other anticoagulant medicine during the week prior to the exploration.

First, the area must be sterilized, for which gel alcohol will suffice. Then, 2% lidocaine local anesthesia is applied to cut the skin and introduce the trocar. We must know the distance of the second cut (usually 2 cm) to take a good sample and avoid the risk of pneumothorax if located far behind the lesion (Figs. 15.6 and 15.7).

The puncture for the biopsy can be ultrasound-guided if a nodule is being examined or guided

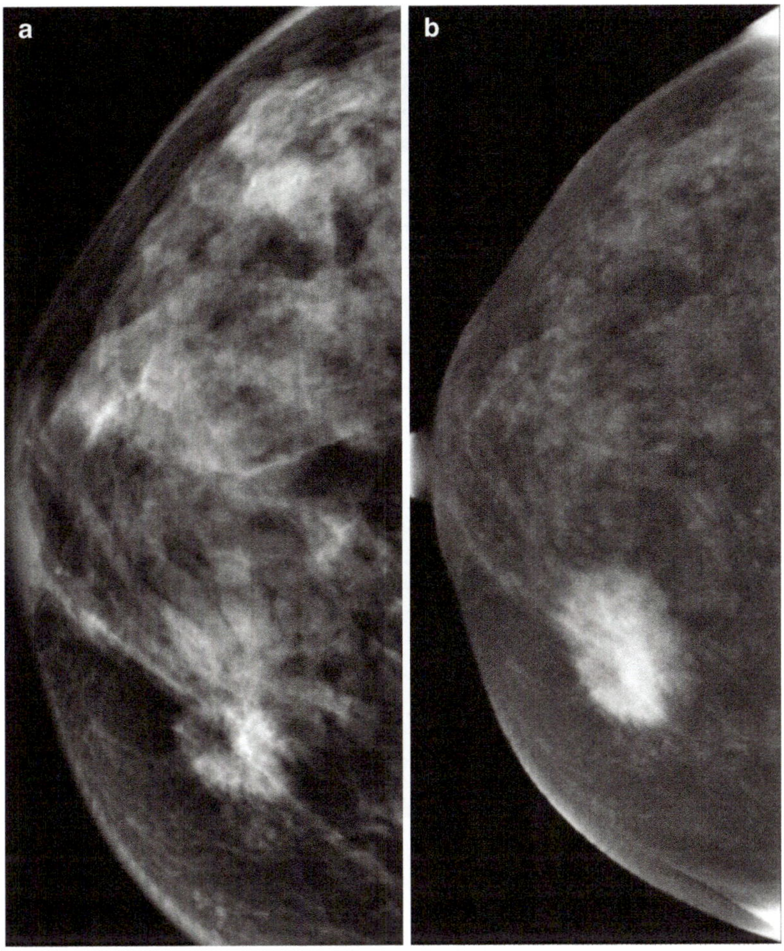

Fig. 15.4 (**a**, **b**) Real size of the lesion

by a mammogram if microcalcifications are being studied, in which case we would be performing a stereotactic biopsy.

Ultrasound-guided biopsies are simpler and faster, so this option will always be tried first.

Stereotactic biopsies are used with lesions that were diagnosed solely by mammogram. The exploration is carried out on a special table where the patient is placed face down. It has an opening for the breast where the biopsy will be performed so that the patient will not be able to see the procedure.

During the procedure, the breast is restricted so as to avoid movement. After finding the area where the biopsy will take place, different projections regarding different angles are carried out, and, through a coordinated calculation system, the equipment calculates the trajectory of the needle. After sterilizing the area, local anesthesia is applied to prevent pain, and samples are extracted with a thick needle. Once the procedure is over, the area is compressed to prevent the appearance of hematoma.

When the material is extracted, it is important to verify if we have included microcalcifications in the sample. For this reason, we currently have a high-definition closed system (Fig. 15.8) that allows us to carry out a high-definition mammogram of the obtained samples.

The difference in the procedure of the study of biopsies is that cylindrical tissue samples are placed, before being submerged in formaldehyde, in small plastic trays, which are provided with the equipment. These are

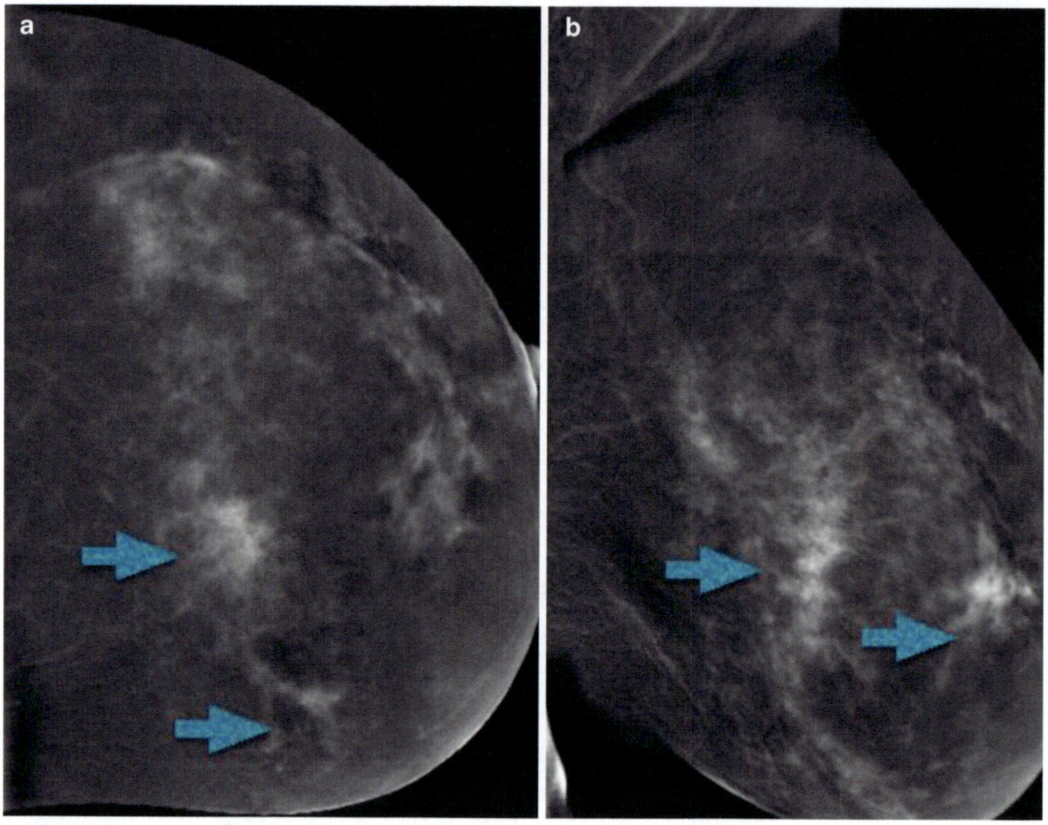

Fig. 15.5 (**a**, **b**)

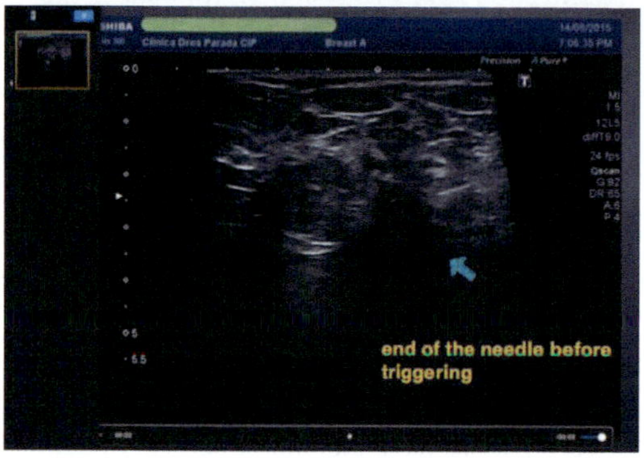

Fig. 15.6 End of thick needle positioned before triggering

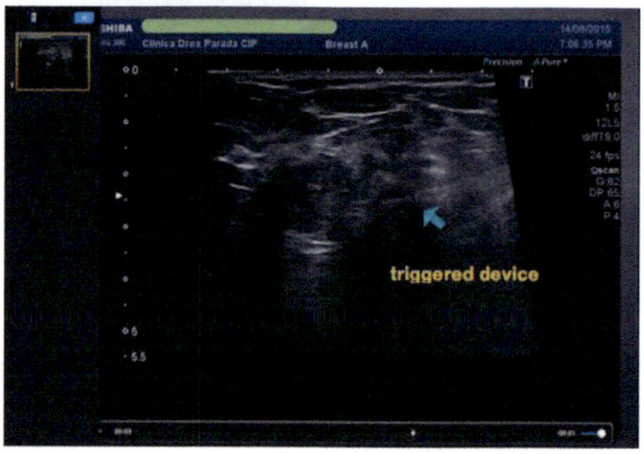

Fig. 15.7 Triggered device piercing the lesion

introduced in a duly shielded compartment where they are submitted to high-definition and magnification x-rays so as to determine the existence of microcalcifications in the tissue fragments.

Paraffin blocks can be documented if a pathologist requires them, as long as the blocks are small and able to fit in the compartment.

In conclusion, we can establish that *when the breast is explored with ductal ultrasound and small images of under 5 mm corresponding to*

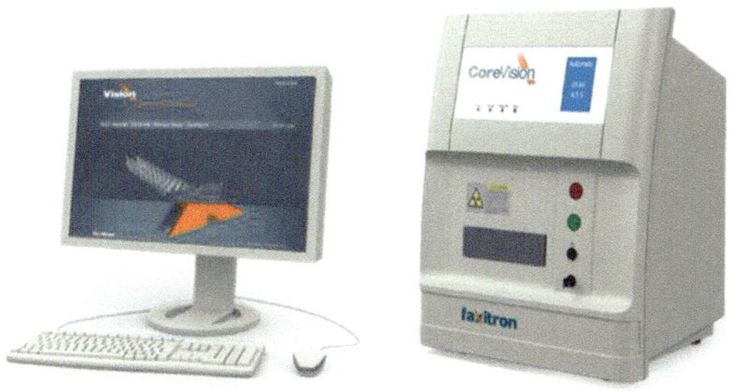

Fig. 15.8 System to document biopsies

multicentric neoplasms are detected, we advise that a fine needle puncture be performed in those small nodules, the results of which must be interpreted by an experienced cytologist.

It is also worth noting that *histologic punctures are recommended as long as the size of the lesion allows it, as they will provide us with better information. Not only do they determine the malignancy of the lesion, but they also provide information regarding its immunohistochemistry.*

Lobar Surgery and Pathological Correlations

16

Giancarlo Dolfin and Giovanni Botta

Key Remarks

- Breast cancer is not a lump but a lobar disease.
- Involvement of the breast lobe is often patchy or diffuse (multifocal or extensive DCIS).
- Breast conservative surgery to be radical must excise the whole lobe (lobar surgical approach).
- Lobar ultrasound is a useful tool to assist and guide breast surgeon.

16.1 Introduction

Breast-conserving surgery is the treatment of choice for women with relatively small breast cancers. The long-term survival rate among women who undergo breast-conserving surgery is the same as that among women who undergo radical mastectomy [1].

In the era of breast-conserving surgery, the problem is local recurrence. Conservative surgery with radiotherapy has been widely accepted as an alternative to mastectomy in the management of early-stage breast cancer, with a long-term local recurrence rate of approximately 10–20%. This number is much higher if postoperative irradiation is omitted. The cumulative incidence of recurrent tumor in the ipsilateral breast was 14.3% in the women who underwent lumpectomy followed by breast irradiation compared with 39.2% in the women who underwent lumpectomy without irradiation ($P < 0.001$) [2].

A considerable number of patients still experience local recurrence, even in some of the cases when the surgical margins of the resection have been judged to be cancer free.

Although several studies have shown no significant difference in distant disease-free survival (DFS) between women who did and did not have a breast recurrence after conservation therapy, a local failure can destabilize the patient's psychological balance. Besides, a re-excision after lumpectomy often causes an unsatisfactory cosmetic outcome.

Working together with other colleagues has proved to be particularly interesting and stimulating, insofar as each of us has come to the same conclusion via different routes: that, in order to battle against breast tumors, we all have to recognize, from within his/her own field, that the functional anatomical unity of the breast is in fact the lobe.

G. Dolfin, M.D. (✉)
Gynecologist, Oncologist,
c. Cosenza 35, Torino 10137, Torino, Italy
e-mail: giancarlodolfin@gmail.com

G. Botta, M.D.
Department of Pathology, Sant' Anna Hospital,
Torino, Italy
e-mail: giovanni.botta@unito.it

D. Amy (ed.), *Lobar Approach to Breast Ultrasound*, https://doi.org/10.1007/978-3-319-61681-0_16

For several decades, Dolfin [3] has performed breast surgery and concurrently utilized ultrasound diagnosis, following directives used in the school led by his friend Michel Teboul [4]. The pathological contribution has always also proved indispensable; indeed, Drs. Botta and Dolfin have always compared correspondences between data as outlined either by microscope, by ultrasound, or by surgical evidence.

Botta has scrutinized such correspondences between ultrasound data and anatomical pathology by utilizing lobar dissection with macrosection, a technique introduced by Dr. Tibor Tot [5], a contributor to the present volume.

Other surgical groups—and Prof. Durante [6] at the University of Ferrara in particular—have used the lobar approach in their surgical interventions in order to obtain better oncological and aesthetic outcomes. Like us, these other circles have obtained a dramatic reduction in the rate of recurrence in women suffering from this pathology, limiting the extension of surgical interventions, whenever allowed by the pathological criteria. Throughout Europe, courses have been offered based on the experiences accrued from the collaboration of diverse specialists in senology. Among the most enthusiastic organizers of these courses, we would like to mention in particular our recently deceased Spanish friend, Javier Amoros Oliveros [7].

Surgery should achieve both acceptable cosmetic results and negative margins [8], which require a preoperative study and localization of lesions.

The surgeon must have a thorough knowledge of the anatomical and functional changes of the mammary gland, the neoplastic and preneoplastic modifications, their origin, and their location; the pathologist must check that the surgeon has removed all the suspected areas, included in a halo of healthy tissue.

Today we know that the disease is not limited to an identified breast node but is extended to the whole breast lobe where that node arose [9].

The "sick lobe" is born genetically misshapen, during embryonic development, carrying some kind of genetic instability that implies an increased sensitivity to endogenic and exogenic oncogenic stimuli.

The number of the transformed cells, their location within the sick lobe, and the time difference in their transformation determines the morphology of the individual cancer and its biological potential [10].

The following parameters could influence the surgical approach and the patient's prognosis:

1. Multiple localization (either in situ or invasive)
2. Tumor extension
3. Lobe extension
4. Skin/fascia/areola/nipple involvement

16.2 Multiple Localization

In their early phase, almost all breast carcinomas seem to affect only one sick lobe [11]. Breast carcinoma is a lobar disease in that the tumor foci (appearing simultaneously or asynchronously, in situ or invasively) develop within a single sick lobe and the cancerous structures are confined to the area of the sick lobe at the early stage of the disease.

For this reason, most breast carcinomas exhibit complex subgross morphology and frequently multiple locations.

The prevalence of multicentric (MC) and multifocal (MF) tumors varies from 5% to 44% in published series [12], depending on the definition used, the method of histological examination of mastectomy specimens, and the type of imaging used for diagnosis.

Different diagnostic criteria for multifocality have deeply influenced the various studies, causing these results to be hardly comparable to each other.

MF carcinomas are usually defined by the presence of several invasive tumors in the same quadrant of the breast within a distance inferior to 5 cm.

MC carcinomas are defined by the presence of at least two invasive tumors in two different quadrants of the breast or in the same quadrant but at least 5 cm apart [13].

Related to lobar breast anatomy and physiology, multifocality means the presence of several tumor foci within a single lobe and multicentricity the presence of two or more sick lobes within the same breast.

Most of these definitions focus on invasive tumor foci, ignoring the in situ component of the tumor [12, 14–16].

Mammography and ultrasound are the standard imaging tools for the diagnosis of breast cancer and are also used to determine the extent of the disease within the affected breast.

Magnetic resonance imaging is increasingly used. However, the impact of breast MRI on breast cancer management is debated, due to a large number of additional benign lesions that could be detected and could incorrectly influence clinical decisions [17, 18].

The histopathologic method used is also an important factor influencing the results in studies of multifocality and everyday diagnostic routine.

Large-section histopathology substantially increases both the proportion of detected multiple tumor foci and their number for each case [19]. Regular use of large sections in diagnostic pathology results in 25–37% multifocality regarding the invasive component [20].

Combining the distribution of the in situ and invasive components results in up to 60% to 65% nonunifocal subgross distribution of the lesions. Such a high level of multifocality seems to be independent of tumor size and histologic type and was observed in a series of smaller than 15-mm invasive carcinomas [10, 11, 21–23].

Approximately half the invasive cases are unifocal (only one invasive focus could be observed in the large sections, which may or may not have contained an in situ component close to the invasive focus.

A quarter of the cases are characterized by the presence of a multifocal invasive lesion characterized by the presence of multiple, well-delineated invasive tumor foci separated from each other by uninvolved breast tissue containing normal tissue, benign lesions, or in situ carcinoma.

The final quarter of the cases exhibit tumors dispersed over a large-section area with no distinct tumor mass, like a spider's web. In situ or invasive breast carcinomas of diffuse type often represent extensive disease, limiting the success of breast-conserving surgery [11, 23].

16.3 Tumor and Lobar Extension

Lobar ultrasound examination allows us to study the ductal tree of the sick lobe and map out the diseased part(s) which is essential in guiding adequate surgical intervention. Breast carcinomas of limited extent (<4 cm), whether unifocal or multifocal, are proper candidates for breast-conserving surgery. Adequacy of breast conservation in more extensive tumors should be carefully judged preoperatively in every individual case.

The dimensions of the breast lobes are very different within the same breast and also individually [24, 25]. The largest lobe appearing in one of the very few related studies comprised 25% of the breast volume, the smallest only 1% of the breast volume. Lobes are larger in the upper outer quadrant of the breast than in the medial parts. In addition, the dimensions of the lobes are also age related; they are larger in younger women and undergo involution around and after the menopause. The lobes in the medial quadrants of the breast develop later and undergo involution earlier than the lobes in the lateral quadrants. During the malignant transformation of the structures of the sick lobe, new cancerous TDLUs and ducts may develop and increase the dimension of the involved lobe [11].

Young age strongly correlates with a high risk of local recurrence after breast-conserving surgery, whether or not radiotherapy is given. This relationship is associated with the dimensions of the sick lobe, which is an important factor in determining the success of breast-conserving surgery.

16.4 Skin/Fascia Involvement

Equally important, both from the oncological point of view and for the surgical planning, is the distance of the tumor from the skin. We need a careful study of the subcutaneous tissue and the areas corresponding to Cooper's ligaments. Through these ligaments, in fact, it has been demonstrated that tumor cells can spread to upper areas. This migration can increase the relapses [24].

16.4.1 Presurgical Cytohistological Examination of Breast Lesions

Presurgical cytohistological examination of breast lesions integrated by palpatory exam and diagnostic imaging (ultrasound and radiological) would minimize the proportion of excision biopsies of benign lesions for diagnostic purposes and would maximize the preoperative diagnosis of cancer (Table 16.1)

Cytological investigation is applicable:

- *On secretion from the nipple*: The examination is indicated when the secretion is the only clinical sign and especially if it is hematic. The prevalence of cancer in the presence of each other type of secretion and in the absence of other clinical findings is irrelevant.
- *On liquid inside a cyst*: The examination is indicated in the presence of bloody or siero-hematic liquid. The prevalence of cancer in the presence of another type of content is irrelevant.
- *On material obtained by abrasion of erosive lesions of the nipple*: The examination is indicated whenever it poses the minimal suspicious for cases of the nipple Paget unaccompanied by mass clinically or radiologically appreciable, a very rare lesion.
- *On material obtained by fine needle aspiration of solid palpable or non palpable breast lesion (FNA)* [26, 27].

Table 16.1 Goals of presurgical cytohistological examination of breast lesions

Select patients with breast abnormalities in preclinical stage to be subjected to surgical biopsy
Improve the preoperative diagnosis of cancer
Reduce the proportion of excision biopsies for diagnostic purposes
In advanced lesions to obtain a cytohistological diagnosis and prognostic factors for neoadjuvant chemotherapy

16.4.1.1 Cytopathological Report (Secretion, Scraping, or FNA)

The descriptive diagnosis is optional. In this case, the cytopathological report must be clear and succinct and, if possible, have reference to the corresponding histopathology. The diagnostic conclusion is obligatory according to one of the following formulas:

C1: Inadequate

Reason must be indicated:

Cellularity poor or absent
Artefactual cellular distortions by unsuitable sample
Cellularity obscured by blood and/or inflammation

The presence of only fat tissue cannot be considered in any case as an "inadequate diagnosis" because in some cases may be the expected finding.

C2: Benign. No evidence of malignancy

If there is sufficient cytological features, a specific diagnosis may be indicated (e.g., fibroadenoma).

C3: Atypical/probably benign

The basic framework of cytology is benign, but there are one or more of the following characteristics:

Increased cellularity
Polymorphism cyto-nuclear
Loss of initial or focal cell cohesion

C4: Suspicious/probably malignant

The cytological features are suggestive but not diagnostic of malignancy. In this category may fall a number of lesions "borderline" or ductal low-G (cribriform, papillary, tubular) when there is insufficient cytologists criteria for belonging to the next category or the presence of atypical elements indicative of malignant lesion in a small amount for the "application of the higher category"

C5: Malignant

The cytological features are diagnostic of malignancy, when it is possible it is preferable to mention the nuclear grade (G) and to specify the presence or absence of microcalcifications.

16.4.1.2 Diagnostic Performance Indices of Cytological Investigation (FNA)

In major centers, the sensitivity for cancer (positive + suspicious, inadequate excluded) is 90–95%. The specificity of a positive outcome is less than 1% and its predictive value greater than 99%. The rate of inadequate in the case of cancer is less than 10%. In the presence of a positive report, verified the high predictability, intraoperative biopsy can be omitted. In the presence of a suspicious report, verified his prediction that ranges in literature between 40% and 80%, surgical biopsy is mandatory, regardless of the clinical evidence. In the presence of a negative report, given the possible false negative, the opportunity to suggest a biopsy indicated by other diagnostic tests is not denied. Rates of sensitivity, specificity, and predictive value not compatible with those observations call for a critical review of the sequence collection/treatment/reading and possibly a comparison with an experienced center. The overall sensitivity and specificity of fine needle aspiration depend on variables intrinsic to the technique as well as related to radiological/clinical and histological features [28].

16.4.1.3 Sampling Techniques for FNA Cytology

According to the guide line of the Royal College of Pathologist of Australia (www.nbcc.org.au) [29], we describe a recommended approach to taking the tissue sample using FNA cytology under clinical guidance (palpable lesion):

- The woman is placed in supine position.
- First disinfect the skin over the lesion.
- The lesion is immobilized between two fingers of one hand, and the needle is introduced with the other hand. Depending on operator preference, the needle may be introduced on its own or directly with the syringe (and its holder) attached. We suggest to use needles from 22G to 27G (2–4 cm long), however, giving preference to small caliber needles.
- When the needle tip is felt to be at the edge of the lesion, negative pressure is applied while entering the lesion.
- Rapid multiple passes are made through the lesion, varying the angling of the sampling.
- If blood is seen in the hub, sampling should be ceased as excessive blood reduces the quality of the sample.
- The negative pressure is released while the needle is still in the lesion. The needle is then withdrawn.
- The material is expelled from the needle onto a labeled glass slide using the syringe
- Using another clean glass slide, smear the material to obtain a thin/uniformed distributed sample followed by a rapid fixation (alcohol 95 or methanol). This is a critical point to obtain a high-quality sample (an appropriate and well-fixed smear).
- If a pathologist is available an immediate examination of the slides after a rapid staining (Blue Toluidine) allow to recognize if aspirated material is sufficient. If an immediate examination is not possible, at least three passes are taken. Typically, any further sampling has little additional yield.

The cells can be also sampled without aspiration (cytopunction) taking advantages of spontaneous rising capillary action. This method offer qualitative advantages (less cell distortion) but usually scant material compare to aspiration technique.

It is preferable to perform FNA by ultrasound guide (this approach it is mandatory in a non-palpable lesion) [28]. The operator holds the ultrasound probe with one hand and introduces the needle with the other. The needle should be introduced so its long axis is in line with the long axis of the probe face. With this approach, the full length of the needle, including the tip, is visualized at all times. The needle angle should be kept as parallel to the probe face and chest wall as possible, so as to aid visualization and reduce the risk of accidental pneumothorax. A hard copy image may be taken to record the position of the tip of the needle inside the lesion. It is also advisable that in the palpable lesions, especially if large and inhomogeneous, an ultrasound examination is preliminarily performed in order to be sure that the needle has reached the diagnostic component of the lesion (Fig. 16.1).

In particular, in the lesions of extension of greater dimensions than or equal to 20 mm, mammographically connoted by hypodense central core, the sampling should be carried out on the marginal areas of the lesion, the more likely mobile and free from phenomena of sclerosis (Fig. 16.2).

FNA cytology requires training in the preparation of quality smears and a considerable cytology expertise for sample interpretation.

Liquid-based cytology applied to FNA of breast lesions allows to reduce unsatisfactory samples giving increased attention to nuclear details [30].

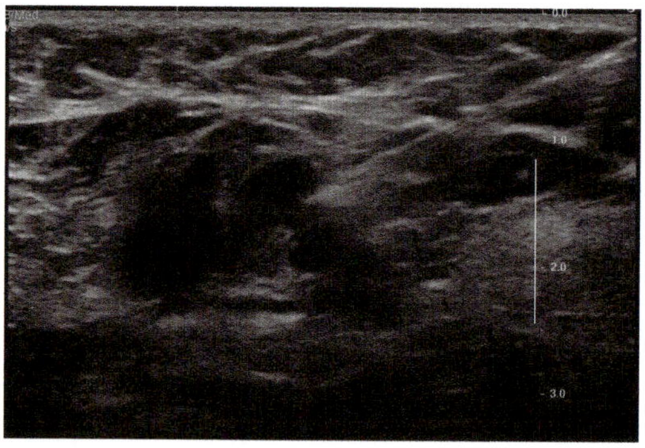

Fig. 16.1 US examination of the pathological area of the lobe and visualization of needle tip (arrow) during the biopsy

16.5 Percutaneous Microbiopsy (Core Biopsy) (CB): Sampling Procedure

According to the guideline of the Royal College of Pathologist of Australia [29], the following description represents one approach to taking the tissue sample using core biopsy under ultrasound guidance (www.nbcc.org.au):

- Patient positioning, skin cleansing, and lesion fixation are the same as for a cytology procedure. However, local anesthesia is always used in the skin and in immediate subcutaneous tissue.
- Using a scalpel blade, a small cut is made at the selected entry point, and the needle is introduced through this entry point.

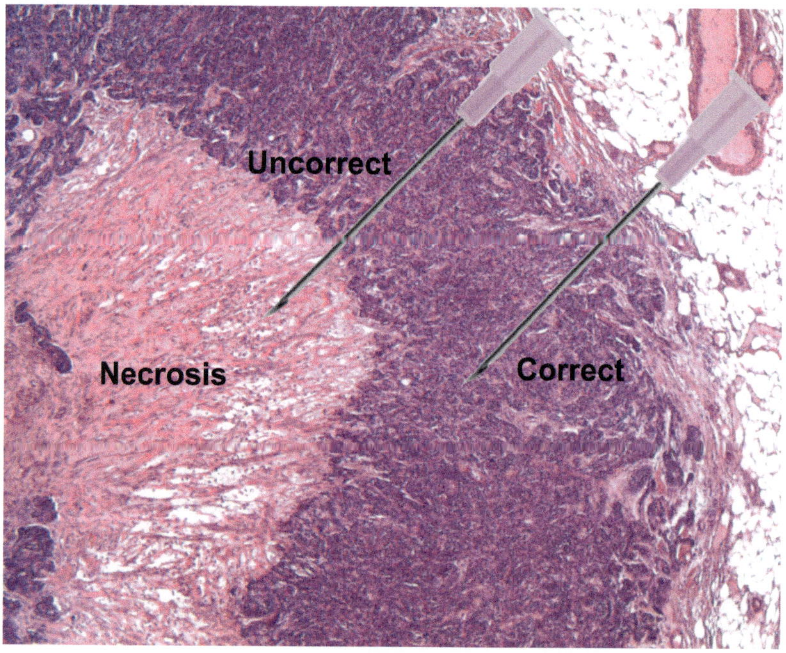

Fig. 16.2 Under ultrasound guide, the needle tip have to reach the breast lump where it is more rich of cells and with no necrosis

- The needle needs to be introduced so its long axis is in line with the long axis of the probe and as parallel to the chest wall as possible. The area beyond the needle tip should be visualized prior to firing to reduce the risk of a pneumothorax, because the needle is typically thrown forward 15–22 mm.
- When the tip of the needle is felt to be at the leading edge of the lesion, the firing mechanism is released and the sample taken.
- The needle is removed and the sample extracted.
- The procedure is then repeated. Typically three to five samples are taken through different parts of the lesion to ensure adequacy of sampling.
- The number of cores will be the result of various issues, including lesion characteristics, imaging findings, ability to localize, guidance modality, patient tolerance, and the confidence in the adequacy of the sample. Generally, between three and five cores will be taken.
- The sample must be fixed immediately; the formaldehyde-based fixatives are the most used but may lead to the dissolution of microcalcifications when the fixing is prolonged beyond 24 h; alcoholic fixatives do not have this problem but cause greater tissue coarctation; a good one is given by the Carnoy's fixative, which does not dissolve the calcifications, narrows slightly the fabric, and allows good preservation of tissue antigens by immunocytochemical investigations; however, it does not allow the radiography of the sample fixed to the radiopacity of its components. After inclusion, it is appropriate to set up immediately additional sections for the possible biological characterization of the tumor, to avoid losing the fabric during the cutting operations.
- The use of snap needles 18G provides frustules usually of 5 mm long with a volume of tissue removed (per withdrawal) of about 6 mm^3 while needles from 14G for taking cores of length up to 10 mm with a volume of tissue that varies from 20 to 35 mm^3. Currently, most of the published series refers to the use of needles from 14G.

16.5.1 Histopathological Report

It is recommended that the classification is divided into five diagnostic categories, with a pattern similar to that used for the needle aspiration cytology; however, it is stressed that the categories do not have the same meaning of the cytological and possess different clinical application outcomes. It is essential to compare the histological picture with the X-ray to ensure the representativeness of the biopsy.

The diagnostic conclusion is obligatory according to one of the following formulas:

- B1: (a) normal tissue, (b) only stroma, or (c) cannot be interpreted for artifacts. The presence of dystrophic calcification in the absence of stromal epithelium, where compatible with the radiological picture, must be classified as BENIGN.
- B2: benign lesion. It is recommended a concise text description.
- B3: benign lesion, but of uncertain biological behavior. It indicates lesions that are associated with increased risk of developing a carcinoma or are often associated with carcinomas in situ or invasive, for example, papillary lesions and scleroelastosis lesions. It is recommended that, where possible, a concise text description.
- B4: suspect. The category should be used when observing with compatible carcinoma in situ lesions or invasive, but when the final diagnosis is not formulated for artifacts for the presence of atypia or borderline. It is recommended that, where possible, a concise text description.
- B5: malignant. It indicates the undeniable presence of malignancy or invasive carcinoma in situ. In the case of diagnosis of carcinoma (B5), must indicate the presence or absence of infiltrating carcinoma or if the invasion is possible but not certain. If you suspect the presence of metastatic cancer, the data needs to be specified with a text description.

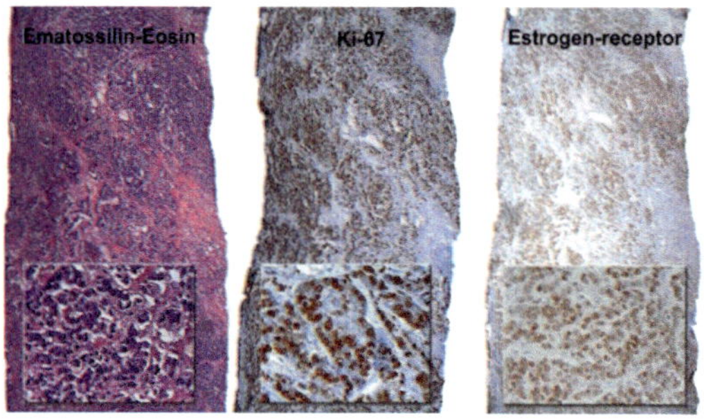

Fig. 16.3 Different markers of the specimens

In case of carcinoma in situ, histological type (ductal or lobular), nuclear grade and presence of associated calcifications must be indicated, if possible.

In case of invasive cancer, histological type, histological grade, the presence of in situ component, and eventually the presence of associated calcifications must be specified.

In cases of locally advanced tumors that will be submitted to neoadjuvant chemotherapy, it is often required to assess the state receptor and the expression of c-erb (Fig. 16.3).

16.5.2 Core Biopsy (CB) Diagnostic Accuracy

According to the literature, the sensitivity and specificity of CB are, respectively, 85–98% and 96–100%, with differences attributable to the experience of the pickup, and the type of breast lesions is investigated. CB produces an inadequate rate less than the FNA (0–17% vs. 5–24%) especially if multiple samples are done and if it is performed with 14G needle. CB can reduce 50–64% of surgical biopsies of benign lesions and increases the diagnosis of invasive carcinoma preoperative up to 92% (only with multiple samples) [27, 31].

Core biopsy (CB) compared to fine needle aspiration (FNA) has higher sensitivity and specificity and a lower rate of samples reported as unsatisfactory particularly for image-detected lesions. Most importantly, core biopsy but not FNA cytology differentiate invasive cancer from in situ lesion and distinguish in a high proportion of cases atypical ductal hyperplasia from low-grade in situ carcinoma. However, core biopsy requires local anesthesia and may result in more discomfort post-procedure, and its results usually take longer to be obtained. Disposables and equipment required to perform FNA are less expensive than for core biopsy. Taking into account the benefits and limitations of both techniques (Tables 16.2 and 16.3), we argue that CB is to be preferred over FNA for the diagnosis of breast lesions [27, 31–33] (Fig. 16.4) (Tables 16.2 and 16.3).

Vacuum-assisted breast biopsy (VABB) is a more recent technique. VABB has proven clinical

Table 16.2 FNA compared to CB

	Fine needle aspiration (FNA)	Core biopsy (CB)
False positive (specificity)	High (91–100%)[a]	Very high (96–100%)[a]
False negative (sensibility)	Discrete (77–100%)[a]	High (85–98%)[a]
Inadequate	Present <25%[a]	Low <15%
Cost	Very low	Higher
Time to get result	Few minutes to hours	1 day
Level of pathological experience required	High	Average
Technique	No anesthetic/training in smear required	Local anesthetic/careful pickup of core biopsies
Complication rate	Low	Low

[a]Many factors may influence the accuracy of FNA cytology and core biopsy:

- The characteristics of the breast lesion being investigated (patient selected by screening or by diagnostic procedure)
- The experience of the clinician performing the procedure
- To perform sample by ultrasound guidance
- To check immediately after fine needle aspiration the sample adequacy
- The availability of pathologists with experience in cytology

Table 16.3 FNA and CB accuracy

Type of lesion	Fine needle aspiration (FNA)	Core biopsy (CB)
Palpable lesion	High	High
Non-palpable tumor (US guide)	Moderate–low	High
Accessibility of deep sites	Yes	No (or with particular attention)
Diagnosis of preinvasive lesions	Low	High
Area of microcalcifications	Low	High
Grading neoplasia	Low	Moderate–high
ER/PR assessment	Low	High
HER2 assessment	Low	High
Proliferation assessment	Low	High

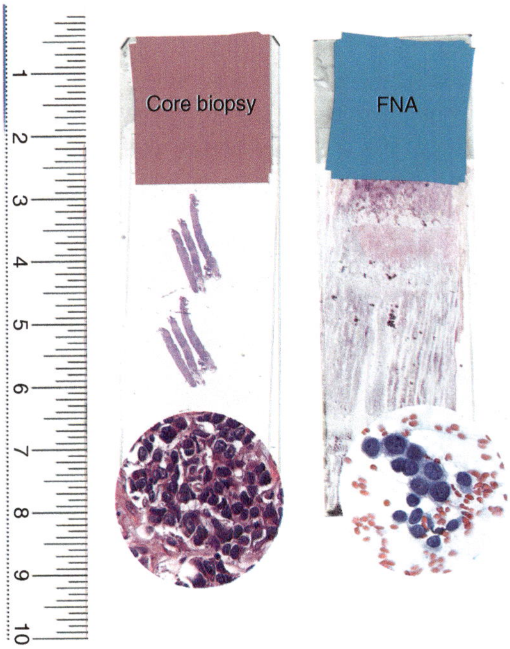

Fig. 16.4 Comparison between two methods of presurgical evaluation of the same breast lump: a specimen with core biopsy (at left) and a specimen of fine needle aspiration (FNA) at right. In the circle specimen's high-power vision (400×)

value and can be used under sonographic, mammographic, and magnetic resonance imaging guidance. The main indication for the use of VABB is for biopsies of clustered microcalcifications, which are usually performed under stereotactic guidance. This method has been proven reliable and should replace surgical biopsies. For masses that are likely benign or indeterminate, we attempt to completely remove the lesion to eliminate uncertainty on later follow-up images. VABB offers the best possible histological sampling and aids avoidance of unnecessary operations. VABB complications include bleeding or pain during the procedure, as well as postoperative pain, hemorrhaging, and hematomas. But, these hemorrhaging could be controlled by the post-procedural compression and bed resting. Overall, VABB is a reliable sampling technique with few complications, is relatively easy to use, and is well-tolerated by patients. The larger amount of extracted tissue reduces sampling error [34].

16.6 A Lobar Surgical Approach

Surgery is only a part of the therapeutic process in the fight against breast cancer. The set of diagnostic tools, the different associated therapies (medical and surgical), and the ultimate control of the removed area by the pathologist allow us to have a good chance against breast cancer and to have the best therapy with the best aesthetic results and the minimum percentage of tumor recurrence.

The problem of breast cancer is old. The first historical references to the treatment of this pathology [7] are found in the Egyptian papyri, in the schedules of Nineveh (2250 BC) and in an Indian treaty of 2000 BC (Yajiur Veda), where it is recommended to burn with acid rather remove with a blade. Starting from destructive surgery as they did with the intervention of William Stewart Halsted (who describes his technique on his series of patients with breast cancer, operated at Johns Hopkins Hospital from 1889 to 1894) or Urban, passing through less destructive surgery according to Patey or Madden, only in recent decades, thanks to the Milan school (Veronesi)

[1], we reach a conservative surgical approach with quadrantectomy.

Equally important is the attempt to overcome the problem of scars, immediately aroused by the operated women, mutilated by such destructive therapies. Good results were obtained by various techniques, including the very old but valid and still relevant one described by Tansini in 1896.

Today, where possible, we can perform a much more limited intervention, lobectomy, thanks to the knowledge and histopathologic confirmation of the concept of lobar disease, now almost universally acknowledged [21, 35].

We know for sure that the tumor propagation can occur in many cases along the milk ducts, so we have strong doubts about the type of intervention called "lumpectomy" [36]. According to us, most recurrences would be eliminated by careful removal of the most central part of the milk duct, which drains the pathological lobe [16].

As early as 1988, Durante introduced the concept of "sectoriectomy": in other words, conservative surgery is based on the concept of integration of image diagnosis and excision of a breast sector, according to the anatomical and pathological knowledge of the mammary gland (Fig. 16.5a). He makes an incision following Langer's lines (Fig. 16.5b, c); he carries on by severing the glandular tissue both from the subcutaneous plane and from the fascia (removed only when it is likely to be affected), with resection of healthy tissue at least 10 mm away from the tumor [37] (Fig. 16.5d).

The result is that relapses are drastically reduced in percentage, under 1% of the operated women (Durante's percentage is 0.6%, the testimony of a perfect radical surgery) [9].

Sometimes with this method you can have a strain of the nipple-areola complex, with the possible presence of annoying scars.

From the experience gained by Durante, we mediated a technique to minimize the scarring

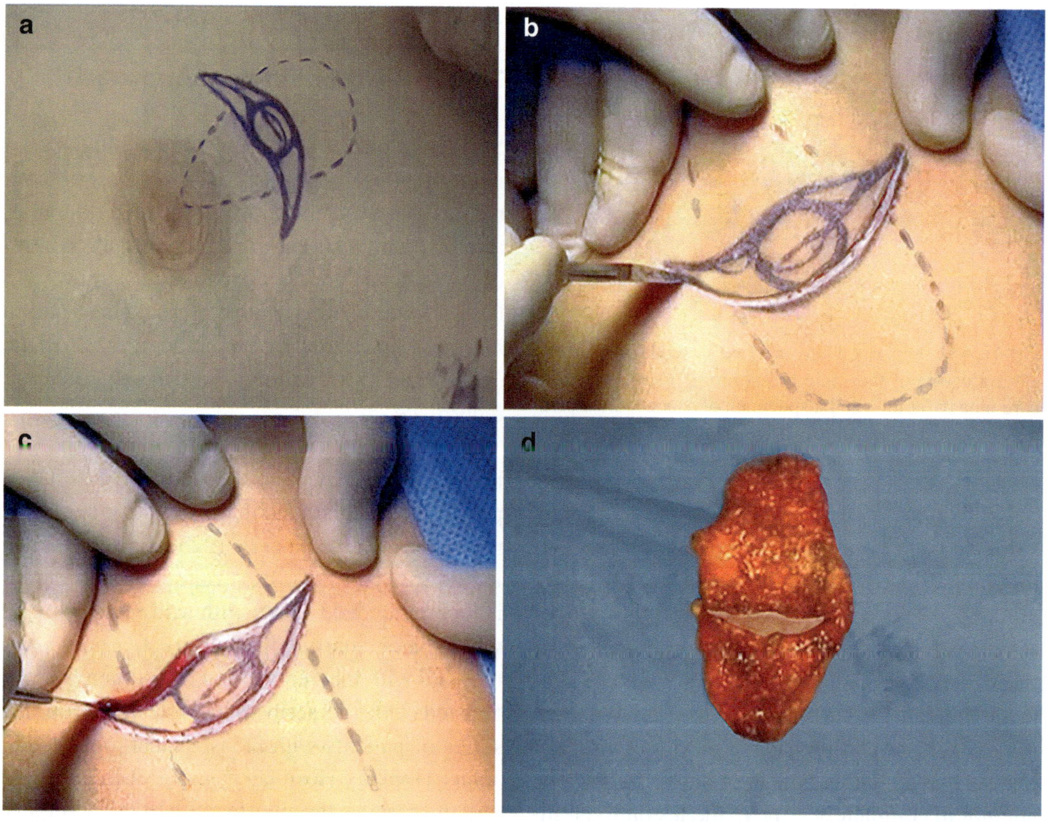

Fig. 16.5 (**a**) Drawing the surgical incisions before starting the lobectomy according to Durante technique. (**b**, **c**) Distal and proximal incision of the skin area to get out. (**d**) Sick lobe resected to be sent to the pathologist's examination

consequences and to reconstruct the shape and volume of the operated breast, so that it can be as similar as possible to the contralateral breast, even on oncological request.

In 1975, Hinderer introduced the "periareolar access to the mammary gland" in breast surgery, and, in 1989, Benelli made a further improvement to the previous methodology.

With the introduction of the technique, called "round block," it has become much more possible to perform a skin reduction while maintaining the same shape and the size of the areola and, at the same time, remodeling the breast cone. Such a contrivance makes use of a "bag of tobacco" simple suture around the areola level, after removal of a circular crown of the periareola epidermis, sufficiently wide to compensate for the area corresponding to the removed glandular tissue, so as to reduce the tension on margins and prevent a gross enlargement of the nipple due to excessive tissue stretching.

This method, modified for this particular indication, seems the most suitable to obtain an excellent surgical field, so as to allow a wide vision, an easy excision of the tumor (and the surrounding tissue), and the recovery of the breast cone after suitable remodeling of the remaining glandular tissue. Now about 60–80% of breast cancers are treated conservatively. To summarize these concepts, here are some key points for a correct approach to the problem [38].

Conservative treatment needs the combination of surgical therapy with radiotherapy. The distance of the tumor from the margins of resection should be more than 10 mm. Mobilization and detachment of the glandular flaps adjacent to the removed lobe, both under the skin and in the prefascial plane, should be carried out by limiting the damage to the vasculature of the flaps, to aim at a structural and functional satisfactory reconstruction. We always make a careful hemostasis, and we limit the use of drainages, so as not to affect the cosmetic result. The use of absorbable materials, the realization of a valid reinforcement under skin, and a dressing with a particular bandaging improve the quality of the scar area.

The possibility of removing the tumor while at the same time maintaining the normal conformation of the breast with scarring reduced to the minimum or almost invisible determines, in addition to the reduction of the negative impact of mutilation, a better tropism in the tissues for radiotherapy, a better therapeutic approach, a better quality of life, and a more active participation of the patient.

After the above assumptions, in this careful and surgically aware planning context, we have tried to make an intervention that associates radical surgery to a minimal mutilating impact. We started from the idea that, for a complete removal of the suspected area, you must always resort to excision of a "slice" of the gland including the ducts of the affected lobe, in order to reduce the possibilities of recurrence, reaching just below the nipple. The rationale for this chapter is to arrive, after a careful selection of the patients, to a valid oncological result, minimizing the aesthetic and psychological negative impact on the modification of the patient's own body image. This allows a better acceptance of the problematic cancer and its indispensable complementary therapies.

Choosing the surgical treatment, you must take into account the following elements:

- Size of the neoplasm
- If it is a single node or if it is multifocal or multicentric [15]
- Measure of the lesion diameters, its distance from the skin, from the fascia, and from the nipple
- Evaluation of the lymph node condition
- Localization of the lesions
- Relations with the surrounding tissues, with the exclusion of the presence of not previously assessed abnormal areas

Here is the reason why in patients with early breast cancer affecting a single lobe radical surgery must be associated with a good aesthetic and functional result.

In palpable tumors, surgeons usually perform blind surgery trusting preoperative mammography and their tactile skills, which can be problematic, especially in dense breasts. This surgical approach implies a high incidence of pathological surgical margins or an over-excision of healthy tissue in the effort to obtain adequate margins.

Lobar structures, usually invisible to the clinician and to mammographic control, become highly visible with ultrasound. Using the ductal method, cancerous structural irregularities, including indirect surrounding signs, highlight the suspected areas.

Due to the development of imaging techniques and screening programs, the incidence of non-palpable breast cancer has increased with up to one third of the diagnosed breast cancers being non-palpable. In this group, DCIS represents a challenging problem for breast-conserving surgery given that it is typically non-palpable and non-contiguous. Different management procedures are used to remove the non-palpable tumor with optimal resection margins: wire-guided localization, radio-guided localization, or intraoperative ultrasound-guided surgery. We suggest the use of ultrasound-guided surgery in order to localize tumors in their lobar context. Only a few reports have been published of the use of ultrasound-guided surgery in breast cancer but with good results.

Ultrasound-guided surgery is an accurate, simpler, and less invasive procedure compared to wire-guided localization. The breast lesion can be easily visualized on ultrasound. The only problem is that ultrasound-guided surgery is not very accurate for lesions appearing as a cluster of microcalcifications. The surgeon needs an ultrasound training; otherwise, a preoperative assisting radiologist is mandatory in performing ultrasound-guided surgery.

This echographic control helps the surgeon to localize the lesions and to visualize the whole lobe around. As the sick lobe may represent the risk tissue for cancer development within the breast, excision of whole lobe before development of malignant lesions within it reduces the local recurrence incidence.

The integration of all the different diagnostic methods (mammography, MRI in some cases, lobar echography) enables the surgeon to make a highly precise resection based also on his knowledge (anatomical, genetic, endocrinological, etc.).

We know very well that the breast is related to the sexual and relational life and to well-being: always in the foreground of advertising spots (on papers, on TV, etc.), the breast has become an organ with specific aesthetic standards in form and volume.

Current knowledge allows us to limit the surgical treatment, avoiding the large mammary mutilations of a few decades ago.

Preoperative ultrasound study allows us to confirm the location of the pathological area with the possibility of removing only the functional unit affected by the disease. An immediate initial assessment of the anatomo-pathologist will provide us with further confirmatory elements of the complete removal of all the pathological functional units.

We remember that all progress and every improvement that you can get in medicine are nothing but the sum of the experiences of the previous study groups, the technical equipment used for the diagnosis and in the operating theater.

Thus with regard to our surgical technique in case of localized and limited breast cancer, we have to be aware of the progress in the individual fields and the importance of their final combination.

The ultrasonic techniques are particularly refined and have reached very advanced diagnostic levels, as demonstrated by many doctors all around the world.

The study of lobar morphology, started by Michel Teboul, is now integrated with the use of elastography (evaluation of the rigidity of the structures) and Doppler (evaluation of vascularity by Doppler method).

16.7 Casuistry

From 1990 to 2010, we carried out 425 operations of lobectomy or quadrantectomy in women with diagnosis of breast carcinoma, with a previous echographic mapping of the lesions.

Five years on, only five patients had a new diagnosis of carcinoma (probably recurrences) in the same operated breast.

In literature we find a much higher recurrence percentage, as previously reported.

The reduction of the problems of cancer recurrence in the same breast seems to be correlated with the understanding that cancer is a lobar disease and that lumpectomy is not, in the light of current knowledge, ontologically correct, because it doesn't take into account either the anatomy or the physiology or the natural history of the tumor.

No doubt radiotherapy and chemotherapy performed after surgery may have perfectly sterilized the mammary gland, but this is also true for what concerns the rates reported in the literature with any other technique.

On the other hand, we never know if a new neoplastic disease in the same area is due to a new disease beginning in another lobe of the same breast or if it is due to a focus asynchronously appearing from the same lobe.

In our opinion, a very close collaboration with the pathologist is essential to improve the surgical discourse as required. The possibility of evaluating the microscopic framework through immediate acquisitions and insights executed confirms the validity and usefulness of what we propose. Today, where possible, you carry out a much more limited intervention, lobectomy, thanks to the knowledge and histopathologic confirmation of the concept of lobar disease now almost universally acknowledged.

Evaluation of your patient, in the same position as in the operating theater with lobar echography, is essential. The main duct should be identified since it corresponds to the longitudinal axis of the lobe; the duct should be followed from the nipple to the end of the lobe. The localization of the cancer and the evaluation of the nearby tissues are performed with radial and antiradial scans (Fig. 16.6). The design of the ductal axis and the associated abnormalities is then drawn on the overlying skin with a marker. The duct is traced from the nipple-areola border to the distal end.

A transverse evaluation of the lobe is then performed. This marks the lateral borders of the resection, inclusive of a 10-mm security distance from the suspect area. The glandular area to remove is assimilated to a triangular area. It is important to remember that one should remove an area of periareolar epidermis (circular sector) corresponding to the area above the lobe to be removed. Mark the border of the areola. Evaluate the skin area to be removed around the areola. It must be equal to an annulus of epidermis with the inner circumference already marked (see note). This area of redundant skin must be removed in order to balance the deficit of glandular tissue removed in the lobar resection, so you can keep a normal morphology of the breast cone (Fig. 16.7a).

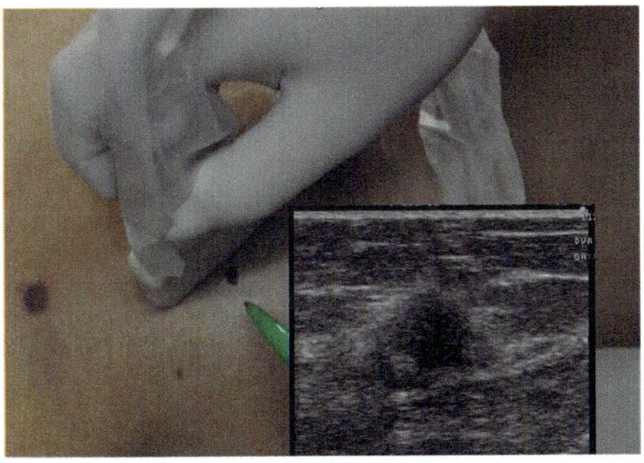

Fig. 16.6 Presurgical time. US examination of the pathological area in the lobe

Explanatory notes:

Triangle area = outer circle area − internal circle area.

Triangle area (half of base × height or 1/2 $B \times H$) + internal circle area (PI Greek × r^2) = outer circle area (PI Greek × R^2).

R = square root of (triangle area + internal circle area) divided by PI Greek.

Surgical steps:

After another control on the operating bed, an axillary evaluation is generally required.

The nipple and the breast cone must be kept in tension to easily remove the epithelial strip in the marked zone between the two circles, keeping the vascular plexus undamaged (Fig. 16.7b).

This is essential for a good feeding of the areola-nipple complex. The dermis is incised on the outside perimeter along the outlined length to expose the breast parenchyma in order to proceed with the resection of the sick lobe. A subcutaneous dissection of the whole lobe and of the nearest areas is then carried out. Grasp the zone 2–3 mm under the nipple with a forceps, to mark the central point of resection (Fig. 16.7c).

Cut the gland as far as the muscular fascia following the marked lines.

Proceed to cut the segment from the surface deep toward the fascia (Fig. 16.7d).

Pulling up on the top of the lobe, you carry on cutting as far as the end of the lobe, and then you remove it (Fig. 16.8a).

If the tumor is close to the muscular fascia, this must be removed with the specimen. A perfect hemostasis must be always achieved.

Real-time ultrasound is now used to study the dissected specimen at both longitudinal and transverse orientation, in order to evaluate the margin around the cancer [36, 39–41] (Fig. 16.8b).

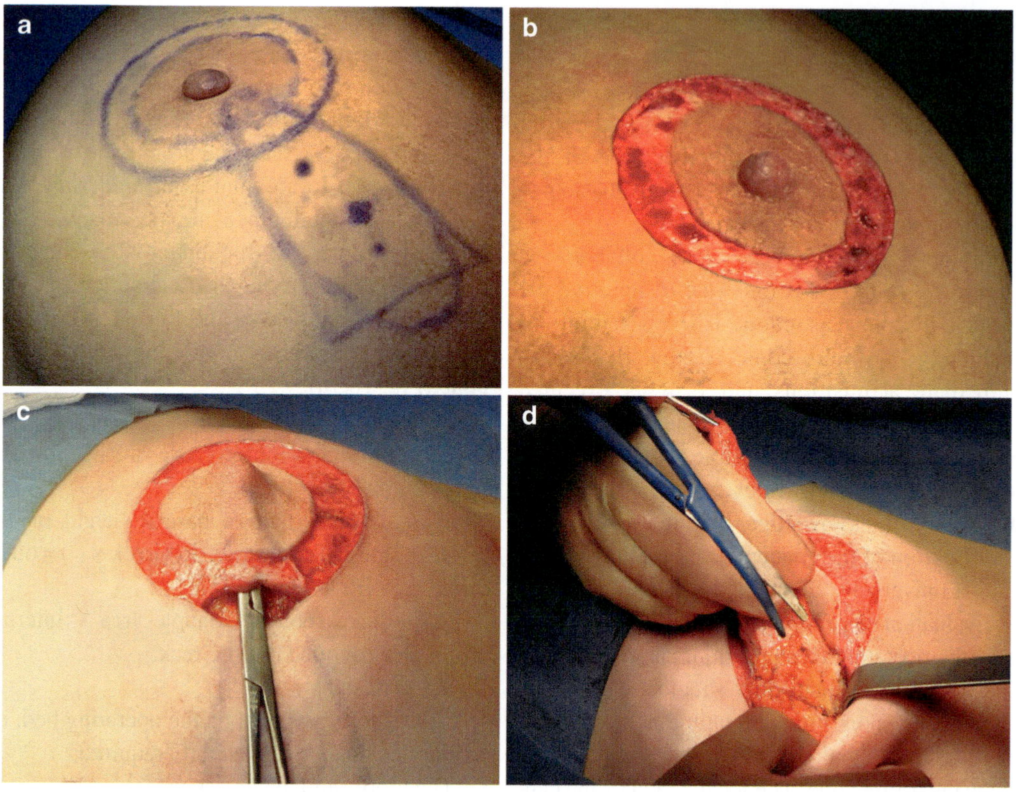

Fig. 16.7 (**a**) Design of the affected lobe and of periareolar circular ring. (**b**) Removed epithelium of the circular ring. (**c**) Forceps under the nipple. (**d**) Distal edge of the lobe

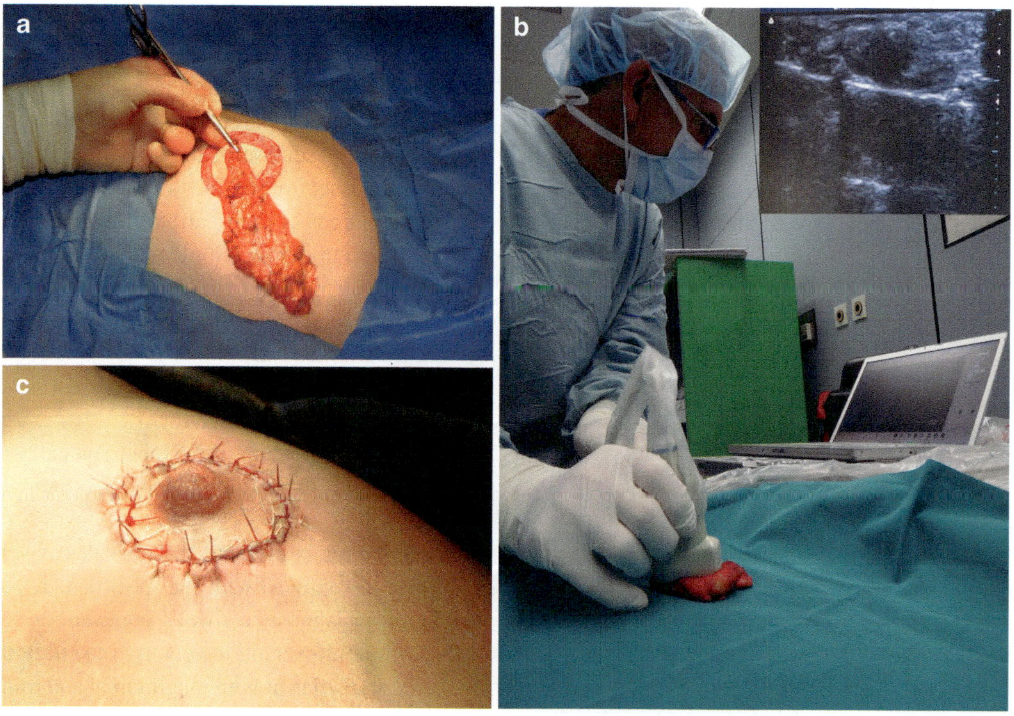

Fig. 16.8 (**a**) End of lobectomy. (**b**) Postsurgical US control of the lobe. (**c**) Final result of lobectomy

Compare the resected images with the preoperative images.

You can place one or two titanium clips on the fascial surface, at the precise location of the cancer, to facilitate the work of the radiotherapist.

An anatomic reconstruction of the breast cone must be performed by the mobilization and detachment of the gland borders close to the resected specimen, using oncoplastic technique. Then proceed with the periareolar "tobacco pouch" suture to remodel the skin and suture the areola mucosal border to epidermis (Fig. 16.8c).

Drains should be avoided if possible to assure better functional and aesthetic results. Absorbable materials, attention to skin closure, and compression bandages are primary factors for an enhanced cosmetic result.

16.8 Surgical Margins Evaluation

The primary goal of breast-conserving surgery is to remove the whole tumor mass with minimal surrounding healthy tissue in order to obtain tumor-free resection margins. Margins positive or focally positive for tumor cells are associated with a high risk of local recurrence, and in these cases, re-excision after lumpectomy or even mastectomy are sometimes needed to achieve definite clear margins.

16.8.1 Intraoperatory Tumor-Free Surgical Margins Diagnosis

The immediate goal of specimen examination is to confirm that the lesion has been completely excised. Ideally, this should be determined intraoperatively. If the lesion is not present in the specimen or if the cut margin is too close to the tumor, the surgeon may immediately re-excide the surgical margins on one or both sides of the specimen.

If the lesion was ultrasound undetectable, you must use RX to mark the zone with a wire guide. After the surgical removal, an RX examination of the whole surgical specimen must be made comparing with the corresponding mammogram. The presence of calcifications associated with a lesion provides an intrinsic marker that can be visualized in clinical and specimen radiographs.

Pathological margin assessment requires an inking of the specimen and multiple section perpendicular to its long axis.

Frozen sections of margins are not indicated unless the tumor appears grossly close to a margin, and confirming this intraoperatively will have an immediate impact on treatment [24].

It is recommended that non-palpable mammographically detected lesions be processed solely for permanent sections and that frozen sections be performed only in exceptional situations.

Despite improved intraoperative techniques, no assessment can ensure clear lumpectomy margins during surgery.

A positive margin is associated with increased risk of local recurrences after BCT for invasive breast cancer and DCIS. There is no cutoff for the margin width, and the significance of a close margin remains controversial. The surgeon needs to balance the risk of local recurrence against cosmetics in planning BCT so that prognosis is not compromised.

16.8.2 Postsurgical Specimen Examination to Confirm Tumor-Free Margins

Ideally, the intact excisional biopsy specimen should be promptly delivered unfixed to the pathology laboratory. It is not possible for a pathologist to accurately orient the margins of an excisional biopsy specimen without appropriate guidance from the surgeon (it is preferable to mark with a suture at the apex of the lobe toward the nipple and with a different suture at the deep margin toward fascia).

Because the contours and orientation of tissue slices may be altered in the course of preparing histologic sections, it is necessary to mark surfaces corresponding to the margin so that they can be identified microscopically. Various colors can be used to designate specified margins. If applied carefully, the ink does not strain into crevices in the tissue surface.

There is no standard method of margin evaluation for breast specimens, and there is no standard number of histologic sections examined from each margin surface. Margins can be evaluated (a) by a radial method, (b) by a shaved method, or (c) by shaving the walls of the lumpectomy cavity.

All specimens were prepared using large-section histopathology (Fig. 16.9a). The accurate method accurate for assessing the extent of carcinoma and feasible for routine diagnosis is to use large-format (10 × 8 cm) contiguous histology sections. This kind of histological approach enhances mammographic pathologic correlation, documents the lesion for adequate and reproducible analysis of the extent and distribution of the disease, and preserves the relation of the lesions to each other and to the circumferential surgical margin [42] (Fig. 16.9b).

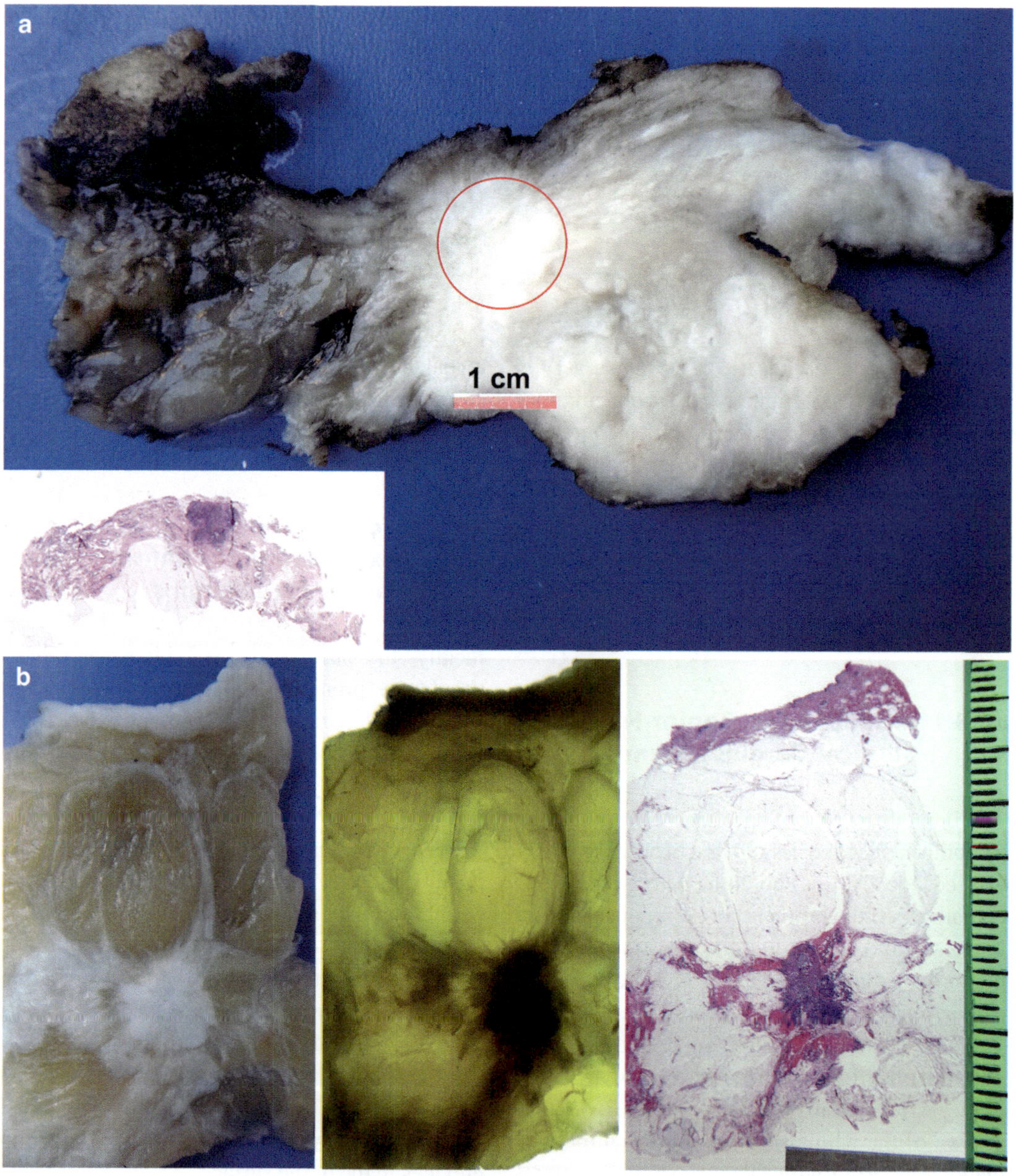

Fig. 16.9 (**a**) Anatomopathological control. (**b**) Macro of the unifocal lesion

Table 16.4 When to consider re-excision

Tumor at the inked margin
Tumor dispersed growing pattern (see text)
Significant discrepancy between radiographic/ ultrasound and pathologic tumor size

The possible scenarios of margin assessment encountered at the microscope are broadly positive margin, focally positive margin, close margin, and negative margin. As previously mentioned, there is a lack of standardization in the pathological methods of margin evaluation, which yields little consensus regarding what constitutes an adequate negative margin. Patient management varies widely based on the threshold that surgeons accept for adequate margins and the subsequent need for re-excision.

Adoption of no ink on tumor as the standard negative margin definition has clear potential to decrease the use of both re-excision and large quadrantectomy-type resections which often necessitate additional surgery on the affected breast for reshaping and on the contralateral breast for symmetry [43–48] (Table 16.4).

Conclusion

Oncological evaluation must be based on the anatomical, endocrinological, and functional knowledge of breast, taking into account the embryological development as well as the natural means of presentation of breast cancer. A full imaging analysis of the breast in question, including ductal echography, is requisite prior to any surgical decision. Because of the use of ductal echography, a better anatomo-pathological assessment of the extent of disease is now available.

A positive surgical margin after breast-conserving surgery correlate closely to local recurrence. Nevertheless, there are other risk factors for local recurrence after breast-conserving surgery, such as tumor growing pattern (unifocal, multifocal, or diffuse) (Fig. 16.10).

Considering that breast cancer is frequently a multifocal/diffuse disease, the finding of negative margins does not necessarily mean that we did not leave in situ or invasive tumor foci in the residue breast. These residual tumor foci are usually localized in the “sick lobe.”

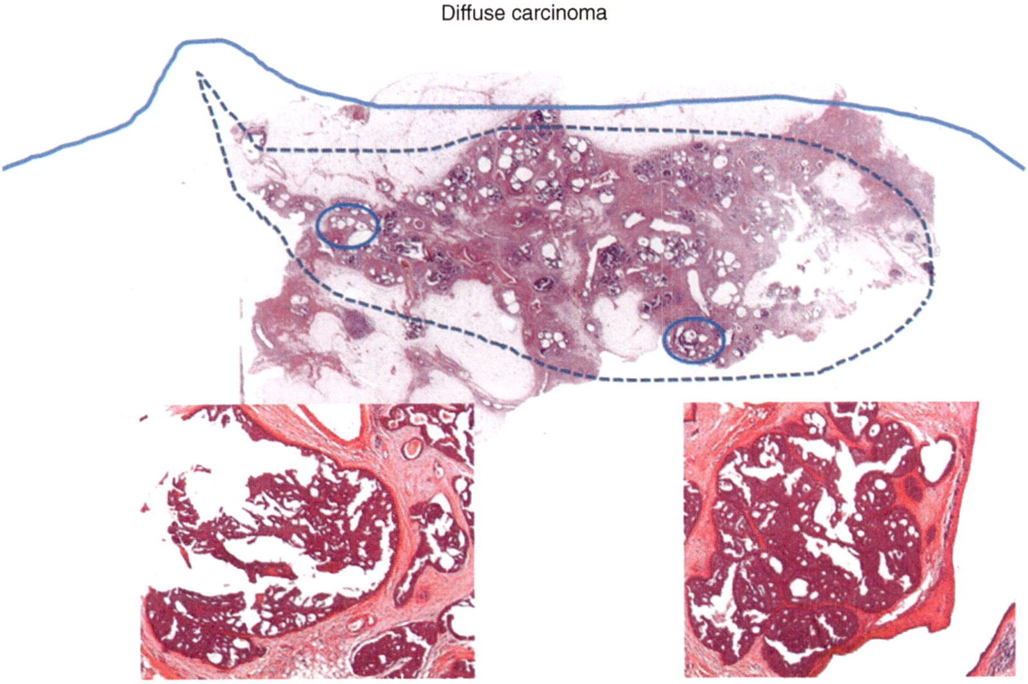

Fig. 16.10 Picture of a lobar carcinoma. Diffuse pattern

Breast cancer develops not as a single tumor but as a lobar disease.

Only a lobar surgical approach allows to excise the whole "sick lobe" which may include any other tumor lesions or in any case the risk tissue for future cancer development.

Lobar resection of the breast is a readily mastered surgical technique that can be performed by every breast surgeon with the appropriate sonographic skills. In this way we will obtain a great (the best?) oncological radicality, with a lower percentage of recurrences, according to Durante and other surgeons' experience. We also obtain a reduction of scars, with a good aesthetic and functional result (Fig. 16.11). This surgical approach needs lobar ultrasound as a useful tool to assist and guide the breast surgeon at each step of the operation [36, 39–41] preoperatively. The radial imaging approach provides better display of the anatomy and the lesions within the ductal system, as well as their relation to fascia and skin during surgery. Intraoperative radial ultrasound examination guides the surgeon to delineate the "sick lobe" during postoperative examination of the excised surgical specimen. Ultrasound examination of the removed specimen enables the surgeon and the pathologist to control the presence of the lesion within the specimen and its distance from the surgical margins.

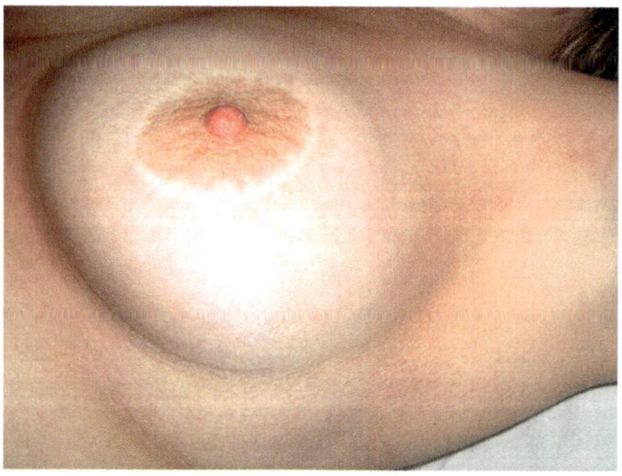

Fig. 16.11 Control of the patient after 5 years from surgery

Acknowledgment Thanks to doctors Anna Maria Dolfin for providing the images and for the help in writing this chapter; Paolo Tagliabue, fellow surgeon; and Riccardo Arisio, pathologist. Thanks to Silvia Botta for pathological drawings.

References

1. Veronesi U, Mariani L, Greco M, Saccozzi R, Luini A, Aguilar M, Marubini E. Twenty-year follow-up of a randomized study comparing breast-conserving surgery with radical mastectomy for early breast cancer. N Engl J Med. 2002;347(16):1227–32.
2. Fisher B, Anderson S, Bryant J, Margolese RG, Deutsch M, Fisher ER, Jeong JH, Wolmark N. Twenty-year follow-up of a randomized trial comparing total mastectomy, lumpectomy, and lumpectomy plus irradiation for the treatment of invasive breast cancer. N Engl J Med. 2002;347(16):1233–41.
3. Dolfin G, Tagliabue P, Dolfin AM, Indelicato S. Chirurgia conservativa: cosa possiamo fare per evitare la mutilazione? Riv It Ost Gin. 2007;14:66370.
4. Teboul M. Practical ductal echography. Madrid, Spain: Medgen. S.A; 2004.
5. Tot T. The clinical relevance of the distribution of the lesions in 500 consecutive breast cancer cases documented in large-format histological sections. Cancer. 2007;110:2551–60.
6. Durante E. Multimodality imaging and interventional techniques. Ferrara, Italy: IBUS Course Abstracts; 2006.
7. Amoros J, Dolfin G, Teboul M. Atlas de Ecografia de la Mama. Torino: Ananke; 2009.
8. Hunt KK, Sahin AA. Too much, too little, or just right? Tumor margins in women undergoing breast-conserving surgery. J Clin Oncol. 2014;32:14–8.
9. Amy D, Durante E, Tot T. The lobar approach to breast ultrasound imaging and surgery. J Med Ultrasound. 2015;42(3):331–9.
10. Tot T. The theory of the sick breast lobe and the possible consequences. Int J Surg Pathol. 2007;15:369.
11. Tot T, Gere M, Pekár G, Tarján M, Hofmeyer S, Hellberg D, Lindquist D, Chen TH-H, Yen AM-F, Chiu SY-H, Tabár L. Breast cancer multifocality, disease extent, and survival. Hum Pathol. 2011;42:1761–9.
12. Coombs NJ, Boyages J. Multifocal and multicentric breast cancer: does each focus matter? J Clin Oncol. 2005;23:7497–502.
13. La Parra RF, De Roos WK, Contant CM, Bavelaar-Croon CD, Barneveld PC, Bosscha K. A prospective validation study of sentinel lymph node biopsy in multicentric breast cancer: SMMaC trial. Eur J Surg Oncol. 2014;40:1250–5.
14. Donker M, Straver ME, van Tienhoven G, van de Velde CJ, Mansel RE, Litière S, Werutsky G, Duez NJ, Orzalesi L, Bouma WH, van der Mijle H, Nieuwenhuijzen GA, Veltkamp SC, Helen Westenberg A, Rutgers EJ. Comparison of the sentinel node pro-

cedure between patients with multifocal and unifocal breast cancer in the EORTC 10981-22023 AMAROS Trial: identification rate and nodal outcome. Eur J Cancer. 2013;49:2093.
15. Yerushalmi R, Tyldesley S, Woods R, Kennecke HF, Speers C, Gelmon KA. Is breast-conserving therapy a safe option for patients with tumor multicentricity and multifocality? Ann Oncol. 2012;23:876–81.
16. Holland R, Veling SH, Mravunac M, Hendriks JH. Histologic multifocality of Tis, T1-2 breast carcinomas. Implications for clinical trials of breast-conserving surgery. Cancer. 1985;56:979–90.
17. Turnbull L, Brown S, Harvey I, Olivier C, Drew P, Napp V, Hanby A, Brown J. Comparative effectiveness of MRI in breast cancer (COMICE) trial: a randomised controlled trial. Lancet. 2010;375:563–71.
18. Peters NH, van Esser S, van den Bosch MA, Storm RK, Plaisier PW, van Dalen T, Diepstraten SC, Weits T, Westenend PJ, Stapper G, Fernandez-Gallardo MA, Borel Rinkes IH, van Hillegersberg R, Mali WP, Peeters PH. Preoperative MRI and surgical management in patients with nonpalpable breast cancer: the MONET - randomised controlled trial. Eur J Cancer. 2011;47:879–88627.
19. Biesemier KW, Alexander C. Enhancement of mammographic-pathologic correlation utilizing large format histology for malignant breast disease. Semin Breast Dis. 2005;8:152–62.
20. Tot T. The role of large-format histopathology in assessing subgross morphological prognostic parameters: a single institution report of 1000 consecutive breast cancer cases. Int J Breast Cancer. 2012;2012: 395–415.
21. Foschini MP, Flamminio F, Miglio R, et al. The impact of large sections on the study of in situ and invasive duct carcinoma of the breast. Hum Pathol. 2007;38:1736–43.
22. Tot T, Pekár G, Hofmeyer S, et al. The distribution of lesions in 1-14-mm invasive breast carcinomas and its relation to metastatic potential. Virchows Arch. 2009;455:109–15.
23. Tot T. DCIS, cytokeratins, and the theory of the sick lobe. Virchows Arch. 2005;447:1–8.
24. Osen R, et al. Rosen's breast pathology. 4th ed. Philadelphia: Wolters Kluwer Health; 2015.
25. Lobar AD. Ultrasound of the breast. In: Tot T, editor. Breast cancer. London: Springer; 2011. p. 153–62.
26. Lavoué V, Fritel X, Antoine M, Beltjens F, Bendifallah S, Boisserie-Lacroix M, Boulanger L, Canlorbe G, Catteau-Jonard S, Chabbert-Buffet N, Chamming's F, Chéreau E, Chopier J, Coutant C, Demetz J, Guilhen N, Fauvet R, Kerdraon O, Laas E, Legendre G, Mathelin C, Nadeau C, Naggara IT, Ngô C, Ouldamer L, Rafii A, Roedlich MN, Seror J, Séror JY, Touboul C, Uzan C, Daraï E, French College of Gynecologists and Obstetricians (CNGOF). Clinical practice guidelines from the French College of Gynecologists and Obstetricians (CNGOF): benign breast tumors - short text. Eur J Obstet Gynecol Reprod Biol. 2016;200:16–23.
27. Mitra S, Dey P. Fine-needle aspiration and core biopsy in the diagnosis of breast lesions: a comparison and review of the literature. Cytojournal. 2016;13:18.
28. Wesoła M, Jeleń M. The diagnostic efficiency of fine needle aspiration biopsy in breast cancers - review. Adv Clin Exp Med. 2013;22(6):887–92.
29. National Breast Cancer Centre. Breast fine needle aspiration cytology and core biopsy: a guide for practice. 2004. This book can also be downloaded from the National Breast Cancer Centre website www.nbcc.org.au.
30. Feoli F, Ameye L, Van Eeckhout P, Paesmans M, Marra V, Arisio R. Liquid-based cytology of the breast: pitfalls unrecognized before specific liquid-based cytology training - proposal for a modification of the diagnostic criteria. Acta Cytol. 2013;57(4):369–76.
31. Willems SM, van Deurzen CH, van Diest PJ. Diagnosis of breast lesions: fine-needle aspiration cytology or core needle biopsy? A review. J Clin Pathol. 2012;65(4):287–92.
32. Nassar A. Core needle biopsy versus fine needle aspiration biopsy in breast--a historical perspective and opportunities in the modern era. Diagn Cytopathol. 2011;39(5):380–8.
33. Rageth CJ, O'Flynn EA, Comstock C, Kurtz C, Kubik R, Madjar H, Lepori D, Kampmann G, Mundinger A, Baege A, Decker T, Hosch S, Tausch C, Delaloye JF, Morris E, Varga Z. First International Consensus Conference on lesions of uncertain malignant potential in the breast (B3 lesions). Breast Cancer Res Treat. 2016;159(2):203–13.
34. Park HL, Hong J. Vacuum-assisted breast biopsy for breast cancer. Gland Surg. 2014;3(2):120–728.
35. Tot T, Ibarra JA. Examination of specimens from patients with ductal carcinoma in situ of the breast using large-format histology sections. Arch Pathol Lab Med. 2009;133(9):1361.
36. Fisher CS, Mushawah FA, Cyr AE, Gao F, Margenthaler JA. Ultrasound-guided lumpectomy for palpable breast cancers. Ann Surg Oncol. 2011;18:3198–203.
37. Luini A, Gatti G, Zurrida S, Caldarella P, Viale G, Rosali dos Santos G, Frasson A. The surgical margin status after breast-conserving surgery: discussion of an open issue. Breast Cancer Res Treat. 2009;113(2):397–402.
38. Dolfin G, Chebib A, Amy D, Tagliabue P. Carcinoma mammarie et Chirurgie Conservatrice. 30° Seminare Franco-Syrien d'Imagerie Médicale. Tartous, Syrie; 2008.
39. Volders JH, Haloua MH, Krekel NM, Meijer S, van den Tol PM. Current status of ultrasound-guided surgery in the treatment of breast cancer. World J Clin Oncol. 2016;7(1):44–53.
40. Krekel N, Zonderhuis B, Muller S, Bril H, van Slooten HJ, de Lange de Klerk E, van den Tol P, Meijer S. Excessive resections in breast-conserving surgery: a retrospective multicentre study. Breast J. 2011;17:602–9.
41. Pan H, Wu N, Ding H, Ding Q, Dai J, Ling L, Chen L, Zha X, Liu X, Zhou W, et al. Intraoperative ultrasound guidance is associated with clear lumpectomy

margins for breast cancer: a systematic review and meta-analysis. PLoS One. 2013;8:e74028.
42. Tot T, Tabár L. Mammographic pathologic correlation of ductal carcinoma in situ of the breast using two- and three-dimensional large histologic sections. Semin Breast Dis. 2005;8:144–51.
43. Tomoka H, Masataka S, Junko I, et al. Impact of intraoperative specimen mammography on margins in breast-conserving surgery. Mol Clin Oncol. 2016;5:269–72.
44. Chiappa C, Rovera F, Corben AD, Fachinetti A, De Berardinis V, Marchionini V, Rausei S, Boni L, Dionigi G, Dionigi R. Surgical margins in breast conservation. Int J Surg. 2013;11(Suppl 1):S69–72.
45. Houssami N, Morrow M. Margins in breast conservation: a clinician's perspective and what the literature tells us. J Surg Oncol. 2014;110(1):2–7.
46. Moehrle M, Breuninger H, Röcken M. A confusing world: what to call histology of three-dimensional tumour margins? J Eur Acad Dermatol Venereol. 2007;21(5):591–5.
47. Dolfin G, et al. The surgical approach to the "sick lobe" in breast cancer: a new era in management. New York: Springer; 2014.
48. Tot T. Subgross morphology, the sick lobe hypothesis, and the success of breast conservation. Int J Breast Cancer 2011;2011: Article ID 634021.

Lobar Resection Under Ultrasound Guide

17

Enzo Durante

Take-Home Message
The sick lobe concept and our guidelines for application to conserving surgery, i.e., lobar resection represent a great deviation from recent traditional lumpectomy.

We stress the surgeons to consider this proposal and to realize a lobar and ductal anatomy in order to motivate surgical innovations following anatomical and imaging guidelines and realize a multicenter prospective randomized trial to test the validity of these concepts and surgical approach that would fundamentally change local therapy. The use of US is continuously evolving as occurs for every equipment due to technological improvement. In the same way, physicians should be able to improve their capacities in the utilization of the new equipment with enlarged indications and outstanding principles. We should know and we should use the imaging techniques in a real gold standard in order to perform the best procedure for each single case.

Ultrasound is the first-line and most cost-effective methods to stage the breast becoming increasingly important for guiding adequate surgical treatment.

The role of surgery in the management of breast cancer has changed markedly reflecting the innovations in breast imaging with the question: Why not combine the concept of the sick lobe with the use of ultrasound guiding the surgeon according to the anatomy of the lobe?

E. Durante, M.D.
University of Ferrara, Ferrara, Italy
e-mail: enzo.durante@unife.it, edurante@ibus.org

17.1 Introduction

Surgery of the organ and not surgery of the lump means surgery according to the anatomy of the organ where the disease is harbored and not a surgery based on the simple removal of the macroscopically visible disease. Treatment for breast cancer has evolved over time and now consists of a multidisciplinary approach that includes surgery, radiation, and systemic therapy, but we are forgetting that local therapy cannot disregard the anatomy and that the breast anatomy is lobar. Now, if surgery is an essential component of local treatment, we cannot ignore the concept of multifocality and the concept of the sick lobe. In this way, surgery still remains crucial and, in many cases, fundamental for the local control that grants an improved quality of life and survival benefit. Adequate surgery following the lobar anatomy and the concept of the sick lobe is a simple, quick technique that eliminates the tumor at the primary site. Image-guided surgery under ultrasound guide according to the lobar anatomy should be seen as a keystone of modern surgery. Intraoperative imaging technique has become a fundamental tool for breast surgeons especially for the most early-stage non-palpable cancer. For these lesions, the surgeon needs an intraoperative

D. Amy (ed.), *Lobar Approach to Breast Ultrasound*, https://doi.org/10.1007/978-3-319-61681-0_17

imaging guide in order to visualize and localize the lesion; to evaluate its extension; to measure the distance from the skin, from the fascia, and from the nipple; to evaluate the tumor-to-breast relation in order to decide if conservative surgery is cosmetically adequate; to choose the best incision site according to the Langer's lines; to select the margin resection; and to evaluate the resected specimen. Intraoperative ultrasound seems to be the method of choice for guiding all the abovementioned procedures, thanks to its handiness; moreover, there is a benefit of greater surgical autonomy in performing all these procedures in the operating room with the patient in supine position and under anesthetic [6, 18, 19, 28, 36, 39, 43].

17.2 Theoretical Principles

Back to the past, Townsend and Craig in 1980 [58] described the concept of the lobar anatomy, and we adopted the principle of lobar anatomy and also the concept of sick lobes [17, 50, 51, 52, 53, 54, 55] not only from the anatomical and diagnostic point of view but also from the pathological and surgical point of view so that we started to perform a comparison of an ultrasound image with a macrosection of surgical specimen (Fig. 17.1a–c). Another clear concept was that the breast is composed of 15–20 lobes as many as the ducts, each lobe is a sector or a segment, major ducts come from periphery to

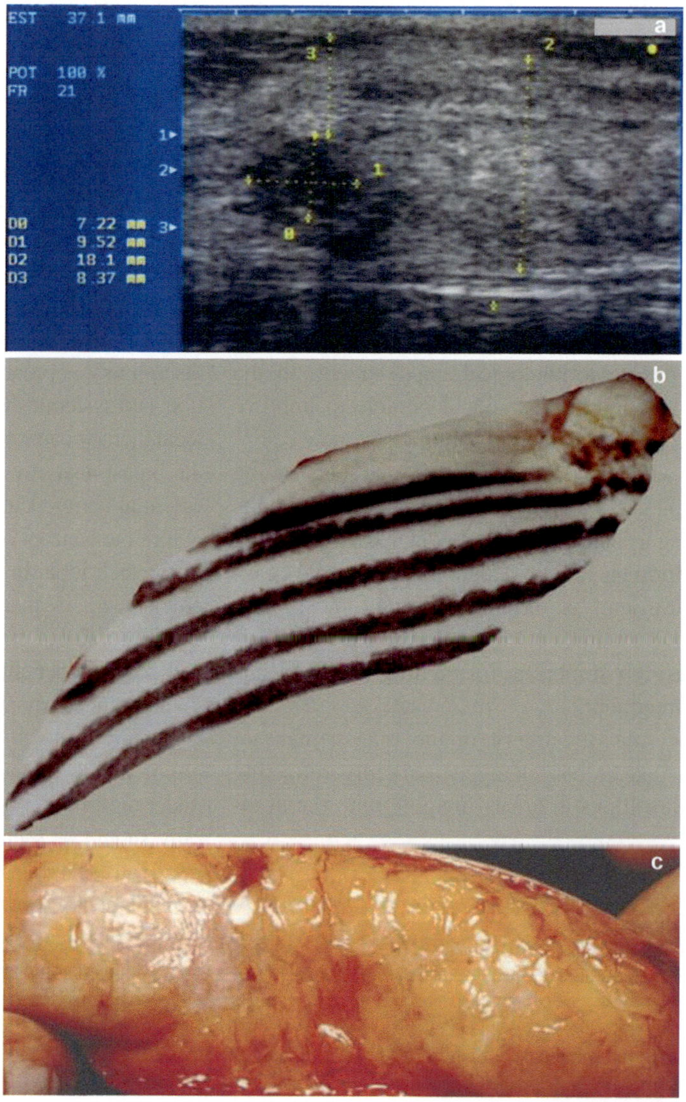

Fig. 17.1 Ultrasound image (**a**), scan draft (**b**), specimen macrosection (**c**)

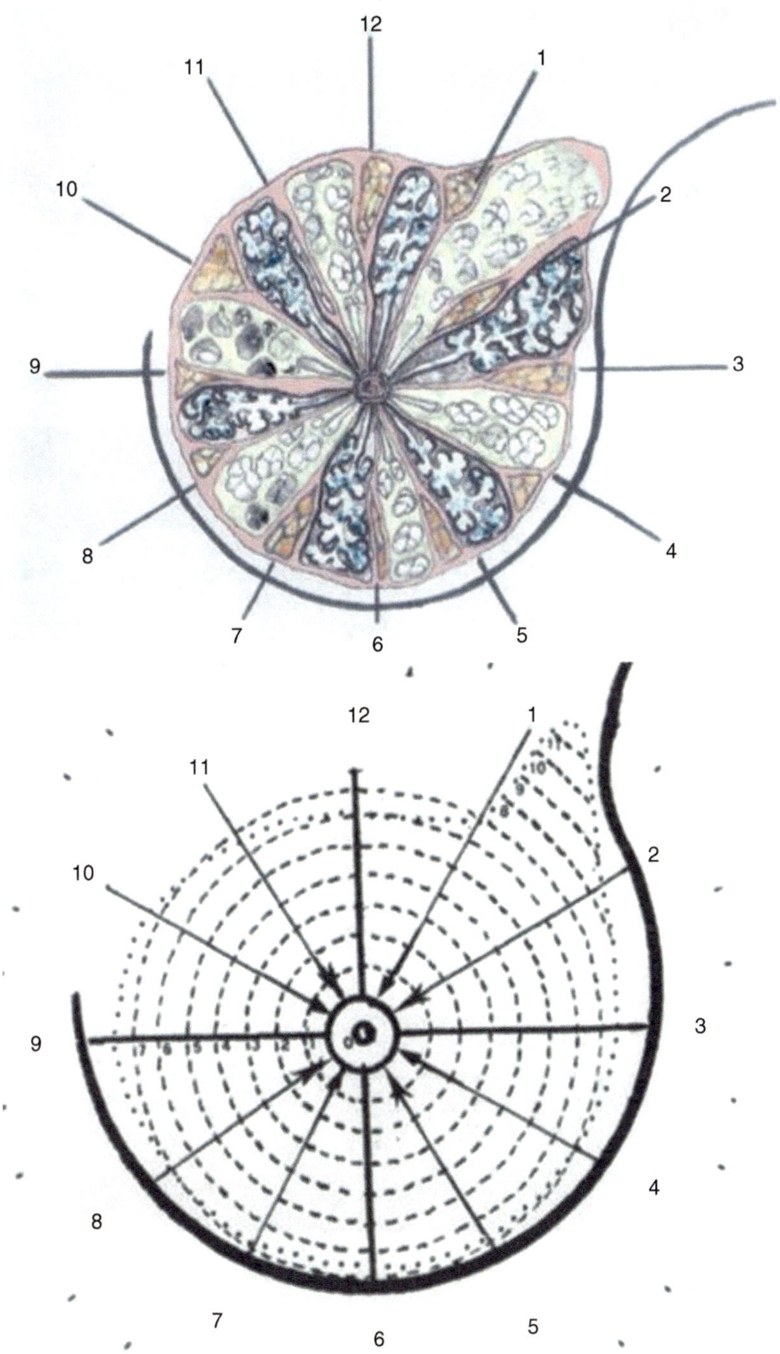

Fig. 17.2 Representation of lobar segmentation in clockwise fashion

the nipple, and breast diseases are diseases of the epithelium of TDLU [25]. For this reason, we arranged a pictorial representation of the lobar segmentation in clockwise fashion and with distance from the nipple using the Langer's lines (Fig. 17.2). After the publication of the paper "Histologic multifocality of Tis, T1–2 breast carcinomas implications for clinical trials of breast-conserving surgery" by Holland [21], we realized that radial scanning is the most suitable technique allowing a clear display of the anatomic structures. Afterwards we started to

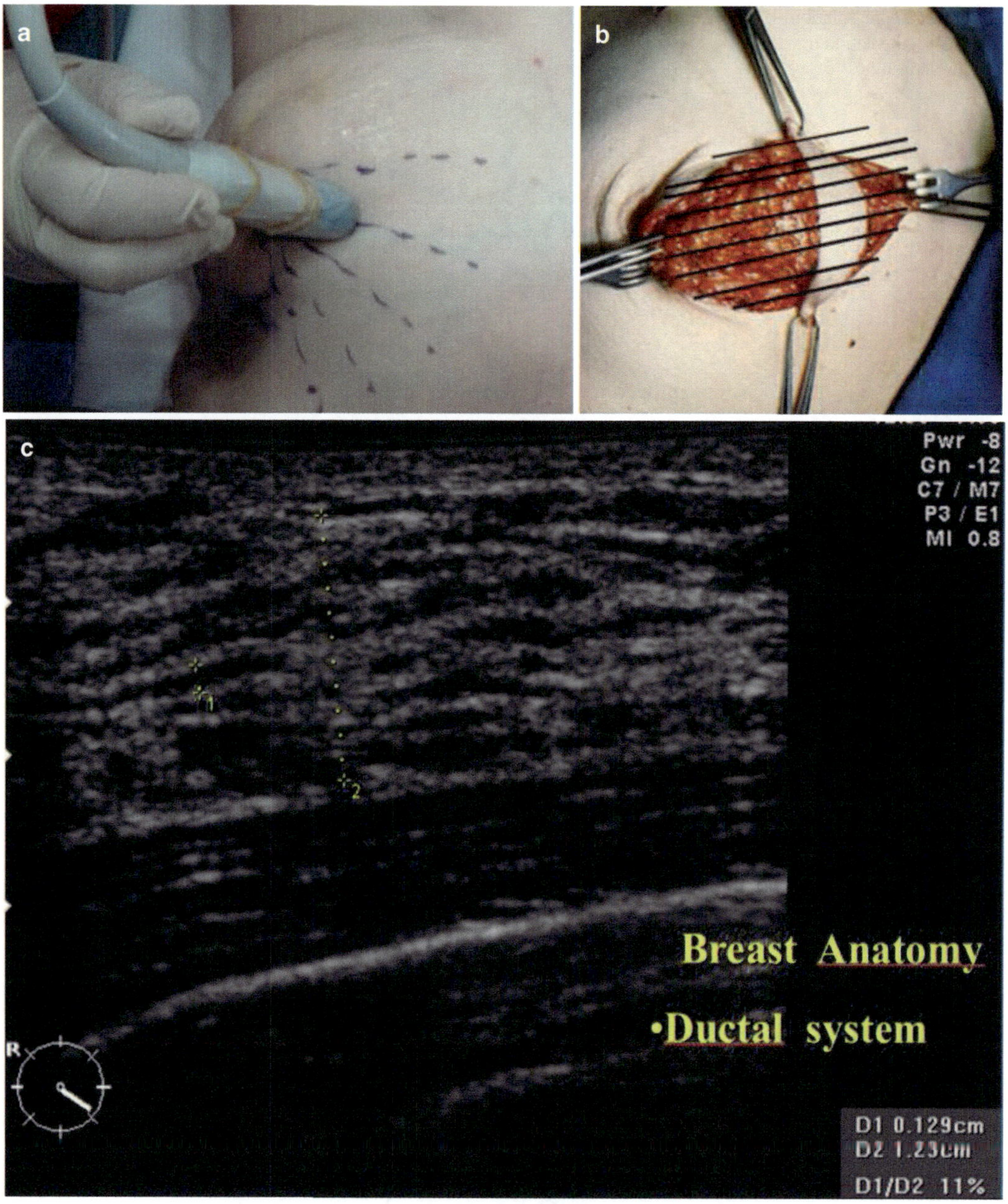

Fig. 17.3 Ultrasonic radial scanning (**c**) with small duct and representation of section in vivo (**a**) and on specimen (**b**)

perform systematically the ultrasound examination in radial and antiradial fashion in order to observe the ductal system along the major axis (Fig. 17.3a–c). The indication of every scan is performed according to the clockwise fashion using a special draft (Fig. 17.4) where lesion and distance from the nipple, skin, and fascia, multifocality, and multicentricity are pointed out. Considering that the human breast is a subcutaneous organ lying completely within the superficial and deep layer of the superficial pectoral fascia, and that only when we have a clear and constant visualization of all anatomical structures we have the possibility to plan an anatomical approach for an oncological radical resection, with all these concepts in mind, we

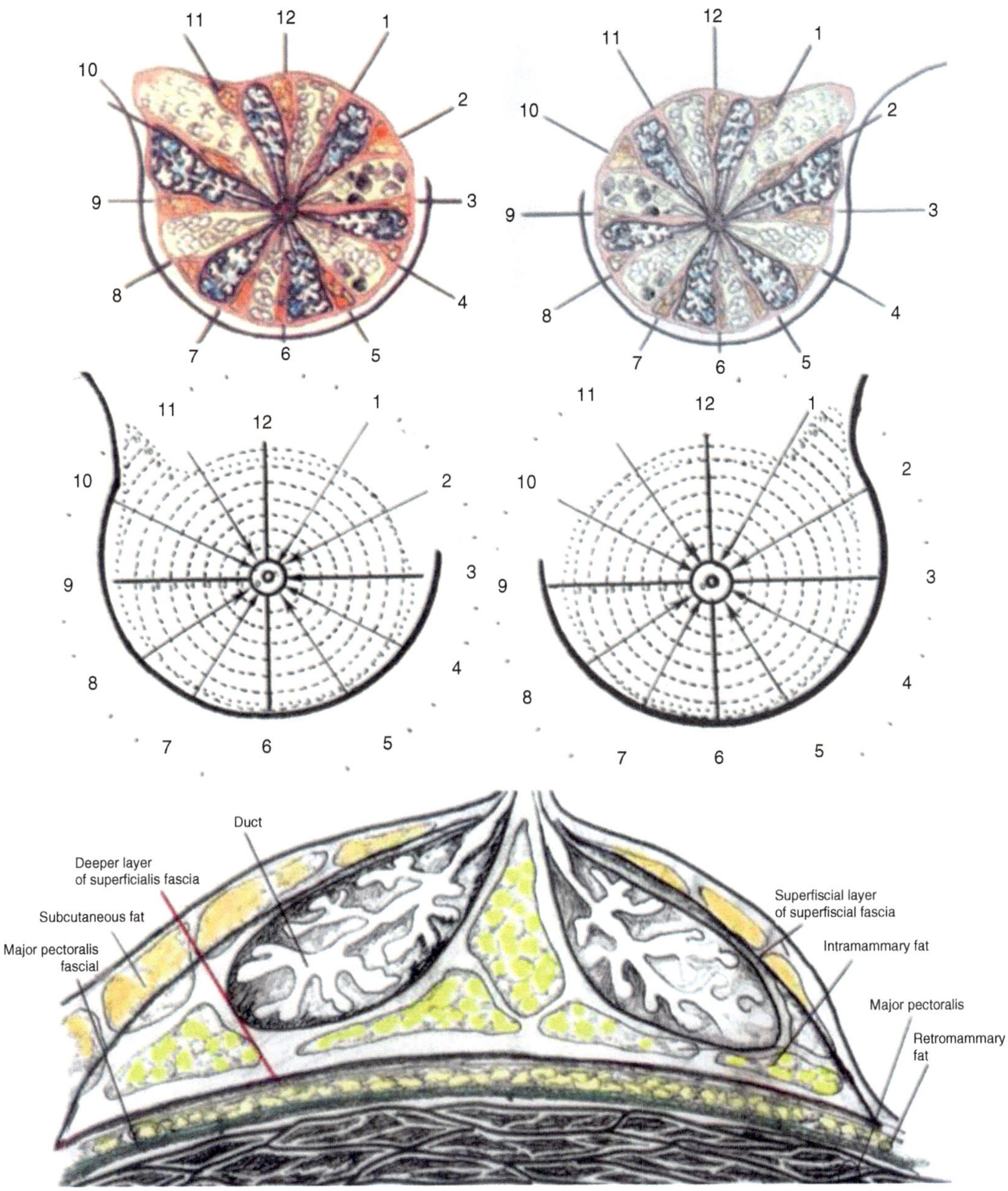

Fig. 17.4 Indication of every scan in clockwise fashion

decided to apply them in surgical technique, planning a lobar resection under ultrasound guide considering also that the rate of multifocality is present in about 40% of cases, and consequent failure of surgery may result in local recurrence which is an emotionally devastating event for the patient and is an independent factor associated with a poor outcome.

17.3 Patient Selection

After the diagnosis of cancer, careful preoperative evaluation is crucial in order to adequately plan the best treatment for the individual patient. Breast cancer staging involves dimensions, extent of disease, ductal extension, multifocality, multicentricity, lymph nodes, vascularity, and minimally invasive pathologic diagnosis of every displayed lesion. In the description sheet, there are indications for site in clockwise fashion, size in mm in 3D, spread (multifocal, multicentric), ductal extension along the major axis, relation (with skin, fascia, nipple, lymph nodes), and bilaterality of lymphatics (Fig. 17.4) [1, 2, 12, 13, 14]. Secondary parameters for conservative, oncologically radical, cosmetic surgery are distance from the skin and pectoralis fascia. The distance from the skin is important in order to decide if it is to be removed, if close or involved, or not. It is to consider that tumors, close to the skin and particularly to the lymphatics subdermal rich plexus, have a diffuse network with general lymph vessels resulting in an increased risk of lymphatic dissemination.

The distance from the fascia of the major pectoral muscle is also an important parameter in order to evaluate the involvement by the deeper tumors. We must remember that pectoralis fascia is a different anatomic entity from the deeper layer of superficial fascia that envelopes the breast tissue. Behind this, there is a retromammary fat layer and then the pectoralis fascia. The distortion or clear involvement requests the sacrifice of the underlying fascia and positioning of titanium clips.

The distance from the nipple is important in order to decide if sectoriectomy is adequate from the oncological point of view considering the more frequent possibility of multifocal, multicentric cancer in this site and diffusion through the lymphatics. Minimal distance considered adequate is 1 cm. If the tumor is behind the nipple, we do not perform a conservative treatment. One of the greatest dilemmas for surgeons today is the margins but, at the moment, there is not a standard definition of negative margin, and for this, we strongly support the lobar resection considering the origin of cancer.

All the parameters achievable by ultrasonic examination are obtained with transducer perpendicular to the skin without compression and methodically in three-dimensional fashion, radial and antiradial, using clockwise location. The parameters are always recorded in a breast ultrasound examination archiving software. The reporting protocol is delivered to the patients with the draft mentioned in this chapter. The software has been realized in 1988 and presented at the Sixth International Congress on the Ultrasonic Examination of the Breast held in Paris in June 1989 (Fig. 17.5).

17.4 Implication for Surgery

Intraoperative ultrasound enables the surgeon to operate under direct vision of the anatomy evaluating the three-dimensional shape of lesion within the dense tissue in surgical position. The primary objective of breast surgeons is to remove lesions with adequate margins but in a radical way and preserving the patient's aesthetic good looks. Another objective for the surgeons is to perform surgical intervention and axillary stag-

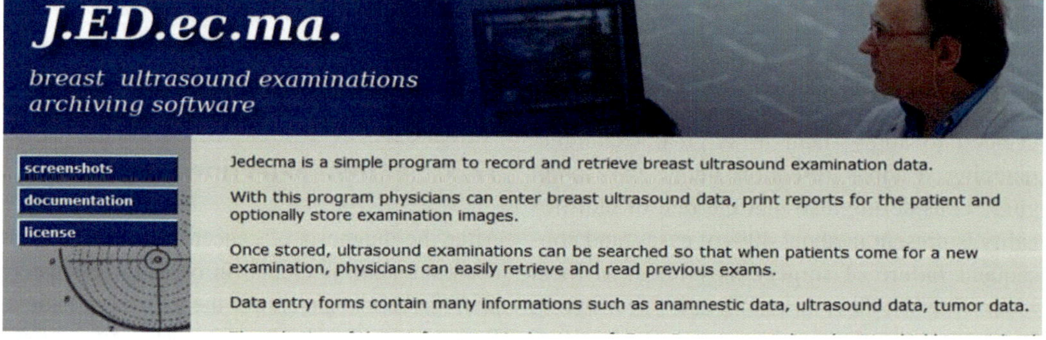

Fig. 17.5 Entry page of breast ultrasound examination archiving software

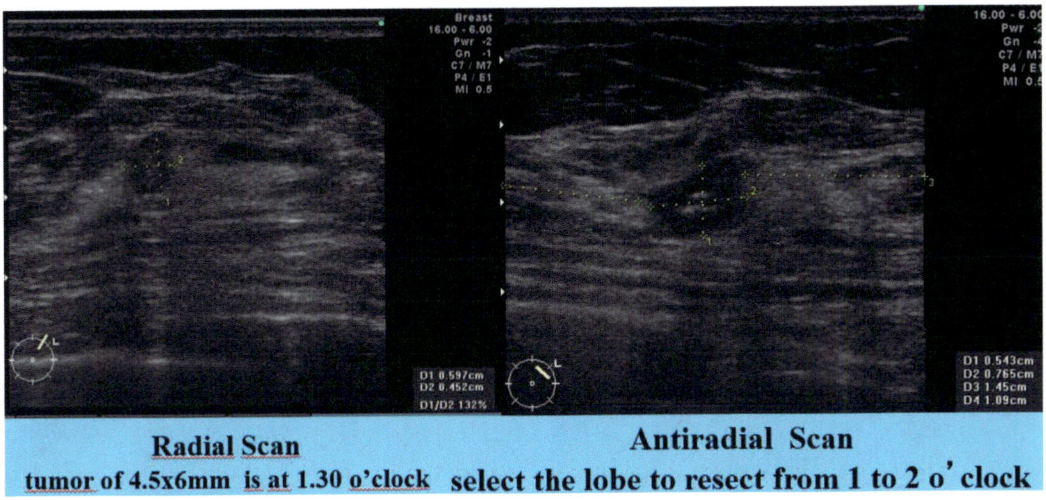

Fig. 17.6 Radial and antiradial scanning in order to define the amount of tissue to resect

ing in one single definitive procedure. One of the advantages of intraoperative localization is that the surgeon visualizes the lesion personally in the surgical position and evaluates the three-dimensional shape of the lesion within the breast, and supine position shortens the distance between the skin and lesion (Fig. 17.6). In doing so, it is appropriate to use a radial approach according to the lobar anatomy. Intraoperative ultrasound localization is more comfortable for the patient; it is time- and cost-efficient. We prefer wire localization, which is more useful and more visible for intraoperative specimen ultrasound and digital X-ray examination and for pathologist workup.

17.5 Surgical Lobar Resection

Surgical planning is based on the echographic assessment of lesion and adjacent tissue in radial scans with multifrequency transducer operating at 8–18 MHz and with 3D–4D scans with transducer operating at 7–14 MHz. An antiradial scan gives the possibility to decide the extension of resection of tissue [3, 15].

We draw on the skin the extension of the lobe in radial-segmental fashion and plan the most advantageous incision always according to the Langer's lines and the resection of breast tissue according to the lobar anatomy (Fig. 17.7a–d). Single or double curvilinear incision depends on the distance of tumor from the skin. If the tumor is far from the skin more than 5 mm and the superficial layer of the superficial fascia is free of distortion or disruption, we don't remove the skin; instead, we perform a single curvilinear incision (Fig. 17.8a, b), and always when it is possible, we perform a periareolar incision even if this requires more time to dissect the tissue until the periphery (Fig. 17.9a, b). When the skin is very near to the tumor, we remove the skin in front of the tumor mostly using a double curvilinear incision according to the Langer's lines (Fig. 17.10a–d).

Broad dissection of breast parenchyma in all directions needs to be performed. Fibroglandular tissue mobilization from periphery to the nipple and in both sides is wider than the resected sector so that the reconstruction of the breast parenchyma is facilitated. Mobilization is performed superficially in the subcutaneous fatty layer (Fig. 17.11a–d), while deep dissection is made behind the deep layer of the superficial fascia in the retromammary fatty layer. Small breasts need more mobilization of tissue as in the inferior quadrants. If the tumor is very near to the major pectoralis muscle's fascia, this is removed.

The resection of breast tissue may involve one or more lobes according to the dimensions of tumor and is performed from the periphery to the

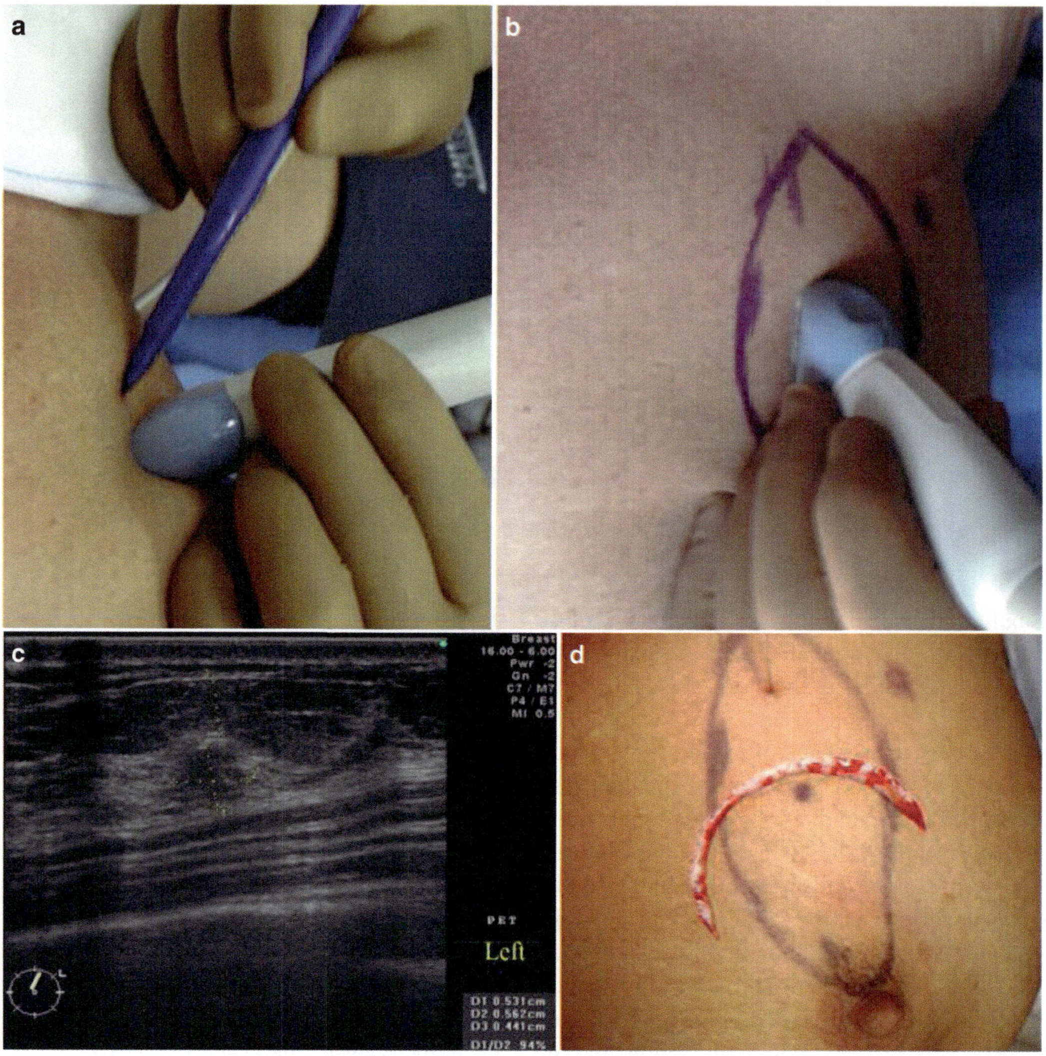

Fig. 17.7 Plan of lobar resection (**a**, **b**) for a T1b tumor (**c**) with skin incision according Langer's line

rear-nipple region where the major ducts are closed by reabsorbable suture No 2/0 after introflexion of the nipple in order to remove all the ducts tributary of the lobe (Fig. 17.12a–f).

After removal of specimen, surgical margins of the breast tissue are examined by an 8–18 MHz transducer enveloped by a sterile disposable cover. An ultrasound image of the resected specimen immediately allows the surgeon to visualize the presence of lesion, the adequate lateral margins that may benefit, eventually, from immediate re-excision (Fig. 17.13a–d) [34].

Precise orientation of specimen is of vital value, and margins are tagged with a number of clips according to a pathologist agreement in clockwise fashion starting from the retro-areolar region one clip, inferior two clips, lateral three clips, superior four clips, deep layer five clips, and superficial layer six clips. One stitch is placed on the terminal duct (Fig. 17.14a–c).

The specimen is then placed in a transparent square box if X-ray is needed. Intraoperative digital X-ray examination is performed on every specimen containing microcalcifications in order

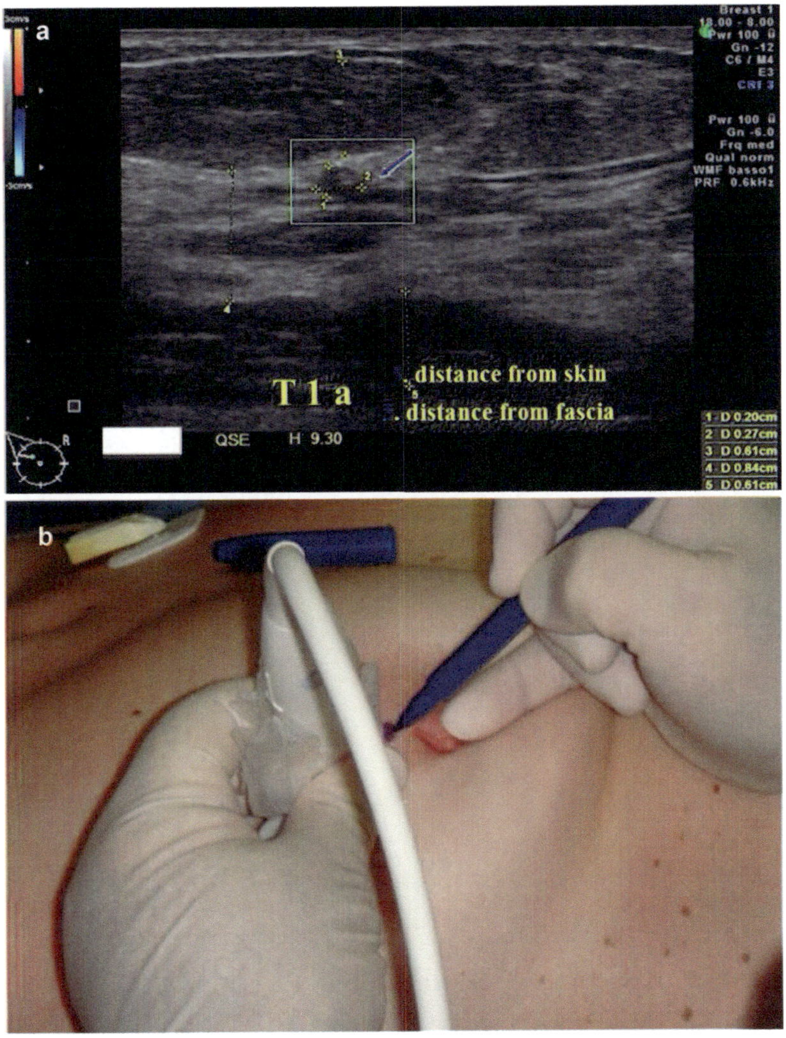

Fig. 17.8 Ultrasonic image of T1a tumor at 6 mm from the skin and 8 mm from the fascia (**a**) and drawing of the sector on the skin (**b**)

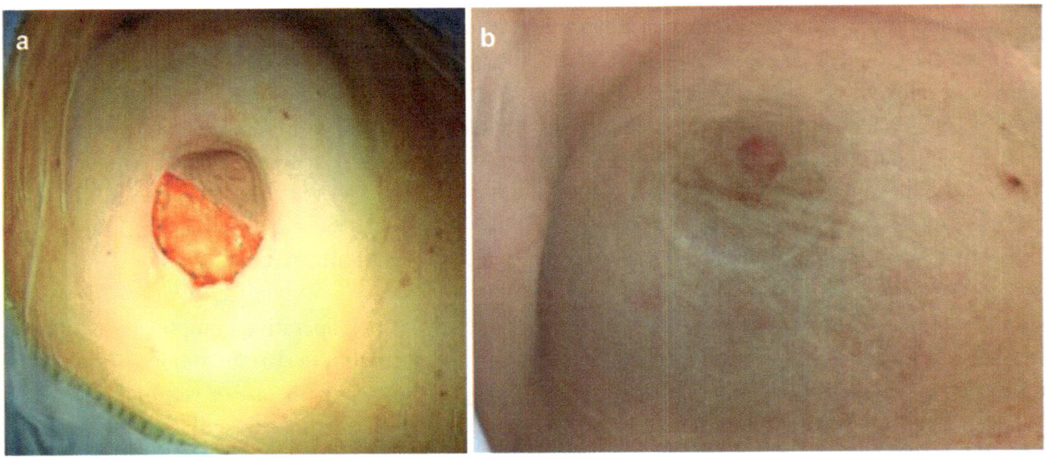

Fig. 17.9 Periareolar incision (**a**) and long distance outcome (**b**)

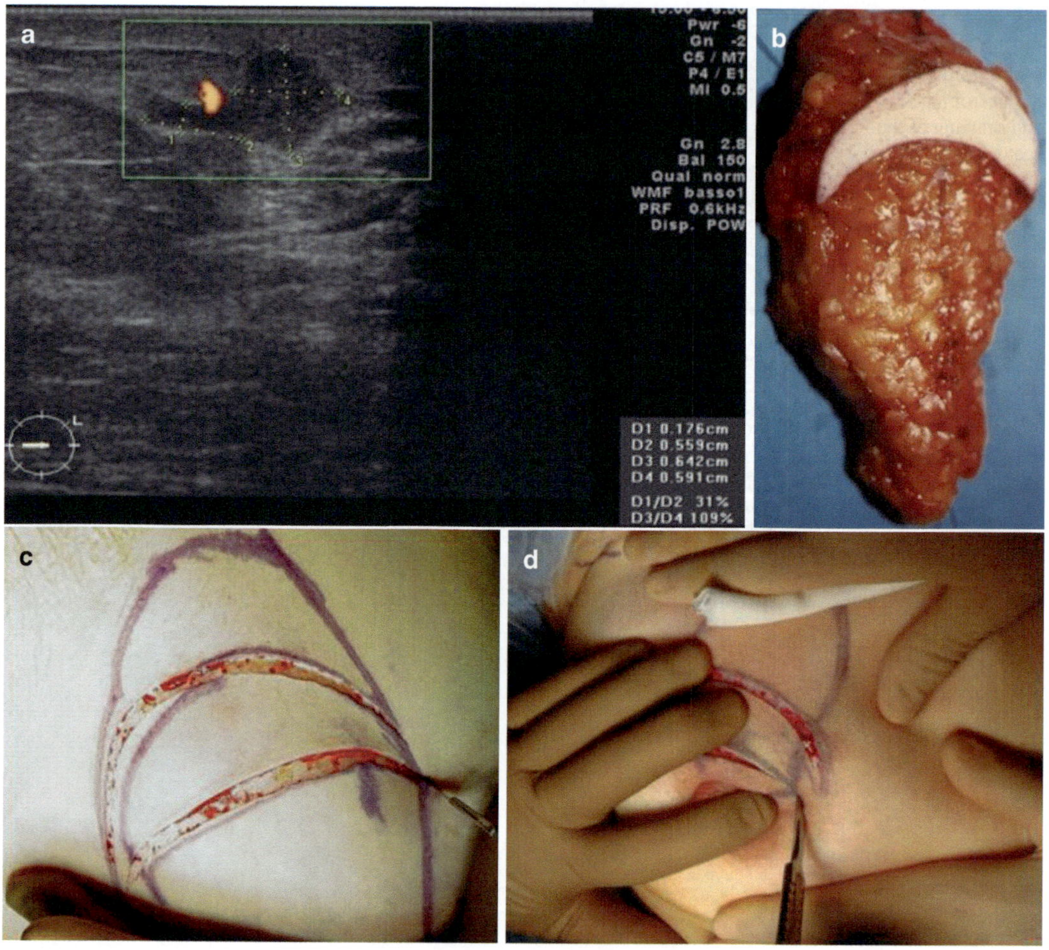

Fig. 17.10 Double curvilinear incision for tumor (**a**) close to skin with resection of skin (**b**, **c**) and sector specimen (**d**)

to ensure the correct targeting and margin situation (Fig. 17.15a, b) [27].

Mobilization of both margins, their advancement, rotation, and transposition must be sufficiently developed without being too extensive in order to avoid damage to the blood supply of the remaining tissue. The reconstruction of the breast tissue is made by reabsorbable thread No 0/1; suture is performed from the rear-nipple region to the periphery with a deeper and superficial plane in continuous fashion (Fig. 17.16a, b).

Intradermal suture is made by 4/0 reabsorbable thread in continuous fashion (Fig. 17.16c).

In order to avoid cosmetically undesirable displacement of the nipple-areola complex, repositioning of the same complex is done by removing a thin strip of skin around the areola, a de-epithelialization like half a donut, in the opposite region of conservative surgery, and suturing the dermis with a 4/0 intradermal reabsorbable thread. This technique is of great usefulness if the resection is realized in the inferior quadrants where unfavorable results due to lack of tissue can be expected (Fig. 17.17a–d).

17.6 Complications

One of the postoperative complications may be the fat necrosis due to the mobilization of the fatty tissue, subcutaneous or retromammary, but preserving an adequate vascularity and avoiding to handle the tissues roughly, we are able to avoid this.

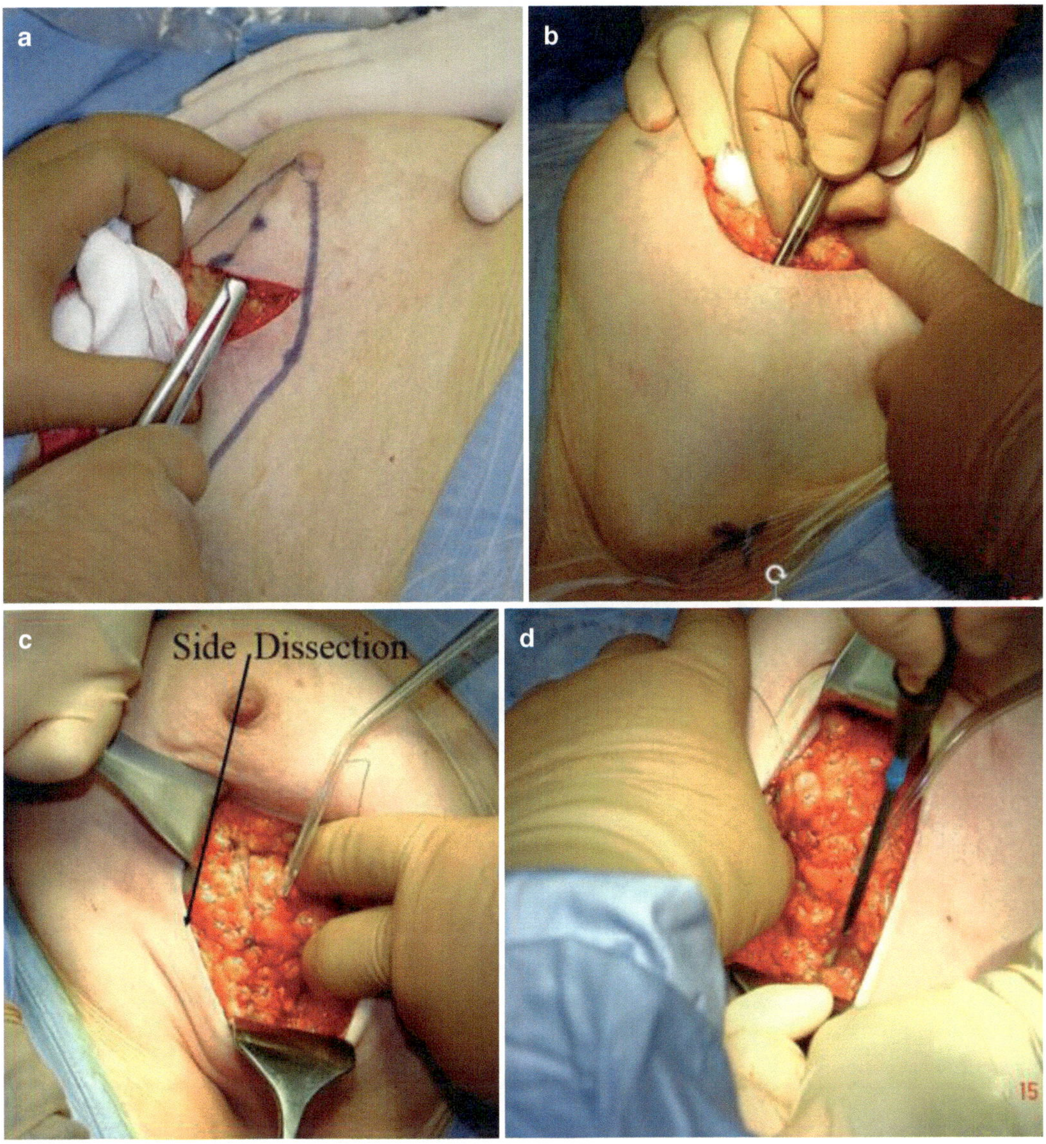

Fig. 17.11 Subcutaneous dissection to the nipple (**a**), to the periphery (**b**), in boths (**c**, **d**)

Another complication may be the skin retraction. This may be due to the inadequate mobilization of the parenchyma or to the adhesion of the dermis to the subcutaneous fat. The first option cannot be overcome without a re-intervention. The second option may be avoided by performing an adequate massage of skin detachment.

Seroma formation may be eliminated by ultrasonically guided aspiration.

The last postoperative complication may be the presence of skin and subcutaneous tissue edema, particularly during the radiotherapy. For this, it is very helpful to use a special bra able to hold the breasts suspended. The final result is highly satisfactory.

17.7 Experience and Discussion

We started the regular use of lobar resection under the definition of "sectoriectomy" at the beginning of 1988 using at the beginning a 7.5 MHz trans-

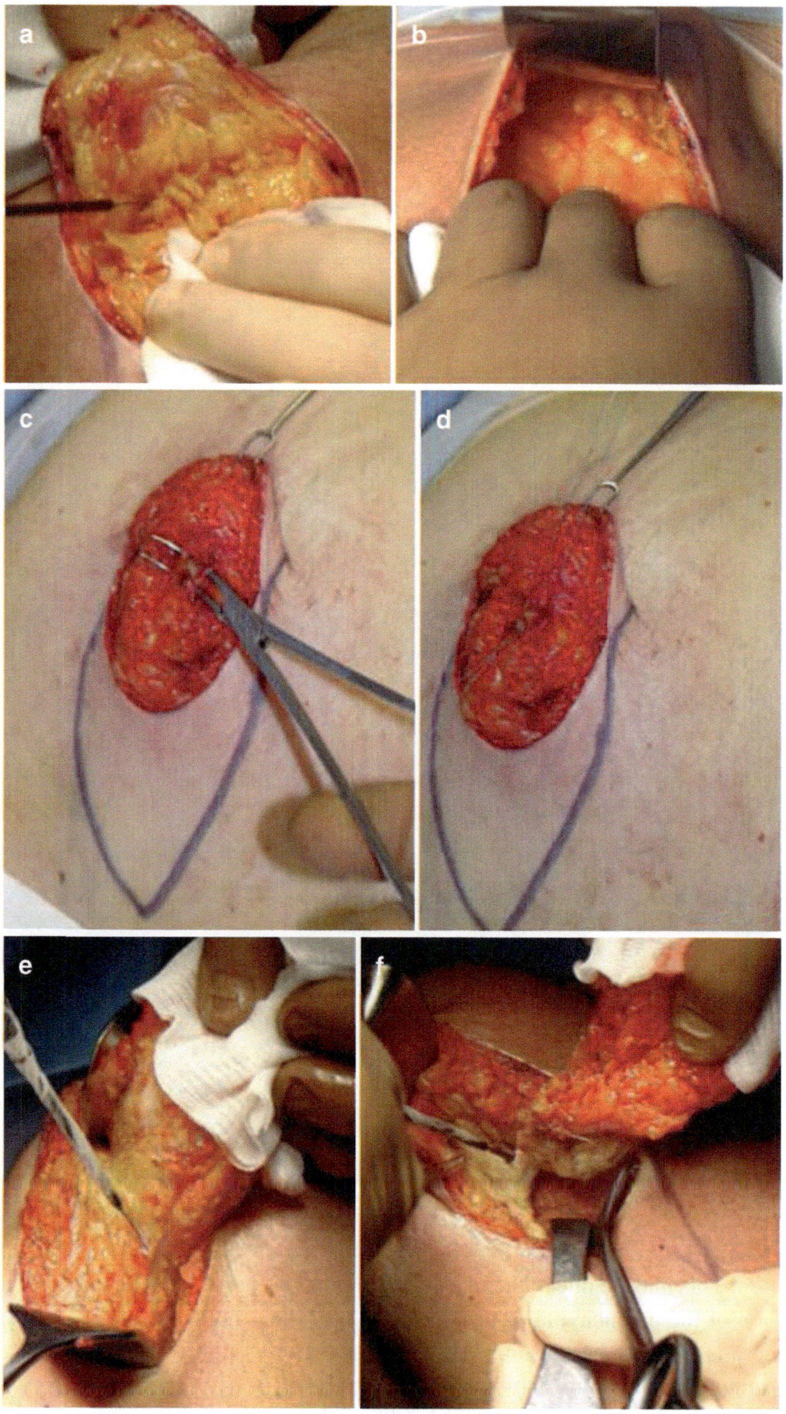

Fig. 17.12 Dissection in subcutaneous layer (**a**, **b**), closure of terminal duct behind the nipple (**c**, **d**), resection of the lobe (**e**, **f**)

ducer moving very quickly to 13 MHz and at last to 8–18 MHz broadband transducer. Our experience is based on 1582 cases from 1988 to 2010 with a follow-up from 6 to 28 years. We have considered a true recurrence, those observed from 1 to 6 years from the first surgery considering that after this interval, we may regard all the incoming tumors in different quadrants as a new tumor. We

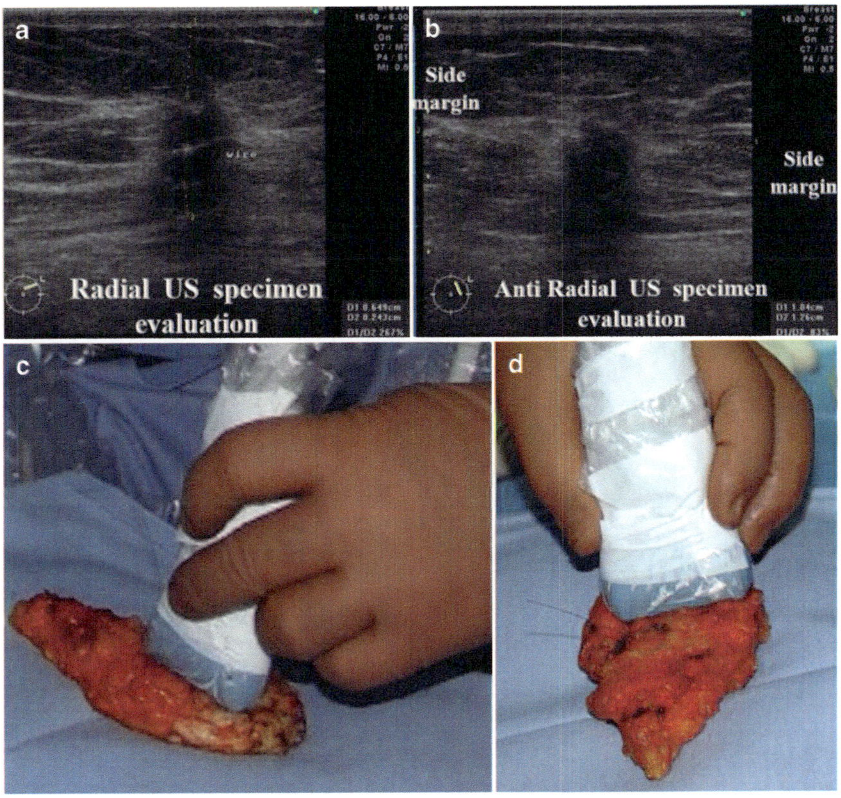

Fig. 17.13 Ultrasonic scanning of the specimen in radial (**a**, **c**) and antiradial (**b**, **d**) allowing a precise dimension of lesion and margins

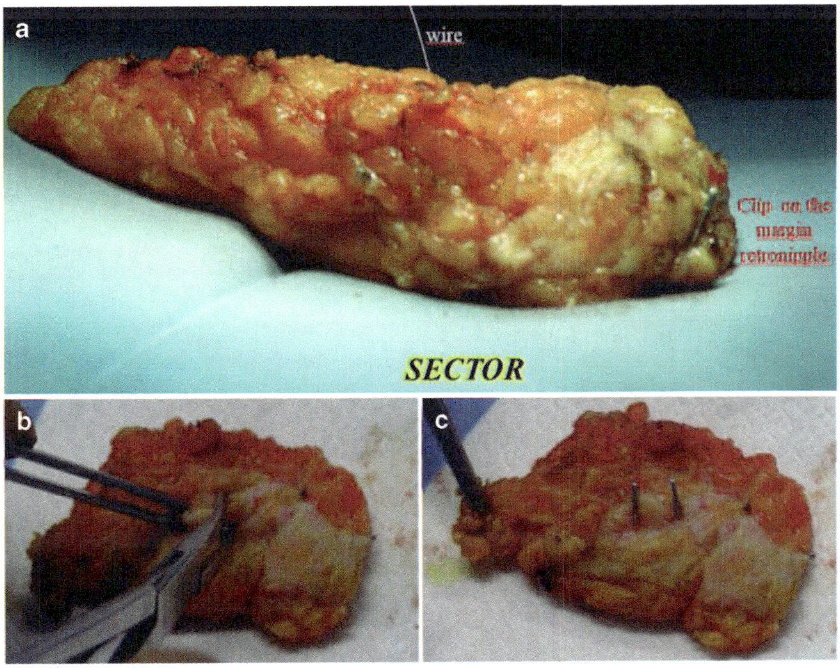

Fig. 17.14 (**a**–**c**) Orientation of specimen tagged with clips in clockwise according the pathologist

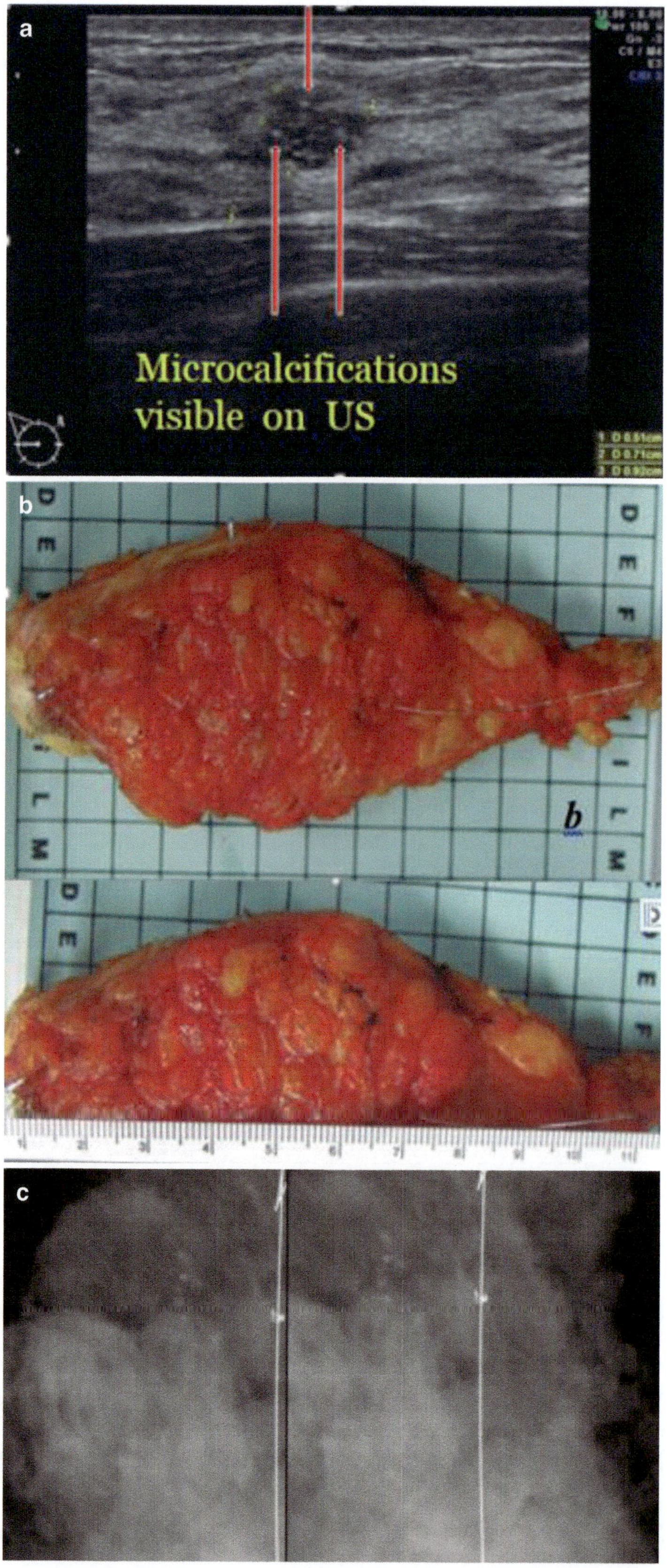

Fig. 17.15 Specimen with microcalcifications (**a**) introduced in a box (**b**) for digital X-ray examination (**c**)

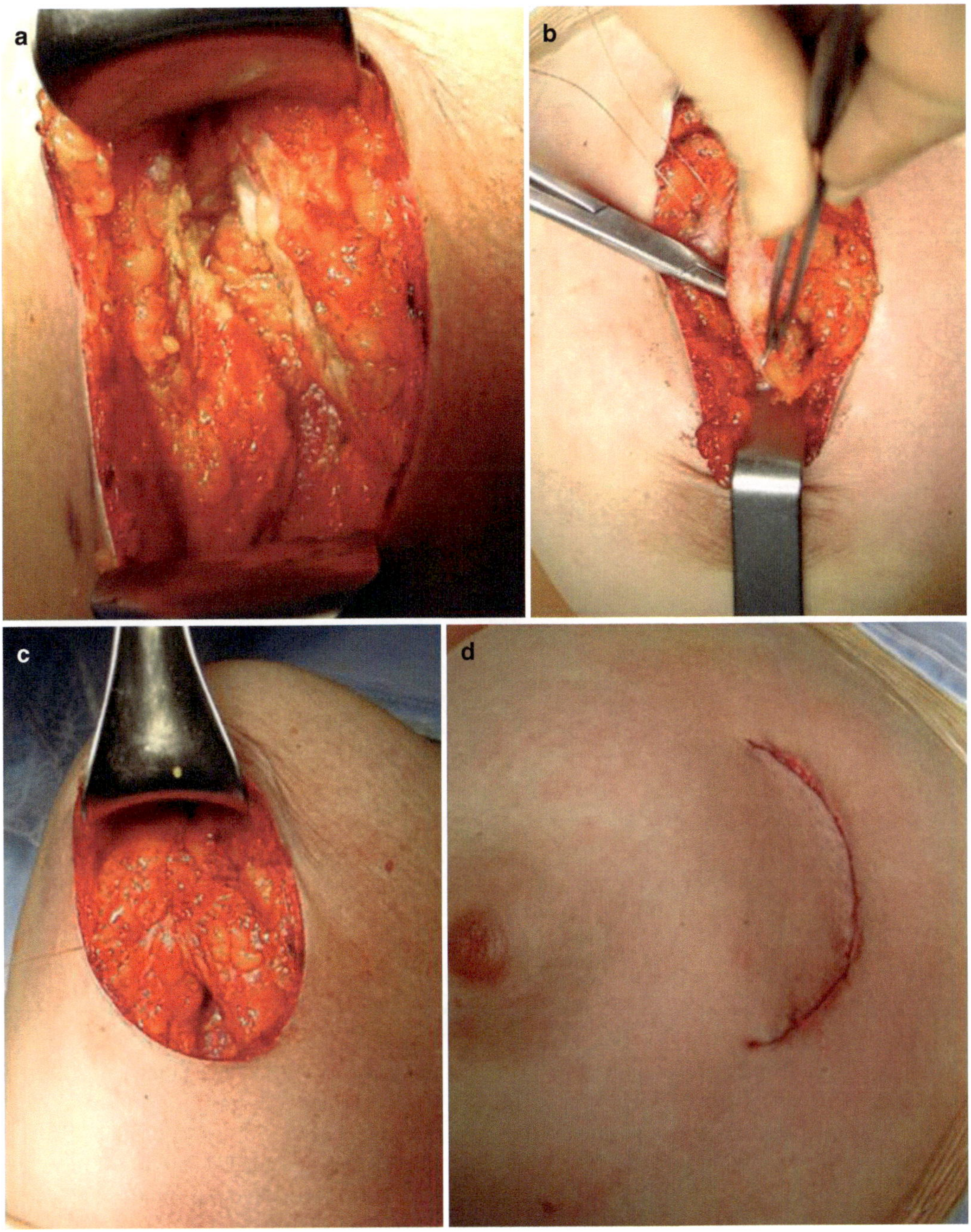

Fig. 17.16 Reconstruction of the breast tissue (**a–c**) and intradermal suture (**d**)

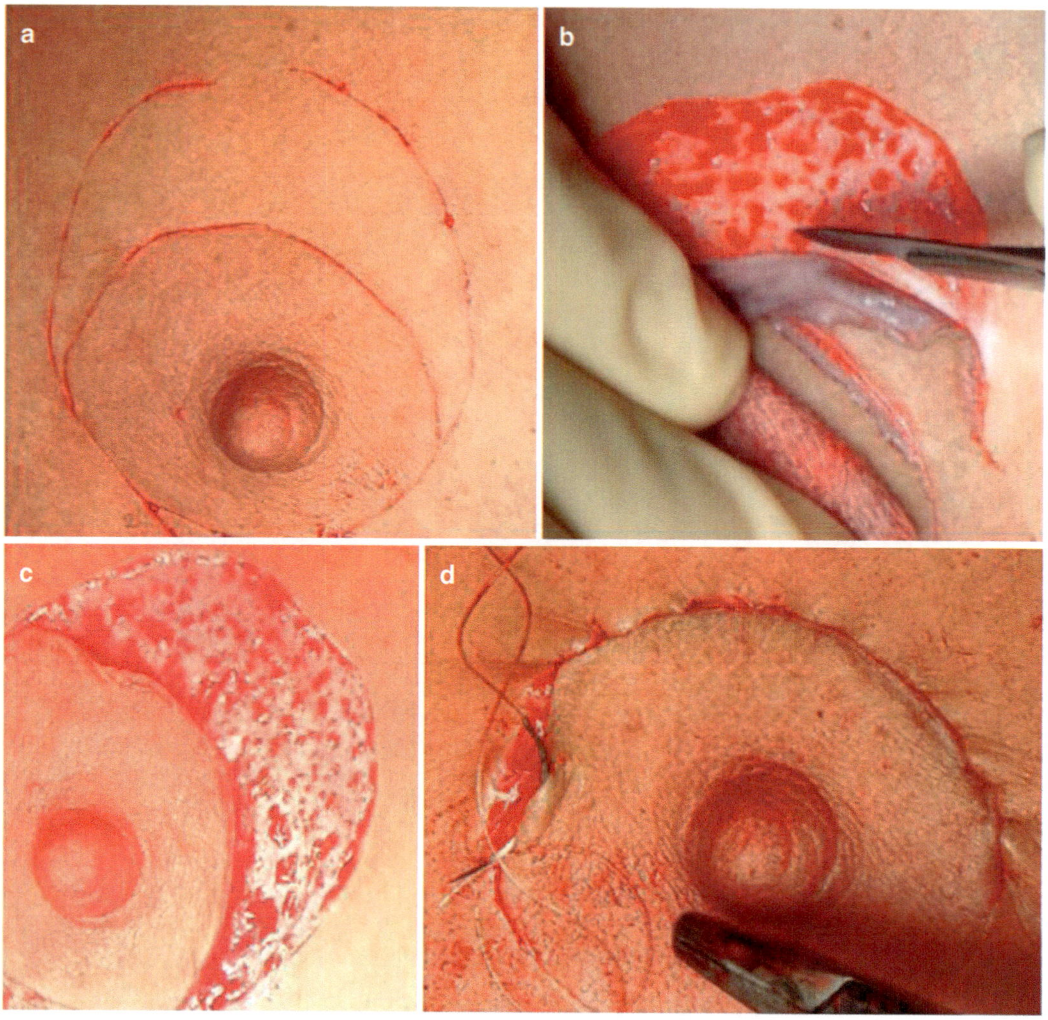

Fig. 17.17 De-epithelialization of periareolar skin (**a–c**) with intradermal suture (**d**)

observed 11 recurrences amounting to 0.7% in a time interval ranging from 2 to 5.8 years. The recurrences in the same quadrant have been five, respectively, after:

- 1.3 years intraductal papillary in situ carcinoma at 9 o'clock the first 53 years old, ductal invasive T1b + DCIS at 11 o'clock the second, 54 years old; no RT after first. Free margins. Alive. F-U 10 years.
- 2.3 years papillary intracystic in situ carcinoma at 12.30 o'clock the first, 76 years old, papillary invasive carcinoma T1a at 2 o'clock the second, 78 years old. Free margins. Concurrent heart and lung failure, no RT. Dead for concurrent diseases.
- 3.8 years ductal invasive carcinoma T1b at 9 o'clock the first, ductal invasive T1a in the scar site the second; close 1 margin; 50 years. Alive. F-U 11 years.
- 5.8 years ductal invasive T1b at 12 o'clock the first, ductal invasive dermo-hypodermic the second; 1 margin involved. 45 years. Alive F-U 15 years
- 5.8 years ductal invasive T1c at 12 o'clock the first 83 years, ductal invasive in the scar site the second, 89 years. Free margins. Dead for heart failure after 7 years.

- Another patient, 39 years old, developed carcinomatous mastitis during chemotherapy and died in the fourth year for the disease.
- All the other five patients who had recurrence are still alive with the longest follow-up of 20 years.

The advantages of ultrasound-guided surgery are:

- Independent planning of surgery according to the lobar anatomy in supine position.
- Intraoperative localization with radial insertion of wire useful particularly for the pathologist who may follow the direction of wire to reach the lesion in dense tissue and considering that localization is performed just before starting surgery, there is absence of needle dislocation.
- Precise planning of incision considering the site and distance regarded as landmarks in our protocol.
- Better anatomic orientation according to the clockwise fashion.
- Less resection of breast health tissue in antiradial section.
- Less hospitalization of every single patient that has been of about 24 h with admission at 7 in the morning of operation and discharge from the hospital the following day.
- Patient is able to return to a normal lifestyle sooner.
- Cosmesis is improved with a great psychological advantage.
- Better cost/benefit ratio of total management of each patient decreases the need for re-interventions.

For intraoperative localization, one of the advantages is that the surgeon visualizes the lesion personally in the surgical position and evaluates the three-dimensional shape of the lesion within the breast. In doing so, it is appropriate to use a radial approach according to the lobar anatomy. Another advantage is that it is more comfortable for the patient and is time- and cost-efficient [19, 38, 42, 46, 48].

Contrary to the literature where a number of disadvantages are reported, the procedure is not technically difficult, particularly in dense breast, using a 20 gauge needle for insertion; wire cannot be displaced since its placement is realized immediately before surgery; procedure cannot be painful considering that the patient is under anesthesia; surgical excision cannot be technically difficult because of wire-guided resection by ultrasound; and the risk of pneumothorax is completely avoided by using the radial approach and adequate needle inclination according to the site of lesion and the thickness of tissue. The published series of positive margin rates after wire-guided localization varying from 14% to 47% is not dependent on the wire but on the surgeon.

In our last 915 ultrasound wire localizations, 753 cancers (Tis and T1) and 162 benign lesions, we did not have any of these inconvenients.

Intraoperative digital specimen radiography allows surgeons to immediately evaluate the resected specimen and margins in the operating room with a great advantage on the operating time and direct interpretation of images [27].

17.8 Comment

Surgical treatment of cancer has evolved from classical quadrantectomy to lumpectomy or wide excision all considered as "conserving surgery" [20] but in many cases completely different and no one remembers that 63% of mastectomy specimens shows additional sites of disease within the same breast, 20% within 2 cm of the primary tumor, and 43% more than 2 cm from the index lesion [21]. Patients with multifocal disease, defined as two or more malignant foci within the same quadrant of the breast, may be candidates for breast conservation surgery but not for lumpectomy. Most parts of cancers can be excised with good cosmetic results, but first oncologic radical resection [26, 32] and intraoperative ultrasound must be performed under the principles of lobar anatomy to avoid leaving in place small foci of cancer along the major axis of the affected lobe. This is true also if we perform IORT (intraoperative radiotherapy) (Fig. 17.18a–d). Intraoperative ultrasound-guided lobar resection significantly improves not only the cosmetic

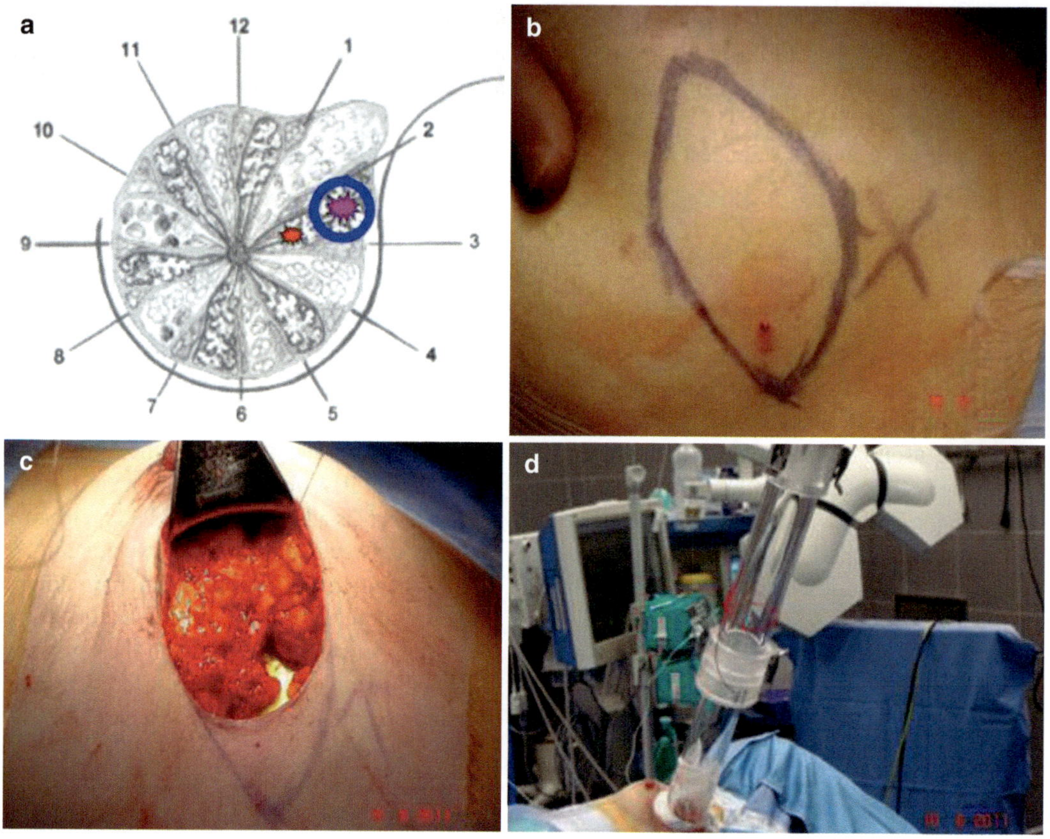

Fig 17.18 Representation of risk to leave in the same lobe a small foci of tumor not included in the resection only around the tumor (**a**) and intraoperative radiotherapy becomes the only possible cure (**b**–**d**)

outcome but also the correct anatomical resection not only in rounded fashion but following the lobar ductal anatomy. Anatomical resection leads to a reduced and more precise volume tissue removal without compromising the reconstruction (Fig. 17.19a–f).

We believe that planning the resection according to the lobar anatomy even if we perform excision of more tissue along the major axis of the duct containing the lesion, we do not lose the possibility of an adequate volume replacement with broad dissection of the breast parenchyma and with its advancement, rotation, and transposition. Another advantage of intraoperative ultrasound-guided surgery is the chance to evaluate immediately the surgical specimen and verify that the tumor or tumors are in the middle of the specimen resected as visualized during the surgical procedure. Ex vivo measurement of distance of index lesion from the margins and visualization of the texture of the margins with high-frequency high-resolution transducer is of great importance and becomes more and more effective with the advent of new generations of high-frequency transducers. The evaluation of specimen by ultrasound greatly reduces the need for re-intervention in the second attempt.

Margin status is a key factor in assessing the adequacy of resection. But the optimal margin distance for breast cancer excision remains an area of controversy, particularly in the setting of renewed interest in maximizing local control. Negative margins can be obtained only if the surgeon has resected a sufficient parenchyma, but is a block only around the tumor without any respect of the ductal anatomy whose epithelium gave rise to the tumor enough? The local recurrence after lumpectomy is from 26% to 39.2%, and with postopera-

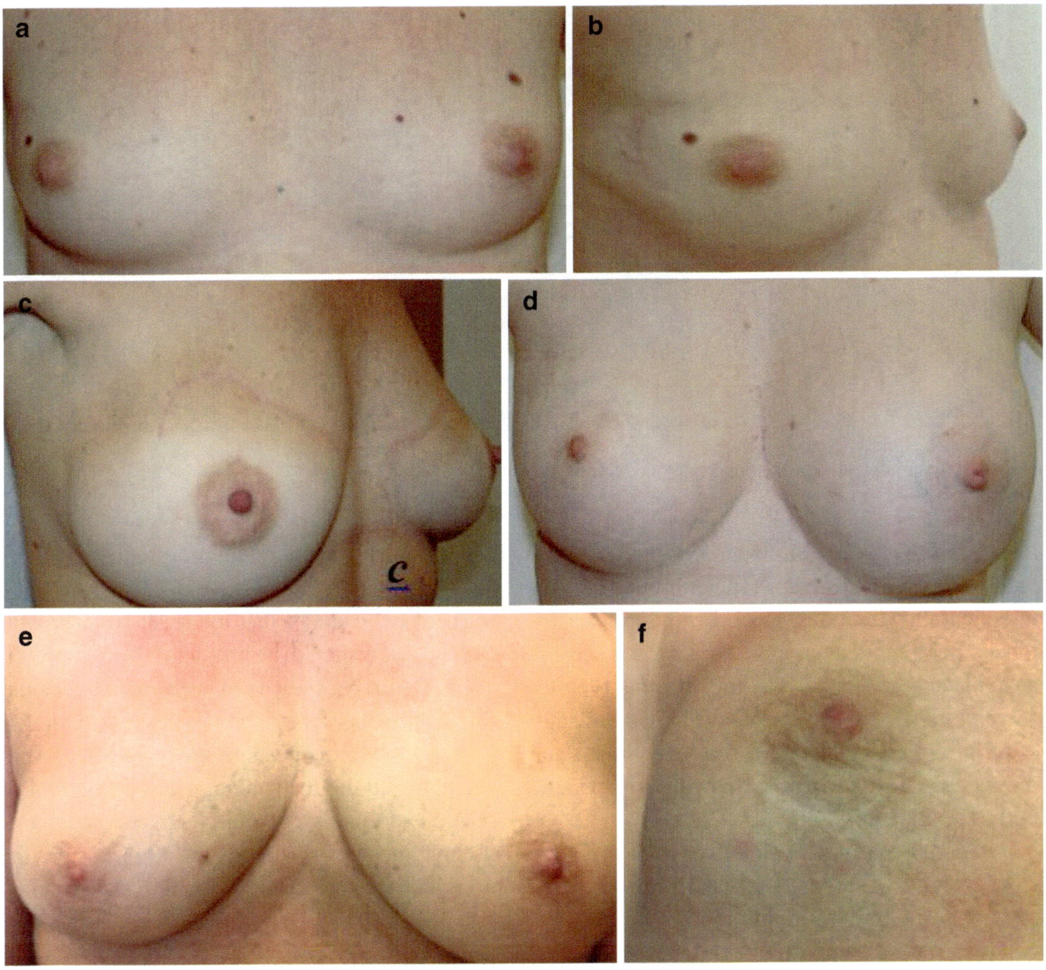

Fig. 17.19 Distant cosmetic outcome in breast of different volume. Small breast (**a**, **b**), medium breast with Langer's line incision (**c**), and periareolar (**d**) and inferior periareolar incision (**e**, **f**)

tive radiation, the risk is reduced to 7–14.3% with negative margin resection. Is it really adequate and correct from the anatomical point of view to resect less? Numerous factors are considered in literature as a cause of recurrences but not the type of resection [5, 10, 16, 22, 35, 49]. But with data showing the highest risk of local recurrence occurring in the same quadrant, near the primary site of tumor, near the lumpectomy, should we still discuss only about margins? Surgical margins are considered as a marker for residual disease remaining after surgery, but there are many cases in which a rapid local recurrence occurs in patients who had negative margins with a rate ranging from 0 to 13%. In the recent years, great attention has been paid on the volume of excision without any anatomical reference and on what causes the recurrence, according to tests that indicate if radiotherapy may be reduced or not. In up to 60% of patients, Waljee [37, 40, 41, 43, 47, 59, 62] (41.9% two excision, 6.6% three excision, 10.8% mastectomy in 714 cases), who undergo conserving surgery "lumpectomy," requires re-excision to obtain clear margins, and factors correlated with re-excision are the presence of multifocality or multicentricity, tumor position in the breast, and histology; all these should drive the surgeons to consider an alternative technique to lumpectomy [7, 8, 9, 11, 31, 33]. It is useful for surgeons to look into their own work before leaving other therapeutic proce-

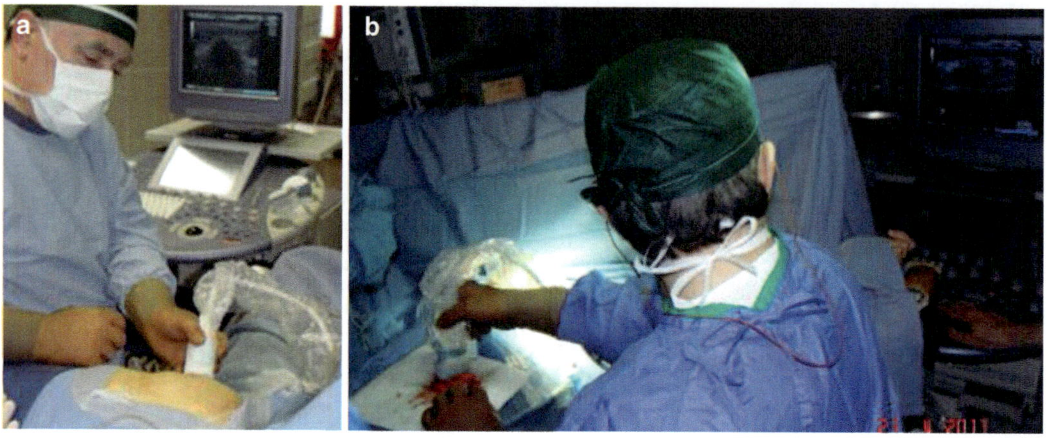

Fig. 17.20 Intraoperative ultrasound guidance of breast surgery

dures to the local care. From an oncologic point of view, the excision of breast cancer through a lobar resection allowing removal of the entire diseased lobe is not a more aggressive surgery, but it is an anatomical resection. If we perform this type of surgery, maybe we can image a trial without subsequent aggressive therapies that have important distant side effects which are now clearly evident in the literature [44].

Image-guided surgery should be seen as a keystone of modern surgery for diagnosing, staging, and planning and for intra- and postoperative control. The surgeon should be autonomous at the highest degree and master technologies. I had the luck to start very early to use US-guided procedures in 1974 after a stage at Hans Holm in Gentofte Hospital with the purpose to improve surgical management of patients, and afterwards I always encouraged the surgeons to become skilled in the use of ultrasound guided procedure not only for breast but also for thyroid and abdominal organs by telling my colleagues that ultrasound transducer should be considered as the third hand of the surgeon. I hope that in the future, all the surgeons become skilled in the use of intraoperative ultrasound-guided breast surgery (Fig. 17.20a, b).

At the end, we must remember that fundamental and mandatory for the success of the conservative, anatomical, and oncological radical surgery is the use of the large-format histopathology that alone gives the possibility to compare anatomy with imaging and real margins [45, 56, 57].

There is no doubt that today all patients with breast cancer should be managed by multidisciplinary teams, but every individual specialist should play his/her relevant autonomous role without delegating to other members of the team his/her specific duty and the recognition that local control of disease is primarily the aim of surgeon and not of systemic therapy; it is necessary to reconsider the surgical treatment integrating surgery and anatomy.

References

1. Akashi-Tanaka S, Sato N, Ohsumi S, et al. Evaluation of the usefulness of breast CT imaging in delineating tumor extent and guiding surgical management: a prospective multi-institutional study. Ann Surg. 2012;256(1):157–62.
2. Akashi-Tanaka S. Preoperative CT evaluation of intraductal spread of breast cancer and surgical treatment. Breast Cancer. 2013;20(1):21–5.
3. Amy D, Durante E, Tot T. The lobar approach to breast ultrasound imaging and surgery. J Med Ultrasonics. 2015;42:331–9.
4. Amy D. Lobar ultrasound of the breast. In: Tot T, editor. Breast cancer, a lobar disease. New York, NY: Springer; 2011. p. 153–62.
5. Anscher MS, Jones P, Prosnitz LR, et al. Local failure and margin status in early stage breast carcinoma treated with conservation surgery and radiation therapy. Ann Surg. 1993;218:22–8.
6. Bennett IC, Greenslade J, Chiam H. Intraoperative ultrasound guided excision of nonpalpable breast lesions. World J Surg. 2005;29:369–74.

7. Bolger JC, Solon JG, Power C, et al. Analysis of margin index as a method for predicting residual disease after breast-conserving surgery in a European Cancer Center. Ann Surg Oncol. 2012;19:207–11.
8. Caughran JL, Vicini FA, Kestin LL, et al. Optimal use of re-excision in patients diagnosed with early-stage breast cancer by excisional biopsy treated with breast-conserving therapy. Ann Surg Oncol. 2009;16:3020–7.
9. Chagpar AB, Martin RCG, Hagendoorn LJ, et al. Lumpectomy margins are affected by tumor size and histologic subtype but not by biopsy technique. Am J Surg. 2004;188:399–402.
10. Clarke DH, Le MG, Sarrazin D, et al. Analysis of loco-regional relapses in patients with early breast cancers treated by excision and radiotherapy: experience of the Institut Goustave-Roussy. Int J Radiat Oncol Biol Phys. 1985;11:137–45.
11. Dillon MF, Hill ADK, Quinn CM, et al. A pathologic assessment of adequate margin status in breast-conserving therapy. Ann Surg Oncol. 2006;13(3):333–9.
12. Durante E, Cavazzini L, et al. Surgical echography as diagnostic and staging tool in breast pathology. Thoracic surgery. Bologna: Monduzzi Ed; 1988. p. 301–8.
13. Durante E. Surgery of impalpable disease. In: Jellins J, Rickard M, Madjar H, editors. Breast ultrasound and mammography seminar. International Breast Ultrasound School Book: Mexico; 1993. p. 88–97.
14. Durante E, Pellegrini F, Carbonell Luna MI. Preoperative local staging of invasive cancer by US. In: Badulescu F, Bondari A, Enachescu V, editors. Syllabus of Euroson School Course Breast Ultrasound (ISBN 973-7757-23-8). Craiova (Romania): Editura Medicala Universitara Craiova; 2004. p. 77–80.
15. Durante E, Pellegrini F, Carbonell Luna MI. US breast conservative surgery and sentinel node. In: Badulescu F, Bondari A, Enachescu V, editors. Syllabus of Euroson School Course Breast Ultrasound (ISBN 973-7757-23-8). Craiova (Romania): Editura Medicala Universitara Craiova; 2004. p. 90–4.
16. Early Breast Cancer Trialists' Collaborative Group (EBCTCG). Local recurrence and breast cancer mortality. Lancet. 2005;366:2087–106.
17. Going JJ, Mohun TJ. Human breast duct anatomy, the 'sick lobe' hypothesis and intraductal approaches to breast cancer. Breast Cancer Res Treat. 2006;97:285–91.
18. Haid A, Knauer M, Dunzinger S. Intra-operative sonography: a valuable aid during breast-conserving surgery for occult breast cancer. Ann Surg Oncol. 2007;14:3090–101.
19. Harlow SP, Krag DN, Ames SE. Intraoperative ultrasound localization to guide surgical excision of nonpalpable breast carcinoma. J Am Coll Surg. 1999;189:241–6.
20. Heimann R, Powers C, Halpem HJ, et al. Breast preservation in stage I and II carcinoma of the breast. The University of Chicago experience. Cancer. 1996;78:1722–30.
21. Holland R, SHJ V, Mravunac M, Hendriks JH. Histologic multifocality of Tis, T1–2 breast carcinomas implications for clinical trials of breast-conserving surgery. Cancer. 1985;56(5):979–90.
22. Huston TL, Simmons RM. Locally recurrent breast cancer after conservation therapy. Am J Surg. 2005;189:229–35.
23. Jellins J, Kossoff G, Buddee FW, Reeve TS. Ultrasonic visualization of the breast. Med J Aust. 1971;1:305.
24. Jellins J, Kossoff G, Reeve TS, Barraclough BH. Ultrasonic grey scale visualization of breast disease. Ultrasound Med Biol. 1975;1:393–404.
25. Jenkinson AD, Al Mufti RA, Mohsen Y, et al. Does intraductal breast cancer spread in a segmental distribution? An analysis of residual tumour burden following segmental mastectomy using tumour bed biopsies. Eur J Surg Oncol. 2001;27:21–5.
26. Khan SA, Eladoumikdachi F. Optimal surgical treatment of breast cancer: implications for local control and survival. J Surg Oncol. 2010;101:677–86.
27. Kaufman CS, Bachman BA, Jacobson L. Intraoperative digital specimen mammography: prompt image review speeds surgery. Am J Surg. 2006;192:513–5.
28. Kaufman CS, Jacobson L, Bachman BA, et al. Intraoperative ultrasound facilitates surgery for early breast cancer. Ann Surg Oncol. 2002;9(10):988–93.
29. Kikuchi Y, Tanaka K, Wagai T. Early cancer diagnosis through ultrasonics. J Acoust Soc Am. 1957;29(7):824–33.
30. Kobayashi T. Present status of differential diagnosis of breast cancer by ultrasound. Jpn J Clin Oncol. 1974;4(2):145–58.
31. Landercasper J, Attai D, Atisha D, et al. Toolbox to reduce lumpectomy reoperations and improve cosmetic outcome in breast cancer patients: the American Society of Breast Surgeons Consensus Conference. Ann Surg Oncol. 2015;22:3174–83.
32. Margenthaler J. A: Optimizing conservative breast surgery. J Surg Oncol. 2011;103:306–12.
33. Merrill AL, Coopey SB, Tang R, et al. Implications of new lumpectomy margin guidelines for breast-conserving surgery: changes in reexcision rates and predicted rates of residual tumor. Ann Surg Oncol. 2016;23:729–34.
34. Mesurolle B, El-Khoury M, Hori D, et al. Sonography of postexcision specimens of nonpalpable breast lesions: value, limitations and description of a method. AJR Am J Roentgenol. 2006;186:1014–24.
35. Mirza NQ, Vlastos G, Meric F, et al. Predictors of locoregional recurrence among patients with early-stage breast cancer treated with breast-conserving therapy. Ann Surg Oncol. 2002;9(3):256–65.
36. Moore MM, Whitney LA, Cerilli L, et al. Intraoperative ultrasound is associated with clear lumpectomy margins for palpable infiltrating ductal breast cancer. Ann Surg. 2001;233:761–8.

37. Mullenix PS, Cuadrado DG, Steele SR, et al. Secondary operations are frequently required to complete the surgical phase of therapy in the era of breast conservation and sentinel lymph node biopsy. Am J Surg. 2004;187:643–6.
38. Ngo C, Pollet AG, Laperrelle J, et al. Intraoperative ultrasound localization of nonpalpable breast cancers. Ann Surg Oncol. 2007;14:2485–9.
39. Paramo JC, Landeros M, McPhee MD, et al. Intraoperative ultrasound-guided excision of nonpalpable breast lesions. Breast J. 1999;5(6):389–94.
40. Park CC, Mitsumori M, Nixon A, et al. Outcome at 8 years after breast-conserving surgery and radiation therapy for invasive breast cancer: influence of margin status and systemic therapy on local recurrence. J Clin Oncol. 2000;18:1668–75.
41. Pleijhuis RG, Graafland M, de Vries J, et al. Obtaining adequate surgical margins in breast-conserving therapy for patients with early-stage breast cancer: current modalities and future directions. Ann Surg Oncol. 2009;16:2717–30.
42. Potter S, Hovindarajulu S, Cawthorn SJ, et al. Accuracy of sonographic localisation and specimen ultrasound performed by surgeons in impalpable screen-detected breast lesions. Breast. 2007;16:425–8.
43. Rahusen FD, Bremers AJ, Fabry HF, et al. Ultrasound-guided lumpectomy of nonpalpable breast cancer versus wire-guided resection: a randomized clinical trial. Ann Surg Oncol. 2002;9:994–8.
44. Sardaro A, Petruzzelli MF, MP D'E, et al. Radiation-induced cardiac damage in early left breast cancer patients: risk factors, biological mechanisms, radiobiology, and dosimetric constraints. Radiother Oncol. 2012;102:133–42.
45. Sabel M. S: Surgical considerations in early-stage breast cancer: lessons learned and future directions. Semin Radiat Oncol. 2011;21:10–9.
46. Schwartz GF, Goldberg BB, Rifkin MD, et al. Ultrasonography: an alternative to x-ray guided needle localization of nonpalpable breast masses. Surgery. 1988;104:870–3.
47. Singletary S. E: Surgical margins in patients with early-stage breast cancer treated with breast conservation therapy. Am J Surg. 2002;184:383–93.
48. Snider HC, Morrison DG. Intraoperative ultrasound localization of nonpalpable breast lesions. Ann Surg Oncol. 1999;6(3):308–14.
49. Soderstrom CE, Harms SE, Farrel SE, et al. Detection with MR imaging of residual tumor in the breast soon after surgery. Am J Roentgenol. 1997;168:485–8.
50. Tot T. DCIS, cytokeratins, and the theory of the sick lobe. Virchows Arch. 2005;447:1–8.
51. Tot T, Tabár L, Dean P. B: The pressing need for better histologic–mammographic correlation of the many variations in normal breast anatomy. Virchows Arch. 2000;437:338–44.
52. Tot T. The limited prognostic value of measuring and grading small invasive breast carcinomas: the whole sick lobe versus the details within it. Med Sci Monit. 2006;12(8):RA170–5.
53. Tot T. The theory of the sick breast lobe and the possible consequences. Int J Surg Pathol. 2007;15:369–75.
54. Tot T, Gere M. Radiological–pathological correlation in diagnosing breast carcinoma: the role of pathology in the multimodality Era. Pathol Oncol Res. 2008;14:173–8.
55. Tot T. Subgross morphology, the sick lobe hypothesis, and the success of breast conservation. Int J Breast Cancer. 2011;2011:634021. https://doi.org/10.4061/2011/634021.
56. Tot T. The role of large-format histopathology in assessing subgross morphological prognostic parameters: a single institution report of 1000 consecutive breast cancer cases. Int J Breast Cancer. 2012;2012:395415.
57. Tot T. Breast cancer subgross morphological parameters and their relation to molecular phenotypes and prognosis. J OncoPathol. 2014;2(4):69–76.
58. Townsend CM, Craig JA. Breast lumps. Clin Symp. 1980;32(2):1–30.
59. Waljee JF, Hu ES, Newman LA, et al. Predictors of re-excision among women undergoing breast conserving surgery for cancer. Ann Surg Oncol. 2008;15:1297–303.
60. Wild JJ, Neal D. Use of high-frequency ultrasonic waves for detecting changes of texture in living tissues. Lancet. 1951;1:655–7.
61. Wild JJ, Reid JM. Further pilot echographic studies on the histologic structure of tumors of the living intact human breast. Am J Pathol. 1952;28:839–61.
62. Wilke LG, Czechura T, Wang C, et al. Repeat surgery after breast conservation for the treatment of stage 0 to II breast carcinoma. A report from the National Cancer Data Base, 2004-2010. JAMA Surg. 2014;149(12):1296–305.

Lobar Surgery for Breast Cancer

18

Mona Tan

18.1 Introduction

The surgical treatment of breast cancer has evolved over the last four decades from performing maximally tolerable operations, represented by radical mastectomy, to minimally effective therapy, exemplified by breast conservation treatment (BCT). Emerging evidence continues to define optimum therapy and the selection criteria for individualised treatment. The "sick lobe" hypothesis has enhanced our understanding of tumour development [1, 2], offering opportunities for refinement of tailored surgical therapy. Such individualised treatment is in contradistinction to mastectomy, a "one-size-fits-all" approach for all tumour types and sizes. Subgross morphology, or large section histopathology, has demonstrated variations in the distribution of disease and provides a deeper appreciation of the nuances of mammary carcinogenesis. While it is known that the breast has a lobar architecture, its distribution has individual anatomic variations. Since each disease presentation is unique in terms of site, multiplicity, distribution and histologic subtype, a preoperative map through comprehensive breast imaging serves as an essential guide to surgery [3].

M. Tan
MammoCare, Singapore, Singapore
e-mail: jabezhopems@gmail.com

The concept of minimally effective surgical therapy in breast cancer began with the pivotal randomised controlled trials (RCTs) comparing breast conservation treatment (BCT) with mastectomy [4, 5]. A sector resection of the diseased area resulted in equivalent survival compared to mastectomy. More recent studies suggest that BCT confers higher breast cancer-specific survival and local control than mastectomy [6–15]. Therefore, de-escalation of surgery comprising wide excision and appropriate adjuvant treatment is not inferior to mastectomy which is the most extensive surgery for breast cancer. These data justify increasing eligibility for BCT. Selection criteria for BCT are evolving, and a balance between expanding indications for BCT and treatment efficacy is required. Surgery predicated on the premise of lobar distribution of disease fulfils these objectives. However, surgery cannot be viewed in isolation but as a cog in the wheel of breast cancer treatment integrating anatomy, pathology, radiology, medical and radiation oncology.

18.2 Lobar Distribution of Disease

Histologic evaluation and careful scrutiny of breast malignancies have identified three main forms of cancer distribution: unifocal, multifocal and diffuse [1, 2]. While it is more common for

D. Amy (ed.), *Lobar Approach to Breast Ultrasound*, https://doi.org/10.1007/978-3-319-61681-0_18

tumorigenesis to occur within a single lobe, the development of carcinoma may occur synchronously in another lobe, distant or close, creating multicentric lesions. Understanding disease on the pathologic basis of its unifocal, multifocal, diffuse or multicentric distribution offers opportunities for improvement in the clinical and surgical therapy.

Imaging is critical for preoperative surgical planning. Standard breast imaging with mammography and sonography can identify suspicious lesions apart from the index tumour. In the preoperative context, it may be impractical to biopsy all suspicious findings. A multidisciplinary approach involving the radiologist, surgeon and pathologist is essential to select the most appropriate lesions to biopsy. Since secondary foci of malignancy apart from the reference tumour may be imaging evident or imaging occult in various permutations, there are several possible clinical scenarios to be considered when planning surgery (Table 18.1). Although every attempt should be made to excise all suspicious lesions on imaging, one should also be mindful of the possibility of imaging-occult tumour foci and take measures to accommodate these.

18.3 Surgical Approach

Mastectomy as described several decades ago continues to have a role in selected clinical scenarios today [16]. The option of BCT is at least equivalent, if not superior, to mastectomy in terms of survival and local control [4–15]. As a consequence, increasing eligibility for BCT may be now considered to be a therapeutic objective. Poor breast-conserving surgery techniques can lead to significant cosmetic deformity in approximately 30% of women [17]. Attempts to increase BCT utility without aesthetic compromise have led to the development of operative techniques known as oncoplastic breast surgery (OBS). There is now a myriad of OBS techniques, which may be broadly classified into volume displacement and volume replacement approaches. Volume displacement often involves reduction mammoplasty techniques, with or without contra-

Table 18.1 Clinical classification of tumour distribution for surgical and pathologic assessment

Nature of disease	Clinical/Imaging	Pathology	Comments	Implications for treatment
True unifocal	Unifocal	Unifocal	Radiologic-clinico-pathologic concordance	None
Apparent unifocal	Unifocal	Multiple lesions	Imaging occult lesions	Possible need for unexpected additional procedures
True multifocal	Multifocal	Multifocal	Radiologic clinico-pathologic concordance	None
Apparent multifocal	multifocal	Unifocal/confluent lesions	Parts of tumour imaging occult	None if accounted for during surgical resection
Apparent multifocal	multifocal	Unifocal	False positive imaging	Possible treatment delay or overtreatment
Apparent multicentric	multicentric	Unifocal/multifocal	False positive imaging	Possible treatment delay or overtreatment
True multicentric	multicentric	multicentric	Radiologic-clinico-pathologic concordance	None

lateral symmetrisation. Volume displacement uses the interposition of either implants or autologous flaps to fill the void created by resection. While these are now commonly used, they are associated with longer operating times and higher complication rates without significantly better local control compared with standard breast-conserving surgery [18–21]. In contrast, conventional lumpectomy is associated with lower complication rates, shorter operating times and improved patient satisfaction scores [18, 19, 21]. A reductionist approach, built on the principles of conventional lumpectomy, optimises BCT in terms of utilisation and cosmesis without mammoplasty, symmetrisation or volume replacement procedures [22].

An appreciation of disease distribution in the breast facilitates the use of this reductionist approach where surgical treatment is tailored according to lesion extent. Preoperative mapping of lesion extent for accurate resection not only avoids overtreatment, but it also spares tissue for defect closure, an essential component of minimising deformity. A balance needs to be struck to achieve the threefold objective of tumour resection with adequate margins, good cosmetic results and avoidance of overtreatment. Emphasising one over another could lead to unfavourable outcomes in the other domains. Routinely applying OBS has been proposed by some, but in view of the absence of improved local control [19], it may be more appropriate to tailor surgical treatment according to disease extent and distribution, information which can be obtained from clinical and imaging data. A reductionist approach aims to excise the disease lobe adequately without excessive tissue loss. This also the added advantage of retention of the lobar integrity for radiotherapy and application of boost. The significant mobilisation with OBS and mammoplasty may lead to the disruption of this lobar integrity, which may account for the trend towards higher recurrence in a recent study [19]. Careful preoperative mapping and surgical planning enables accurate resection while minimising disruption of the lobar parenchymal tree.

18.4 Preoperative Mapping and Choice of Surgical Approach

18.4.1 Unifocal Breast Malignancies

Unifocal malignancies usually comprise both a unifocal in situ component (that involves a single terminal ducto-lobular unit [TDLU] or several neighbouring TDLUs in close association with the related subsegmental or segmental duct(s)) and a unifocal invasive component (a single well-delineated invasive focus in the same area as the in situ part). Rarely, only the in situ or the invasive component is present. True pathological unifocal cancers are estimated to occur in approximately 40% of cancers [2]. From a clinical and surgical viewpoint, unifocal disease may be true or apparent [23–26]. Regardless, surgery is always planned to accommodate the possibility that there is imaging-occult disease, and resection patterns should conform to the anticipated lobar distribution. Preoperative imaging is essential in determining extent of disease and providing a surgical map. Clinical examination, together with mammography and sonography, is the minimum requisites for preoperative evaluation. Magnetic resonance imaging (MRI) is controversial. While there are advocates of its routine use [27], it appears that current opinion tends towards a selective approach for MRI [28–31]. MRI poses certain challenges, and a suggested solution for these potential difficulties is illustrated in Fig. 18.1.

Since breast disease has been identified to have a lobar distribution [1–3], surgery should be directed accordingly. At present, we are yet unable to delineate the lobar tree, so a guiding principle would be to plan resection in an elliptical or teardrop pattern around the tumour to incorporate a substantial proportion of the affected lobe (Fig. 18.2). The radial dimension of this ellipse, or its length, is usually greater than its breadth or anti-radial dimension. The axis of its length is directed radially towards the nipple. Rather than equidistant margins surrounding the tumour, radial margins are usually

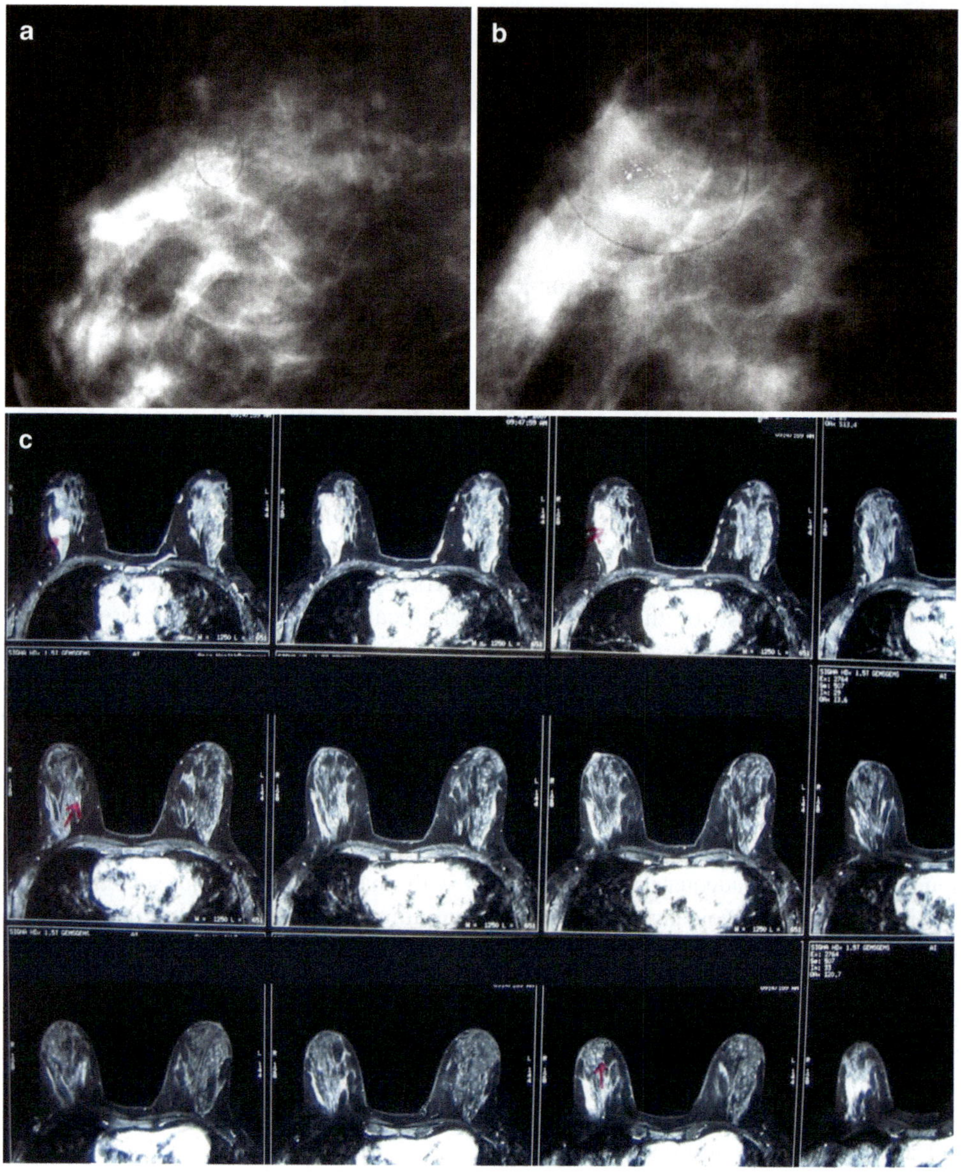

Fig. 18.1 (**a–l**). This 42 year-old woman presented with rapid progression of screen detected microcalcifications which prompted further investigations with ultrasound as well as MRI breast. (**a–c**) MRI demonstrated a true multifocal lesion close to the index palpable tumour and two other suspicious findings in other areas of the breast. The patient elected for multiple MR localisation and wide excision with frozen section analysis to avoid delay. She was prepared for the possibility of a mastectomy. (**d–i**). The two lesions in the upper outer quadrant were approached through an eccentric elliptical incision. This allows for scar lengthening and avoids puckering. An ellipse of tissue is excised for the main tumour. Resection is performed in a perpendicular fashion down to the pectoralis fascia. The other two lesions were approached through separate incisions. After tumour resection, the parenchymal pillars were mobilised and apposed with sutures prior to skin closure. The two lesions in the upper outer quadrant were malignant, but the other two were benign. (**k–l**) The patient's final cosmetic results 4 years after treatment. *Comments*: This is a case demonstrating false positive results with MRI and the possibility of either delay of treatment if she had elected to go for MRI guided biopsy or overtreatment if mastectomy was performed based on MRI findings. Her ultimate surgical treatment would unlikely have differed if MRI had not been performed, as an elliptical tissue resection, representing a substantial portion of the diseased lobe would have been resected and the second focus would have likely been removed en bloc with adequate margins

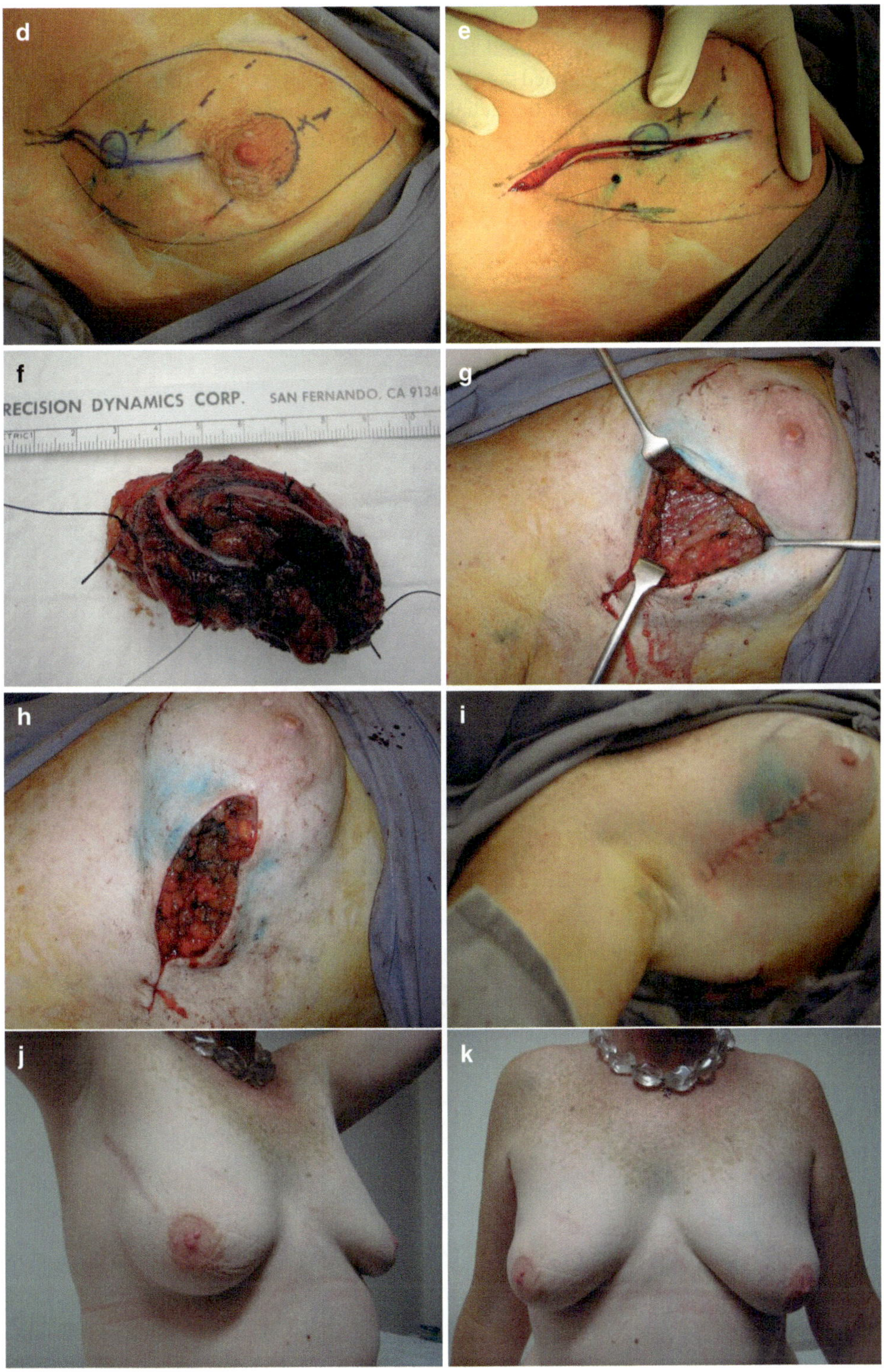

Fig. 18.1 (continued)

greater than anti-radial margins. To facilitate this, a “boomerang” incision may be used for lesions in certain positions, so named as the crescent in a periareolar position and the radial limb forms a shape that resembles a boomerang [32].

18.4.2 Multifocal Breast Malignancies

If multifocal lesions are identified preoperatively, then surgical resection should be mapped to accommodate all lesions within the anticipated involved

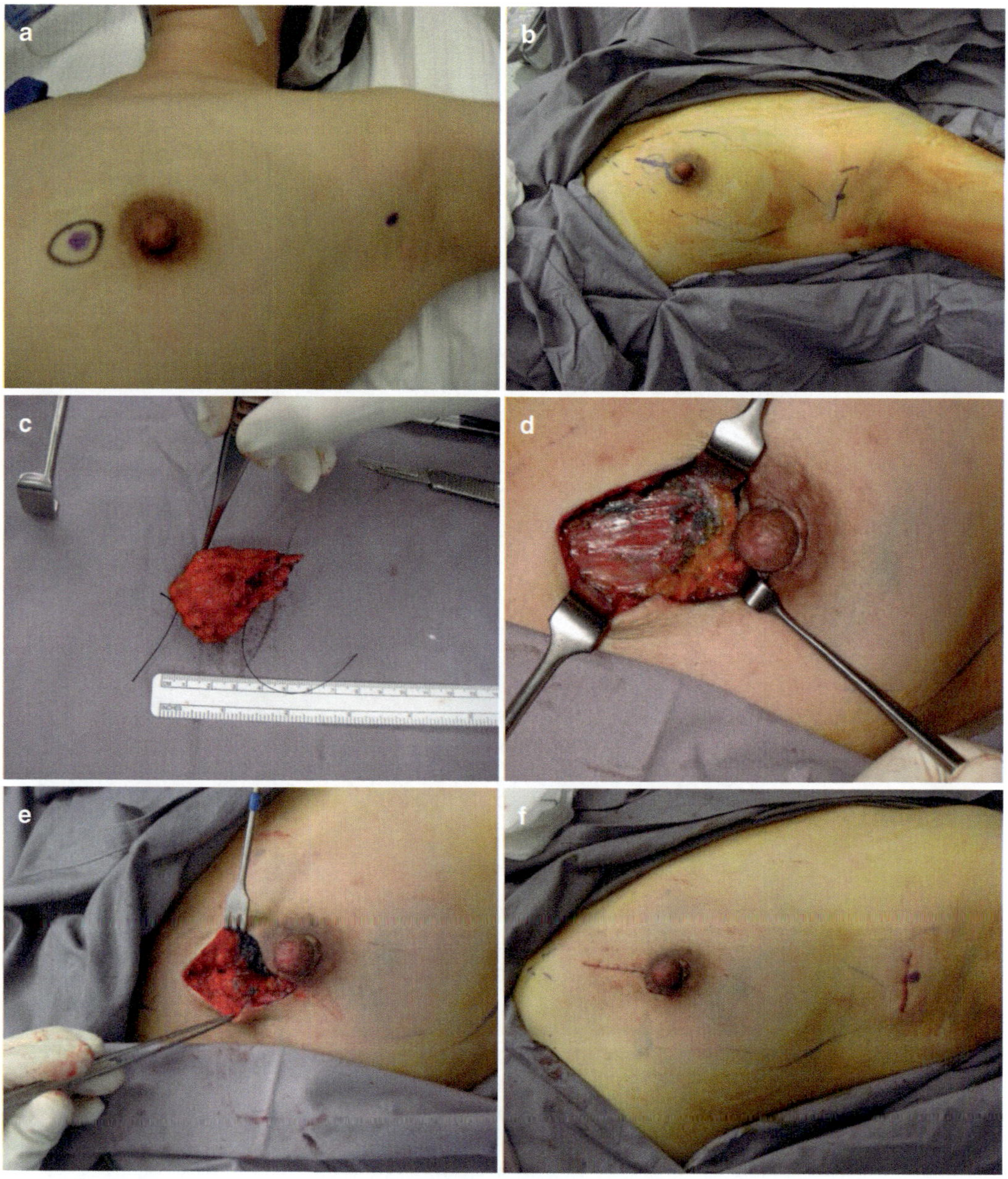

Fig. 18.2 (**a**–**h**) This 39 year old patient presented with a palpable left breast lump and surgery for her true (clinic-radiologic-pathologically concordant) unifocal tumour is illustrated. A boomerang incision is used and a tear-drop tissue resection is performed to achieve clear margins. After clearance down to the muscle, tissue apposition is performed, followed by skin closure. (**g** and **h**) illustrate her cosmetic outcome 1 year after surgery. *Comment*: This approach allows surgery to be distilled to its irreducible elements, yet achieving adequate resection of the diseased lobe and avoiding the ‘bird-beak’ deformity 40

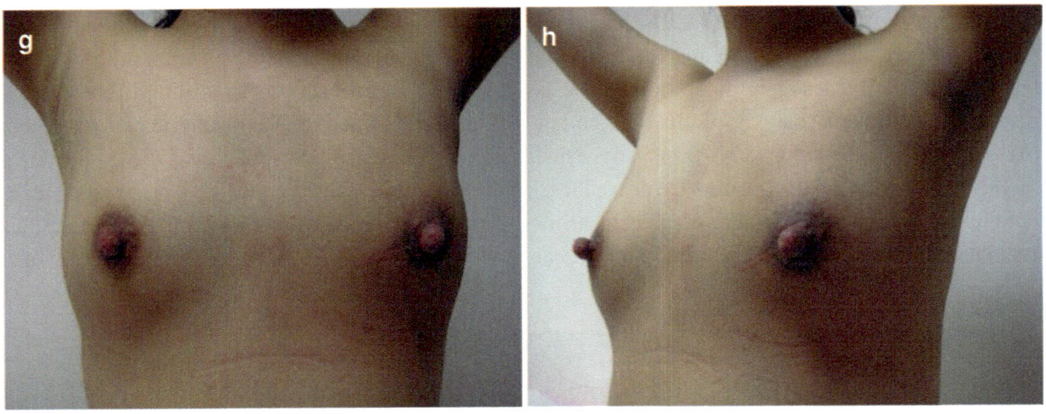

Fig. 18.2 (continued)

lobe. As for a clinical unifocal lesion, preoperative mapping with lobar anatomy in mind often leads to an elliptical or teardrop resection pattern to excise the diseased lobe, although total volume resected is usually slightly greater [3] (Fig. 18.3). The shape of the resultant cavity allows direct apposition of the tumour cavity walls, which is a requisite for good cosmetic outcomes. This surgical approach also retains lobar integrity, which has implications for radiotherapy [33].

OBS techniques may be applicable in multifocal tumours as they allow larger resection volumes and minimise deformity. However, one of the objectives of OBS is to achieve wide margins around the tumour, which can result in excessive tissue loss, and lead to the necessity of volume replacement or contralateral symmetrisation to correct for significant reduction in ipsilateral breast volume. OBS techniques are also associated with significant mobilisation of tissue, potentially disrupting the residual and neighbouring ducto-lobular anatomy. In contrast, minimising the amount of tissue loss to the bare essentials has the potential to reduce the extent of operation, operative time and possible complications [18, 20, 21].

Although there were initial concerns regarding the presence of occult tumour foci retained after partial mastectomy [23–25], local control rates with BCT in the NSABP-B06 trial [5], as well as more recent studies, suggest that radiotherapy can eradicate the minute residual foci of tumour [6–15]. Results of large studies on BCT for multifocal and multicentric disease reporting acceptable local control support this phenomenon [34–38]. Since radiotherapy boost to the tumour bed has an impact on local control [33], retention of the positional integrity of the lobar anatomy of the breast becomes essential. Concerns regarding this positional disruption with OBS have been raised by radiation oncologists as clips placed to mark the tissue edges have been displaced outside the tumour quadrant in 43% of cases [33, 39], potentially compromising accurate delivery of a boost [33]. As opposed to commonly used incisions for OBS which may not correlate to tumour position, thoughtful placement of incisions over main tumour site(s) allows adequate surgical access for full-thickness wide excisions and apposition of parenchymal pillars, preferably directly beneath the scar to retain lobar integrity. Radio-opaque clips may be placed to identify the most distant point of the cavity, if it is more than 2 cm from the scar. Such an approach would accommodate the possibility clinically apparent multifocal disease turns out to be pathologically unifocal or extensively diffuse (Fig. 18.4).

18.4.3 Multicentric Breast Malignancies

Mastectomy was the quondam standard for the surgical treatment of multicentric breast cancer until about a decade ago when data from several large studies demonstrated acceptable local control with BCT [34–38]. Experts recently endorsed the use of BCT for multifocal and multicentric breast cancers (MFMCBC) provided clear margins were obtained and radiotherapy was administered [40, 41]. Even so, multicentric disease is often excluded from analysis of BCT outcomes [42–44]. Extreme oncoplasty is a suggested method of achieving BCT for multicentric cancer, but the nomenclature used to denote multicentricity in these reports could in fact refer to multifocal disease in a single sick lobe with a broad radial front [45, 46]. To date, there are no reports on the use of OBS for lesions that are in different quadrants or separated in a hemispheric manner. There are, however, reports of non-OBS procedures through separate incisions [33, 47], but such techniques may violate well-established guidelines which stipulate that women with lesions which

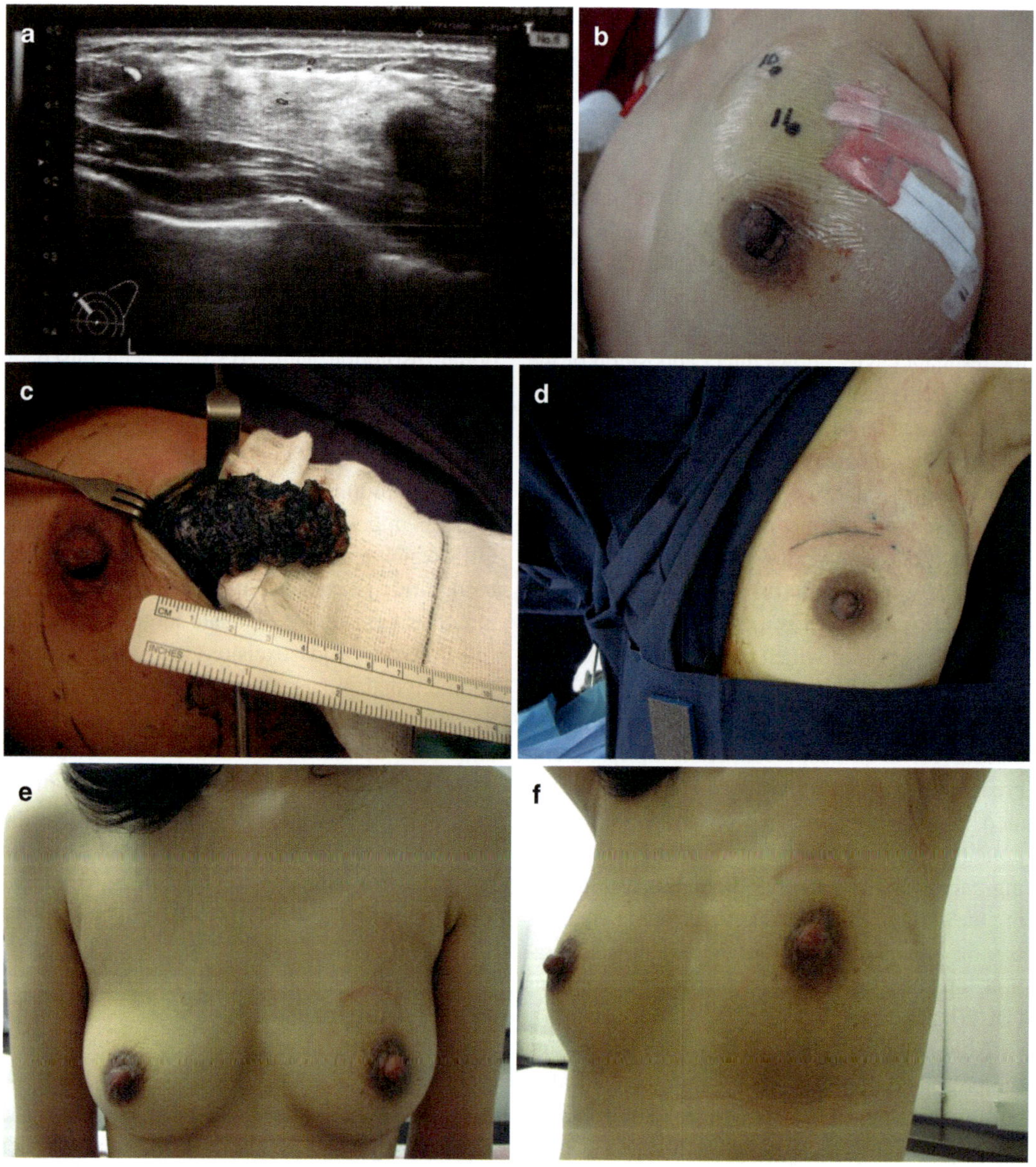

Fig. 18.3 (**a**–**f**) Concordant or true multifocal disease which is a distance away from the nipple can be approached through a skin crease incision. However, the principle of lobar or segment resection is unchanged. Histology revealed a superior 7 mm and inferior 15 mm infiltrating ductal carcinomata, separated by 15 mm of normal tissue

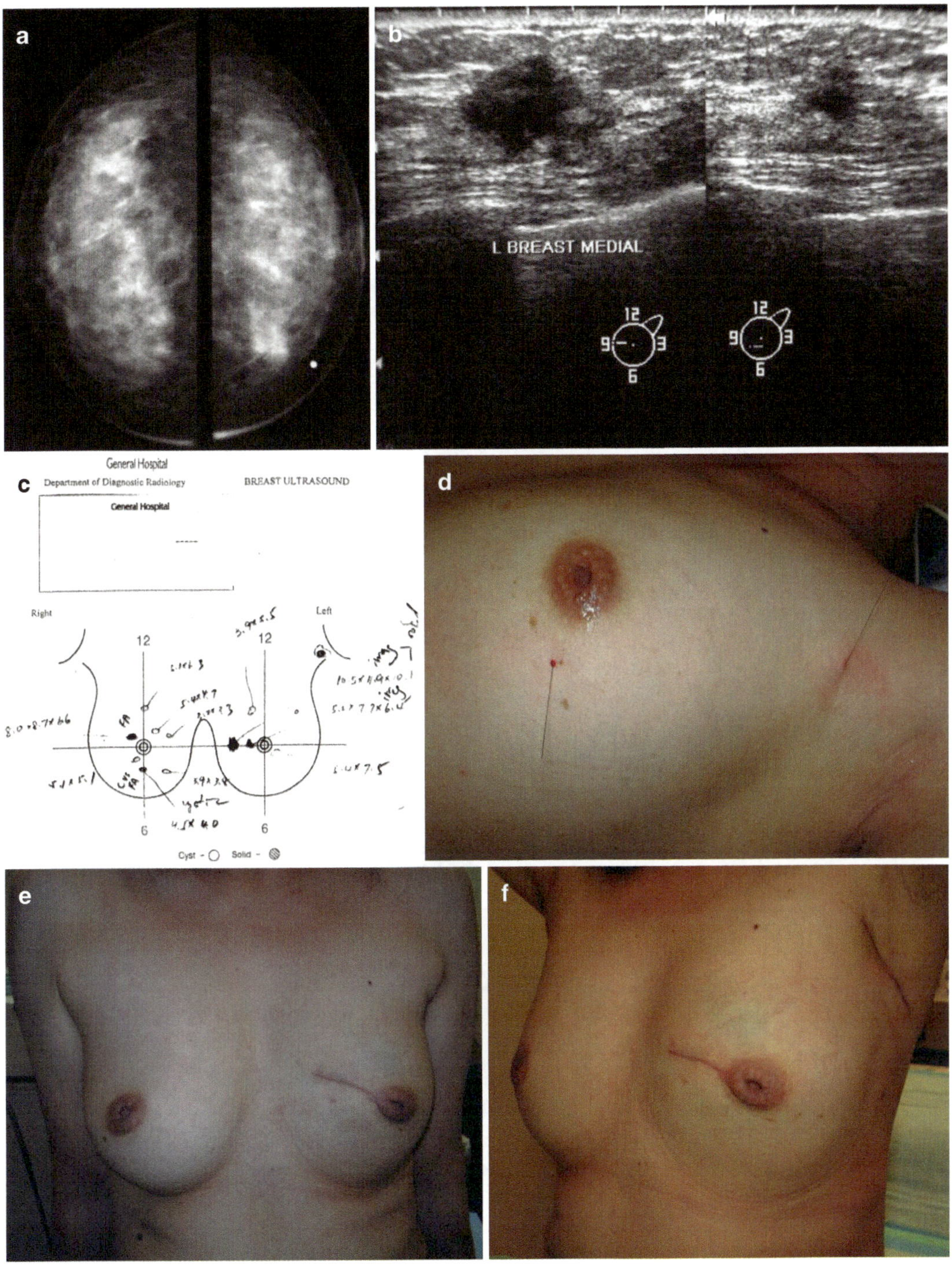

Fig. 18.4 (**a–f**) This 45 year-old patient was diagnosed with what was thought to be multifocal invasive ductal carcinoma at another facility following core biopsy. Mastectomy was originally recommended at the first centre due to the presence of multifocal disease. Following a second opinion at the authors' facility, she elected for a "trial of BCT". Localisation of the impalpable periareolar lesion and of the suspicious axillary lymph node was performed. She underwent an en bloc wide excision of the two *left* breast lesions through a boomerang incision, and axillary staging through a separate axillary incision. Histology was reported as a 40 mm invasive ductal carcinoma, with no intervening normal tissue between the clinical lesions. Three of sixteen axillary lymph nodes were involved. She had an "apparent" multifocal disease which was proven to be extensive diffuse disease on histology. Her final cosmetic outcome is illustrated in **e** and **f**

cannot be excised with clear margins through a single incision are not candidates for BCT [48].

To surmount these challenges of multicentric disease, a segment classification has been proposed [49]. This combines preoperative mapping with the lobar anatomy in mind and a multilobular or multisegment surgical resection fashioned according to the diseased lobes [49]. A clear distinction between multifocal and multicentric disease is sometimes challenging. Nevertheless, accurate tumour extirpation can be achieved through a single incision regardless of its true anatomy and pathologic distribution with optimum preoperative mapping and surgical planning (Figs. 18.5 and 18.6). The objective is to excise all clinical and imaging evident foci within

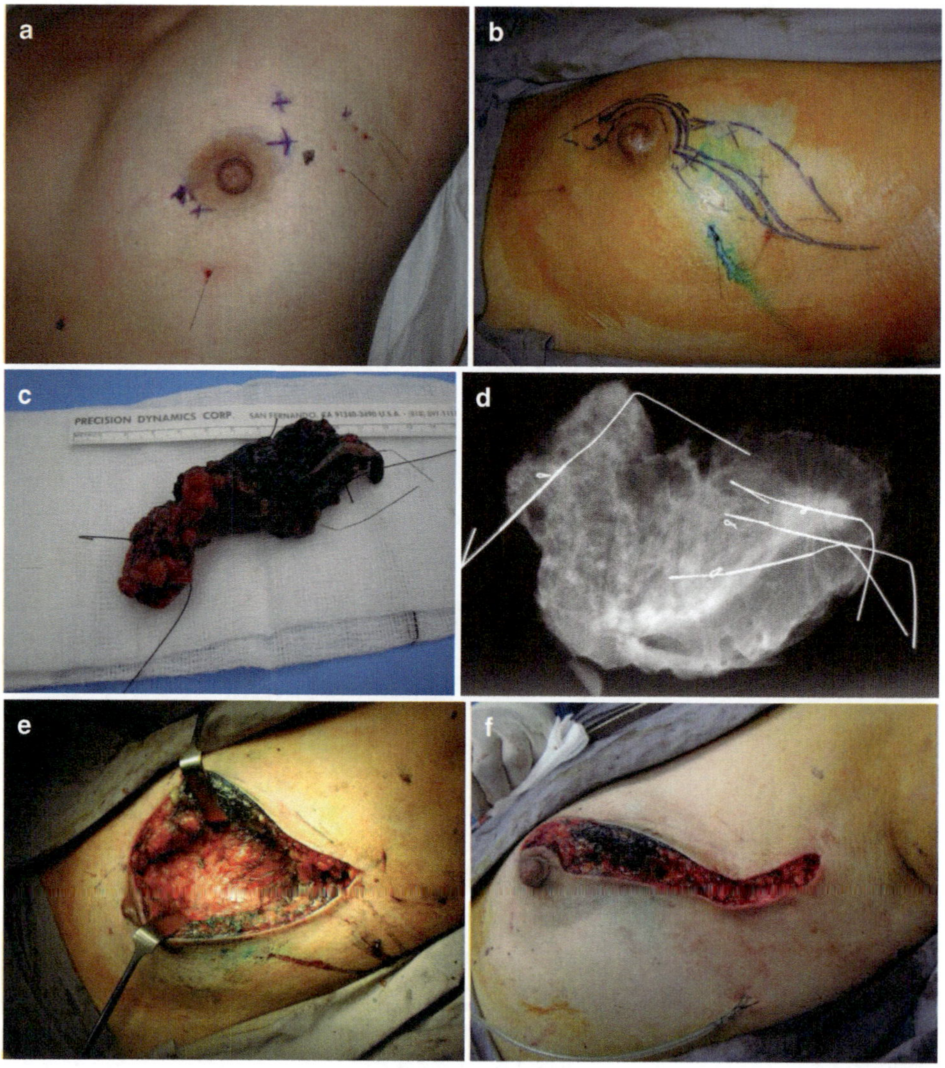

Fig. 18.5 (**a**–**h**) This patient was diagnosed with multicentric breast cancer at a tertiary oncology centre and offered mastectomy, which she declined. Having undergone neoadjuvant chemotherapy, a modified boomerang incision was used with a dual-pronged segment resection joined centrally (*dotted lines*). (**b**) En bloc resection for lesions in opposite quadrants across the nipple-areolar complex through a single incision was performed. After extirpation of all identified residual lesions, parenchymal pillars were mobilised, followed by direct apposition with sutures. (**f**) Her cosmetic outcome 2 years after completion of treatment is shown in (**h**). *Comment*: The use of a modified boomerang incision allows multi-lobar or multisegment resections through a single incision which fulfils guideline recommendations

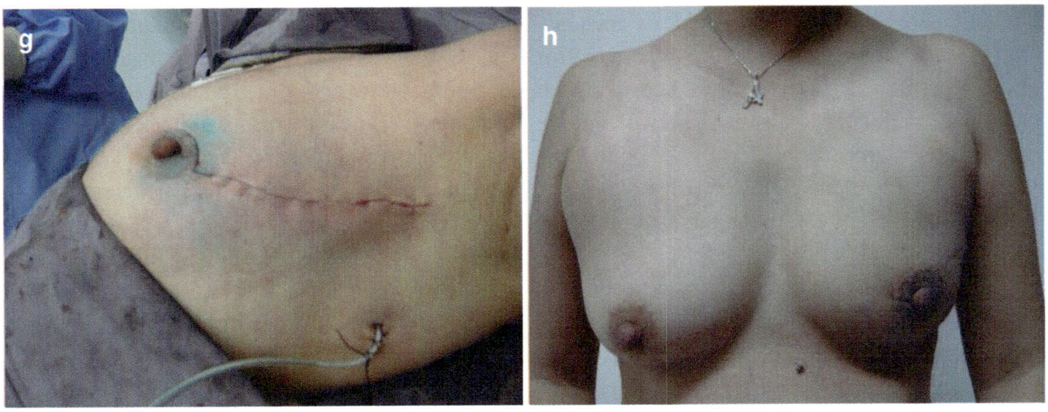

Fig. 18.5 (continued)

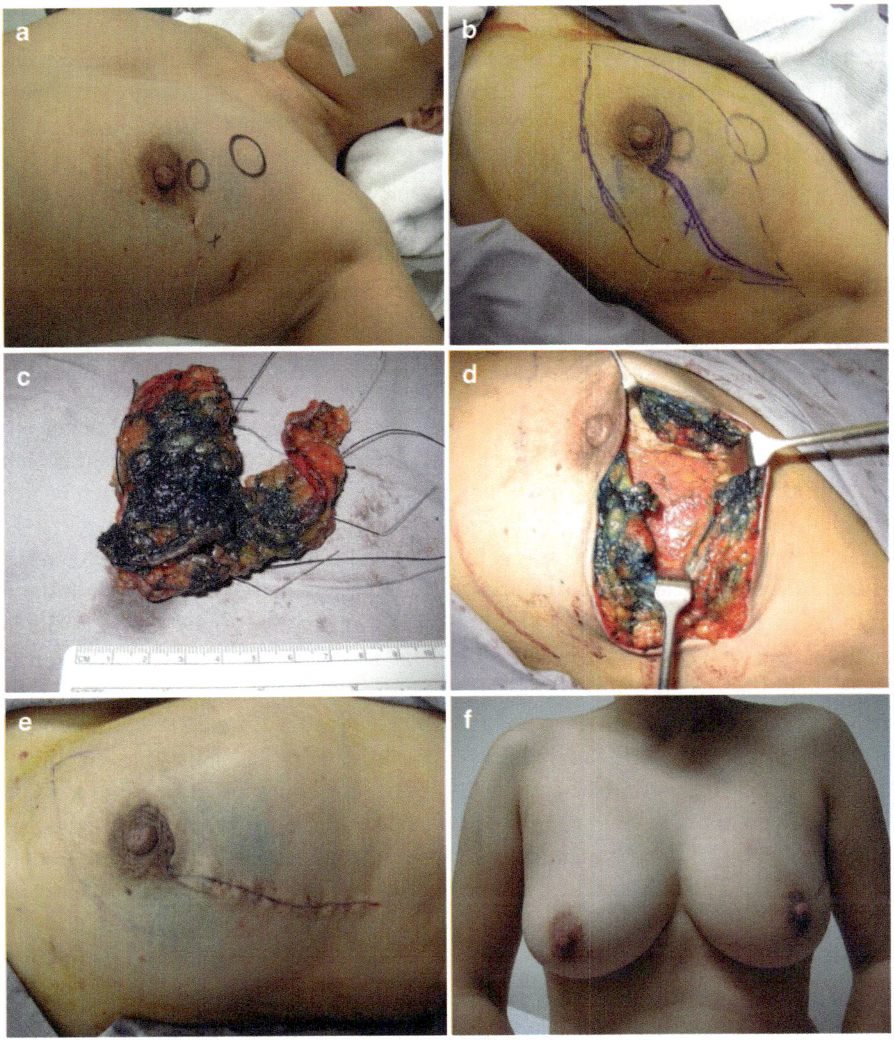

Fig. 18.6 (**a–h**) The same incision may be used for this patient who had multicentric lesions at the 12 & 2 o'clock positions. The dual segment resection specimen is shown in (**c**). The defect has been repaired through apposition of full thickness parenchymal flaps, followed by skin closure (**d**, **e**). Her cosmetic outcome a year after treatment is shown in (**f**)

the anticipated diseased lobe, achieve adequate margins and yet retain sufficient parenchyma for tissue repair to avoid deformity. The resection pattern for multicentric disease has two or three tissue ellipses connected centrally, much like the petals of an incomplete flower (Figs. 18.5 and 18.6). This analogy of the lobar anatomy has been previously described [50]. Since the volume of tissue resection can be significant, a proportion of women with multicentric disease will benefit from neoadjuvant chemotherapy for downstaging to increase eligibility for BCT. Marker clips at the time of diagnostic biopsy facilitate identification of the original tumour sites and accuracy of excision. In fact, there is data indicating that in patients who have good response to neoadjuvant chemotherapy, both overall survival and disease-free survival are not significantly different whether BCT or mastectomy was performed [38]. This therapeutic strategy may surmount previously suggested limitations of multicentricity or tumours in excess of 20 mm for BCT [42–44].

18.4.4 Diffuse Malignant Disease of the Breast

Diffuse in situ cancers involve the larger ducts [2] in a confluent fashion and commonly present as widespread tumours. These extensive tumours occur in approximately 25% of breast cancer patients. Diffuse invasive carcinomas comprise about 5% of invasive cancers [51]. Due to the distinct characteristics of natural progression for non-invasive and invasive disease, therapeutic strategies differ accordingly. Nevertheless, one common feature is that diffuse disease in excess of 40 mm for either form is associated with poorer prognosis and may represent the eligibility threshold for BCT [2, 51]. At present, there is no therapeutic regimen for DCIS which allows preoperative downstaging, and non-invasive lesions need to be excised with clear margins based on size at presentation. Bracketing the radiologic extent of disease may aid successful BCT. The principles of sector resection for BCT applies, where the objective is to excise a clear margin around the tumour is obtained concomitantly with as much of the estimated involved sick lobe as would allow a reasonable cosmetic outcome. While BCT can still be achieved when DCIS involves almost the entire radial dimension (length) of a sick lobe with a narrow anti-radial dimension (breadth) (Fig. 18.7a–d), extensive involvement of a diseased lobe with a broad anti-radial width may preclude BCT.

In large and advanced cases of diffuse invasive disease, infiltration may extend beyond the borders of the sick lobe, making its true expanse difficult, if not impossible, to determine. A significant proportion of these cases would require mastectomy for adequate tumour extirpation and local control. One advantage that invasive disease has over non-invasive disease is the potential for response to neoadjuvant chemotherapy. However, there are certain histologic subtypes, like invasive lobular carcinoma, which are associated with therapeutic non-response with neoadjuvant chemotherapy [52]. Approximately 75% of diffuse invasive cancers are lobular and may form a barrier to adequate downstaging for BCT. In this respect, there is potential for further refinement of case selection for the optimal administration of neoadjuvant chemotherapy for lesions 40 mm or larger [52]. Nonetheless, based on current evidence, neoadjuvant chemotherapy may be administered as an attempt to improve eligibility for BCT [53–57]. Variability in institutional practice may lead to differences in BCT rates, postulated to be based both on size [58] and surgeon philosophy [59–63]. The threshold size for BCT in the case of diffuse invasive carcinoma is a function of the tumour to breast volume ratio; the former factor being potentially modifiable by neoadjuvant therapy. As with DCIS, the entire radial length of a diseased lobe can be sacrificed without much impact on the ability to perform BCT, if the anti-radial dimension does not exceed 20% of its circumference. Depending on breast tissue volume, 40 mm could represent the 'breadth' restriction for BCT with acceptable cosmesis. On the basis that the original footprint of the cancer does not need to be excised, good clinical and radiological response with neoadjuvant therapy minimises

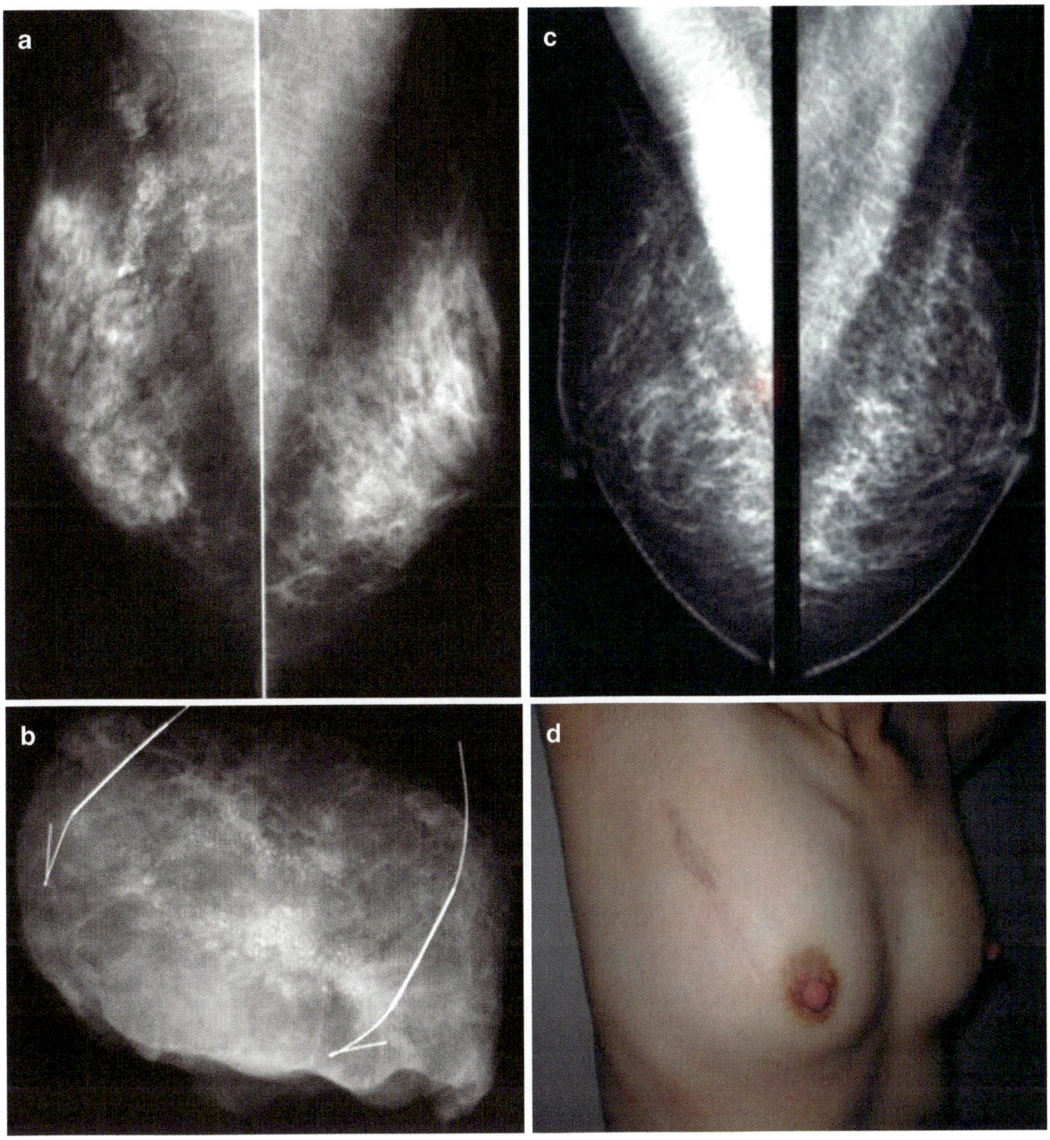

Fig. 18.7 This patient had high grade ductal carcinoma in situ of the right breast in the upper outer quadrant, 7 cm at the longest dimension. As the maximal extent was distributed in a radial fashion, with the anti-radial dimension measuring 2.5 cm, it was possible to perform breast conserving surgery after using localisation techniques to localise the furthest separation points. Resection was done using a radial incision with an eccentric ellipse and volume displacement techniques were used to close the resultant tissue defect. (**a**–**d**) shows sequential images comprising her preoperative mammographic bracketing, specimen radiograph demonstrating the clear margin, postoperative mammogram and cosmetic outcome 4 years after surgery, respectively. She remains recurrence-free more than 12 years after treatment

tissue loss at surgery and increases eligibility for BCT for larger cancers [40, 54–58]. Hence, a tumour extent of 40 mm may represent a survival-related negative prognostic parameter and a relative rather than absolute contraindication to BCT, especially when lobar surgery is applied (Fig. 18.8a–h). Nevertheless, poor response to neoadjuvant in the presence of large diffuse invasive cancer remains an indication for mastectomy.

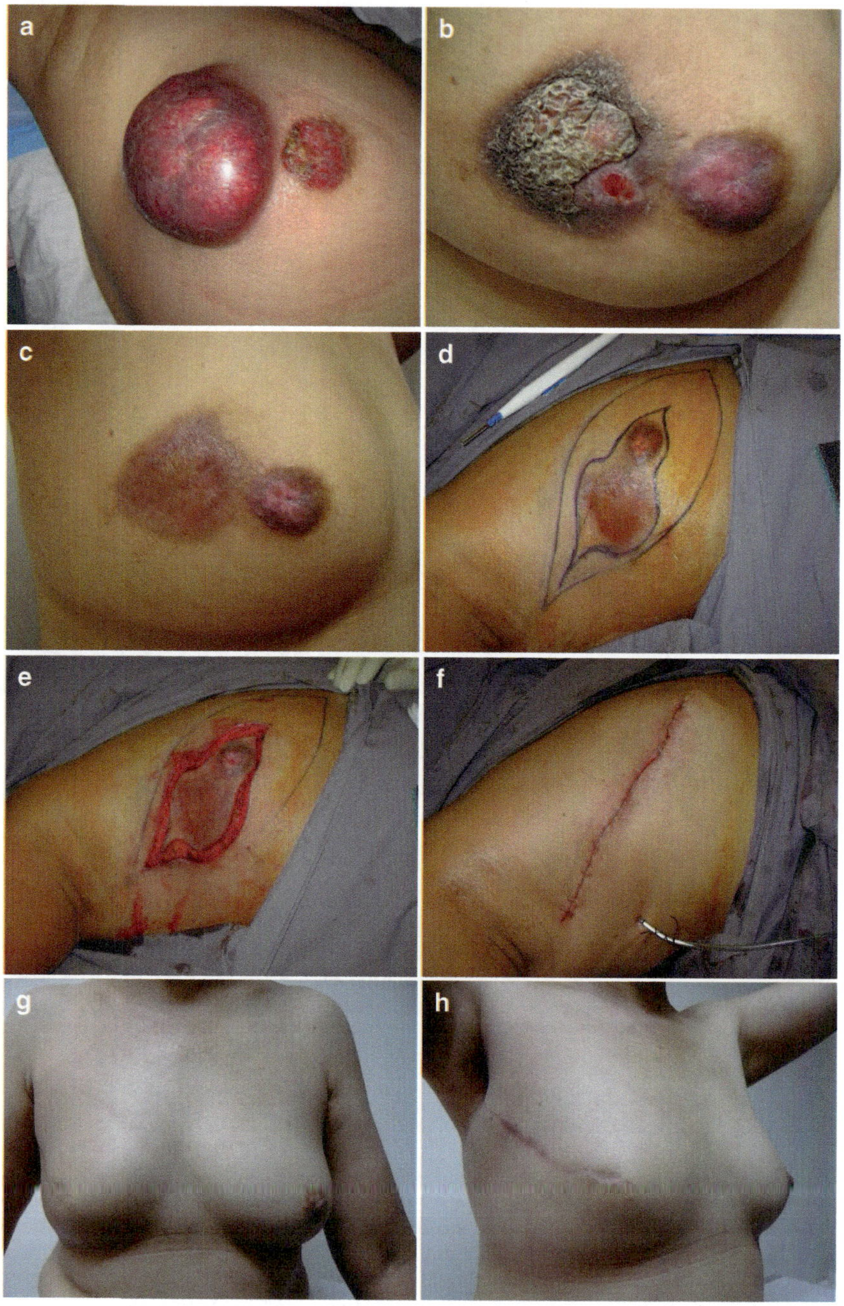

Fig. 18.8 (**a**–**h**) This 54 year old patient presented with T4 tumour associated with Paget's disease. Neoadjuvant chemotherapy was administered which allowed BCT with sacrifice of the nipple-areolar complex. Her cosmetic result after completion of treatment is illustrated in **e** and **f**. She is disease-free more than 5 years after treatment. *Comment*: Extensive and diffuse tumours larger than 40 mm may be downstaged with neoadjuvant chemotherapy and they respond favourably, can be treated with BCT

In all cases of breast cancer, whether unifocal, multifocal, multicentric or diffuse, large section or subgross histology is the optimum form of breast tumour distribution and margin assessment [2]. On the other hand, intraoperative frozen section analysis reduces the need for a reoperation and ameliorates patient anxiety and dissatisfaction [64–66]. A possible compromise to these competing demands is to perform a lobar resection based on the principles detailed above, with the main specimen reserved for comprehensive pathologic assessment, followed by a shave margin which may be used for either frozen section or paraffin analysis [65]. If shave margins are assessed to be extensively or persistently positive, one can proceed directly to mastectomy. This offers a patient the benefit of a trial of BCT and adequate tissue evaluation for tumour extent and minimises re-excisions.

18.5 Discussion

As alluded to earlier, superior breast cancer-specific survival and local control have been reported with BCT when compared to mastectomy, where BCT rates were in excess of 50% [6–15]. In one study, it was estimated that for every 1 percentage point increase in mastectomy rates, there would be a reduction in 7-year survival by 0.1% [14]. Survival differences between those undergoing BCT and mastectomy is consistent with this analysis, and data suggests that BCT rates lower than 30% would not result in any observable survival benefit [7, 8]. By reasonable extrapolation, therefore, any strategy which raises BCT rates would have a positive impact on survival. As an illustration, BCT rates in Asian populations have been recently reported to be low, approximately 40% or less, even for women with Stage I and II disease [67, 68]. Performing lobar surgery allows higher eligibility and utility of BCT among Asian women, in spite of smaller volume breasts [62, 69]. In one study analysing women with symptomatic Stage 0–IV breast cancer, BCT rates of less than 32% resulted in 5-year overall and disease-free survival of 84.3% and 76.6%, respectively [70]. Women with screen-detected malignancies were reported to have 5-year disease-free survival of 83.3% [70]. In contrast, where a BCT rate of 85% was achieved through the use of lobar surgery in an Asian cohort of patients with Stage I–III treated for MFMCBC, 5-year overall survival and disease-free survival were 95.7% and 92.7%, respectively [71]. While these statistics may not be directly comparable, it does suggest that higher BCT rates using the lobar surgical techniques as described in the foregoing discussion could be associated with improved survival, consistent with previously reported instrument variable estimates [14]. The impact of lobar surgery specifically on breast cancer-specific survival is an area of future research.

The existence of MFMCBC was documented before the start of the pivotal RCTs comparing BCT and mastectomy, together with warnings that partial mastectomy resulted in residual cancer in the retained breast [23–25]. However, the results of the RCTs showed that radiotherapy can eradicate occult foci of disease, rendering them impotent for a significant impact on survival [4, 5, 25]. Based on early studies, up to 63% of women with clinically unifocal cancers have other disease foci within the breast [25]. However, modern therapy combining surgery, radiotherapy and appropriate medical treatment has resulted in superior survival and improved local control with BCT compared with mastectomy for clinically unifocal cancers. Furthermore, there is a growing body of evidence that BCT for MFMCBC does not result in inferior local control or survival [34–38, 72, 73]. The current philosophy of breast cancer treatment embraces the concept of reducing tumour burden rather than complete surgical eradication [74]. The ultimate goal for the treatment of breast cancer is to optimise survival and local control while minimising morbidity [21, 75, 76]. This philosophy would favour a reductionist surgical approach offering minimum effective treatment rather than an expansive one resulting in higher complication rates [22, 45, 77]. Progress on predictive factors relating to tumour biology and molecular signatures can enhance opportunities for individualised surgical therapy in the future, refining selection criteria for patients who require extensive surgical resection and those who need minimalist, reductionist treatment.

References

1. Tot T. The theory of the sick lobe and the possible consequences. Int J Surg Pathol. 2007;15(4):369–75.
2. Tot T. Subgross morphology, the sick lobe hypothesis, and the success of breast conservation. Int J Br Cancer. 2011;2011:8. https://doi.org/10.4061/2011/634021.
3. Amy D, Durante E, Tot T. The lobar approach to breast ultrasound imaging and surgery. J Med Ultrason. 2015;42:331–9.
4. Veronesi U, Cascinelli N, Nariani L, et al. Twenty-year follow-up of a randomized study comparing breast-conserving surgery with radical mastectomy for early breast cancer. N Engl J Med. 2002;347:1227–32.
5. Fisher B, Anderson S, Bryant J, et al. Twenty-year follow-up of a randomised trial comparing mastectomy, lumpectomy, and lumpectomy plus irradiation for the treatment of invasive breast cancer. N Engl J Med. 2002;347:1233–41.
6. Hwang ES, Lichtensztajn DY, Gomez SL, Foeble B, Clarke CA. Survival after lumpectomy and mastectomy for early stage invasive breast cancer: the

effect of age and hormone receptor status. Cancer. 2013;119:1402–11.
7. Agarwal S, Pappas L, Neumayer L, et al. Effect of breast conservation therapy vs mastectomy on disease-specific survival for early-stage breast cancer. JAMA Surg. 2014;149(3):267–74. https://doi.org/10.1001/jamasurg2013.3049.
8. van Hezewijk M, Bastiaannet E, Putter H, et al. Effect of local therapy on locoregional recurrence in postmenopausal women with breast cancer in the Tamoxifen Exemestane adjuvant multinational (TEAM) trial. Radiother Oncol. 2013;108:190–6.
9. Abdulkarim BS, Cuartero J, Hanson J, Deschenes J, Lesniak D, Sabri S. Increased risk of locoregional recurrence for women with T1-2N0 triple-negative breast cancer treated with modified radical mastectomy without adjuvant radiation therapy compared with breast –conserving therapy. J Clin Oncol. 2011;29:2852–8.
10. Keating NL, Landrum MB, Brooks JM, et al. Outcomes following local therapy for early-stage breast cancer in non-trial populations. Breast Cancer Res Treat. 2001;125(3):803–13.
11. Schonberg MA, Marcantonio ER, Li DL, et al. Breast cancer among the oldest old: tumour characteristics, treatment choices and survival. J Clin Oncol. 2010;28:2038–45.
12. Martin MA, Meyricke R, O'Neill T, Roberts S. Breast-conserving surgery versus mastectomy for survival from breast cancer: the western Australian experience. Ann Surg Oncol. 2007;14:157–64.
13. Hofvind S, Holen A, Aas T, Roman M, Sebuødegård S, Akslen LA. Women treated with breast conserving surgery do better than those with mastectomy independent of detection mode, prognostic and predictive tumour characteristics. Eur J Surg Oncol. 2015;41(10):1417–22. https://doi.org/10.1016/j.ejso.2015.07.002.
14. Brooks JM, Chrischilles EA, Landrum MB, et al. Survival implications associated with variation in mastectomy rates for early-staged breast cancer. Int J Surg Oncol. 2012;2012:9. https://doi.org/10.1155/2012/127854.
15. van der Heiden-van der Loo M, Siesling S, Wouters MWJM, van Dalen T, Rutgers EJT, Peeters PHM. The value of ipsilateral breast tumour recurrence as a quality indicator: hospital variation in the Netherlands. Ann Surg Oncol. 2015;22(Supplement 3):522–8. https://doi.org/10.1245/s10434-015-4626-9.
16. George WD. Management of early breast cancer. Langenbecks Arch Chir. 1977;345:111–3.
17. Baildam AD. Oncoplastic surgery of the breast. Br J Surg. 2001;89:532–3.
18. Eichler C, Kolsch M, Sauerwald A, Bach A, Gluz O, Warm M. Lumpectomy versus mastopexy–a post-surgery patient survey. Anticancer Res. 2013;33:731–6.
19. De Lorenzi F, Hubner G, Rotmensz N, et al. Oncological results of oncoplastic breast-conserving surgery: long term follow-up of a large series at a single institution: a matched-cohort analysis. Eur J Surg Oncol. 2015;42(1):71–7. https://doi.org/10.1016/j.ejso.2015.08.160.
20. Clough KB, Benyahi D, Nos C, Charles C, Sarfati I. Oncoplastic surgery: pushing the limits of breast-conserving surgery. Breast J. 2015;21:140–6.
21. Chatterjee A, Pyfer B, Czerniecki B, Rosenkranz K, Tchou J, Fisher C. Early postoperative outcomes in lumpectomy versus simple mastectomy. J Surg Res. 2015;198:143–8.
22. Tan M. Toward a reductionist approach to the surgical treatment of breast cancer. J Am Coll Surg. 2016;222:967.
23. Rosen PP, Fracchia AA, Urban JA, Schottenfeld D, Robbins GF. "residual" mammary carcinoma following simulated partial mastectomy. Cancer. 1975;35:739–47.
24. Lagios MD. Multicentricity of breast carcinoma demonstrated by routine correlated serial subgross and radiographic examination. Cancer. 1977;40:1726–34.
25. Holland R, Veling SHJ, Mravunac M, Hendriks JHCL. Histologic multifocality of Tis, T1-2 breast carcinomas: implications for clinical trials of breast-conserving surgery. Cancer. 1985;56:979–90.
26. Tot T, Gere M. Radiologically unifocal invasive breast carcinomas: large section histopathology correlate and impact on surgical management. J Cancer Sci Ther. 2016;8:050–4. https://doi.org/10.4172/1948-5956.1000389.
27. Iacconi C, Galman L, Zheng J, et al. Multicentric cancer detected at breast MR imaging and not ar mammography: important or not? Radiology. 2015;25:150796.
28. McLaughlin S, Mittendorf EA, Bleicher RJ, McCready DR, King TA. The 2013 society of surgical oncology Susan G Komen for the cure symposium: MRI in breast cancer: where are we now? Ann Surg Oncol. 2014;21:28–36.
29. Menezes GLG, Knuttel FM, Stehouver BL, Pijnappel RM, van den Bosch MSSJ. Magnetic resonance imaging in breast cancer: a literature review and future perspectives. World J Clin Oncol. 2014;5:61–70.
30. Dershaw DD. Preoperative MRI. Breast J. 2016;22:141–2.
31. Tan MP. An algorithm for the integration of breast magnetic resonance imaging into clinical practice. Am J Surg. 2009;197:691–4.
32. Tan MP. The boomerang incision for periareolar breast malignancies. Am J Surg. 2007;194:690–3.
33. Pezner RD. The oncoplastic breast surgery challenge to the local radiation boost. Int J Radiat Oncol Biol Phys. 2011;79:963–4.
34. Gentilini O, Botteri E, Rotmensz N, et al. Conservative surgery in patients with multifocal/multicentric breast cancer. Breast Cancer Res Treat. 2009;113:577–83.
35. Ustaalioglu BO, Bilici A, Kefeli U, et al. The importance of multifocal/multicentric tumour on the disease-free survival of breast cancer patients. Am J Clin Oncol. 2012;35:580–6.
36. Lynch SP, Lei XD, Hsu LM, et al. Breast cancer multifocality and multicentricity and locoregional recurrence. Oncologist. 2013;18:1167–73.

37. Wolters R, Wockel A, Janni W, et al. Comparing the outcome between multicentric and multifocal breast cancer: what is the impact on survival, and is there a role for guideline-adherent adjuvant therapy? A retrospective multicentre cohort study of 8,935 patients. Breast Cancer Res Treat. 2013;142:579–90.
38. Ataseven B, Lederer B, Blohmer JU, et al. Impact of multifocal of muliticentric disease on surgery and locoregional. Distant and overall survival of 6.134 breast cancer patients treated with neoadjuvant chemotherapy. Ann Surg Oncol. 2014;22(4):1118–27. https://doi.org/10.1245/s10434-014-4122-7.
39. Eaton BR, Losken A, Okwan-Diodu D, et al. Local recurrence patterns in breast cancer patients treated with oncoplastic reduction mammoplasty and radiotherapy. Ann Surg Oncol. 2014;21:93–9.
40. Coates AS, Winer EP, Goldhirsch A, et al. Tailoring therapies–improving the management of early breast cancer: St Gallen international expert consensus on the primary therapy of early breast cancer 2015. Ann Oncol. 2015;26:1533–46.
41. Nijenhuis MV, Rutgers EJ. Conservative surgery for multifocal/multicentric breast cancer. Breast. 2015;24:S96–9.
42. Jochelson MS, Lampen-Sachar K, Gibbons G, et al. Do MRI and mammography reliably identify candidates for breast conservation after neoadjuvant chemotherapy? Ann Surg Oncol. 2015;22:1490–5.
43. Clough KB, Gouveia PF, Benyahi D, et al. Positive margins after oncoplastic surgery for breast cancer. Ann Surg Oncol. 2015;22:4247–53.
44. Dolfin G. The surgical approach to the 'sick lobe'. In: Francescatti DS, Silverstein MJ, editors. Breast cancer: a new era in management. New York: Springer; 2014. p. 113–32.
45. Silverstein MJ. Radical mastectomy to radical conservation (extreme oncoplasty): a revolutionary change. J Am Coll Surg. 2016;222:1–9.
46. Savalia NB, Silverstein MJ. Oncoplastic breast reconstruction: patient selection and surgical techniques. J Surg Oncol. 2016;113(8):875–82. doi: 10.1002/jso.24212
47. Kapoor NM, Chung A, Huynh K, Giuliano AE. Preliminary results: double lumpectomies for multicentric breast cancer. Am Surg. 2012;78: 1345–8.
48. NCCN. http://www.nccn.org/professionals/physician_gls/f_guidelines.asp Accessed 25 Feb 2016.
49. Tan MP. A novel segment classification for multifocal and multicentric breast cancer to facilitate breast-conservation treatment. Breast J. 2015;21:410–7.
50. Amy D. Lobar ultrasound of the breast. In: Tot T, editor. Breast cancer. London: Springer-Verlag; 2011. p. 153–62.
51. Tot T. Diffuse invasive breast carcinoma of no special type. Virchows Arch. 2016;468:199–206.
52. Balmativola D, Marchio C, Maule M, et al. Pathological non-response to chemotherapy in a neoadjuvant setting of breast cancer: an inter-institutional study. Breast Cancer Res Treat. 2014;148: 511–23.
53. Redden MH, Fuhrman GM. Neoadjuvant chemotherapy in the treatment of breast cancer. Surg Clin N Am. 2013;93:493–9.
54. King TA, Morrow M. Surgical issues in patients with breast cancer receiving neoadjuvant chemotherapy. Nat Rev Clin Oncol. 2015;12:335–43. https://doi.org/10.1038/nrclinonc.2015.63.
55. Golshan M, Cirrincione CT, Sikov WM, et al. Impact of neoadjuvant chemotherapy in stage II-III triple negative breast cancer on eligibility for breast-conserving surgery and breast conservation rates. Ann Surg. 2015;262:434–9.
56. Bollet MA, Savignoni A, Pierga JY, et al. High rates of breast conservation for large ductal and lobular invasive carcinomas combining multimodality strategies. Br J Cancer. 2008;98:734–41.
57. Criscitiello C, Azim HA, Agbor-tarh D, et al. Factors associated with surgical management following neoadjuvant therapy in patients with primary HER2-positive breast cancer: results from the NeoALTTO phase III trial. Ann Oncol. 2013;24:1980–5.
58. Bleicher RJ, Ruth K, Sigurdson ER, et al. Breast conservation versus mastectomy for patients with T3 primary tumours (>5 cm): a review of 5685 Medicare patients. Cancer. 2016;122:42–9.
59. Garcia-Etienne CA, Tomatis M, Heil J, et al. Mastectomy trends for early-stage breast cancer: a report from the EUSOMA multi-institutional European database. Eur J Cancer. 2012;48: 1947–56.
60. Mahmood U, Hanlon AL, Koshy M, et al. Increasing national mastectomy rates for the treatment of early stage breast cancer. Ann Surg Oncol. 2013;20:1436–43.
61. Arrington AK, Jarosek SL, Virnig BA, Haberman EB, Tuttle TM. Patient and surgeon characteristics associated with increased use of contralateral prophylactic mastectomy in patients with breast cancer. Ann Surg Oncol. 2009;16:2697–704.
62. Tan MP, Sitoh NY, Sim AS. Evaluation of eligibility and utilisation of breast conservation treatment in an Asian context. Asian Pac J Cancer Prev. 2014;15:4683–8.
63. Molenaar S, Oort F, Sprangers M, Rutgers E, Luiten E, Mulder J, de Haes H. Predictors of patients' choices for breast-conserving therapy or mastectomy: a prospective study. Br J Cancer. 2004;90: 2123–30.
64. Esbona K, Li ZH, Wilke LG. Intraoperative imprint cytology and frozen section pathology for margin assessment in breast conservation surgery: a systemic review. Ann Surg Oncol. 2012;19(10):3236–45. https://doi.org/10.1245/s10434-012-2492-2.
65. Tan MP, Nadya NY, Sim AS. The value of intraoperative frozen section analysis for margin status in breast conservation surgery in a non-tertiary institution. Int J Breast Cancer. 2014;2014:7. https://doi.org/10.1155/2014/715404.
66. Jeevan R, Cromwell DA, Trivella M, Lawrence G, Kearins O, Pereira J, et al. Reoperation rates after breast conserving surgery for breast cancer among

women in England: retrospective study of hospital episode statistics. BMJ. 2012;345:e4505. doi: 10.1136bmj.e4505
67. Woon YY, Chan MYP. Breast conservation surgery-the surgeon factor. Breast. 2005;14:131–5.
68. Chan SW, Cheung C, Chan A, Cheung PS. Surgical options for Chinese patients with early invasive breast cancer: data from the Hong Kong breast cancer registry. Asian J Surg. 2016. https://doi.org/10.1016/j.asjsur.2016.02.003.
69. Yau TK, Soong IS, Sze H, et al. Trends and patterns of breast conservation treatment in Hong Kong: 1994–2007. Int J Radiat Oncol Biol Phys. 2009;74:98–103.
70. Wang WV, Tan SM, Chow WL. The impact of mammographic breast cancer screening in Singapore: a comparison between screen-detected and symptomatic women. Asian Pac J Cancer Prev. 2011;12:2735–40.
71. Tan MP, Sitoh NY, Sitoh YY. Perspectives of cosmesis following breast conservation for multifocal and multicentric breast cancers. Int J Br Cancer. 2015;2015:9. doi: 10/1155/2015/126793
72. Vera-Badillo FE, Napoleone M, Ocana A, et al. Effect of multifocality and multicentricity on outcome in early stage breast cancer: a systematic review and meta-analysis. Breast Cancer Res Treat. 2014;146:235–44.
73. Neri A, Marellu D, Megha T, et al. Clinical significance of multifocal and multicentric breast cancers and choice of surgical treatment: a retrospective study on a series of 1158 cases. BMC Surg. 2015;15:1.
74. Morrow M, Van Zee KJ. Margins in DCIS: does residual disease provide an answer? Ann Surg Oncol. 2016;23(11):3423–5. https://doi.org/10.1245/s10434-016-5255-7.
75. Marescaux J, Diana M. Inventing the future of surgery. World J Surg. 2015;39:615–22.
76. Morrow M. Progress in the surgical management of breast cancer: present and future. Breast. 2015;24:s2–5.
77. Jagsi R, Jiang J, Momoh AO, et al. Complications after mastectomy and immediate breast reconstruction for breast cancer. Ann Surg. 2016;263:219–27.

19 Automatic Breast Ultrasound Scanning

Dominique Amy

There is no doubt that the future of mammary ultrasound is linked to the development of automated equipment effecting a scanning of the whole breast (like what could be obtained with a CT scan or MRI).

For a number of years since the brief appearance of the ancestor of automated equipment, the Australian Ultrasound Institute's Octoson 36 years ago, various teams throughout the world have been trying to tackle such an issue. At present, there are six machines on the market using different techniques: Sofia, Invenia Abus, S 2000 Abus, Awbus, Softvue and Episonica iABUS.

After a brief analysis of this equipment and the presentation of a few clinical cases, we'll map out the ideal equipment suitable for a lobar approach of the breast.

Two main techniques are presented:

Prone position examination: Sophia, Softvue and Episonica
Supine position examination: Invenia, S 2000 and Awbus

The three machines using the patients' supine position make use of a compression system.

D. Amy
Centre du sein, Aix-en-Provence, France
e-mail: domamy@wanadoo.fr

The three using the prone position make use of immersion for one and of a cone slightly compressing the breast for the other.

Characteristics of the various machines:

- 5–15 Mhz transducers depending on the trademarks.
- Straight or slightly curved linear transducers.
- Transducers' field of view from 38/50 mm to 200 mm. The transducer ring allows a coronal coverage of the whole breast.
- Number of acquisition volumes per breast: one volume for the prone position equipment and two to five volumes for the others.
- Time length of volume acquisition per breast: from one minute to a maximum of fifteen minutes (15 min for the Awbus system only).
- Total duration of the examination per patient: from 10 to 30 min and over 45 min for Awbus.
- Operator variability for each examination: only for the three machines using the supine position.
- Duration of analysis by the radiologist: from 2 to 15 min.
- Number of slices effected: from 120 or 480 or 5,000 to 15,000 slices maximum.
- Possible slicing planes: 2D or 3D with MPR, coronal, axial and sagittal according to the machines (none of them can carry out the whole range of these options).

D. Amy (ed.), *Lobar Approach to Breast Ultrasound*, https://doi.org/10.1007/978-3-319-61681-0_19

- Dicom compatibility: Sophia alone has compatible Dicom images.
- Optional workstation depending on the trademark.
- The Softvue or ultrasound coronal tomography with a transducer ring is specific with a study of transmitted, reflected and attenuated ultrasonic beam.
- All the equipment available is either linked to a manufacturer or to a type of transducer (except one); their prices vary from the cheapest (EpiSonica) to 200.000 USD for four machines and 500.000 USD (Softvue).

Problems encountered in the use of this equipment:

- The patients experience some pain depending on the degree of strength and discomfort with the supine machines.
- The characteristic operator dependent for the choice and adjustment of the acquisition of the various volumes except for the prone equipment.
- Too long a duration of the acquisition and reading of the volumes.
- Problem of adaptation to the sizes of too small or too big breasts.
- Impossibility to scan the whole breast and more specifically the axillary fossa in prone position.
- No examination of the nipple and the zone behind it with Sophia.
- Too high a number of slices to be examined for each breast.
- Expense for setting up contact membranes ensuring compression.
- High cost of this equipment difficult to write off with complementary examinations in breast exploration.
- Problems avoided by EpiSonica: compatible with any commercial system and probe, no limitation of breast size, double ring of radial scans for whole-breast acquisition, good correlation to nipple position, short time of acquisition or review and minimal number of slices. Plus they advocate that the prone position gives more privacy (shy Asian population and Muslim women) less compression (adequate after breast surgery, implants and neoadjuvant chemotherapies).
- Presentation of a few examinations carried out in both prone and supine positions.

A. Screening mammogram in a 45-year-old woman (Figs.19.1, 19.2, 19.3 and 19.4)

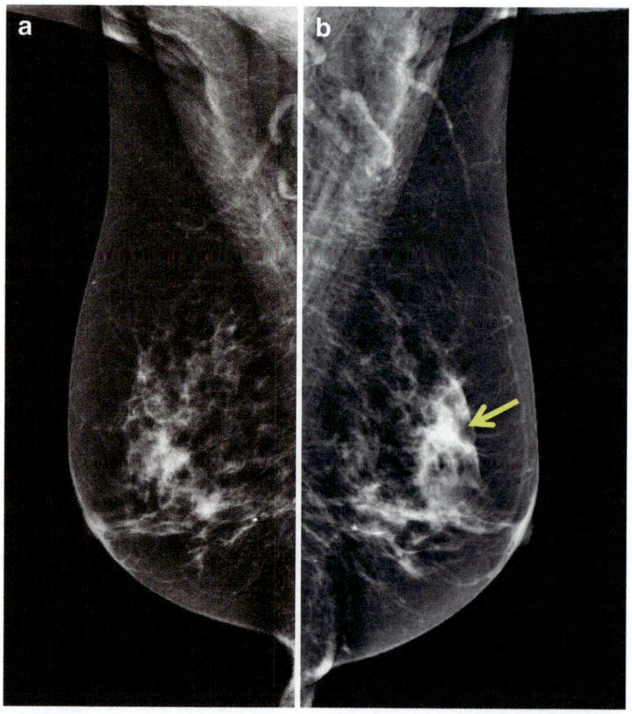

Fig. 19.1 (**a–d**) Mediolateral (**a, b**) and craniocaudal projections (**c, d**) show a subtle architectural distortion identified only at the mediolateral projection of the left breast (*arrow*) (courtesy of Dr A.Vourtsi Greece)

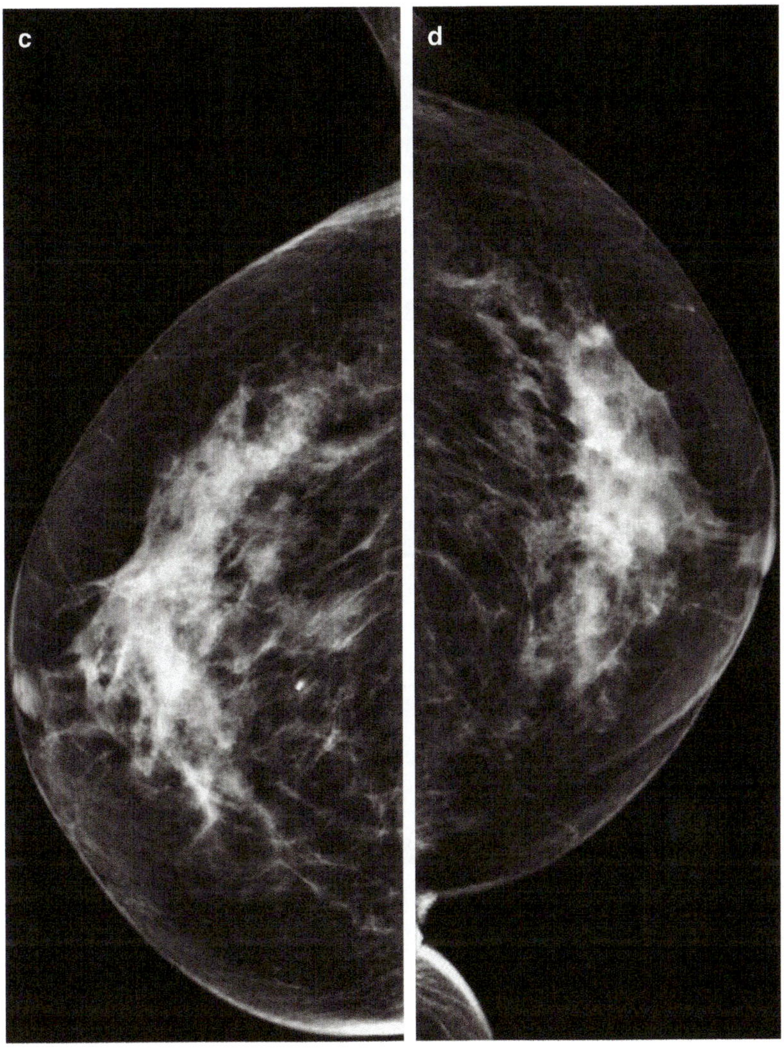

Fig. 19.1 (continued)

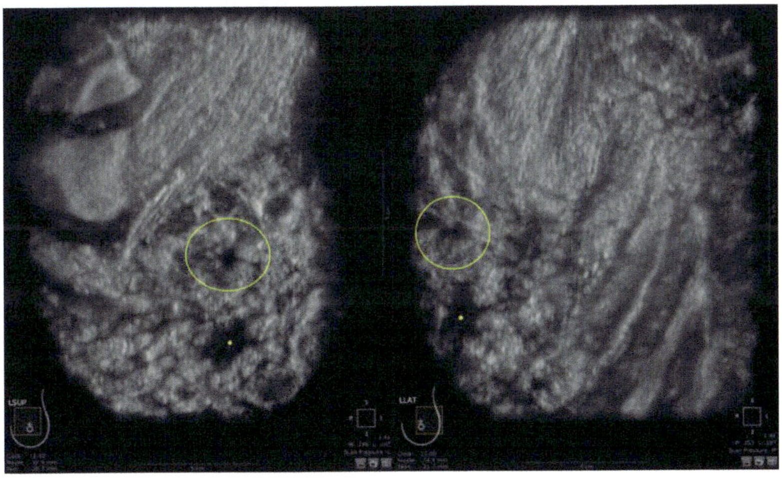

Fig. 19.2 Automated breast ultrasound (ABUS), *left breast*. A small defect is identified on the coronal and transverse volumes of the left superior and left lateral acquisitions, indicating the presence of a suspicious finding (courtesy of Dr A.Vourtsi Greece)

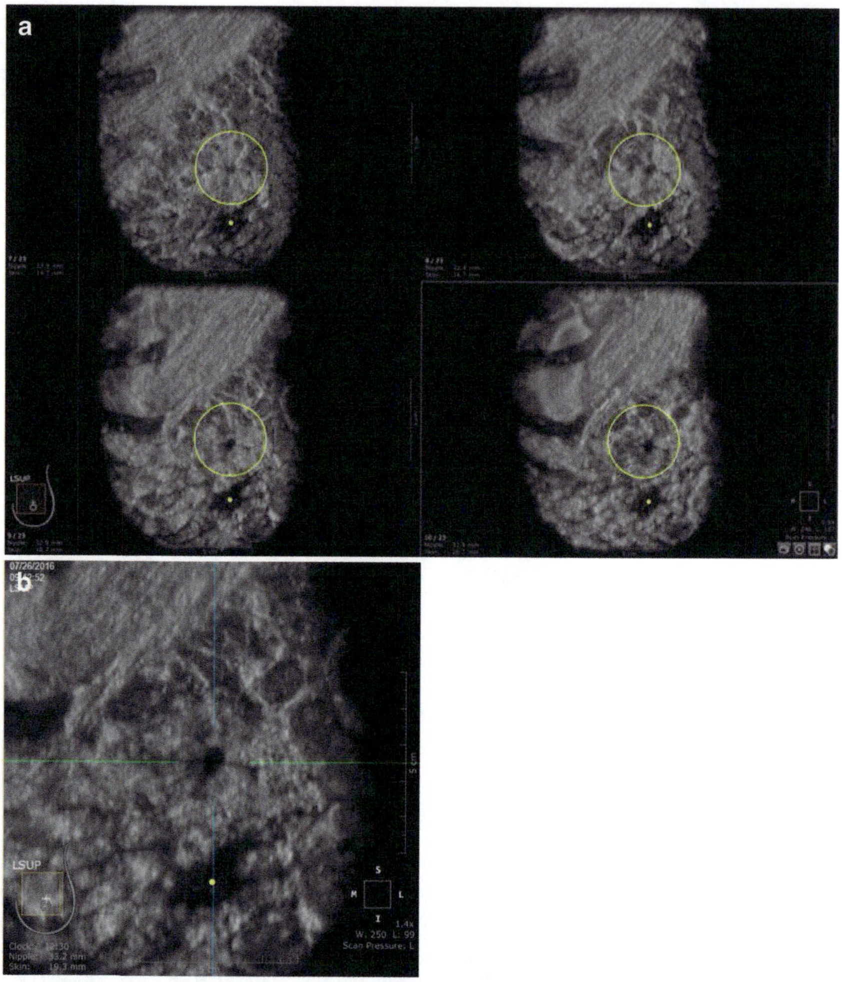

Fig. 19.3 (**a, b**) Automated breast ultrasound (ABUS), *left breast*. On coronal 2 mm consecutive slices tissue defect is clearly identified (courtesy of Dr A.Vourtsi Greece)

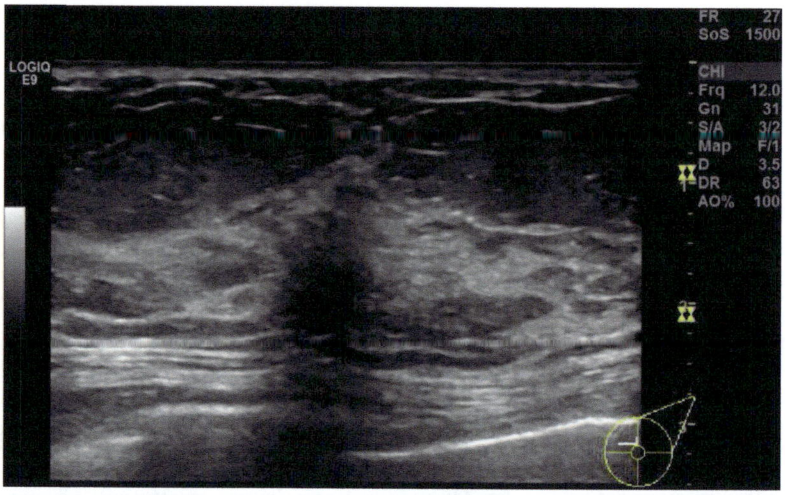

Fig. 19.4 Hand-held breast ultrasound shows a suspicious lesion. Histology revealed a 9 mm invasive ductal carcinoma (courtesy of Dr A.Vourtsi Greece)

B. Screening mammogram in a 57-year-old woman (Figs.19.5, 19.6, 19.7, 19.8, 19.9, 19.10, 19.11 and 19.12)

Theorical 3D representation of a breast (Fig. 19.3):

Analysis of the results:

Necessary criteria for an ideal complete checkup:

1. Respect of breast anatomy.
2. If possible, use of radial scanning linked to the anatomic reality of the acini-ductal axes of each lobe.
3. The direct radial technique is very precise and reproducible. It is fast and does not depend on electronic reconstruction. Furthermore, it allows 2D/3D exploration in the three planes (coronal, axial and digital).
4. Absolute necessity of a thorough trans-nipple and retro-nipple study since 12–15 % of the cancers are localized there (data from Perkins et al. 2004).
5. Avoiding an excessive compressing of the cutaneous and subcutaneous tissues (cf. Chap. 3: Anatomy) and in particular the Cooper's ligaments.
6. Possibility to localize and reposition the transducer directly and immediately on a suspect zone and avoid to call back for 'a second look with HHUS' (hand-held ultrasound).
7. Possibility to move rapidly onto Doppler and elastography.
8. Posttreatment and reconstruction, storage and comparison with previous examinations, with mammography and MRI (this is already largely on offer from the manufacturers).
9. Limitation and sparing of the duration of examination/acquisition and rereading.
10. Lastly offering a selling price for this equipment lower than the current one with systems independent from the trademarks and adaptable to various echographs [1, 2].

The present goal of automated breast ultrasound units is principally the examination of breasts said to be "dense" radiologically, the breasts of young women, after operation and treatment, and the follow-up of patients with previously detected lesions. Given the not insignificant number of radio-transparent cancers, of multifocal and multicentric cancers, the use of this automated equipment must become more

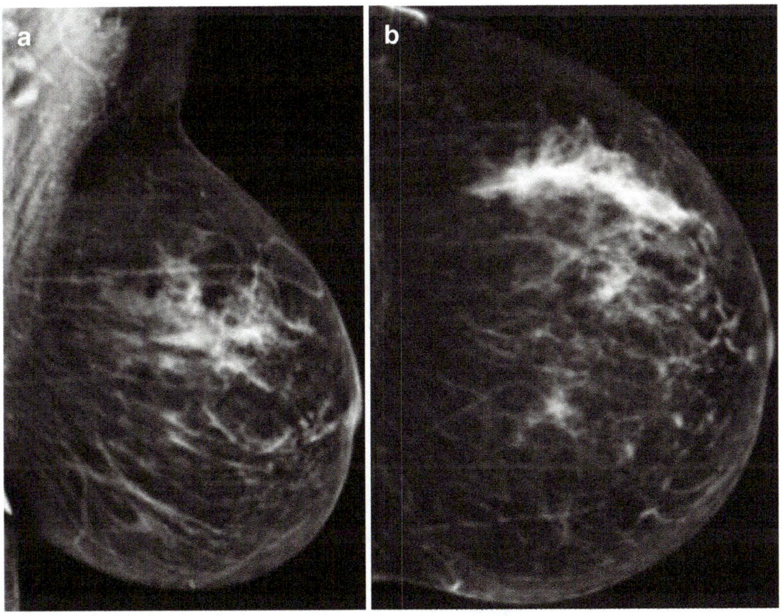

Fig. 19.5 (**a, b**) Mediolateral and craniocaudal projections of the *left breast* (**a, b**) does not show any suspicious finding (courtesy of Dr A. Vourtsi Greece)

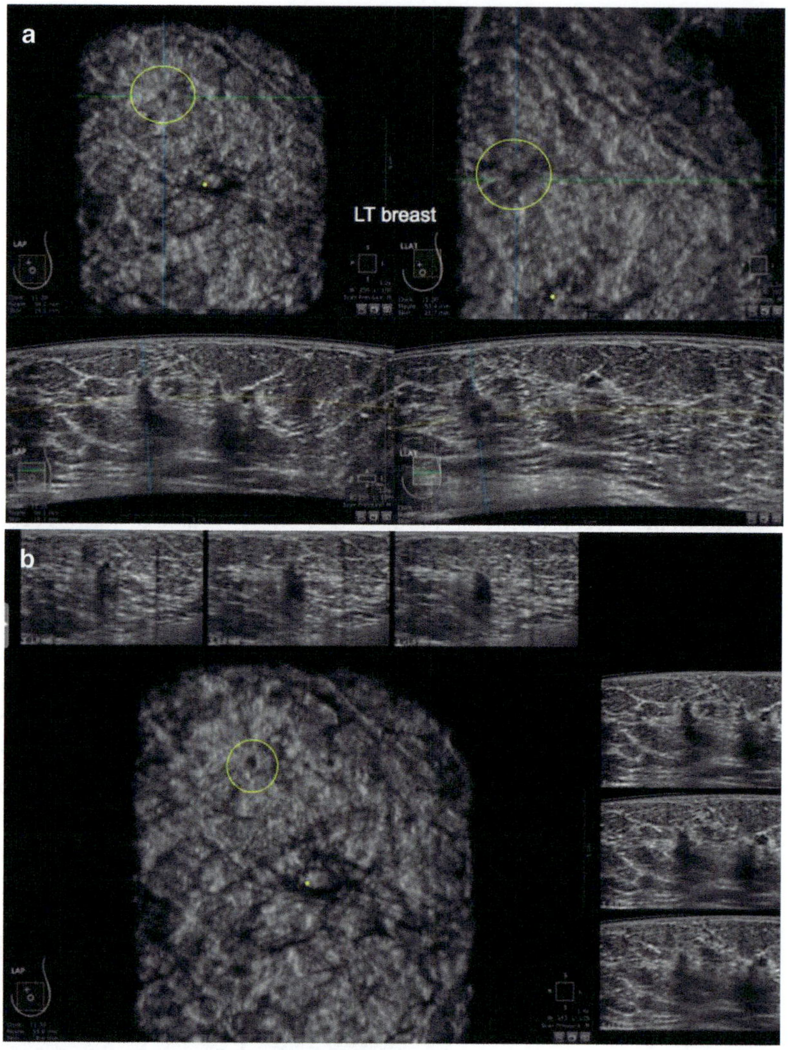

Fig. 19.6 (**a**, **b**). Automated breast ultrasound (ABUS), *left breast*. A defect is identified on the coronal and transverse volumes of the left AP and left lateral acquisitions, indicating a suspicious finding (courtesy of Dr A.Vourtsi Greece)

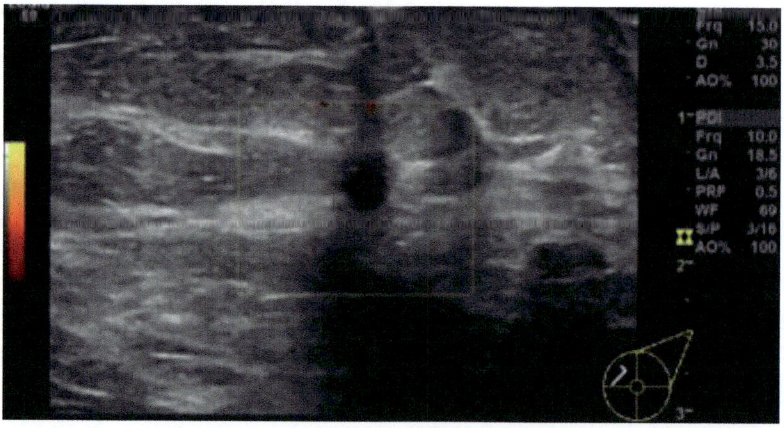

Fig. 19.7 Hand-held ultrasound shows the suspicious lesion. Histology revealed a 5 mm tubular carcinoma Grade I (courtesy of Dr A.Vourtsi Greece)

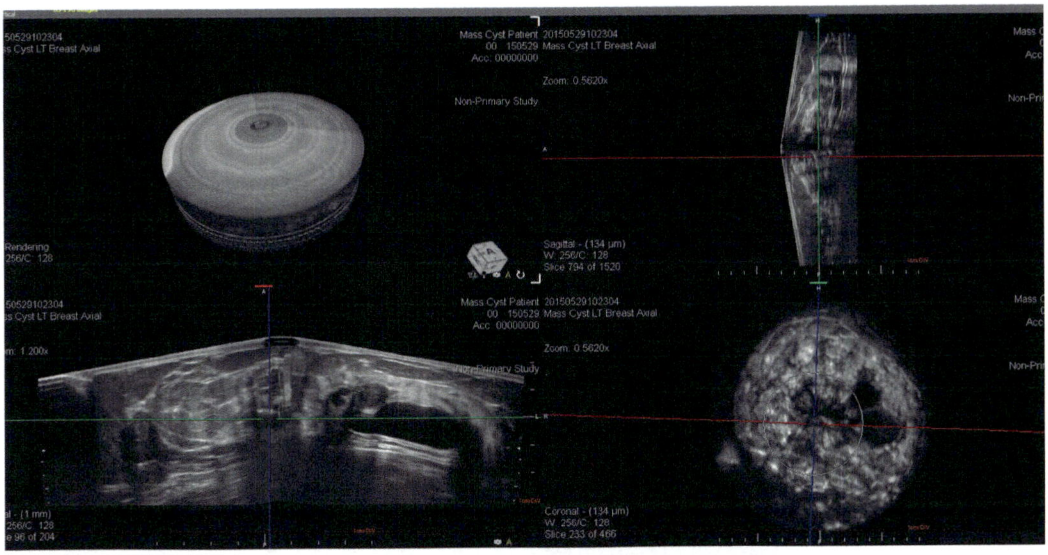

Fig. 19.8 Cystic mass on a left breast: axial, radial and coronal sections (courtesy of iVu imaging Corporation, USA)

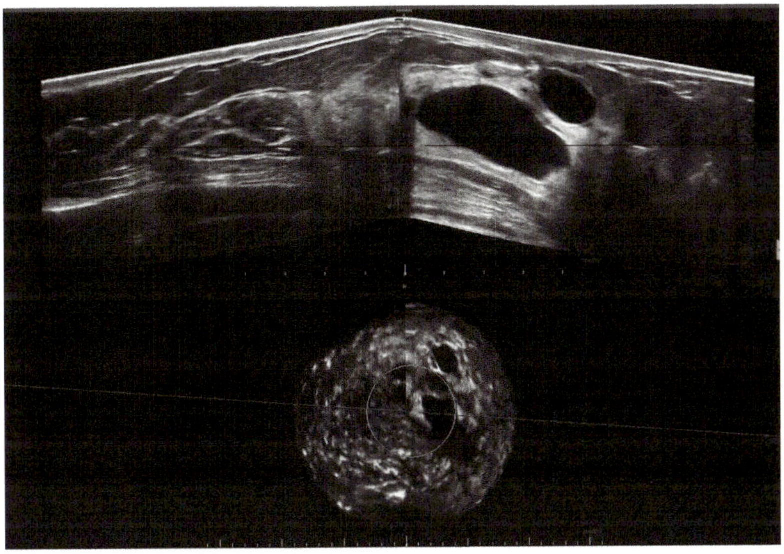

Fig. 19.9 Details of the radial and coronal sections of the different cysts (courtesy of iVu imaging Corporation, USA)

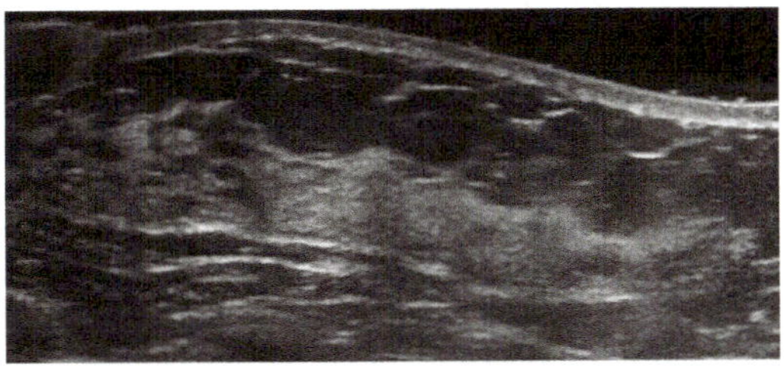

Fig. 19.10 Strict radial analysis of a lobe (nipple on the upper left part, the lobe development toward the right part of the image) (courtesy of EpiSonica Taiwan)

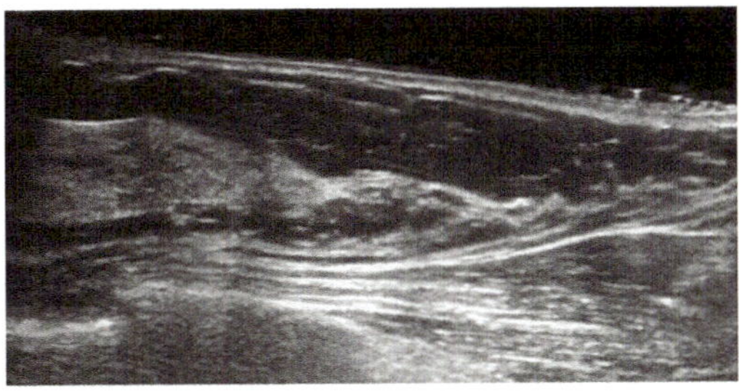

Fig. 19.11 Strict radial lobar extremity analysis with terminal cooper ligaments (courtesy of EpiSonica Taiwan)

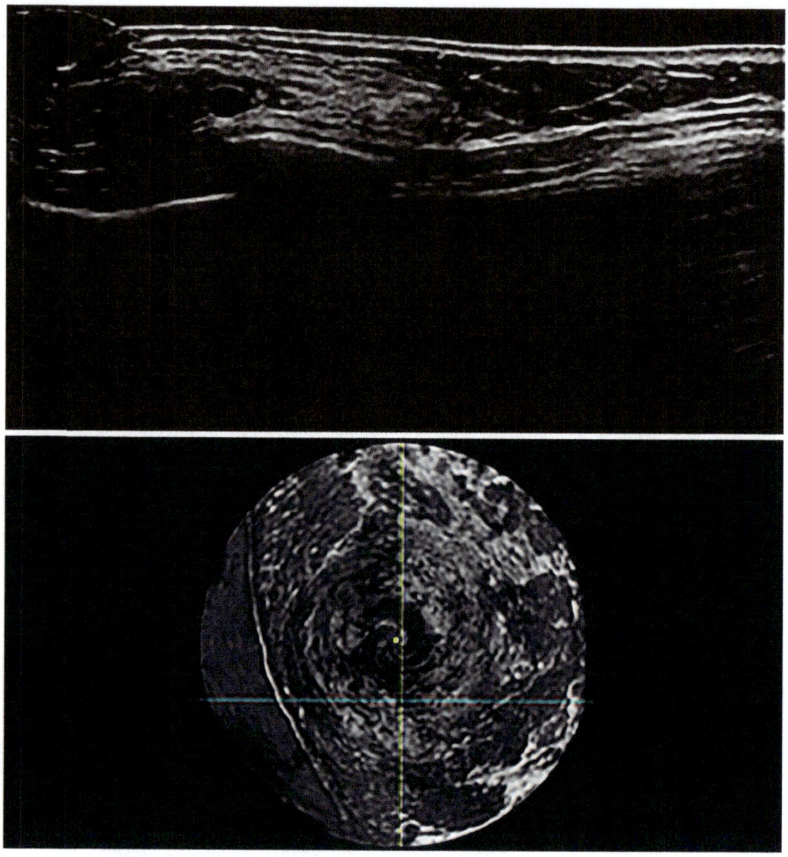

Fig. 19.12 Radial and coronal 3D breast ultrasound reconstruction: millimetric micro-cyst beneath the areola (courtesy of EpiSonica Taiwan)

widespread and be a screening technique for an unlimited population [3]. According to the SomoInsight study [4] for dense breast tissue, increase the cancer detection but increase the number of false-positive results. It has been estimated that 30% of breast cancers depend on breast density in comparison with less than 10% associated with BRCA ½ mutations.

The number of radiologically dense breasts is 74% at the age of 40, 57% at the age of 50, 44% at the age of 60 and 36% at the age of 70, according to a Swedish study. Dense breasts (if more than 50% of the tissue is fibro-glandular) are linked with a 4–6 times increased risk of breast cancer. By using the combination of mammography and automated technique, 1.9 additional breast cancers per 1000 women screened were detected (Ref. [5–9]. Most of them were invasive but with an increased recall rate. The combination of mammography and automated ultrasound increases the rate of detection without substantially affecting the specificity. In the case of dense breasts, 1/3 of all the cancers are not detected at an early stage by mammography. The recent contribution of tomo-synthesis will reduce this rate of false negatives but also increase the rate of recall examination for additional diagnostic testing (false-positive call back); a rate of about 20% indeterminate findings corresponds to very dense breasts for which other breast imaging modalities should be considered. The technical quality of premium ultrasound is now highly satisfactory, the resolution is sufficient for the diagnosis of small millimetric lesions. The already offered technique of reconstruction is compatible with a good tridimensional analysis; it now becomes essential to define the reproducible study protocols.

The techniques used at present do not however fully satisfy the users who demand stricter usage protocols and regret the lack of standardization of diagnostic criteria and the absence of suitable

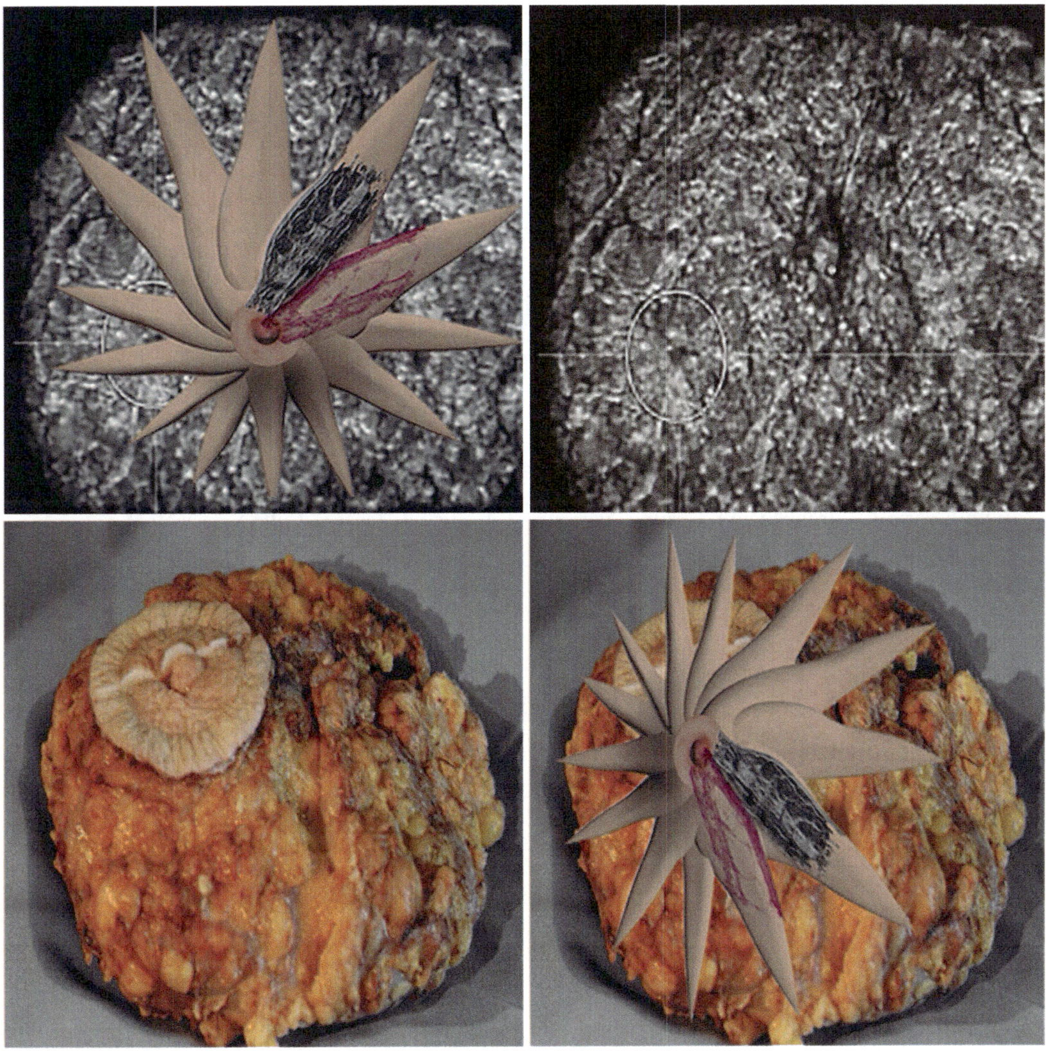

Fig. 19.13 Theoretical 3D superimposition of the different lobes within the block of mastectomy: the lobes are surrounded by the fatty tissue—such a lobe location renders the surgical identification very difficult during surgery in the operating room without ultrasonic complementary exam. The mastectomy specimen appearance is very similar to the coronal ABVS section

clinical instructions. Some authors are beginning to refuse to recommend the use of automated equipment before its validation by extensive studies [10–13].

They ask for the elaboration of a software programme to detect lesions automatically when reading [14, 15].

The duration of the examination is also an essential criterion for the users. The improved quality of the images (although it is satisfactory at present) must also be a factor of improvement.

Conclusion

What the ideal choice must be as concerns automated equipment:

- Since there is a demand for the systematization of automated examination and since the breast has a clearly defined lobar organization, the choice of a radial technique must be privileged.
- The selected EpiSonica technic seems adequate (among the six different machines), but some improvements are required.

- The technique of "supine" available equipments necessitates too much compression, and the radial anatomic reconstruction must be privileged above all 3D studies.
- The transducer ring does not foster the anatomic lobar study of the breast. Adapted software must be on offer in the future.
- The size of the transducer being limited, a double concentric radial examination is needed: a central one around the nipple and a peripheral one for the upper part of the breast including the axillary area.
- Longest possible probe, longer than 7 cm, linear transducers are desirable.
- The ideal is to have equipment compatible with various transducers from various manufacturers, which limits the dependence on a type of echographer for a greater adaptability.
- The price of that system has to be more reasonable so as to make a greater diffusion possible.
- The reading station must be included in the cost of the equipment.
- The direct radial lobe acquisition considerably limits the number of slices needed and therefore the duration of time/acquisition and of course of time/reading for the radiologist.
- The examination is no longer operator dependent and can in time of follow-up be reproduced perfectly.
- There is a significant reduction in the irradiation of the breast, which is a sensitive issue nowadays for the screening of a selected feminine population.

  The ideal choice of equipment is the one which respects the lobar approach of the breast.
- There are teams already working on the automatic specific development of such equipment which will soon be available on the market.
- The patient (in a next future with a new machine) should be in supine position without compression, with a good positioning in relation to the different quadrants examined.
- Therefore, the automated whole-breast ultrasonic unit should be perfectly adapted to the screening of the population.

References

1. Wojcinski S, Farrokh A, Hille U, Wiskirchen J, Gyapong S, Soliman AA, Degenhardt F, Hillemanns P. The automated breast volume scanner (ABVS) initial experiences in lesion detection compared with conventional handheld B-mode ultrasound: a pilot study of 50 cases. Int J Womens Health. 2011;3:337–46.
2. Giger ML, Inciardi MF, Edwards A, Papaioannou J, Drukker K, Jiang Y, Brem R, Brown JB. Automated breast ultrasound in breast cancer screening of women with dense breasts: reader study of mammography-negative and mammography-positive cancers. AJR Am J Roentgenol. 2016;206:1341–50.
3. Berg WA, Bandos AI, Mendelson EB, Lehrer D, Jong RA, Pisano ED. Ultrasound as the primary screening test for breast cancer: analysis from ACRIN 6666. J Natl Cancer Inst. 2016;108:djv367. PMID: 26712110
4. Brem R, Tabar L, Duffy S, Inciardi M, Guingrich J, Hashimoto B, Lander M, Lapidus R, Petreson M, Rapelyea J, Roux S, Schilling K, Shah B, Torrente J, Wynn R, Miller D. Assessing improvement in detection of breast cancer with three-dimensional automated breast US in women with dense breast tissue : the Somolnsight study. Radiology. 2015;274(3):663–73.
5. Wilczek B, Wilczek Henryk E, Leifland K, Rasouliyan L. Adding 3D automated breast ultrasound to mammography screening in women with heterogeneously and extremely dense breasts. Eur J Radiol. 2016;85:1554–63.
6. Duric N, Boyd N, Littrup P, Sak M, Myc L, Li C, West E, Minkin S, Martin L, Yaffe M, Schmidt S, Faiz M, Shen J, Melnichouk O, Li Q, Albrecht T. Breast density measurements with ultrasound tomography: a comparison with film and digital mammography. Med Phys. 2013;40:013501. PMID: 23298122
7. Chen JH, Lee YW, Chan SW, et al. Breast density analysis with automated whole breast ultrasound: comparison with 3D magnetic resonance imaging. Ultrasound Med Biol. 2016;42:1211.
8. Chen JH, Chan S, Lu NH, et al. Opportunistic breast density assessment in women receiving low dose chest computed tomography screening. Acad Radiol. 2016;23:1154.
9. Scheel JR, Lee JM, Sprague BL, Lee CI, Lehman CD. Screening ultrasound ' as an adjunct to mammography in women with mammographically dense breasts. Am J Obstet Gynecol. 2015;212:9–17.
10. Moon WK, Shen Y-W, Huang CS, Chiang LR, Chang RF. Computer-aided diagnosis for the classification of breast masses in automated whole breast ultrasound images. Ultrasound Med Biol. 2011;37:539–48.
11. Shin HJ, Kim HH, Cha JH, Park JH, Lee KE, Kim JH. Automated ultrasound of the breast for diagnosis : interobserver agreement on lesion detection and characterization. AJR Am J Roentgenol. 2011;197:474–754.

12. Shin H, Kim HH, Cha JH. Current status of automated breast ultrasonography. Ultrasonography. 2015;34:165–72. PMID: 25971900
13. Golatta M, Baggs C, Schweitzer-Martin M, Domschke C, Schott S, Harcos A, Scharf A, Junkermann H, Ranch G, Rom J, Sohn C, Heil J. Evaluation of an automated breast 3D-ultrasound system by comparing it with hand-held ultrasound (HHUS) and mammography. Arch Gynecol Obstet. 2015;291:889–95. PMID: 25311201
14. Van Zelst JC, Platel B, Karssemeijer N, Mann RM. Multiplanar reconstructions of 3d automated breast ultrasound improve lesion differentiation by radiologists. Acad Radiol. 2015;22:1489–96. PMID: 26345538
15. Van Zelst JC, Platel B, Karssemeijer N, Mann RM. Multiplanar reconstructions of 3d automated breast ultrasound improve lesion differentiation by radiologists. Acad Radiol. 2015;22:1489–96. (PMID: 26345538)

20 Conclusion

Dominique Amy

It is absolutely clear that the presentation of the lobar approach in the diagnosis of breast cancer at an early stage leads to some calling into question in the management of benign or malignant lesions, as regards the diagnosis and surgical techniques as well as the therapeutic management.

A few remarks must be made in conclusion, which correspond to what the majority of the coauthors in this volume agree on. These remarks are the fruit of years of research and analyses by different pluri-disciplinary (anatomo-pathologists, oncologists, radiologists, surgeons, therapists, etc.) teams. They follow up to numerous publications which all converge towards the new concept, the new lobar approach in the detection of breast cancers.

The understanding of the precise anatomy of the breast with its radial-lobar organisation is an essential improvement brought forth by radial echography. Even if, in certain cases, the radiologist or the surgeon may find it difficult to identify it, it nevertheless forms the basis of a systematic, logical and reproducible analysis of the mammary structures.

If the lobar notion of anatomy is, at first, not very obvious to colleagues not trained in it, the investigation of the intra-lobar ductal axes soon becomes easier and more precise, and that is precisely what we are aiming at. The lobar analysis allows us to understand the development of the breast, the physiological modifications and the early modifications in the case of benign or malignant pathology.

This lobar approach makes it necessary to achieve a closer collaboration between the anatomo-pathologists, the breast imagers (radiologists for the most part), the surgical teams, the oncologists and also the designers of ultrasound equipment who must adapt their machines to the lobar analysis of the breast. In the near future, the use of fully automated machines for the patients' screening will only be successful through the adoption of the concept of lobar anatomy and of the cancerous disease of the breast.

The understanding of the anatomy, the investigation of the epithelial structures and the confrontation with the results of gross-section histology has allowed us to achieve an earlier detection of mammary pathology. Pr. E. UENO's remarkable diagrams presented here are essential in the understanding of the development of the cancerous disease of the breast.

D. Amy, M.D.
Centre du sein, Aix-en-Provence, France
e-mail: domamy@wanadoo.fr

D. Amy (ed.), *Lobar Approach to Breast Ultrasound*, https://doi.org/10.1007/978-3-319-61681-0_20

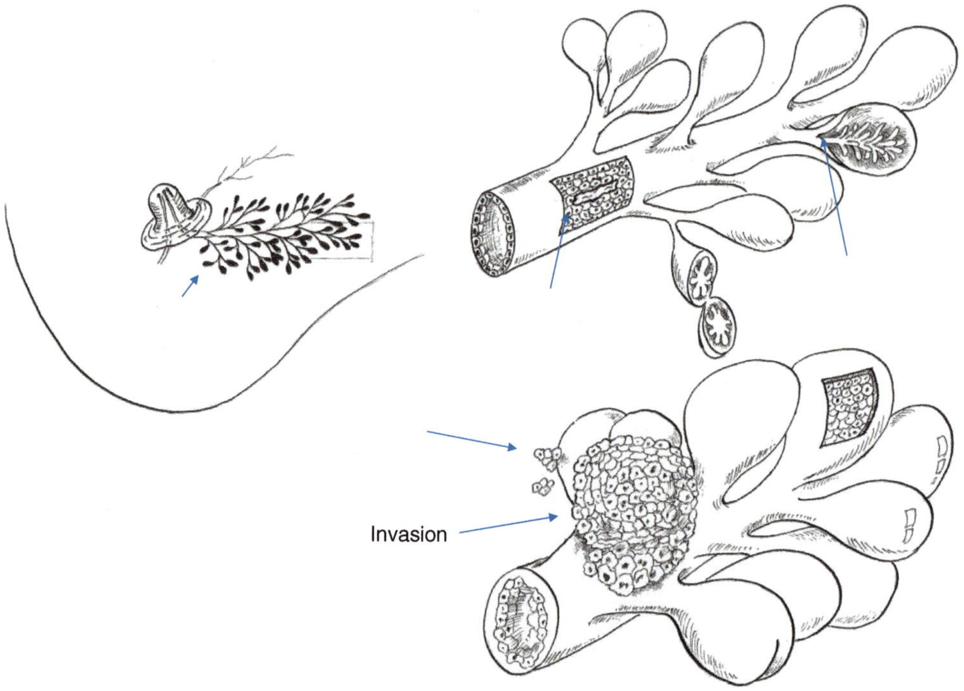

Diagram 1. Termino-ducto-lobular unit and breast cancer early development

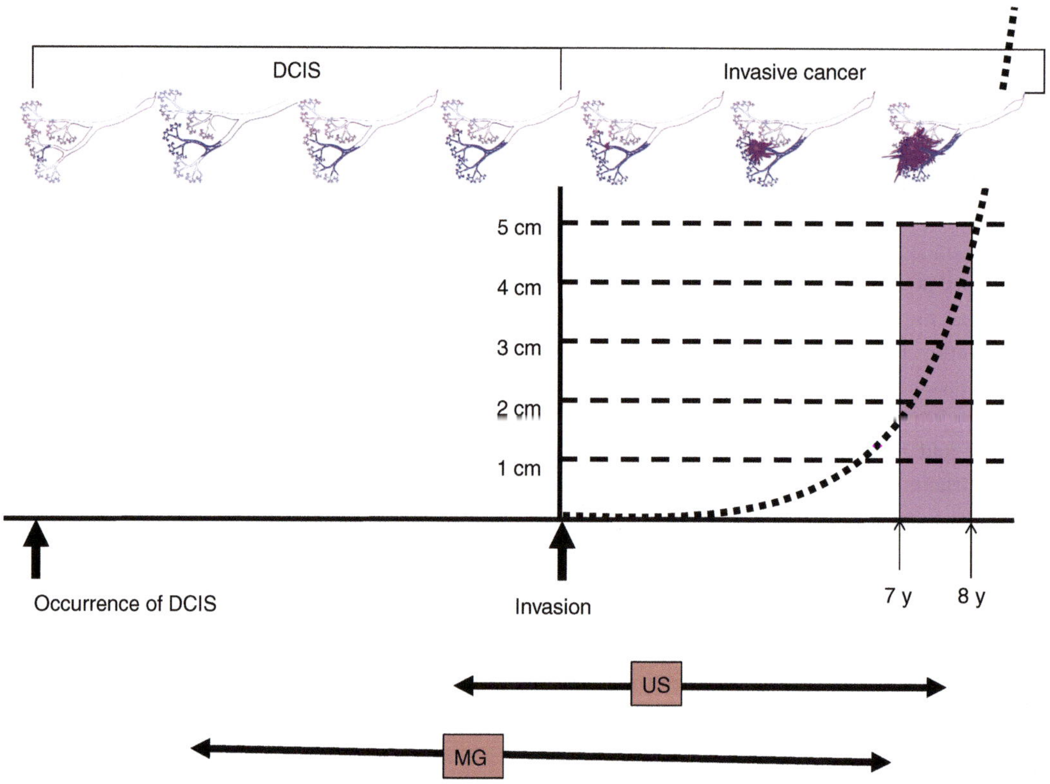

Diagram 2. Chronological breast cancer development: 7/8 years evolution

The concept of the lobar disease of the breast and its ultrasound analysis cannot, of course, at this stage in 2017, answer all the queries or all the controversies and oppositions which will crop up. There are nevertheless a few assertions that we can spell out.

1. Breast cancer must no longer be considered as a simple tumour but as a breast disease (Tot, Going, Teboul, Francescatti, Dolfin, etc.). Some coauthors have raised the issue of the exact definition of such words as tumour and disease. The essential point is to understand and conceive breast cancer as a lobar and sometimes pluri-lobar attack.
2. Over half the cohort of patients will suffer from a multifocal disease. To this day, no technique of breast imaging is able to reach such a rate of detection (over 50%). The large histological sections (10 × 10 cm gross sections) confirm the lobar diffusion of malignant cells: according to Tot, about a third of breast carcinomas have a multifocal invasive component and another third a multifocal in situ component, which leaves a clearly unifocal group of about 30–40%. Unfortunately even ducto-radial echography is unable to visualise such a rate of lesions.
3. It is necessary to redefine the notions of multifocality and multicentricity in cancer. The word 'multifocal' corresponds to the contamination of a single lobe and 'multicentric' to the contamination of several adjacent lobes within the same quadrant or in various quadrants. Hence the notion of the 4 cm wide 'in sano' safety zone around a focal lesion must also be rediscussed.
4. Echography allows us to distinguish between ductal and lobular lesions; this is not absolutely accurate as cancer develops in the TDLU (termino-ducto-lobular unit), and, because of this, in echography we are able to differentiate cancer in the ducts from cancer in the lobules which may both have ductal or lobular characteristics.
5. Epithelial cell proliferation in the ducts and lobules can be detected through ultrasound. This proliferation modifies the volume of ducts and lobules and their acoustic impedance and thus allows us to identify it on the echographic sections.
6. It is quite impossible to differentiate epithelial proliferation from ductal carcinoma in situ (DCIS). In the future, given the technical improvements in the new generations of echographic and elastographic machines, such a distinction may prove to be feasible in some cases. For the time being, the frontiers between these various evolutive stages are not echographically obvious. The only real bonus is that a category of women on the danger list can be identified for whom a careful, regular follow-up monitoring will be required. Likewise, 'radial scar'-type lesions, sclerosing adenosis, proliferative change with or without atypia or such types of lesions as mucinous or medullar cancers often have a misleading appearance and require further investigation.
7. The ducto-radial approach of the lobes will no doubt lead to overdiagnosis since the distinction between the initial stages of development is not always obvious. This is nevertheless a low risk which will be partly limited with the fast-growing development of such techniques as elastography or molecular biology and the improvement of echographic probes. One must accept that the smaller the lesions one tries to analyse, the greater the difficulty to analyse them, the echographic lesional signs being indeed hardly specific and clearly different from those one notes in centimetre or pluricentimetre large lesions. All the techniques of breast imaging are likely to induce either underdiagnosis or overdiagnosis. It seems preferable to us not to underestimate the risk of the development of a breast cancer; given the time a lesion takes to increase twice its size (Ueno's diagram), it is essential to come to a diagnosis at the earliest possible stage.
8. In order to help in this early detection, the lobar anatomic approach of the breast and the understanding of the morphotypes and the initial variations is a major decisive improvement.
9. The diagnostic imagery of the breast (combining radiology, MRI and above all ducto-

radial echography) is a perfect guide to the surgical intervention. An excellent correlation between anatomo-pathology and echography provides an analytical, topographic and prognostic (elastography) precision and a help to the management of the oncological therapy, which was impossible with the traditional imaging techniques.

10. The future of mammary echography is linked to the development of automated machines. The presence on the market of six different machines demonstrates the interest of the designers and their advisers in the echographic screening of the breast. Only the machines integrating the lobar approach with direct acquisition of the sections and secondary 3D reconstruction will be competitive. Benefiting from the systematisation of ducto-radial anatomy, the perfect reproducibility of the examinations as well as the fast-growing improvements in I.T., these machines are going to modify the screening of breast cancers completely.
11. An important part has been given to fine needle aspiration in interventional echography. Without denying the more traditional techniques of core biopsy or mamotome, the authors have been eager to reassert that breast fine-needle aspiration is a precise, quick, inexpensive method, which is very useful in the case of a small multicentric lesion or small adenopathy. Furthermore, in many developing countries, this inexpensive technique can be used easily.

To conclude, many other points will have to be dealt with in complementary studies and analyses involving larger statistics. For example, is there a benefit in long-term survival linked to the early detection of the breast disease? We do not claim to give an answer to all these questionings. We are convinced that the adoption of the concept of the lobar disease of the breast corresponds to an important stage in the fight against breast cancer. Allow us to reassert that it is important to understand what we visualise, to identify women on the danger list and to limit the number of unnecessary interventions. Our hope is that the concept offered here will lead to more enthusiastic approval than reproval, to more vocations than sterile criticisms.

We hope we will prove Niccolo Machiavelli wrong who wrote in *The Prince* published in 1513:

> It must be remembered that there is nothing more difficult to plan, more doubtful of success, nor more dangerous to manage, than the creation of a new system. For the initiator has the enmity of all who would profit by the preservation of the old institutions and merely lukewarm defenders in those who would gain by the new ones

Aix en Provence January 2017

Index

D. Amy (ed.), *Lobar Approach to Breast Ultrasound*, https://doi.org/10.1007/978-3-319-61681-0

C

G

H

I

GPSR Compliance

The European Union's (EU) General Product Safety Regulation (GPSR) is a set of rules that requires consumer products to be safe and our obligations to ensure this.

If you have any concerns about our products, you can contact us on ProductSafety@springernature.com

In case Publisher is established outside the EU, the EU authorized representative is:

Springer Nature Customer Service Center GmbH
Europaplatz 3
69115 Heidelberg, Germany

Batch number: 09635481

Printed by Printforce, the Netherlands